Apley & Solomon's Concise System of Orthopaedics and Trauma

Apley & Solomon's Concise System of Orthopaedics and Trauma

Fifth Edition

David Warwick DM MD BM FRCS FRCS(Orth) Eur Dip Hand Surg
Honorary Professor and Consultant Hand Surgeon
University Hospital Southampton
Southampton, UK

Ashley Blom MBChB MD PhD FRCS(Tr&Orth)
Head of Bristol Medical School
and
Professor of Orthopaedic Surgery
University of Bristol
Bristol, UK

Michael Whitehouse PhD MSc(Ortho Eng) BSc(Hons)
PGCert(TLHE) FRCS(Tr&Ortho) FHEA
Professor of Trauma and Orthopaedics
University of Bristol
and
Bristol Medical School
University of Bristol
Bristol, UK

International Editor

Richard Gardner FRCS(Tr&Orth)
Orthopaedic Surgeon
CURE Children's Hospital of Zimbabwe
and
Chief Medical Officer
CURE International, Zimbabwe

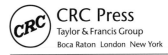

CRC Press
Taylor & Francis Group
Boca Raton London New York

CRC Press is an imprint of the
Taylor & Francis Group, an **informa** business

Fifth edition published 2022
by CRC Press
6000 Broken Sound Parkway NW, Suite 300, Boca Raton, FL 33487-2742

and by CRC Press
2 Park Square, Milton Park, Abingdon, Oxon, OX14 4RN

CRC Press is an imprint of Taylor & Francis Group, LLC

ISBN: 9780367198954 (hbk)
ISBN: 9780367198770 (pbk)
ISBN: 9780429243974 (ebk)

DOI: 10.1201/9780429243974

Typeset in ITC Galliard Std
by Nova Techset Private Limited, Bengaluru & Chennai, India.

Access the companion website: www.routledge.com/cw/apley

Printed in Great Britain by Bell and Bain Ltd, Glasgow

CONTENTS

Preface   vii
Preface to the First Edition   ix
Acknowledgements   xi
Abbreviations   xiii

SECTION 1: GENERAL ORTHOPAEDICS

1	Diagnosis in orthopaedics	3
2	Infection	23
3	Inflammatory rheumatic disorders	51
4	Crystal deposition disorders	67
5	Osteoarthritis	75
6	Osteonecrosis and osteochondritis	87
7	Metabolic and endocrine bone disorders	97
8	Genetic disorders, dysplasias and malformations	129
9	Tumours	161
10	Neuromuscular disorders	199
11	Peripheral nerve injuries	227
12	Orthopaedic operations	247

SECTION 2: REGIONAL ORTHOPAEDICS

13	The shoulder and pectoral girdle	273
14	The elbow	297
15	The wrist	309
16	The hand	325
17	The neck	345
18	The back	359
19	The hip	393
20	The knee	421
21	The ankle and foot	453

SECTION 3: TRAUMA

22	The management of major injuries	485
23	Principles of fractures	513
24	Shoulder and upper arm injuries	551
25	Elbow and forearm injuries	565
26	Wrist injuries	589
27	Hand injuries	607
28	Spine and thorax injuries	625
29	Pelvic injuries	643

30   Hip and femur injuries   653
31   Knee and leg injuries   675
32   Ankle and foot injuries   697

Index   717

PREFACE

We are confident that the spirits of Alan Apley and Louis Solomon are kept alive with this new edition. Yes, we are now able to perform tests and imaging studies that were unknown in years gone by and it is true that there are now more shortcuts to diagnosis than before. Even so, the most useful and important tools to assist in an understanding of our patients and the management of their problems are our own hands and our clinical acumen. That has always been the focus of the book that arose out of Apley's teachings. Alan Apley was then joined by Louis Solomon who continued with this system of teaching. Sadly, they have both passed on, but it is our honour as the new editors to carry this flame into the future.

Why do we call it a 'system' of orthopaedics and not simply a textbook? What Alan Apley had in mind when he set up his famous courses in orthopaedics over 60 years ago was to imbue his listeners – the orthopaedic surgeons of the future – with not only the theory of this subject but also the clinical habits that would lead them to all the observations and connections from which they could construct a credible diagnosis and a reliable plan of treatment. *Look–Feel–Move* became not merely a mantra for those who had been at his classes but a constant reminder that diagnosis is more than inspired guesswork; it is the result of a systematic consideration of all the appearances and issues (the trivial as well as the obviously unusual) from which the alert mind will choose what is truly relevant. It is that approach which we have tried to preserve, however many clever instruments come into play during this repeatedly exciting enterprise.

As in previous editions, the book is divided into three sections.

General Orthopaedics comprises the main categories of clinical examination, special investigations and individual chapters on the most common groups of musculoskeletal disorders such as infection, arthritis, metabolic bone disease, developmental abnormalities, tumours, central neurological conditions and peripheral nerve disorders. This section ends with a chapter on the principles of operative orthopaedics and other methods commonly used in treating patients with musculoskeletal complaints.

Regional Orthopaedics examines the specific manifestations and treatment of these conditions in each of the major bodily regions.

Trauma covers the principles of trauma surgery. It begins with a chapter on the emergency management of the severely injured patient, which is followed by a chapter on the principles of fracture management and then individual chapters on the management of fractures and dislocations in each anatomical region.

A hallmark of the book has been the liberal spread of pictures, illustrations and diagrams, which, together with their captions, provide an instant summary of the accompanying text. In this edition, we have also added summary boxes, alert boxes that emphasize crucial points, and a sports icon has been introduced alongside those topics which are of particular relevance in sports medicine to represent this growing specialty. We have also added many additional images to the companion website, which are indicated in the text by a laptop icon in the margin. Finally, the text has been reviewed by Rick Gardner to ensure that it maintains its relevance to those practising in low- and middle-income countries, for whom we are honoured to provide this book as a resource.

For this book, we have relied on the work of many others. Some of the text dates back to the classic teachings of the original editions; the updated text relies on our own experience and on that of the host of expert co-authors who contributed to the larger 10th edition of *Apley & Solomon's System of Orthopaedics and Trauma*, to whom we are so grateful.

A question that crops up repeatedly is, 'To whom have we aimed this book?' Most obviously, medical students, trainees in orthopaedic surgery, and even their consultant teachers who want a concise review of subjects with which they are already familiar. Then many others as well: trainees in related surgical specialties; doctors and nurses working in accident and emergency units; experienced general practitioners; physiotherapists, occupational therapists and paramedics who deal with physical abnormalities. We hope that they will enjoy these pages as much as we have enjoyed their preparation.

David Warwick
Ashley Blom
Michael Whitehouse
August 2021

PREFACE TO THE FIRST EDITION

For many years a course in orthopaedics and fractures, designed primarily for FRCS candidates, has been held at Pyrford. As the course grew and developed, so did the desire to cover the field as comprehensively as possible. Eventually, as a prophylactic against writer's cramp, lecture notes were issued. Re-written and amplified, these form the basis of the present book. The aim has been to prepare a text comprehensive enough for postgraduates, yet simple enough for undergraduates.

Many students, whether postgraduate or undergraduate, are not lacking in factual knowledge so much as in a methodical approach. The presentation used is designed to overcome this handicap and to inculcate method. Physical signs are described in a constant sequence throughout and as far as possible, a standard system of headings is used both for orthopaedic disorders and for fractures.

In practice, the same doctor usually deals with orthopaedics and with fractures; and rightly so, for they share many principles in common. Consequently, a book dealing with both subjects may be appropriate and convenient. To this end, brevity was important. I have tried to avoid wordiness and to present facts concisely. Illustrations have not been included; their value is not denied but, if the reader keeps the patient constantly in mind, and punctiliously follows the precept of 'LOOK, FEEL, MOVE', illustrations should not be indispensable. Their absence has been accepted as a challenge to provide unambiguous verbal descriptions instead.

The combination of method and compactness will, it is hoped, help the busy house surgeon, casualty officer, or the doctor who only occasionally practises orthopaedics, to find his way quickly in a large and complex subject.

In preparing this book I have leaned heavily on others. Many of their ideas have made such instant appeal that I have absorbed them and can no longer recall their source or adequately acknowledge my indebtedness. An immeasurable debt is, however, due to my teacher George Perkins, whose influence has, I hope, pervaded both my work and my teaching.

On many occasions I have sought the help of my colleague Mr F.A. Simmonds, who has never failed to give sound advice. I am greatly indebted to Dr I. Churchill-Davidson for his ungrudging and detailed help in writing the sections on radiotherapy. Mr Gordon Hadfield read through the entire text and his many valuable suggestions are deeply appreciated. It is a pleasure to pay tribute to the diligence and skill of my secretary, Miss L. Freeland, and to acknowledge the constructive suggestions and friendly co-operation of the publishers.

A. Graham Apley
January 1959

ACKNOWLEDGEMENTS

Advances in medical research and practice during the last three decades have led to ever greater specialization and the need for multi-authorship in modern textbooks. The Apley System was no exception: the 10th edition of the main textbook, published three years ago, involved three Principal Authors and 42 Contributing Authors. They were duly acknowledged in that edition and we express our gratitude to them again with the appearance of this new 5th edition of the concise version, which is based on the more extensive publication. In particular, we acknowledge the contribution of Selvadurai Nayagam.

In addition, we have enlisted Rick Gardner as International Editor whose remit has been to provide an international perspective in the present *Concise System* and to ensure its global relevance. Our sincere thanks to Rick for his considerable help with updating the text and for supplying many new photographs.

No textbook would see the light of day without the help of its publishing editors and copy editors. We have had the good fortune to work with Dr Joanna Koster, Publisher at CRC Press (Taylor & Francis Group), our eagle-eyed Project Manager Nora Naughton of Naughton Project Management, and Copy Editor Becky Freeman. We pay them our sincere thanks.

We never forget that writing a textbook is not a single-handed job. Behind the individuals pounding the computer keyboards there are our partners and families: some take part in organizing the work, some offer helpful comments, others offer a ready ear to listen to the problems that beset every author; all of them endure the long periods of silence around us, the writers. We can never thank them enough for the many ways in which they help us in our somewhat selfish endeavours.

Finally, we owe a huge debt of gratitude to the many patients who have allowed us to intrude upon their suffering and use their stories to populate our book.

David Warwick
Ashley Blom
Michael Whitehouse

ABBREVIATIONS

 highlights those topics which are of particular relevance in sports medicine.

 indicates where additional images are available on the companion website www.routledge.com/cw/apley

^{99m}Tc-HDP	^{99m} technetium hydroxymethylene diphosphonate
ABC	aneurysmal bone cyst
ABG	arterial blood gas
ABPI	ankle brachial pressure indices
ACI	autologous cartilage implantation
ACL	anterior cruciate ligament
ACPA	anti-citrullinated peptide antibody
ADI	atlantodental interval
AIDS	acquired immunodeficiency syndrome
AJCC	American Joint Committee on Cancer
ALIF	anterior lumbar interbody fusion
ALP	alkaline phosphatase
ALS	advanced life support
AO/ASIF	Arbeitsgemeinschaft für Osteosynthesefragen/ Association for the Study of Internal Fixation
AP	anteroposterior
APBI	ankle-brachial pressure index
APC	anteroposterior compression
ARDS	acute respiratory distress syndrome
ARMD	adverse reaction to metal debris
AS	ankylosing spondylitis
ASCT	autologous stem cell transplantation
ASIS	anterior superior iliac spine
ATFL	anterior talofibular ligament

ATLS	Advanced Trauma Life Support
AVN	avascular necrosis
BCP	basic calcium phosphate
BMD	bone mineral density
BMI	body mass index
BMP	bone morphogenetic protein
BOA	British Orthopaedic Association
BSA	body surface area
BUN	blood urea nitrogen
BVM	bag–valve–mask
CC	cartilage calcification
(anti-)CCP	(anti-)cyclic citrullinated peptide (antibody)
CCP	calcium pyrophosphate
CKD-MBD	chronic kidney disease mineral bone disorder
CMC	carpometacarpal
CNS	central nervous system
CPPD	calcium pyrophosphate dehydrate
CRP	C-reactive protein
CRPS	complex regional pain syndrome
CSF	cerebrospinal fluid
CT	computed tomography
CVP	central venous pressure
DDH	developmental dysplasia of the hip
DEXA	dual-energy X-ray absorptiometry
dGEMRIC	delayed gadolinium-enhanced MRI of cartilage
DIP	distal interphalangeal
DISI	dorsal intercalated segment instability

DLC	discoligamentous complex	ICU	intensive care unit
DLIF	direct lateral interbody fusion	IMRT	intensity-modulated radiotherapy
DMARD	disease-modifying antirheumatic drug	INR	international normalized ratio
DNA	deoxyribonucleic acid	IO	intraosseous
DRUJ	distal radioulnar joint	IP	interphalangeal
DVT	deep vein thrombosis	IT	information technology
ECG	electrocardiography	IV	intravenous
ECU	extensor carpi ulnaris	JIA	juvenile idiopathic arthritis
EDF	elongation–derotation–flexion	LBC	low back pain
EDS	Ehlers–Danlos syndrome	LCL	lateral collateral ligament
EEG	electroencephalography	LCPD	Legg–Calvé–Perthes disease
eFAST	extended focused assessment with sonography in trauma	LDH	lactate dehydrogenase
		LHB	long head of biceps
eGFR	estimated glomerular filtration rate	LLD	leg length discrepancy
		LMIC	low to middle-income country
EMG	electromyography	LMN	lower motor neuron
ESR	erythrocyte sedimentation rate	LMWH	low molecular weight heparin
$EtCO_2$	end-tidal carbon dioxide	MARS	metal artifact reduction sequences
FAB	foot abduction brace		
FAI	femoroacetabular impingement	MCL	medial collateral ligament
FAST	Focussed Assessment Sonography for Trauma	MCP	metacarpophalangeal
		MED	multiple epiphyseal dysplasia
		MEN	multiple endocrine neoplasia
FBC	full blood count	MHC	major histocompatibility complex
FDP	flexor digitorum profundus		
FDS	flexor digitorum superficialis		
FGFR3	fibroblast growth factor receptor 3	MODS	multiple organ failure or dysfunction syndrome
FHH	familial hypocalciuric hypercalcaemia	MoM	metal-on-metal
		MPFL	medial patellofemoral ligament
FNCLCC	Federation Nationale des Centres de Lutte Contre le Cancer	MPS	mucopolysaccharidoses
		MRC	Medical Research Council
FPE	fatal pulmonary embolism	MRI	magnetic resonance imaging
GAG	glycosaminoglycan	MRSA	methicillin-resistant *Staphylococcus aureus*
GCS	Glasgow Coma Score		
GCT	giant-cell tumour	MSSA	methicillin-sensitive *Staphylococcus aureus*
GCTTS	giant-cell tumour of tendon sheath		
		MTP	metatarsophalangeal
GH	growth hormone	NF	neurofibromatosis
GPI	'general paralysis of the insane'	NICE	National Institute for Health and Care Excellence
HA	hydroxyapatite		
HIV	human immunodeficiency virus	NOF	non-ossifying fibroma
HLA	human leucocyte antigen	NP	nasopharyngeal
HMSN	hereditary motor and sensory neuropathy	NSAID	non-steroidal anti-inflammatory drug
HR	hip resurfacing	OA	osteoarthritis
HRT	hormone replacement therapy	OCD	osteochondritis dissecans
ICP	intracerebral pressure	OI	osteogenesis imperfecta

ONJ	osteonecrosis of the jaw	SERM	selective oestrogen receptor modulators
OP	oropharyngeal		
OTA	Orthopaedic Trauma Association	SIJ	sacroiliac joint
		SLAC	scapholunate advanced collapse
PA	posteroanterior	SLAP	superior part of the glenoid labrum anteriorly and posteriorly
$PaCO_2$	arterial carbon dioxide tension		
PACS	Picture Archiving and Communication System	SLE	systemic lupus erythematosus
		SLIC	Subaxial Cervical Spine Injury Classification
PAO	periacetabular osteotomy		
PaO_2	arterial oxygen tension	SPECT	single-photon emission computed tomography
PCL	posterior cruciate ligament		
PCR	polymerase chain reaction	SSEP	somatosensory-evoked response
PDB	Paget's disease of bone	STIR	short-tau inversion recovery
PE	pulmonary embolism	STT	soft-tissue tumour
PEA	pulseless electrical activity	SUA	serum uric acid
PET	positron emission tomography	SUFE	slipped upper femoral epiphysis
PH	Pavlik harness	TB	tuberculosis
PIP	proximal interphalangeal	TDR	total disc replacement
PJI	periprosthetic joint infection	TED	thromboembolus deterrent
PLC	posterior ligamentous complex / posterolateral corner	TFCC	tears of the triangular fibrocartilage complex
PMMA	polymethylmethacrylate	THA	total hip arthroplasty
PMR	posteromedial release	TLIF	transforaminal lumbar interbody fusion
PNS	peripheral nervous system		
PPE	personal protective equipment	TMT	tarsometatarsal
pQCT	peripheral quantitative computer tomography	TNF	tumour necrosis factor
		TNM	tumour–node–metastasis (staging)
PRP	platelet-rich plasma		
PSA	prostate-specific antigen	TSH	thyroid-stimulating hormone
PTH	parathyroid hormone		
PTHrP	parathyroid hormone-related peptide	UHMWPE	ultra-high molecular weight polyethylene
PVNS	pigmented villonodular synovitis	UICC	Union for International Cancer Control
QCT	quantitative computed tomography	ULT	urate-lowering therapy
		UMN	upper motor neuron
RA	rheumatoid arthritis	US	ultrasound
RF	rheumatoid factor	VAC	vacuum-assisted closure
RICE	rest, ice, compression and elevation	VISI	volar intercalated segment instability
SAC	space available for the cord	VMO	vastus medialis oblique
SBC	simple bone cyst	VP	ventriculoperitoneal
SCFE	slipped capital femoral epiphysis	V/Q	ventilation–perfusion
SCIWORA	spinal cord injury without obvious radiographic abnormality	VTE	venous thromboembolism
		WALANT	wide awake local anaesthetic no tourniquet
SE	spin echo	WBC	white blood cell
SED	spondyloepiphyseal dysplasia	WHO	World Health Organization

Section 1

General Orthopaedics

1 Diagnosis in orthopaedics 3

2 Infection 23

3 Inflammatory rheumatic disorders 51

4 Crystal deposition disorders 67

5 Osteoarthritis 75

6 Osteonecrosis and osteochondritis 87

7 Metabolic and endocrine bone disorders 97

8 Genetic disorders, dysplasias and malformations 129

9 Tumours 161

10 Neuromuscular disorders 199

11 Peripheral nerve injuries 227

12 Orthopaedic operations 247

Diagnosis in orthopaedics

1

- History   3
- Examination   6
- Terminology   8
- Neurological examination   9
- Examining infants and children   12
- Variations and deformities   12
- Diagnostic imaging   16
- Bone biopsy   20
- Electrophysiological studies   21

Diagnosis begins with the systematic gathering of information – from the patient's history, the physical examination, X-ray appearances and special investigations. It should, however, never be forgotten that every orthopaedic disorder is part of a larger whole – a patient who has a unique personality, a job and hobbies, a family and a home; all have a bearing upon, and are in turn affected by, the disorder and its treatment.

HISTORY

'Taking a history' is a misnomer. The patient tells a story; it is we, the listeners, who construct a history. The history has to be systematic. Carefully and patiently compiled, it is more informative than examination or laboratory tests.

Certain key words will inevitably stand out: *injury, pain, stiffness, swelling, deformity, instability, weakness, altered sensibility* and *loss of function*. Each symptom must be pursued for more detail.

> **QUESTIONS TO ASK WHEN ASSESSING SYMPTOMS**
>
> When did it begin?
> Did it start suddenly or gradually?
> Did it begin spontaneously or after some specific event?
> How has it changed or progressed?
> What makes it worse?
> What makes it better?

While listening, consider if the story fits some recognizable pattern that might suggest a possible diagnosis.

SYMPTOMS

Pain

Pain is the most common symptom. Its precise location is important, so ask the patient to point to where it hurts. But don't assume that the site of pain is always the site of pathology; '*referred*' pain and '*autonomic*' pain can be very deceptive.

REFERRED PAIN

Pain arising in or near the skin is usually localized accurately. Pain arising in deep structures is more diffuse and is sometimes of unexpected distribution; thus, hip disease may manifest with pain in the knee (but so might an obturator hernia!). This is not because sensory nerves connect the two sites; it is due to inability of the cerebral cortex to distinguish between sensory messages from embryologically related sites (**1.1**).

AUTONOMIC PAIN

Pain that does not fit the usual pattern is often dismissed as 'inappropriate' (i.e. psychologically determined). But pain can also affect the autonomic nerves that accompany the peripheral blood vessels and this is much more vague, more widespread and often associated with vasomotor and trophic changes. It is poorly understood, often doubted, but nonetheless real.

Stiffness

Stiffness may be generalized (typically in rheumatoid arthritis and ankylosing spondylitis) or localized to a particular joint. Patients often have difficulty distinguishing stiffness from painful movement; limited movement should never be assumed until verified by examination.

Ask when the stiffness occurs.

- *Regular early morning stiffness* of many joints is one of the cardinal features of rheumatoid arthritis.
- *Transient stiffness* of one or two joints after periods of inactivity is typical of osteoarthritis.

Locking is a term used to describe the sudden inability to complete a certain movement; it suggests a mechanical block, for example due to a loose body or a torn meniscus becoming trapped between the articular surfaces. Unfortunately, patients use the term for any painful limitation of movement; much more reliable is a history of 'unlocking' when the offending body suddenly moves out of the way.

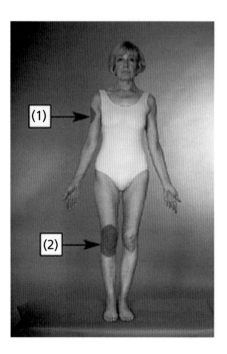 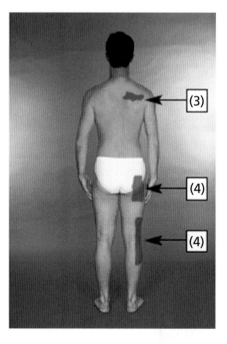

1.1 Referred pain Common sites of referred pain: (1) from the shoulder; (2) from the hip; (3) from the neck; (4) from the lumbar spine.

Swelling

Swelling may be in the soft tissues, the joint or the bone; to the patient they are all the same. It is important to establish whether the swelling followed an injury, whether it appeared rapidly (probably a haematoma or a haemarthrosis) or slowly (soft-tissue inflammation or a joint effusion), whether it is painful (acute inflammation, infection – or a tumour!), whether it is constant or comes and goes, and, most importantly, whether it is increasing in size.

Deformity

The common deformities are well described in terms such as round shoulders, spinal curvature, knock knees, bow legs, pigeon toes and flat feet. Some 'deformities' are merely variations of the normal (e.g. short stature or wide hips); others disappear spontaneously with growth (e.g. flat feet or bandy legs in an infant). However, if the deformity is progressive, or if it appears on only one side of the body, it may be serious (**1.2**).

Weakness

Generalized weakness is a feature of all chronic illness and any prolonged joint dysfunction will inevitably lead to weakness of the associated muscles. However, weakness affecting a single group of muscles suggests a more specific neurological disorder. Try to establish precisely which movements are affected; this may give an important clue to the site of the lesion.

Instability

The patient complains that the joint 'gives way' or 'jumps out'. If this happens repeatedly, it suggests ligamentous deficiency, recurrent subluxation or some internal derangement such as a loose body.

Change in sensibility

Tingling or numbness signifies interference with nerve function: pressure from a neighbouring structure (e.g. a prolapsed intervertebral disc), local ischaemia (e.g. nerve entrapment in a fibro-osseous tunnel) or a peripheral neuropathy.

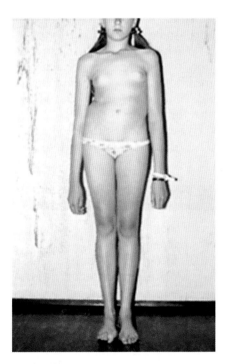 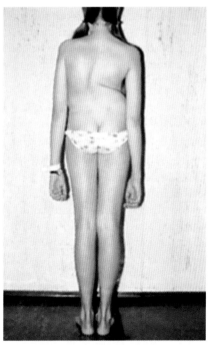

1.2 Deformity This young girl complained of a prominent right hip; the real deformity was scoliosis.

It is important to establish its exact distribution; from this we can tell whether the fault lies in a peripheral nerve or in a nerve root.

Loss of function

Functional disability is more than the sum of individual symptoms and its expression depends upon the needs of the patient. The patient may say 'I can't sit for long' rather than 'I have backache', or 'I can't put my socks on' rather than 'My hip is stiff'. Moreover, what to one patient is merely inconvenient may, to another, be incapacitating. Thus, a lawyer or a teacher may readily tolerate a stiff knee provided it is painless and does not impair walking; but to a plumber, the same disorder might spell economic disaster.

PREVIOUS DISORDERS

Patients should always be asked about previous accidents, illnesses, operations and drug therapy. They may give vital clues to the present disorder.

FAMILY HISTORY

Patients often wonder (and worry) about inheriting a disease or passing it on to their children. To the doctor, information about musculoskeletal disorders in the patient's family may help with both diagnosis and counselling.

SOCIAL BACKGROUND

No history is complete without enquiry about the patient's background: details about work, travel, recreation, home circumstances and the level of support from family and friends. These always impinge on the assessment of disability; occasionally a particular activity (at work, on the sports field or in the kitchen) is responsible for the entire condition.

EXAMINATION

In Conan Doyle's story 'A Case of Identity', Sherlock Holmes has the following conversation with Dr Watson:

Watson: You appeared to read a good deal upon [your client] which was quite invisible to me.
Holmes: Not invisible but unnoticed, Watson.

Some disorders can be diagnosed at a glance: who would mistake the facies of acromegaly or the hand deformities of rheumatoid arthritis for anything else? Nevertheless, even in these cases a systematic approach is rewarding; it provides information about the patient's particular disability, it keeps reinforcing good habits and the patient feels that he or she has been properly attended to.

The examination actually begins from the moment we set eyes on the patient. We observe their general appearance, posture and gait. Are they walking freely or do they use a stick? Are they in pain? Do their movements look natural? Can you spot any distinctive features immediately: a characteristic facial appearance; a spinal curvature; a short limb; any type of asymmetry? They may have a telltale gait suggesting a painful hip, an unstable knee or a foot drop. The clues are endless and the game is played by everyone (qualified or lay) at each new encounter throughout life. In the clinical setting the assessment needs to be more focused.

When we proceed to the structured examination, the patient must be suitably undressed; no mere rolling up of a trouser leg is sufficient. If one limb is affected, both must be exposed so that they can be compared.

We examine first the good limb, then the bad. The student is often inclined to rush in with both

---

ROUTINE FOR EXAMINATION

1 *Look* – at the patient's general appearance.
2 *Feel* – the skin, soft tissues, bones and joints, and for tenderness.
3 *Move* – testing active, passive and abnormal movement.
4 If necessary, add *special manoeuvres* to assess neurological integrity or test for joint instability.

See **Table 1.1**.

Table 1.1 Usual sequence for examination

1 Look	At the patient's general shape, posture and gait	Is there any obvious deformity?
	At the skin, with noteworthy areas suitably exposed	Are there any old scars (1.3)?
	At the local shape	Is there swelling? Is there wasting? Is there a lump? Is there any local deformity?
	At the local posture	Is it unusual? Nerve lesions may cause characteristic changes in normal posture.
2 Feel	The skin	Is it warm or cold? Is it moist or dry? Is sensation normal?
	The soft tissues	Is there a lump and where does it arise? Are the pulses normal?
	The bones and joints	Are the outlines normal? Is there excessive fluid in the joint?
	For tenderness	Where is it? If you know precisely *where* the trouble is, you're halfway to knowing *what* it is.
3 Move	*Active movement*	Ask the patient to move the joint and test for power.
	Passive movement The examiner moves the joint in each anatomical plane (1.4).	Express the range of movement in degrees, starting from zero, which is the neutral or anatomical position of the joint. Is movement painful? Is movement associated with crepitus?
	Abnormal movement	Is the joint unstable?
4 Special manoeuvres Special tests for conditions such as joint instability are described in the relevant chapters.	*Provocative movement*	One of the most telling clues to diagnosis is reproducing the patient's symptoms by applying a specific, *provocative movement*. Shoulder pain due to impingement of the subacromial structures may be 'provoked' by moving the joint in a way that is calculated to produce such impingement; the patient recognizes the similarity between this pain and his or her daily symptoms.
	Apprehension test	Likewise, a patient who has had a previous dislocation can be so vividly reminded of that event, by stressing the joint in a way that it again threatens to dislocate, that he or she goes rigid with anxiety at the anticipated result. This is aptly called the *apprehension test*.

hands – a temptation that must be resisted. Only by proceeding in a purposeful, orderly way can we avoid missing important signs. The routine we normally use is simple but comprehensive.

Obviously, the sequence may sometimes have to be changed because a patient is in pain or severely disabled; you would not try to 'move' a limb with a suspected fracture when an X-ray can provide the answer. Furthermore, resuscitation will always take priority and in severely injured patients the detailed local examination may have to be curtailed or deferred.

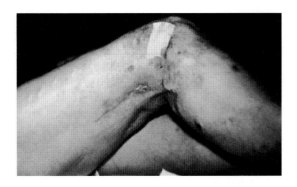

1.3 Look Scars often give clues to the previous history. The faded scar on this patient's thigh is an old operation wound - internal fixation of a femoral fracture. The other scars are due to postoperative infection; one of the sinuses is still draining.

TERMINOLOGY

Bodily surfaces, planes and positions are described in relation to the anatomical position: standing erect, facing the viewer, legs together with the knees pointing directly forwards and arms held by the sides with the palms facing forwards.

The principal planes of the body are named *sagittal*, *coronal* and *transverse*; they define the direction across which the body (or body part) is viewed in any description (**1.5**). Sagittal planes, parallel to each other, pass vertically through the body from front to back; the midsagittal or median plane divides the body into right and left halves. Coronal planes are also orientated vertically, corresponding to a frontal view, at right angles to the sagittal planes; transverse planes pass horizontally across the body.

- *Anterior* (or *ventral*) signifies the frontal aspect and *posterior* (or *dorsal*) the rear aspect of the body or a body part. In the foot, the upper surface is called the *dorsum* and the sole is called the *plantar* surface.
- *Medial* means facing towards the midline of the body and *lateral* away from the midline. These terms are usually applied to a limb, the clavicle or one half of the pelvis. Thus, the inner aspect of the thigh lies on the medial side of the limb and the outer part of the thigh lies on the lateral side. We could also say that the little finger lies on the medial or ulnar side of the hand and the thumb on the lateral or radial side of the hand.
- *Proximal* and *distal* are used mainly for parts of the limbs, meaning respectively the upper

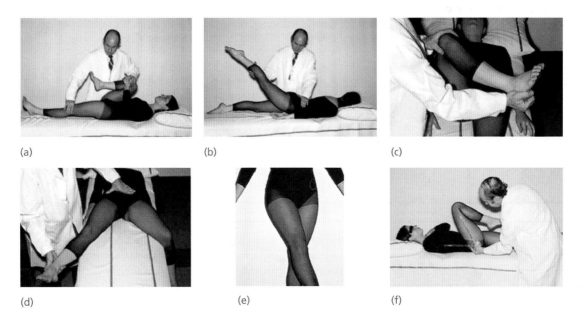

(a)   (b)   (c)

(d)   (e)   (f)

1.4 Testing for movement (a) Flexion; (b) extension; (c) rotation; (d) abduction; (e) adduction. The range of movement can be estimated by eye or measured accurately using a goniometer (f).

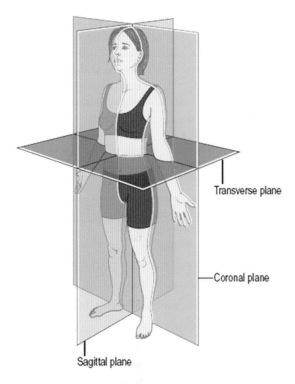

1.5 The principal planes of the body Diagram showing planes as viewed in the anatomical position: sagittal, coronal and transverse.

end and the lower end as they appear in the anatomical position. Thus, the knee joint is formed by the distal end of the femur and the proximal end of the tibia.

- The longitudinal arrangements of adjacent limb segments are also named: for example the knees and elbows are normally angulated slightly outwards (*valgus*) while the opposite – 'bow-legs' – is more correctly described as *varus*. Tortile arrangements of segments of a long bone (or an entire limb) are named *lateral* (or *external*) rotation and *medial* (or *internal*) *rotation*. *Pronation* and *supination* are also rotatory movements, but the terms are applied only to movements of the forearm and the foot.
- *Flexion* and *extension* are joint movements in the sagittal plane, most easily imagined in hinge joints such as the knee, the elbow and the joints of the fingers and toes. Flexion means bending the joint and extension means straightening it. In the ankle flexion is also called *plantarflexion* (pointing the foot

downwards) and extension is called *dorsiflexion* (drawing the foot upwards).

- *Abduction* and *adduction* are movements in the coronal plane, away from or towards the midline. Not quite for the fingers and toes, though: here abduction and adduction mean away from and towards the longitudinal midline of the hand or foot!
- *Specialized movements*, such as opposition of the thumb, lateral flexion and rotation of the spine and inversion or eversion of the foot, will be described in the relevant chapters.

NEUROLOGICAL EXAMINATION

If the symptoms include weakness or incoordination or a change in sensibility, or if they point to any disorder of the neck or back, a complete neurological examination of the related part is mandatory.

Once again, we follow a systematic routine (see Chapter 10 for further details).

ROUTINE FOR NEUROLOGICAL EXAMINATION

1 *Look* – at the patient's general appearance.
2 *Assess motor function* – muscle tone, power and reflexes.
3 *Test for sensory function* – both skin sensibility and deep sensibility.

Appearance

Some neurological disorders result in postures that are so characteristic as to be almost diagnostic. Examples include the claw hand of an ulnar nerve lesion or a wrist drop due to radial nerve palsy (**1.6**). Usually, however, it is when the patient moves that we can best appreciate the type and extent of motor disorder (e.g. the 'spastic' movement of cerebral palsy and the flaccid posture of a lower motor neuron lesion).

Concentrating on the affected part, we look for trophic changes that signify loss of sensibility: the smooth, hairless skin that seems to be

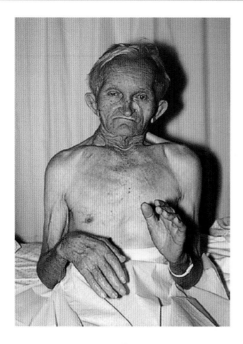

1.6 Posture Posture is often diagnostic. This patient's 'drop wrist' – typical of a radial nerve palsy – is due to carcinomatous infiltration of the supraclavicular lymph nodes on the right.

stretched too tight; atrophy of the fingertips and the nails; scars that tell of accidental burns; and ulcers that refuse to heal. Muscle wasting is rapidly assessed by comparing the two limbs.

Tone and power

Tone in individual muscle groups is tested by moving the nearby joint to stretch the muscle. Increased tone (spasticity) is characteristic of upper motor neuron disorders such as cerebral palsy and stroke. It must not be confused with rigidity (the 'lead-pipe' or 'cogwheel' effect) which is seen in Parkinson's disease. Decreased tone (flaccidity) is found in lower motor neuron lesions such as poliomyelitis. Muscle power is diminished in all three states; it is important to recognize that a 'spastic' muscle may still be weak.

Testing for power is not as easy as it sounds; the difficulty is making ourselves understood. The simplest way is to place the limb in the 'test' position, then ask the patient to hold it there as firmly as possible and resist any attempt that you make to change that position. The normal limb is examined first, then the affected limb and the two are compared. Finer muscle actions, such as those of the thumb and fingers, may be reproduced by first demonstrating the movement yourself, then testing it in the unaffected limb and then in the affected one. Muscle power is usually graded on the Medical Research Council (MRC) scale.

MUSCLE POWER: MRC GRADING	
Grade 0	No movement – total paralysis
Grade 1	Only a flicker of movement
Grade 2	Movement with gravity eliminated
Grade 3	Movement against gravity
Grade 4	Movement against resistance
Grade 5	Normal power

We can also assess the patient's ability to perform complex movements by asking them to perform specific tasks, such as gripping a rod, holding a pen, doing up a button or picking up a pin.

Tendon reflexes

A deep tendon reflex is elicited by rapidly stretching the tendon near its insertion. A sharp tap with the tendon hammer does this well; but all too often this is performed with a flourish and with such force that the finer gradations of response are missed. It is better to employ a series of taps, starting with the most forceful and reducing the force with each successive tap until there is no response. Comparing the two sides in this way, we can pick up fine differences showing that a reflex is 'diminished' rather than 'absent'. In the upper limb we test biceps, triceps and brachioradialis; and in the lower limb the patellar ligament and Achilles tendon.

The tendon reflexes are monosynaptic segmental reflexes, i.e. the reflex pathway takes a 'short cut' through the spinal cord at the segmental level. Depression or absence of the reflex signifies interruption at some point along this pathway. It is a reliable pointer to the segmental level of dysfunction. An unusually brisk reflex, on the other hand, is characteristic of an upper motor neuron disorder (e.g. cerebral palsy, a stroke or injury to the spinal cord); the lower motor neuron is released from the normal central inhibition and there is an exaggerated response to tendon stimulation.

Superficial reflexes

The superficial reflexes are elicited by stroking the skin at various sites to produce a specific muscle contraction; the best known are the abdominal (T7−T12), cremasteric (L1, 2) and anal (S4, 5) reflexes. These are corticospinal (upper motor neuron) reflexes. Absence of the reflex indicates an upper motor neuron lesion (usually in the spinal cord) above that level.

The plantar reflex

Forceful stroking of the sole normally produces flexion of the toes (or no response at all). An extensor response (the big toe extends while the others remain in flexion) is characteristic of upper motor neuron disorders. This is the Babinski sign, which is a type of withdrawal reflex which is present in young infants and normally disappears after the age of 18 months.

Sensibility

Sensibility to touch and to pinprick may be increased (*hyperaesthesia*) or unpleasant (*dysaesthesia*) in certain irritative nerve lesions. More often, though, it is diminished (*hypoaesthesia*) or absent (*anaesthesia*), signifying pressure on or interruption of a peripheral nerve, a nerve root or the sensory pathways in the spinal cord. The area of sensory change can be mapped out on the skin and compared with the known segmental or dermatomal pattern of innervation (see **10.4**). If the abnormality is well defined, it is an easy matter to establish the level of the lesion, even if the precise cause remains unknown.

Brisk percussion along the course of an injured nerve may elicit a tingling sensation in the distal distribution of the nerve (*Tinel's sign*). The point of hypersensitivity marks the site of abnormal nerve sprouting: if it progresses distally at successive visits, this signifies regeneration; if it remains unchanged, this suggests a local neuroma.

Tests for *temperature recognition* and *two-point discrimination* (the ability to recognize two touchpoints a few millimetres apart) are sometimes used in the assessment of peripheral nerve disorders.

Deep sensibility can be examined in several ways. In the vibration test a sounded tuning fork is placed over a peripheral bony point (e.g. the medial malleolus or the head of the ulna); the patient is asked if they can feel the vibrations and to say when they disappear. By comparing the two sides, differences can be noted. Position sense is tested by asking the patient to find certain points on the body with the eyes closed (e.g. touching the tip of the nose with the forefinger). The sense of joint posture is tested by grasping the big toe and placing it in different positions of flexion and extension. The patient is asked to say whether it is 'up' or 'down'. Stereognosis, the ability to recognize shape and texture by feel alone, is tested by giving the patient (whose eyes are closed) a variety of familiar objects to hold and asking them to name each object.

The pathways for deep sensibility run in the posterior columns of the spinal cord. Disturbances are therefore found in peripheral neuropathies and in spinal cord lesions such as posterior column injuries or tabes dorsalis. The sense of balance is also carried in the posterior columns. This can be tested by asking the patient to stand upright with his or her eyes closed; excessive body sway is abnormal (*Romberg's sign*).

Cortical and cerebellar function

A staggering gait may imply drunkenness, an unstable knee or a disorder of the spinal cord or cerebellum. If there is no musculoskeletal abnormality to account for the sign, a full examination of the central nervous system will be necessary.

EXAMINING INFANTS AND CHILDREN

Paediatric practice requires special skills. You may have no first-hand account of the symptoms; a baby screaming with pain will tell you very little and over-anxious parents will probably tell you too much. When examining the child, you should be flexible. If they are moving a particular joint, take your opportunity to examine movement then and there. You will learn much more by adopting methods of play than by applying a rigid system of examination. And leave any test for tenderness until last!

Infants and small children

The baby should be undressed, in a warm room and placed on the examining couch. Look carefully for birthmarks, deformities, and abnormal movements or absence of movement. If there is no urgency or distress, take time to examine the head and neck, including facial features which may be characteristic of specific dysplastic syndromes. Then examine the back and limbs for abnormalities of position or shape. Examining for joint movement can be difficult. Active movements can often be stimulated by gently stroking the limb. When testing for passive mobility, be careful to avoid frightening or hurting the child.

In the neonate and throughout the first 2 years of life, examination of the hips is mandatory, even if the child appears to be normal. This is to avoid missing the subtle signs of developmental dysplasia of the hip (DDH) at the early stage when treatment is most effective.

It is also important to assess the child's general development by testing for the normal milestones which are expected to appear during the first 2 years of life (**Table 1.2**).

Older children

Most children can be examined in the same way as adults, though with different emphasis on particular physical features. Posture and gait are very important; subtle deviations from the norm may herald the appearance of serious abnormalities such as scoliosis or neuromuscular disorders,

Table 1.2 Normal development milestones

Age (months)	Normal development milestone(s)
Newborn	*Grasp reflex:* infant will grasp the examiner's finger *Morrow reflex:* slapping the couch causes the infant to reach arms out and move the legs about *Tonic neck reflex:* if the baby's head is suddenly turned to one side, the elbow and knee on that side will be flexed and the opposite arm and leg extended
4	Newborn reflexes should disappear by 4 months
6–12	*Landau reflex:* when the child is held prone, the head, back and lower limbs are involuntarily extended
3–6	Infant can hold the head up unsupported
6–9	Able to sit up
9–12	Crawling Standing up
9–18	Walking
18–24	Running

while more obvious 'deformities' such as knock knees and bow legs may be no more than transient stages in normal development, similarly with mild degrees of 'flat feet' and 'pigeon toes'. More complex variations in posture and gait patterns, when the child sits and walks with the knees turned inwards (medially rotated) or outwards (laterally rotated), are usually due to anteversion or retroversion of the femoral necks, sometimes associated with compensatory rotational 'deformities' of the femora and tibiae. Seldom need anything be done about this; the condition usually improves as the child approaches puberty and only if the gait is very awkward would one consider performing corrective osteotomies of the femora.

VARIATIONS AND DEFORMITIES

The word 'deformity' is derived from the Latin for 'misshapen', but the range of normality is so wide that variations should not automatically be designated as deformities and some undoubted 'deformities' are not necessarily pathological; for example, the generally accepted cut-off points for 'abnormal' shortness or tallness are arbitrary and people who in one population might be considered abnormally short or abnormally tall could, in other populations, be seen as quite ordinary. However, if one leg is short and the other long, no one would quibble with the use of the word 'deformity'! In any particular case, an assessment of 'deformity' will also depend on additional factors, such as the extent to which the appearance deviates from the norm, any symptoms to which it gives rise and the degree to which it interferes with function.

- *Postural deformity* is something which the patient can, if properly instructed, correct voluntarily (e.g. a 'round back' due to slumped shoulders). However, a postural deformity may also be caused by temporary muscle spasm.
- *Structural deformity* results from a permanent change in anatomical structure which cannot be voluntarily corrected.
- *'Fixed deformity'* seems to mean that a joint is deformed and unable to move, but this is not so. It means that one particular movement cannot be completed. Thus, the knee may be able to flex fully but not extend fully – at the limit of its extension it is still 'fixed' in a certain amount of flexion. This would be called a 'fixed flexion deformity'.

Varus and valgus

It may seem pedantic to replace 'bow legs' and 'knock knees' with *'genu varum'* and *'genu valgum'*. But comparable colloquialisms are not available for deformities of other joints and, in addition, the formality is justified by the need for clarity and consistency. *Varus* means that the part distal to the apex of the deformity is displaced towards the midline, *valgus* away from the midline (**1.7**).

Kyphosis and lordosis

Seen from the side, the normal spine has a series of curves that are *convex* posteriorly in the dorsal region (*kyphosis*) and *concave* posteriorly in the cervical and lumbar regions (*lordosis*). Abnormally marked curvature constitutes a kyphotic or lordotic deformity (also sometimes referred to as *hyperkyphosis* and *hyperlordosis*).

Scoliosis

Seen from behind, the spine is straight. Any curvature in this (coronal) plane is called *scoliosis*. It is important to distinguish *postural scoliosis* from *structural* (*fixed*) *scoliosis*: the former is non-progressive and benign; the latter is usually progressive and may require treatment.

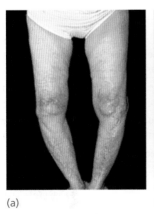 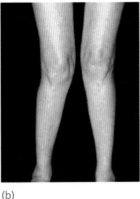 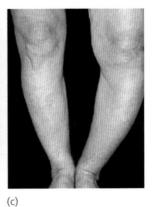

(a)   (b)   (c)

1.7 Varus and valgus (a) Varus knees due to osteoarthritis; **(b)** valgus deformity in rheumatoid arthritis; **(c)** not a varus knee but a varus deformity of the left tibia due to Paget's disease.

COMMON CAUSES OF DEFORMITY

In joints

There are six basic causes of joint deformity (Table 1.3).

In bones

There are six basic causes of bone deformity (Table 1.4).

BONY LUMPS

A bony lump may be due to faulty development, injury, inflammation or a tumour. Although X-ray examination is essential, the clinical features can be highly informative (**1.8**, Table **1.5**).

STIFF JOINTS

It is convenient to distinguish three grades of joint stiffness (Table **1.6**).

LAX JOINTS

Generalized joint hypermobility occurs in about 5% of people and is familial. Hypermobile joints are not necessarily unstable – as witness the controlled performances of acrobats and gymnasts – but they do have a tendency to recurrent dislocation (e.g. of the shoulder or patella).

Table 1.3 Common causes of joint deformity

Cause	Description
Contracture of the overlying skin	Severe scarring across the flexor aspect of a joint is typical.
Contracture of the subcutaneous fascia	The classic example is Dupuytrens contracture in the palm of the hand.
Muscle contracture	Fibrosis and contracture of muscles that cross a joint will cause a fixed deformity of the joint. This may be due to deep infection or fibrosis following ischaemic necrosis (Volkmann's ischaemic contracture).
Muscle imbalance	Unbalanced muscle weakness or spasticity will result in joint deformity which, if not corrected, will eventually become fixed. This is seen typically in poliomyelitis and cerebral palsy.
Joint instability	An unstable joint may look 'deformed' when force is applied.
Joint destruction	Trauma, infection or arthritis may lead to severe deformity.

Table 1.4 Common causes of bone deformity

Cause	Description
Genetic or developmental disorders	Deformities can sometimes be diagnosed *in utero* (e.g. achondroplasia).
	Some become apparent as the child grows (e.g. hereditary multiple exostosis).
	Some become apparent only in adulthood (e.g. multiple epiphyseal dysplasia).
Rickets (in children) and *osteomalacia* (in adults)	These affect the entire skeleton.
Injuries involving the physis may result in asymmetrical growth	The deformity emerges as the bone elongates.
Malunited fractures	These can occur at any age.
Paget's disease	Disease affects older people.
Postoperative iatrogenic deformity	Keep this in mind.

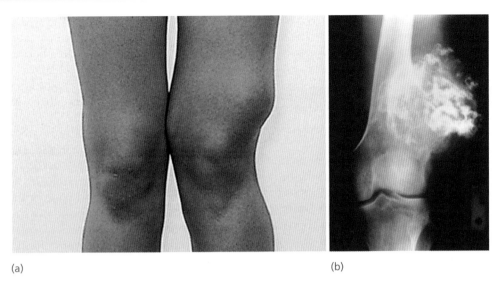

(a)   (b)

1.8 Bony lumps (a) The lump above the left knee is hard, well-defined and not increasing in size. The clinical diagnosis of cartilage-capped exostosis (osteochondroma) is confirmed by the X-ray **(b)**.

Table 1.5 Clinical features of bony lumps

Feature	Possible cause
Size	A lump attached to bone, or a lump which is getting bigger, is nearly always a tumour.
Site	A lump at the metaphysis is most likely to be a tumour. A lump in the diaphysis may be fracture callus, inflammatory new bone or a tumour.
Shape	A benign tumour has a well-defined margin. Malignant tumours, inflammatory lumps and calluses have an ill-defined edge.
Consistency	Benign tumours feel bony hard; a malignant tumour often feels spongy.
Tenderness	Marked tenderness suggests an inflammatory lesion, infection or perhaps even a malignant tumour.
Multiplicity	Multiple bony lumps are uncommon: they occur in hereditary multiple exostosis and in Ollier's disease.

Table 1.6 Grades of joint stiffness

Degree of movement	Possible cause
All movements absent	Surgical fusion of a joint is called *arthrodesis*. Pathological fusion is called *ankylosis*. Acute suppurative arthritis typically ends in *bony ankylosis*. Tuberculous arthritis often heals by fibrosis and causes *fibrous ankylosis*.
All movements limited	Restriction of movement in all directions is characteristic of non-infective arthritis and is usually due to synovial swelling or capsular fibrosis.
One or two movements limited	Limitation of movement in some directions with full movement in others suggests a mechanical block or joint contracture.

SECTION 1 GENERAL ORTHOPAEDICS

Severe joint laxity is a feature of certain rare connective tissue disorders such as Marfan's syndrome and osteogenesis imperfecta.

DIAGNOSTIC IMAGING

Plain film radiography

X-rays are produced by firing electrons at high speed onto a rotating anode. The resulting beam of X-rays is attenuated by the patient's soft tissues and bones, casting what are effectively 'shadows' which are displayed as images on an appropriately sensitized plate or stored as digital information which is then available to be transferred throughout the local information technology (IT) network (**1.9**).

The denser the tissue, the greater the X-ray attenuation and therefore the more blank, or white, the image that is captured. Thus, a metal implant appears intensely white, bone less so and

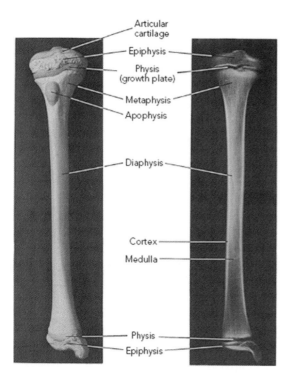

1.9 The radiographic image X-ray of an anatomical specimen to show the appearance of various parts of the bone in the X-ray image.

soft tissues in varying shades of grey depending on their 'density'. Cartilage, which causes little attenuation, appears as a dark area between adjacent bone ends; this 'gap' is usually called the joint space, though of course it is not a space at all, merely a radiolucent zone filled with cartilage. Other 'radiolucent' areas are produced by fluid-filled cysts in bone.

One bone overlying another (e.g. the femoral head inside the acetabular socket) produces superimposed images; any abnormality seen in the resulting combined image could be in either bone, so it is important to obtain several images from different projections in order to separate the anatomical outlines. Similarly, the bright image of a metallic foreign body superimposed upon that of, say, the femoral condyles could mean that the foreign body is in front of, inside or behind the bone. A second projection, at right angles to the first, will give the answer.

Picture Archiving and Communication System (PACS) is the system whereby all digitally coded images are filed, stored and retrieved to enable the images to be sent to work stations throughout the hospital, to other hospitals or to the consultant's personal computer.

How to read an X-ray

Although '*radiograph*' is more correct, the term 'X-ray' (or 'X-ray film') has become entrenched by usage. The process of 'reading an X-ray' should be as methodical as a clinical examination. It is seductively easy to be led astray by some flagrant anomaly; systematic study is the only safeguard against missing important signs (**1.10**).

Start with a general orientation: identify the part, the particular view and, if possible, the type of patient. Then examine, in sequence, the soft tissues, the bones, the joints, the surrounding tissues.

The patient Make sure that the name on the film is that of your patient; mistaken identity is a potent source of error. The clinical details are important; it is surprising how much more you can see on the X-ray when you know the background. For example, when considering a malignant bone lesion, simply knowing the patient's age may provide an important clue: under the age

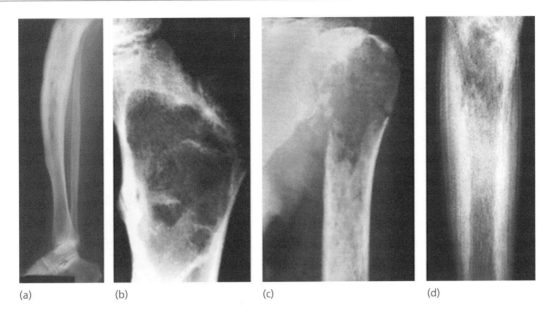

(a)   (b)   (c)   (d)

1.10 X-rays – important features to look for (a) *General shape and appearance:* in this case the cortices are thickened and the bone is bent (Paget's disease). **(b,c)** *Interior density:* a vacant area may represent a true cyst **(b)** or radiolucent material infiltrating the bone, like the metastatic tumour in **(c)**. *Periosteal reaction:* typically seen in healing fractures, bone infection and malignant bone tumours, as in this example of Ewing's sarcoma **(d)**.

of 10 it is most likely to be a Ewing's sarcoma; between 10 and 20 years it is more likely to be an osteosarcoma; and over the age of 50 years it is likely to be a metastatic deposit.

Soft tissues Look for generalized change such as swelling or wasting, then localized changes such as a mass, soft-tissue calcification, ossification, gas (from a penetrating wound or gas-forming organism) or the presence of a radio-opaque foreign body.

Bones Take note of any generalized change in bone 'texture' (osteoporosis and abnormally thin cortices). Is there anything unusual about the shape of the bone? Look for deformity or local irregularities; examine the cortices for areas of destruction or new bone formation; then look for areas of reduced density (osteoporosis or destruction) or increased density (sclerosis). Remember that 'vacant' areas are not necessarily spaces or cysts; any tissue that is radiolucent may look 'cystic'.

Joints The radiographic 'joint' consists of the articulating bones and the 'space' between them. The 'joint space' is, of course, illusory; it is

occupied by radiolucent articular cartilage. Look for narrowing of this 'space', which signifies loss of cartilage thickness, and examine the bone ends for flattening, erosion, cavitation or sclerosis – all features of arthritis. The joint margins may show osteophytes (typical of osteoarthritis) (**1.11**) or erosions (typical of rheumatoid arthritis). Similarly, intervertebral disc 'spaces' are not gaps in the vertebral column; you must imagine the fibrous discs which occupy those 'spaces' and, if a 'disc space' is abnormally flattened or narrowed, it means that the intervertebral disc has collapsed.

OTHER X-RAY TECHNIQUES

Contrast radiography

Radio-opaque liquids may be used to outline cavities during X-ray examination (air or gas can be used in the same way). Common examples are sinography (outlining a sinus), arthrography (outlining a joint) and myelography (outlining the spinal theca).

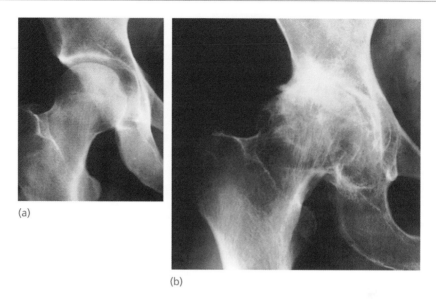

(a)

(b)

1.11 Plain X-rays of the hip (a) *Normal hip:* anatomical shape with joint 'space' (articular cartilage) fully preserved. **(b)** *Advanced osteoarthritis:* joint space markedly decreased; osteophytes at the joint margin.

Computed tomography

Computed tomography (CT) is capable of recording bone and soft-tissue outlines in cross-section. It is particularly useful for showing detailed fracture patterns, for displaying the shape of the spinal canal and for mapping the spread of tumours into the soft tissues. The computed data can also be reconstructed as a 3D image (**1.12**).

A disadvantage of CT is the relatively high radiation exposure. It should, therefore, be used with discretion.

Radionuclide scanning

A bone-seeking radio-isotope compound – usually 99m technetium hydroxymethylene diphosphonate (99mTc-HDP) – is injected intravenously and its presence in the tissues is recorded with a gamma camera or rectilinear scanner. Increased uptake during the blood phase (immediately after injection) signifies hyperaemia; activity during the bone phase (about 3 hours later) suggests new bone formation. This information is valuable in the diagnosis of stress fractures (which

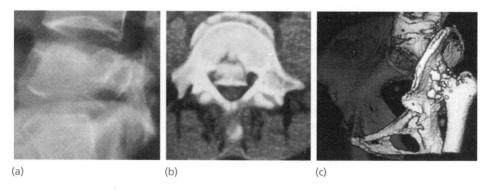

(a)   (b)   (c)

1.12 CT The plain X-ray **(a)** shows a fracture of the vertebral body but one cannot tell precisely how the bone fragments are displaced. The CT **(b)** shows clearly that they are dangerously close to the cauda equina. **(c)** 3D CT reconstruction of a congenital hip dislocation.

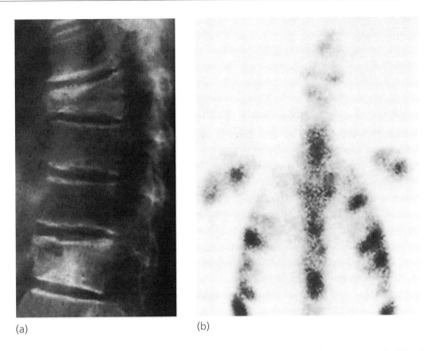

(a)   (b)

1.13 Radionuclide scanning (a) The plain X-ray showed a compression fracture, probably through a metastatic tumour. **(b)** The bone scan revealed generalized secondaries, here involving the spine and ribs.

often do not show on X-ray), bone infection and bone tumours (**1.13**).

MAGNETIC RESONANCE IMAGING

Unlike X-ray imaging, magnetic resonance imaging (MRI) relies upon radiofrequency emissions from atoms and molecules in tissues exposed to a static magnetic field. It does not involve ionizing radiation. The images produced by these signals are similar to those of CT scans, but with even better contrast resolution and more refined differentiation of tissues (**1.14**).

Tissues containing abundant hydrogen (fat, cancellous bone and marrow) emit high-intensity

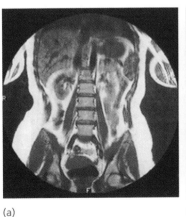
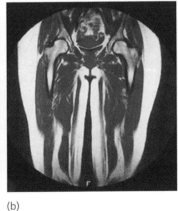
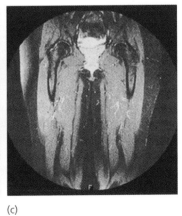

(a)   (b)   (c)

1.14 MRI MRI can define both the shape and the structure of various tissues, thus revealing the presence and the extent of pathological change.

signals and produce the brightest images; those containing little hydrogen (cortical bone, ligament, tendon and air) appear black; intermediate in the grey scale are cartilage, spinal canal and muscle. By adjusting various parameters, different tissues and organs can be displayed with extraordinary clarity. Bone tumours can be shown in their transverse and longitudinal extent and extraosseous spread can be accurately assessed. Moreover, there is the potential for characterizing the actual tissue, thus allowing a pathological as well as an anatomical diagnosis.

Other areas of usefulness are in the early diagnosis of bone ischaemia and necrosis, the investigation of backache and spinal disorders and the elucidation of cartilage and ligament injuries. In the knee, MRI is as accurate as arthroscopy in diagnosing meniscal tears and cruciate ligament injuries. It is also useful for diagnosing rotator cuff tears and labral injuries in the shoulder and ligament injuries around the ankle.

As MRI is so versatile and free of the risks of ionizing radiation, it is tempting to overindulge its use. It is well to remember that it is still only one diagnostic method among many.

Diagnostic ultrasound

High-frequency sound waves, generated by a transducer, can penetrate several centimetres into the soft tissues; as they pass through the tissue interfaces some of these waves are reflected back (like echoes) to the transducer, where they are registered as electrical signals and displayed as images on a screen or plate. With modern equipment, tissues of varying density can be 'imaged' in gradations of grey that allow reasonable definition of the anatomy. Real-time display on a monitor gives a dynamic image, which is more useful than the usual static images on transparent plates. One major advantage of this technique is that the equipment is simple and portable and can be used almost anywhere. Another is that it produces no harmful side effects.

As a result of the marked echogenic contrast between cystic and solid masses, ultrasonography is particularly useful for identifying hidden 'cystic' lesions such as haematomas, abscesses, popliteal cysts and arterial aneurysms. It is also capable of detecting intra-articular fluid.

One of the most useful applications is in screening newborn babies for DDH, where the anatomical outlines can be identified even though they are entirely cartilaginous.

BONE BIOPSY

Bone biopsy is often the only means of establishing a diagnosis or distinguishing between local conditions that closely resemble one another, such as an area of bone destruction that could be due to a compression fracture, a bone tumour or infection. Even if it is obvious that the lesion is a tumour, we need to know what type of tumour, whether benign or malignant, primary or metastatic. Radical surgery should never be undertaken for a suspected neoplasm without first confirming the diagnosis histologically. In bone infection, the biopsy permits not only histological proof of acute inflammation but also bacteriological typing of the organism and tests for antibiotic sensitivity.

Open or closed?

Open biopsy is the most reliable way of obtaining a suitable sample of tissue, but it has several drawbacks.

- It requires an operation, with the attendant risks of anaesthesia and infection.
- Tissue planes are opened up, predisposing to spread of infection or tumour.
- The incision may interfere with subsequent plans for tumour excision.

A carefully performed *closed biopsy*, using a needle or trephine, is the procedure of choice except when the lesion cannot be accurately localized or when the tissue consistency is such that a sufficient sample cannot be obtained.

Precautions

- The biopsy site and approach should be carefully planned with the aid of X-rays or other imaging techniques.
- If there is any possibility of the lesion being malignant, the approach should be sited so that the wound and biopsy track can be excised if later radical surgery proves to be necessary.
- The procedure should be carried out in an operating theatre, under anaesthesia (local or general) and with full aseptic technique.
- For deep-seated lesions, fluoroscopic control of the needle insertion is essential.
- The appropriate size of biopsy needle or cutting trephine should be selected.
- Knowledge of the local anatomy, and of the likely consistency of the lesion, is important. Large blood vessels and nerves must be avoided; potentially vascular tumours may bleed profusely and the means to control haemorrhage should be readily to hand. More than one surgeon has set out to aspirate an 'abscess' only to plunge a wide-bore needle into an aneurysm!
- Clear instructions should be given to ensure that the tissue obtained at the biopsy is suitably processed. If infection is suspected, the material should go into a culture tube and be sent to the laboratory as soon as possible. A smear may also be useful. Whole tissue is transferred to a jar containing formalin, without damaging the specimen or losing any material. Aspirated blood should be allowed to clot and can then be preserved in formalin for later paraffin embedding and sectioning. Tissue thought to contain crystals should not be placed in formalin as this may destroy the crystals; it should either be kept unaltered for immediate examination or stored in saline.
- No matter how careful the biopsy, there is always the risk that the tissue will be too scanty or too unrepresentative for accurate diagnosis. Close consultation with the radiologist and pathologist beforehand will minimize this possibility. In the best hands, needle biopsy has an accuracy rate of over 95%.

ELECTROPHYSIOLOGICAL STUDIES

Nerve and muscle function can be studied by electrical methods. Two types of investigation are employed: nerve conduction and electromyography.

Nerve conduction

The time interval between stimulation of a motor nerve and muscle contraction can be measured accurately. If the test is repeated at two points a fixed distance apart along the nerve, the *conduction velocity* between these points can be determined. Normal values are about 40–60 m/s. Sensory nerve conduction can be measured in a similar way.

Conduction velocity is slowed in peripheral nerve damage or compression, and the site of the lesion can be established by taking measurements in different segments of the nerve.

If the nerve is divided, there is no response to stimulation of the nerve and an abnormal response to galvanic stimulation of the muscle — the '*reaction of degeneration*'. By plotting the voltage against the duration of stimulus necessary to produce contraction, a *strength/duration curve* can be obtained, which reflects the degree of muscle innervation after nerve injury. Serial examinations will show whether recovery is taking place.

Electromyography

Electromyography does not involve electrical stimulation. Instead, an electrode in the muscle is used to record motor unit activity at rest and during attempts to contract the muscle. There is normally no electrical activity at rest, but on voluntary contraction characteristic oscilloscopic patterns appear. Changes in these patterns can identify certain neuropathic and myopathic disorders. After nerve injury there may be typical *denervation potentials*, and with recovery equally typical *reinnervation potentials*.

Infection

2

- General aspects of infection   23
- Acute haematogenous osteomyelitis   24
- Subacute haematogenous osteomyelitis   32
- Post-traumatic osteomyelitis   33
- Chronic osteomyelitis   33
- Periprosthetic joint infection   37
- Acute suppurative arthritis   38
- Gonococcal arthritis   42
- Spirochaetal infections   42
- Tuberculosis   44
- Mycotic infections   47
- Hydatid disease   48
- Final comment   49

Infection is a condition in which pathogenic microorganisms multiply and spread within the body tissues. Microorganisms may reach the musculoskeletal tissues by:

- *direct introduction* through the skin (a pinprick, an injection, a stab wound, a laceration, an open fracture or an operation, particularly when biomaterials are implanted)
- *direct spread from a contiguous focus of infection*
- *indirect spread via the bloodstream* from a distant site such as the nose or mouth, the respiratory tract, the bowel or the genitourinary tract.

Depending on the type of invader, the site of infection and the host response, the result may be a pyogenic osteomyelitis, a septic arthritis, a chronic granulomatous reaction (classically seen in tuberculosis of either bone or joint), or an indolent response to a less aggressive organism (as in low-grade periprosthetic infections) or to an unusual organism (e.g. a fungal infection). Soft-tissue infections range from superficial wound sepsis to widespread cellulitis and life-threatening necrotizing fasciitis.

GENERAL ASPECTS OF INFECTION

Infection usually gives rise to an acute or chronic *inflammatory reaction*, which is the body's way of combating the invaders by destroying them, or at least immobilizing and confining them to a restricted area. The classic signs of inflammation are *redness, swelling, heat, pain* and *loss of function*. Bone infection is called *osteomyelitis*.

Host susceptibility to infection is increased by:

- *local factors*, e.g. trauma, scar tissue, poor circulation, diminished sensibility, chronic bone or joint disease and the presence of foreign bodies including implants
- *systemic factors*, e.g. malnutrition, diabetes, rheumatoid disease, corticosteroid administration and immunosuppression. Resistance is also diminished in the very young and the very old.

SECTION 1 GENERAL ORTHOPAEDICS

Bacterial colonization and resistance to antibiotics are enhanced by the ability of certain microorganisms to adhere to avascular bone surfaces and foreign implants, protected from both host defences and antibiotics by a protein–polysaccharide slime (*glycocalyx* or *biofilm*). Biofilm formation aids the development of a complex bacterial community that protects microorganisms and eradication of biofilm-forming microorganisms becomes impossible without implant removal.

- *Acute pyogenic bone infections* are characterized by the formation of pus – a concentrate of defunct leucocytes, dead and dying bacteria and tissue debris – which is often localized in an abscess. Pressure builds up within the abscess and infection may then extend locally. It may also spread further via lymphatics (causing lymphangitis and lymphadenopathy) or via the bloodstream (bacteraemia and septicaemia). An accompanying systemic reaction varies from a vague feeling of lassitude with mild pyrexia to severe illness, fever, toxaemia and shock. The generalized effects are due to the release of bacterial enzymes and endotoxins as well as cellular breakdown products from the host tissues.
- *Chronic pyogenic infection* may follow unresolved acute infection and is characterized by persistence of the infecting organism in pockets of necrotic tissue. Purulent material accumulates and may be discharged through sinuses at the skin. Factors which predispose to this outcome are the presence of damaged muscle, dead bone (*sequestrum*) or a foreign implant, diminished local blood supply and a weak host response.
- *Chronic non-pyogenic infection* may result from invasion by organisms that produce a cellular reaction leading to the formation of granulomas consisting largely of lymphocytes, modified macrophages and multinucleated giant cells; this type of granulomatous infection is seen most typically in tuberculosis. Systemic effects are less acute but may ultimately be very debilitating, with lymphadenopathy, splenomegaly and tissue wasting.

TREATMENT OF INFECTION

1 Identify the infecting organism and administer effective antibiotic treatment or chemotherapy.
2 Provide analgesia and general supportive measures, including rest of the affected part or splintage of the affected joint.
3 Release pus as soon as it is detected.
4 Eradicate avascular and necrotic tissue.
5 Stabilize the bone if it has fractured and restore continuity if there is a gap in the bone.
6 Maintain or regain soft-tissue and skin cover.

ACUTE HAEMATOGENOUS OSTEOMYELITIS

Aetiology and pathogenesis

Acute haematogenous osteomyelitis is mainly a disease of children. When adults are affected, it is usually because their resistance is lowered. Trauma may determine the site of infection, possibly by causing a small haematoma or fluid collection in a bone, in patients with concurrent bacteraemia. The incidence of acute haematogenous osteomyelitis in Western European children is thought to have declined in recent years, probably a reflection of improving social conditions. Studies from the United Kingdom confirm a low incidence (less than 1 case per 100 000).

The causal organism is *Staphylococcus aureus* in over 70% of cases, and less often one of the other Gram-positive cocci, such as the Group A beta-haemolytic streptococcus (*Streptococcus pyogenes*) which is found in chronic skin infections, as well as Group B streptococcus (especially in newborn babies) or the alphahaemolytic diplococcus *S. pneumoniae*. In children between 1 and 4 years of age, the Gram-negative *Haemophilus influenzae* used to be a fairly common pathogen for osteomyelitis and septic arthritis, but the introduction of *H. influenzae* type B vaccination in the 1990s has been followed by a much reduced incidence. In recent years its place has been taken by the increasing presence of *Kingella kingae*, mainly following upper respiratory infection in young children. Other Gram-negative organisms (e.g. *Escherichia coli*, *Pseudomonas aeruginosa*, *Proteus mirabilis* and the anaerobic *Bacteroides fragilis*) occasionally cause acute bone infection. Curiously, patients with sickle-cell disease are prone to infection by *Salmonella typhi*.

IN CHILDREN AND INFANTS

- *In children*, the infection usually starts in the vascular metaphysis of a long bone, most often in the proximal tibia or in the distal or proximal ends of the femur. Predilection for this site has traditionally been attributed to the peculiar arrangement of the blood vessels in that area: the non-anastomosing terminal branches of the nutrient artery twist back in hairpin loops before entering the large network of sinusoidal veins; the relative vascular stasis and consequent lowered oxygen tension are believed to favour bacterial colonization. The structure of the fine vessels in the hypertrophic zone of the physis may more easily allow bacteria to pass through and adhere to type I collagen in that area.
- *In infants*, in whom there are still anastomoses between metaphyseal and epiphyseal blood vessels, infection can also reach the epiphysis (**2.1**).

IN ADULTS

Haematogenous infection in adults accounts for only about 20% of cases of osteomyelitis. *Staphylococcus aureus* is the commonest organism but *Pseudomonas aeruginosa* often appears in patients using intravenous drugs. Adults with diabetes and vascular disease, who are prone to soft-tissue infections of the foot, may develop contiguous bone infection involving a variety of organisms.

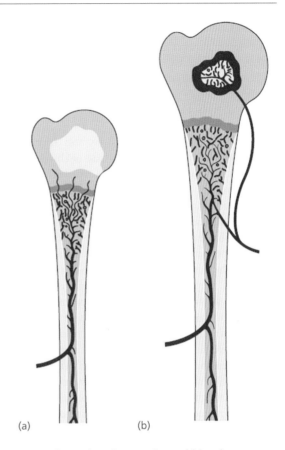

(a)   (b)

2.1 Epiphyseal and metaphyseal blood supply (a) In newborn infants some metaphyseal arterioles from the nutrient artery penetrate the physis and may carry infection directly from the metaphysis to the epiphysis. **(b)** In older children the physis acts as a barrier and the developing epiphysis receives a separate blood supply from the epiphyseal and periarticular blood vessels.

Pathology

ACUTE HAEMATOGENOUS OSTEOMYELITIS: CHARACTERISTIC PROGRESSION
1 Inflammation
2 Suppuration
3 Bone necrosis
4 Reactive new bone formation
5 Resolution and healing or intractable chronicity

SECTION 1 GENERAL ORTHOPAEDICS

IN CHILDREN

The 'classic' picture is seen in children between 2 and 6 years. The earliest change in the metaphysis is an acute inflammatory reaction with vascular congestion, exudation of fluid and infiltration by polymorphonuclear leucocytes. The intraosseous pressure rises rapidly, causing intense pain, obstruction to blood flow and intravascular thrombosis. The bone tissue is threatened by impending ischaemia and resorption due to a combination of phagocytic activity and the local accumulation of cytokines, growth factors, prostaglandin and bacterial enzymes. By the second or third day, pus forms within the bone and forces its way along the Volkmann canals to the surface where it produces a subperiosteal abscess. From the subperiosteal abscess, pus can spread along the shaft, to re-enter the bone at another level or burst into the surrounding soft tissues.

The rising intraosseous pressure, vascular stasis, small-vessel thrombosis and periosteal stripping increasingly compromise the blood supply; by the end of a week there is usually microscopic evidence of bone death. Bacterial toxins and leucocytic enzymes also may play their part in the advancing tissue destruction. With the gradual ingrowth of granulation tissue the boundary between living and devitalized bone becomes defined. Pieces of dead bone may separate as *sequestra*.

Macrophages and lymphocytes arrive in increasing numbers and the debris is slowly removed by a combination of phagocytosis and osteoclastic resorption. A small focus in cancellous bone may be completely resorbed, leaving a tiny cavity, but a large cortical or cortico-cancellous sequestrum will remain entombed, inaccessible to either final destruction or repair.

Another feature of advancing acute osteomyelitis is new bone formation. Initially, the area around the infected zone is porotic, but if the pus is not released, either spontaneously or by surgical decompression, new bone starts forming on viable surfaces in the bone and from the deep layers of the stripped periosteum. This is typical of pyogenic infection, and fine streaks of subperiosteal new bone usually become apparent on radiographs by the end of the second week. With time, this new bone thickens to form a casement, or *involucrum*, enclosing the sequestrum and infected tissue. If the infection persists, pus and tiny sequestrated spicules of bone may discharge through perforations (*cloacae*) in the involucrum and track by sinuses to the skin surface (**2.2**).

If the infection is controlled and intraosseous pressure released at an early stage, this dire progress can be halted. The bone around the zone of infection becomes increasingly dense; this, together with the periosteal reaction, results in thickening of the bone. In some cases, the normal anatomy may eventually be reconstituted; in others, though healing is sound, the bone is left permanently deformed.

If healing does not occur, a nidus of infection may remain locked inside the bone, causing pus and sometimes bone debris to be discharged intermittently through a persistent sinus (or several sinuses). The infection has now lapsed into *chronic osteomyelitis*, which may last for many years.

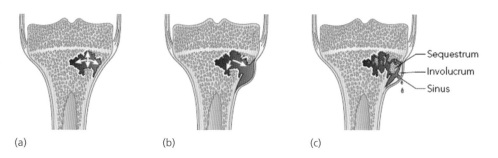

(a)   (b)   (c)

2.2 Acute osteomyelitis (a) Infection in the metaphysis may spread towards the surface, to form a subperiosteal abscess **(b)**. Some of the bone may die and is encased in periosteal new bone as a sequestrum **(c)**. The encasing involucrum is sometimes perforated by sinuses.

IN INFANTS

The early features of acute osteomyelitis in infants are much the same as those in older children. However, a significant difference, during the first year of life, is the frequency with which the metaphyseal infection spreads to the epiphysis and from there into the adjacent joint. In the process, the physeal anlage may be irreparably damaged, further growth at that site is severely retarded and the joint will be permanently deformed.

IN ADULTS

Bone infection in the adult usually follows an open injury, an operation or spread from a contiguous focus of infection (e.g. a neuropathic ulcer or an infected diabetic foot). True haematogenous osteomyelitis is uncommon and, when it does occur, it usually affects one of the vertebrae, a metaphyseal region of a long bone or a small cuboidal bone. A vertebral infection may spread through the end plate and the intervertebral disc into an adjacent vertebral body.

Clinical features

Clinical features of acute osteomyelitis differ in the three described groups.

IN CHILDREN

The patient, usually a child over 4 years, presents with severe pain, malaise and a fever; in neglected cases, toxaemia may be marked. The parents will have noticed that the child refuses to use one limb or to allow it to be handled or even touched. There may be a recent history of infection: a septic toe, a boil, a sore throat or a discharge from the ear. Typically, the child looks ill and feverish; the pulse rate is likely to be over 100 and the temperature is raised. The limb is held still and there is acute tenderness near one of the larger joints. Even the gentlest manipulation is painful and joint movement is restricted ('pseudoparalysis'). Local redness, swelling, warmth and oedema are later signs and signify that pus has escaped from the interior of the bone. Lymphadenopathy is common but non-specific.

 It is important to remember that all the clinical features of acute osteomyelitis may be attenuated if antibiotics have been administered.

IN INFANTS

In children under 1 year old, and especially in the newborn, the constitutional disturbance can be misleadingly mild; the baby simply fails to thrive and is drowsy but irritable. Suspicion should be aroused by a history of birth difficulties, umbilical artery catheterization or a site of infection (however mild) such as an inflamed intravenous infusion point or even a heel puncture. Metaphyseal tenderness and resistance to joint movement can signify either osteomyelitis or septic arthritis; indeed, both may be present, so the distinction hardly matters. Look for other sites: multiple infections are not uncommon, especially in babies who acquire the infection in hospital. Radionuclide bone scans may help to discover additional sites.

> **CARDINAL FEATURES OF ACUTE OSTEOMYELITIS IN CHILDREN**
>
> Pain
> Fever
> Refusal to bear weight
> Elevated white blood cell (WBC) count
> Elevated erythrocyte sedimentation rate (ESR)
> Elevated C-reactive protein (CRP)

IN ADULTS

A common site for haematogenous infection is the thoracolumbar spine. There may be a history of some urological procedure followed by a mild fever and backache. Local tenderness is not very marked and it may take weeks before X-ray signs appear; when they do appear, the diagnosis may still need to be confirmed by fine-needle aspiration and bacteriological culture. Other imaging may be required such as MRI, CT or single-photon emission computed tomography/computed tomography (SPECT/CT).

> *In the very elderly, and in those with immune deficiency, systemic features are mild and the diagnosis is easily missed.*

Diagnostic imaging

PLAIN X-RAY

During the first week after the onset of symptoms, the plain radiograph shows no abnormality of the bone. Displacement of the fat planes signifies soft-tissue swelling, but this could as well be due to a haematoma or soft-tissue infection. By the second week there may be a faint extracortical outline due to periosteal new bone formation; this is the classic X-ray sign of early pyogenic osteomyelitis. Later, the periosteal thickening becomes more obvious and there is patchy rarefaction of the metaphysis; later still, the ragged features of bone destruction appear (**2.3**). An important late sign is the combination of regional osteoporosis with a localized segment of apparently increased density. Osteoporosis

is a feature of metabolically active, and thus living, bone; the segment that fails to become osteoporotic is metabolically inactive and possibly dead.

ULTRASONOGRAPHY

Ultrasonography may detect a subperiosteal collection of fluid in the early stages of osteomyelitis, but it cannot distinguish between a haematoma and pus.

CT

CT offers the advantage of planar bone definition, including bone destruction and soft-tissue mass, such as an abscess, within or surrounding bone. Disadvantages include high radiation dose.

RADIONUCLIDE SCANNING

Radioscintigraphy with ^{99}mTc-HDP reveals increased activity in both the perfusion phase and the bone phase. This is a highly sensitive investigation, even in the very early stages, but it has relatively low specificity and other inflammatory lesions can show similar changes. In doubtful cases, scanning with ^{67}Ga-citrate or ^{111}In-labelled leucocytes can be considered.

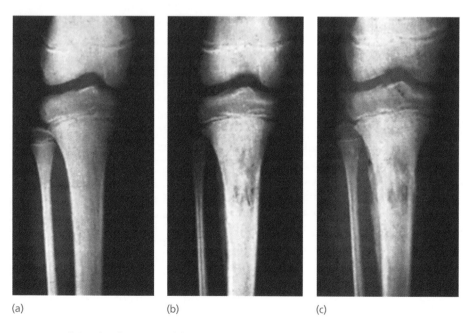

(a)   (b)   (c)

2.3 Acute osteomyelitis The first X-ray **(a)**, 2 days after symptoms began, is normal – it always is; metaphyseal mottling and periosteal changes were not obvious until the second film **(b)**, taken 14 days later; eventually much of the shaft was involved **(c)**.

SPECT/CT

Hybrid SPECT/CT imaging, compared with conventional planar study and SPECT alone, provides improved anatomic localization of infection and more accurate definition of its extent.

MAGNETIC RESONANCE IMAGING

Magnetic resonance imaging (MRI) can be helpful in cases of doubtful diagnosis, and particularly in suspected infection of the axial skeleton. It is the best method of demonstrating bone marrow inflammation. It is extremely sensitive, even in the early phase of bone infection, and it can therefore assist in differentiating between soft-tissue infection and osteomyelitis.

Laboratory investigations

> ### DIAGNOSIS OF ACUTE OSTEOMYELITIS
>
> The most certain way to confirm the clinical diagnosis of acute osteomyelitis is to aspirate and test pus or fluid from the metaphyseal subperiosteal abscess, the extraosseous soft tissues or an adjacent joint.

A simple Gram stain may help to identify the type of infection initially and assist with the early choice of antibiotic, but only until microbiological diagnosis through culture and antibiogram is established. *Aspiration* will give a positive result in over 60% of cases that could be improved in case of open surgery by culture of tissue samples.

Blood cultures should be obtained if fever above 38 °C is detected, even though positive culture is obtained in less than half the cases of proven infection. The CRP values are usually elevated within 12–24 hours and the ESR within 24–48 hours after the onset of symptoms. The *WBC count* rises and the haemoglobin concentration may be diminished.

 In the very young and the very old, blood tests are less reliable and may show values within the range of normal.

Differential diagnosis

Cellulitis   This is often mistaken for osteomyelitis. There is widespread superficial redness, with a clear demarcation between infected and normal skin, and lymphangitis. The source of skin infection may not be obvious and should be searched for (e.g. on the sole or between the toes). If doubt remains about the diagnosis, MRI will help to distinguish between bone infection and soft-tissue infection. The organism is usually a *Staphylococcus* or *Streptococcus*. Mild cases will respond to high-dosage oral antibiotics; severe cases need intravenous antibiotic treatment.

Acute suppurative arthritis   Tenderness is diffuse, and movement at the joint is completely abolished by muscle spasm. In infants, the distinction between metaphyseal osteomyelitis and septic arthritis of the adjacent joint is somewhat theoretical, as both often coexist.

Streptococcal necrotizing myositis   Group A beta-haemolytic streptococci (the same organisms which are responsible for the common 'sore throat') occasionally invade muscles and cause an acute myositis. Although the condition is rare, it should be kept well to the foreground in the differential diagnosis because it may rapidly spiral out of control towards muscle necrosis, septicaemia and death.

 Intense pain and board-like swelling of the limb in a patient with fever and a general feeling of illness are warning signs of a medical emergency.

MRI will reveal muscle swelling and possibly signs of tissue breakdown. Immediate treatment with intravenous antibiotics is essential. Surgical debridement of necrotic tissue – and sometimes even amputation – may be needed to save a life.

Acute rheumatism   The pain is less severe and it tends to flit from one joint to another. There may also be signs of carditis, rheumatic nodules or *erythema marginatum*.

Sickle-cell crisis   The patient may present with features indistinguishable from those of acute osteomyelitis. In areas where *Salmonella* is endemic, it would be wise to treat such patients with suitable antibiotics until infection is definitely excluded.

Gaucher's disease 'Pseudo-osteitis' may occur with features closely resembling those of osteomyelitis. The diagnosis is made by finding other stigmata of the disease, especially enlargement of the spleen and liver.

Treatment

 If osteomyelitis is suspected on clinical grounds, blood and fluid samples should be taken for laboratory investigation and then treatment started immediately, without waiting for final confirmation of the diagnosis.

There are four important aspects to the management of the patient:

• appropriate antimicrobial therapy (first empirical, then specific)
• surgical drainage if required
• splintage and rest of the affected part
• supportive treatment for pain and dehydration.

ANTIBIOTICS

 Blood and aspiration material should be sent immediately for examination and culture, but the *prompt intravenous administration of antibiotics* is so vital that treatment should not await the result.

Initially, the choice of antibiotics is based on the findings from direct examination of the pus smear and the clinician's experience of local conditions – in other words, early empirical antibiotic administration, a 'best guess' at the most likely pathogen. *Staphylococcus aureus* is the most common at all ages, but treatment should provide cover also for other bacteria that are likely to be encountered in each age group.

Neonates and infants up to 6 months of age Initial antibiotic treatment should be effective against penicillin-resistant *Staphylococcus aureus*,

Group B streptococcus and Gram-negative organisms. Drugs of choice are flucloxacillin plus a third-generation cephalosporin such as cefotaxime. Alternatively, effective empirical treatment can be provided by a combination of flucloxacillin (for penicillin-resistant staphylococci), benzylpenicillin (for Group B streptococci) and gentamycin (for Gram-negative organisms).

Children 6 months to 6 years of age Empirical treatment in this age group should include cover against *Haemophilus influenzae*, unless it is known for certain that the child has had an anti-haemophilus vaccination. This is best provided by a combination of intravenous flucloxacillin and cefotaxime or cefuroxime.

Older children and previously fit adults The vast majority in this group will have a staphylococcal infection and can be started on intravenous flucloxacillin and fusidic acid. Fusidic acid is preferred to benzylpenicillin partly because of the high prevalence of penicillin-resistant staphylococci and because it is particularly well concentrated in bone. However, for a known streptococcal infection, benzylpenicillin is better. Patients who are allergic to penicillin should be treated with a polypeptide.

Elderly and previously unfit patients In this group there is a greater than usual risk of Gram-negative infections, due to respiratory, gastrointestinal or urinary disorders and the likelihood of the patient needing invasive procedures. The antibiotic of choice would be a combination of flucloxacillin and a second- or third-generation cephalosporin.

Patients with sickle-cell disease These patients are prone to osteomyelitis, which may be caused by a staphylococcal infection but in many cases is due to *Salmonella* and/or other Gram-negative organisms. Chloramphenicol, which is effective against Gram-positive, Gram-negative and anaerobic organisms, used to be the preferred antibiotic, though there were always worries about the rare complication of aplastic anaemia. The current antibiotic of choice is a third-generation cephalosporin or a fluoroquinolone such as ciprofloxacin.

Heroin addicts and immunocompromised patients Unusual infections (e.g. with *Pseudomonas aeruginosa*, *Proteus mirabilis* or anaerobic *Bacteroides* species) are likely in these patients. Infants with human immunodeficiency virus (HIV) infection may also have picked up other sexually transmitted organisms during birth. All patients with this type of background are therefore best treated empirically with a broad-spectrum antibiotic such as one of the third-generation cephalosporins or a fluoroquinolone preparation, depending on the results of sensitivity tests.

Patients considered to be at risk of methicillin-resistant *Staphylococcus aureus* (MRSA) infection Patients admitted with acute haematogenous osteomyelitis and who have a previous history of MRSA infection, or any patient with a bone infection admitted to a hospital or a ward where MRSA is endemic, should be treated with intravenous vancomycin (or other glucopeptide such as teicoplanin) together with a third-generation cephalosporin.

SURGICAL DRAINAGE

If antibiotics are given early (within the first 48 hours after the onset of symptoms), drainage is often unnecessary. However, if the clinical features do not improve within 36 hours of starting treatment, if there are signs of deep pus (swelling, oedema, fluctuation), and most certainly if pus is aspirated, the abscess should be drained by open surgery under general anaesthesia.

SPLINTAGE

Some type of splintage is desirable, partly for comfort but also to prevent joint contractures. Simple skin traction may suffice and, if the hip is involved, this also helps to prevent dislocation.

GENERAL SUPPORTIVE TREATMENT

The distressed child needs to be comforted and treated for pain. Analgesics should be given at repeated intervals without waiting for the patient to ask for them. Septicaemia and fever can cause severe dehydration and it may be necessary to give fluid intravenously.

Complications

Epiphyseal damage and altered bone growth

In neonates and infants whose epiphyses are still entirely cartilaginous, metaphyseal vessels penetrate the physis and may carry the infection into the epiphysis. If this happens, the physeal growth plate can be irrevocably damaged and the cartilaginous epiphysis may be destroyed, leading to arrest of growth and shortening of the bone.

Suppurative arthritis   This may occur:

- in very young infants, in whom the growth plate is not an impenetrable barrier
- where the metaphysis is intracapsular, as in the upper femur
- from metastatic infection.

In infants, it is so common as almost to be taken for granted, especially with osteomyelitis of the femoral neck. Ultrasound will help to demonstrate an effusion, but the definitive diagnosis is obtained by joint aspiration.

 Be aware of the risk of concurrent septic arthritis.

The *intracapsular metaphyses* are anatomical areas where a focus of osteomyelitis can discharge directly into the joint, resulting in septic arthritis. These are:

- proximal femur (causing septic arthritis of the hip)
- proximal humerus (causing septic arthritis of the shoulder)
- proximal radius (causing septic arthritis of the elbow)
- distal fibula (causing septic arthritis of the ankle).

Metastatic infection   This is sometimes seen – generally in infants – and may involve other bones, joints, serous cavities, the brain or the lung(s).

Pathological fracture   Fracture is uncommon, but it may occur if treatment is delayed and the bone is weakened, either by erosion at the site of infection or by overzealous debridement.

SUBACUTE HAEMATOGENOUS OSTEOMYELITIS

This condition is no longer rare, and in some countries the incidence is equal to that of acute osteomyelitis. Its relative mildness is presumably due to the organism being less virulent or the patient more resistant. Its skeletal distribution is more variable than in acute osteomyelitis, but the distal femur and the proximal and distal tibia are the frequent sites.

Pathology

Typically, there is a well-defined cavity in cancellous bone – usually in the tibial metaphysis – containing seropurulent fluid. The cavity is lined by granulation tissue containing a mixture of acute and chronic inflammatory cells. The surrounding bone trabeculae are often thickened.

Clinical features

The patient is usually a child or adolescent who has had pain near one of the larger joints for several weeks. They may have a limp and often there is slight swelling, muscle wasting and local tenderness. The temperature is usually normal and there is little to suggest an infection. The WBC count and blood cultures usually show no abnormality but the ESR is sometimes elevated.

Imaging

The typical radiographic lesion is a circumscribed, round or oval radiolucent 'cavity' 1–2 cm in diameter. Most often it is seen in the tibial or femoral metaphysis, but it may occur in the epiphysis or in one of the cuboidal bones. The 'cavity' is sometimes surrounded by a halo of sclerosis (the classic *Brodie's abscess*); occasionally, it is less well defined, extending into the diaphysis (2.4).

Metaphyseal lesions cause little or no periosteal reaction; diaphyseal lesions may be associated with periosteal new bone formation and marked cortical thickening. If the cortex is eroded, the lesion may be mistaken for a malignant tumour.

The radioisotope scan shows markedly increased activity.

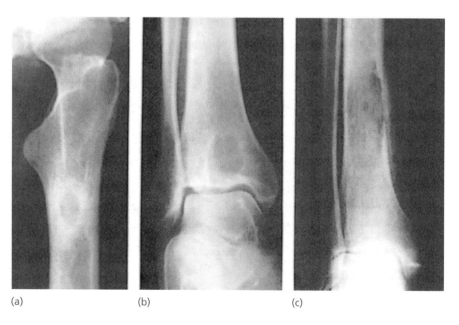

(a)   (b)   (c)

2.4 Subacute osteomyelitis (a,b) The classic Brodie's abscess looks like a small walled-off cavity in the bone with little or no periosteal reaction. **(c)** Sometimes rarefaction is more diffuse and there may be cortical erosion and periosteal reaction.

Diagnosis

The clinical and X-ray appearances may resemble those of cystic tuberculosis, eosinophilic granuloma or osteoid osteoma; occasionally, they mimic a malignant bone tumour such as Ewing's sarcoma. Epiphyseal lesions are easily mistaken for chondroblastoma. The diagnosis often remains in doubt until a biopsy is performed.

If fluid is encountered, it should be sent for bacteriological culture; this is positive in about half the cases and the organism is almost invariably *Staphylococcus aureus*.

Treatment

Treatment may be conservative if the diagnosis is not in doubt. Immobilization and antibiotics (flucloxacillin and fusidic acid) intravenously for 4–5 days and then orally for another 6 weeks usually result in healing. If the diagnosis is in doubt, an open biopsy is needed and the lesion may be curetted at the same time.

POST-TRAUMATIC OSTEOMYELITIS

Open fractures are always contaminated and are therefore prone to infection.

 The most common cause of osteomyelitis in adults is an infected open fracture.

Staphylococcus aureus is the usual pathogen, but other organisms such as *Escherichia coli*, *Proteus mirabilis* and *Pseudomonas aeruginosa* are sometimes involved. Occasionally, anaerobic organisms appear in contaminated wounds.

Clinical features

The patient becomes feverish and develops pain and swelling over the fracture site; the wound is inflamed and there may be a seropurulent discharge. Blood tests reveal leucocytosis, increased CRP levels, and an elevated ESR; it should be remembered, though, that these inflammatory markers are non-specific and may be affected by tissue trauma.

- *X-ray* appearances may be more difficult than usual to interpret because of bone fragmentation.
- *MRI* can be helpful in differentiating between bone and soft-tissue infection.

Microbiological investigation

If the wound is infected, a wound swab should be examined and cultured for organisms which can be tested for antibiotic sensitivity.

 Standard laboratory methods will yield negative results in about 20% of cases of overt infection.

Routine wound swabs of open fracture wounds in the absence of infection is not recommended as cultured organisms are very unlikely to be the same as the organism causing any subsequent infection. Multiple tissue samples taken with clean, sterile instruments are preferred for microbiological investigations.

Treatment

The essence of treatment of open fractures is prophylaxis of infection: thorough cleansing and debridement of open fractures, the provision of drainage by leaving the wound open, immobilization of the fracture and antibiotics. In most cases a combination of flucloxacillin and benzylpenicillin (or sodium fusidate), given 6-hourly for 48 hours, will suffice. If the wound is clearly contaminated, it is wise also to give metronidazole for 4–5 days to control both aerobic and anaerobic organisms.

Advances in external fixation techniques have meant that almost all fractures can, if necessary, be securely fixed by that method, with the added advantage that the wound remains accessible for dressings and superficial debridement.

CHRONIC OSTEOMYELITIS

In adults, this usually occurs after an open fracture or an operation. The commonest organisms are *Staphylococcus aureus*, *Escherichia coli*, *Streptococcus pyogenes*, *Proteus mirabilis* and

Pseudomonas aeruginosa; in the presence of foreign implants, *Staphylococcus epidermidis* (frequently coagulase-negative staphylococci) is the commonest of all. In low-to-middle-income countries (LMICs), chronic osteomyelitis is a common presentation in children and a cause of considerable morbidity.

Predisposing factors

Acute haematogenous osteomyelitis, if left untreated – and provided the patient does not succumb to septicaemia – will subside into a chronic bone infection which lingers indefinitely, perhaps with alternating 'flare-ups' and spells of apparent quiescence. The host defences are inevitably compromised by the presence of scar formation, dead and dying bone around the focus of infection, poor penetration of new blood vessels and non-collapsing cavities in which microbes can thrive. Bacteria covered in a protein–polysaccharide slime (*glycocalyx*) that protects them from both the host defences and antibiotics have the ability to adhere to inert surfaces such as bone sequestra and metal implants, where they multiply and colonize the area. There is also evidence that bacteria can survive inside osteoblasts and osteocytes and be released when the cells die.

Pathology

Bone is destroyed or devitalized, either in a discrete area around the focus of infection or more diffusely along the surface of an implant. Cavities containing pus and sequestra are surrounded by vascular tissue, and beyond that by areas of sclerosis – the result of chronic reactive new bone formation – which may take the form of a distinct bony sheath (*involucrum*). Sequestra act as substrates for bacterial adhesion ensuring the persistence of infection until they are removed or discharged through perforations in the involucrum and sinuses that drain to the skin. A sinus may seal off for weeks or even months, giving the appearance of healing, only to reopen when the tissue tension rises. Bone destruction, and the increasingly brittle sclerosis, sometimes results in a pathological fracture.

In children, chronic osteomyelitis can result in rapid bone necrosis.

Bone necrosis can ensue when the endosteal blood supply is damaged by the intramedullary abscess. Pus can then break through the cortex to form a sub-periosteal collection, thus also compromising the periosteal supply. The resultant necrotic bone (the sequestrum) can be small or may affect the entire bone (**2.5**).

The following *complications* can occur with chronic osteomyelitis in children, each requiring a care management plan:

- a large sequestrum compromising the structural integrity of the limb
- involvement of the growth plate (physis), resulting in growth arrest and leg length discrepancy (**2.6**)
- angular deformity.

Clinical features

The patient presents because pain, pyrexia, redness and tenderness have recurred (a 'flare'), or with a discharging sinus. In long-standing cases, the tissues are thickened and often puckered or folded inwards where a scar or sinus adheres to the underlying bone.

Imaging

- *X-ray examination* will usually show bone resorption – either as a patchy loss of density or as frank excavation around an implant – with thickening and sclerosis of the surrounding bone (**2.7**). A *sinogram* may help to localize the site of infection.
- *Radioisotope scintigraphy* is sensitive but not specific. ^{99}mTc-HDP scans show increased activity in both the perfusion phase and the bone phase. Scanning with ^{67}Ga-citrate or ^{111}In-labelled leucocytes is said to be more specific for osteomyelitis; such scans could be useful for showing up hidden foci of infection, although its low specificity has led to limited use.
- *CT* and *MRI* are invaluable in planning operative treatment: together they will show

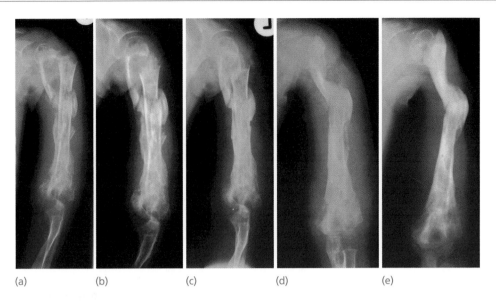

(a)   (b)   (c)   (d)   (e)

2.5 Chronic osteomyelitis (a–e) Radiographs of a 5-year-old child with chronic osteomyelitis affecting the entire humerus. **(a–c)** Over several months the involucrum develops structural integrity, allowing safe removal of the large diaphyseal sequestrum **(d)**. Premature removal of the sequestrum would have resulted in a flail arm.

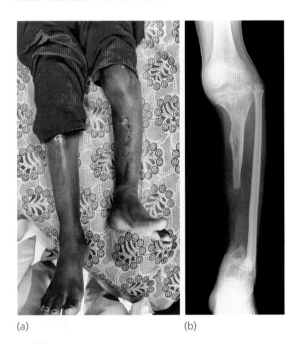

(a)   (b)

2.6 Chronic osteomyelitis (a) The clinical photo and **(b)** the radiograph demonstrate some of the sequelae of chronic osteomyelitis: a proximal and distal tibia physeal arrest causing leg length discrepancy, segmental bone loss following discharge of a diaphyseal sequestrum and ankylosis of the ankle joint.

the extent of bone destruction and reactive oedema, hidden abscesses and sequestra.

- *SPECT/CT* may provide advantages of sensitivity and local definition, and its use may increase in complex cases.

Investigations

During acute flares the CSR, ESR and WBC levels may be increased; these non-specific signs are helpful in assessing the progress of bone infection but they are not diagnostic.

Organisms cultured from discharging sinuses should be tested repeatedly for antibiotic sensitivity; with time, they often change their characteristics and become resistant to treatment. A superficial swab sample may not reflect the really persistent infection in the deeper tissues or may suffer from contamination; sampling from deeper tissues is crucial to understand the bone infection.

Treatment

ANTIBIOTICS

Chronic infection is seldom eradicated by antibiotics alone, yet bactericidal drugs are important: to suppress the infection and prevent its spread to

SECTION 1 GENERAL ORTHOPAEDICS

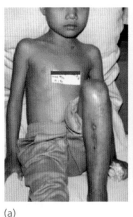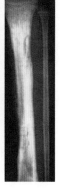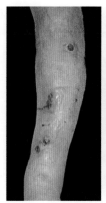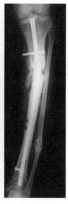

(a) (b)

2.7 Chronic osteomyelitis Chronic osteomyelitis may follow acute. The young boy **(a)** presented with draining sinuses at the site of a previous acute infection. The X-ray shows densely sclerotic bone. **(b)** In adults, chronic osteomyelitis is usually a sequel to open trauma or operation.

healthy bone and to control acute flares. The choice of antibiotic depends on microbiological studies, but the drug must be capable of penetrating sclerotic bone and should be non-toxic with long-term use. Fusidic acid, clindamycin and the cephalosporins are good examples. Vancomycin and teicoplanin are effective in most cases of MRSA.

Antibiotics are administered for 4–6 weeks (starting from the beginning of treatment or the last debridement) before considering operative treatment. During this time, serum antibiotic concentrations should be measured at regular intervals to ensure that they are kept at several times the minimal bactericidal concentration.

LOCAL TREATMENT

A sinus may be painless and need dressing simply to protect the clothing. Colostomy paste can be used to stop excoriation of the skin. An acute abscess may need urgent incision and drainage, but this is only a temporary measure.

OPERATION

A waiting policy, punctuated by spells of bed rest and antibiotics to control flares, may have to be patiently endured until there is a clear indication for radical surgery.

- For *chronic haematogenous infections*, this means intrusive symptoms, failure of adequate antibiotic treatment or clear evidence of a sequestrum or dead bone.

- For *post-traumatic infections*, this means an intractable wound or an infected ununited fracture.
- For *postoperative infection*, similar criteria and evidence of bone erosion are needed.

The presence of a *foreign implant* may prompt surgical intervention to remove the implant.

Debridement At operation, all infected soft tissue and dead or devitalized bone, as well as any infected implant, must be excised. The wound is inspected after 3–4 days and, if there are renewed signs of tissue death, the debridement may have to be repeated, several times if necessary. Antibiotic cover is continued for at least 4 weeks after the last debridement.

Dealing with the 'dead space' There are several ways of dealing with the resulting 'dead space'. *Porous antibiotic-impregnated beads* can be laid in the cavity and left for 2–3 weeks and then replaced with *cancellous bone grafts*. Bone grafts have also been used on their own; in the *Papineau technique* the entire cavity is packed with small cancellous chips mixed with an antibiotic and a fibrin sealant. Where possible, the area is covered by adjacent muscle and the skin wound is sutured without tension.

An alternative approach is to employ a *muscle flap transfer*: in suitable sites a large wad of muscle, with its blood supply intact, can be mobilized and laid into the cavity; the surface is later covered with a split-skin graft. In areas with too little adjacent muscle (e.g. the distal part of the leg), the same objective can be achieved by transferring a myocutaneous island flap on a long vascular pedicle. A free vascularized bone graft is considered to be a better option, provided the site is suitable and the appropriate facilities for microvascular surgery are available.

A different technique is the *Lautenbach approach*, involving radical excision of all avascular and infected tissue followed by closed irrigation and suction drainage, and an appropriate antibiotic solution in high concentration to allow the 'dead space' to be filled by vascular granulation tissue.

In refractory cases it may be possible to excise the infected and/or devitalized segment of bone completely and then close the gap by the *Ilizarov method* of 'transporting' a viable segment from the remaining diaphysis (**2.8**).

Soft-tissue cover   The bone must be adequately covered with skin. For small defects, split thickness skin grafts may suffice; for larger wounds, local musculocutaneous flaps, or free vascularized flaps, are needed. Vacuum-assisted closure (VAC) may help when the deep infection is solved, not before.

PERIPROSTHETIC JOINT INFECTION

Periprosthetic joint infection (PJI) is a specific type of infection related to joint replacement and a dreadful complication, potentially chronic, with significant clinical relevance for the affected patient, the treating surgeon and the health system. With an incidence of about 1–2% in hip arthroplasty, 2–3% in knee arthroplasty, 1–2% in the shoulder and even 3–5% in the elbow, the economic impact may represent a 5- to 10-fold cost increase compared to a primary arthroplasty. Patient risk factors include obesity, diabetes, rheumatoid arthritis and immunosuppressive treatments.

Once in contact with the surface of the implant, microorganisms adhere to and colonize the surface of the implant and form *biofilms*. Biofilms

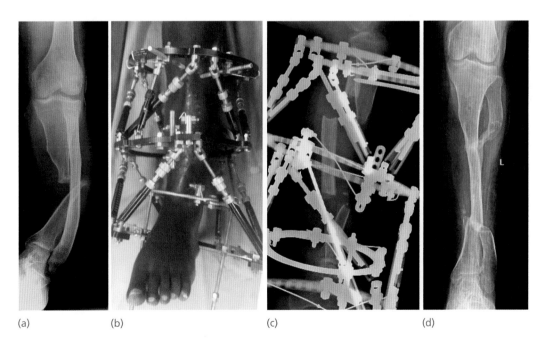

(a)   (b)   (c)   (d)

2.8 Chronic osteomyelitis – operative treatment   Pre- and postoperative clinical images and radiographs of an 18-year-old patient with the sequelae of chronic osteomyelitis of the left tibia. The limb was short and the mid-diaphyseal tibial bone defect resulted in bowing and hypertrophy of the fibula from weight-bearing. Using a circular fixator, the central third of the fibula was 'transported' and the tibia lengthened through the defect. The fibula could then be docked, restoring leg length, alignment and structural integrity.

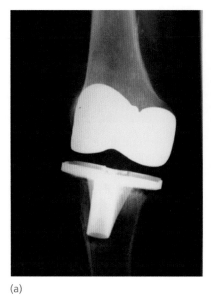
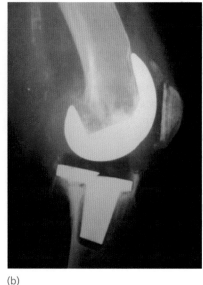

(a)   (b)

2.9 Periprosthetic joint infection Septic loosening surrounding the tibial stem in this case with PJI 3 years after total knee arthroplasty associated with immunodepression due to chemotherapy in the treatment of severe malignancy in **(a)** anteroposterior and **(b)** lateral radiographic views.

are complex communities of microorganisms embedded in an extracellular matrix formed on surfaces. From the attachment of microbial cells to a surface, the biofilm grows and matures until detachment and propagation (**2.9**), protecting microorganisms in a multicellular non-homogeneous structure where microbial cells communicate with one another (e.g. through quorum sensing) as in a multicellular organism protected from antibiotics and the host immune system. Clearing the biofilm requires surgical treatment, frequently with implant removal together with radical debridement of all infected tissues, followed by specific intravenous antibiotics.

The causative microorganism of PJI is most frequently *Staphylococcus aureus*, followed by coagulase-negative *Staphylococcus*. Together, these represent more than 50% of PJIs. *Streptococcus* species, *Enterococcus* species, aerobic Gram-negative bacilli, and some anaerobic (such as *Propionibacterium acnes* in the shoulder) account for 20–30%, while polymicrobial infections occur in 10–20%.

Treatment of PJI usually requires both surgery and medical therapy, including prolonged antibiotic therapy after hospital discharge. The team approach, including surgeons and microbiologists, is strictly required. Surgical treatment options include debridement with prosthesis retention, one-stage arthroplasty exchange, two-stage arthroplasty exchange with or without antibiotic-loaded polymethylmethacrylate spacer, arthroplasty resection without reimplantation, or even suppression treatment consisting of long-term antibiotic treatment alone. Rarely, amputation may be required in case of vital risk for the patient.

ACUTE SUPPURATIVE ARTHRITIS

A joint can become infected by:

- direct invasion through a penetrating wound, intra-articular injection or arthroscopy
- direct spread from an adjacent bone abscess
- blood spread from a distant site.

In infants, it is often difficult to tell whether the infection started in the metaphyseal bone and spread to the joint or vice versa.

The causal organism is usually *Staphylococcus aureus*; however, in children between 1 and

4 years old, *Haemophilus influenzae* is an important pathogen unless they have been vaccinated against this organism. Occasionally other microbes, such as *Streptococcus*, *Escherichia coli* and *Proteus*, are encountered.

PREDISPOSING CONDITIONS FOR ACUTE SUPPURATIVE ARTHRITIS

Rheumatoid arthritis
Chronic debilitating disorders
Intravenous drug abuse
Immunosuppressive drug therapy
Acquired immune deficiency syndrome (AIDS)

Pathology

The usual trigger is a haematogenous infection which settles in the synovial membrane; there is an acute inflammatory reaction with a serous or seropurulent exudate and an increase in synovial fluid. As pus appears in the joint, articular cartilage is eroded and destroyed, partly by bacterial enzymes and partly by proteolytic enzymes released from synovial cells, inflammatory cells and pus (**2.10**).

- *In infants*, the entire epiphysis, which is still largely cartilaginous, may be severely damaged.
- *In older children*, vascular occlusion may lead to necrosis of the epiphyseal bone.

- *In adults*, the effects are usually confined to the articular cartilage, but in late cases there may be extensive erosion due to synovial proliferation and ingrowth.

With *healing* there may be:

- complete resolution and a return to normal
- partial loss of articular cartilage and fibrosis of the joint
- loss of articular cartilage and bony ankylosis
- bone destruction and permanent deformity of the joint.

Clinical features

The clinical features differ somewhat according to the age of the patient.

IN NEWBORN INFANTS

In newborn infants, the emphasis is on septicaemia rather than joint pain. The baby is irritable and refuses to feed; there is a rapid pulse and sometimes a fever. Infection is often suspected, but it could be anywhere! The joints should be carefully felt and moved to elicit the local signs of warmth, tenderness and resistance to movement.

⚠️ *In newborn infants*, special care should be taken not to miss a concomitant osteomyelitis in an adjacent bone end.

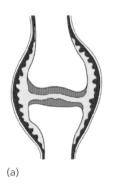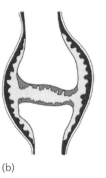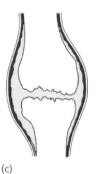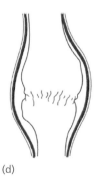

(a)   (b)   (c)   (d)

2.10 Acute suppurative arthritis – pathology In the early stage (a), there is an acute synovitis with a purulent joint effusion. (b) Soon the articular cartilage is attacked by bacterial and cellular enzymes. If the infection is not arrested, the cartilage may be completely destroyed (c). Healing then leads to bony ankylosis (d).

SECTION 1 GENERAL ORTHOPAEDICS

IN CHILDREN

In children, the usual features are acute pain in a single large joint (commonly the hip or the knee) and reluctance to move the limb ('pseudoparesis'). The child is ill, with a rapid pulse and a swinging fever. The overlying skin looks red and in a superficial joint swelling may be obvious. There is local warmth and marked tenderness. All movements are restricted, and often completely abolished, by pain and spasm. It is essential to look for a source of infection.

IN ADULTS

In adults, it is often a superficial joint that is painful, swollen and inflamed. There is warmth and marked local tenderness, and movements are restricted. Patients with rheumatoid arthritis, and especially those on corticosteroid treatment, may develop a 'silent' joint infection. Suspicion may be aroused by an unexplained deterioration in the patient's general condition.

Imaging

- *Ultrasonography* is the most reliable method for revealing a joint effusion in early cases. Both hips should be examined for comparison. Widening of the space between capsule and bone of more than 2 mm is indicative of an effusion, which may be echo-free (perhaps a transient synovitis) or positively echogenic (more likely septic arthritis).
- *X-ray examination* is usually normal early on but signs to be watched for are soft-tissue swelling, loss of tissue planes, widening of the radiographic 'joint space' and slight subluxation (because of fluid in the joint) (2.11). With some infections, there is sometimes gas in the joint. Narrowing and irregularity of the joint space are late features.
- *MRI and radionuclide imaging* are helpful in diagnosing arthritis in obscure sites such as the sacroiliac and sternoclavicular joints.

Investigations

The WBC count, CRP and ESR are raised and blood culture may be positive. However, special

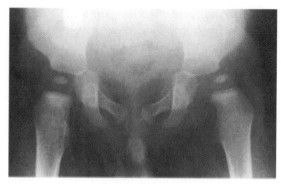

(a)

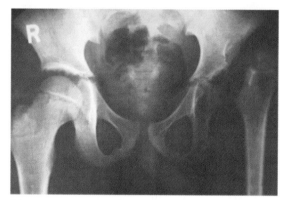

(b)

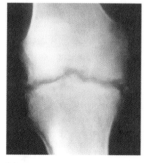

(c)

2.11 Suppurative arthritis – X-rays (a) In this child, the left hip is subluxated and the soft tissues are swollen. **(b)** If the infection persists untreated, the cartilaginous epiphysis may be entirely destroyed, leaving a permanent pseudarthrosis. **(c)** Septic arthritis in an adult knee joint.

investigations take time and it is much quicker (and usually more reliable) to aspirate the joint and examine the fluid. A WBC and Gram stain should be carried out immediately: the normal synovial fluid leucocyte count is under 300 per mL; it may be over 10 000 per mL in non-infective inflammatory disorders, but counts of over 50 000 per mL are highly suggestive of sepsis. Gram-positive cocci are probably *Staphylococcus aureus*; Gram-negative cocci are either *Haemophilus influenzae* or *Kingella kingae* (in children) or *Gonococcus* (in adults). Samples of fluid should also be sent for full microbiological examination and tests for antibiotic sensitivity.

Treatment

 The first priority is to aspirate the joint and examine the fluid.

ANTIBIOTICS

Antibiotic treatment follows the same guidelines as presented for acute haematogenous osteomyelitis.

After aspiration, treatment is started without further delay and follows the same lines as for acute osteomyelitis. Once the blood and tissue samples have been obtained, there is no need to wait for detailed results before giving antibiotics.

DRAINAGE

If the aspirate looks purulent, the joint should be drained without waiting for laboratory results.

Under anaesthesia the joint is opened through a small incision, drained and washed out with physiological saline. A small catheter is left in place and the wound is closed; suction–irrigation is continued for another 2–3 days. For the knee, arthroscopic debridement and copious irrigation may be equally effective. Older children with early septic arthritis (symptoms for less than 3 days) involving any joint except the hip can often be treated successfully by repeated closed aspiration of the joint; however, if there is no improvement within 48 hours, open drainage will be necessary.

SPLINTAGE

The joint should be rested, and for neonates and infants this may mean light splintage; with hip infection, the joint should be held abducted and 30 degrees flexed, on traction to prevent dislocation.

GENERAL SUPPORTIVE CARE

Analgesics are given for pain and intravenous fluids for dehydration.

Complications

Infants under 6 months of age have the highest incidence of complications, most of which affect the hip. The most obvious risk factors are a delay in diagnosis and treatment (more than 4 days) and concomitant osteomyelitis of the proximal femur.

Subluxation and dislocation of the hip, or instability of the knee Prevent by appropriate posturing or splintage (2.12).

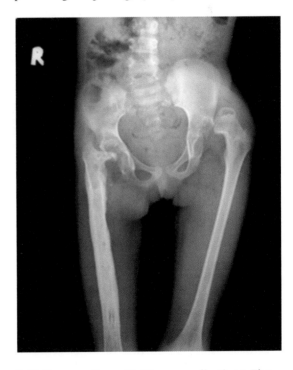

2.12 Suppurative arthritis – complications The radiograph demonstrates some of the complications following untreated bilateral hip sepsis with concurrent femoral osteomyelitis: dislocation of the left hip, avascular necrosis of the right hip, residual sclerosis of the femoral shaft and a small intramedullary sequestrum in the distal diaphysis.

SECTION 1 GENERAL ORTHOPAEDICS

Damage to the cartilaginous physis or the epiphysis In the growing child, this is the most serious complication. Sequelae include:

- *retarded growth*
- *partial or complete destruction of the epiphysis*
- *deformity of the joint*
- *epiphyseal osteonecrosis*
- *acetabular dysplasia*
- *pseudarthrosis of the hip.*

Articular cartilage erosion (chondrolysis) This is seen in older patients and may result in restricted movement or complete *ankylosis of the joint.*

GONOCOCCAL ARTHRITIS

Neisseria gonorrhoeae is the commonest cause of septic arthritis in sexually active adults, especially among poorer populations.

Clinical features

Two types of clinical disorder are recognized:

- *disseminated gonococcal infection* – a triad of polyarthritis, tenosynovitis and dermatitis
- *septic arthritis of a single joint* (usually the knee, ankle, shoulder, wrist or hand).

Both syndromes may occur in the same patient. There may be a slight pyrexia and the ESR and WBC count will be raised. If the condition is suspected, the patient should be questioned about possible contacts during the previous days or weeks and they should be examined for other signs of genitourinary infection (e.g. a urethral discharge or cervicitis).

Treatment

Treatment is similar to that of other types of pyogenic arthritis. Patients will usually respond quite quickly to a third-generation cephalosporin given intravenously or intramuscularly. However, bear in mind that many patients with gonococcal infection also have chlamydial infection, which is resistant to cephalosporins; both are sensitive to quinolone antibiotics such as ciprofloxacin and ofloxacin.

SPIROCHAETAL INFECTIONS

SYPHILIS

Syphilis is caused by the spirochaete *Treponema pallidum*, generally acquired during sexual activity by direct contact with infectious lesions of the skin or mucous membranes. The infection spreads to the regional lymph nodes and thence to the bloodstream. The organism can also cross the placental barrier and enter the fetal blood stream directly during the latter half of pregnancy, giving rise to congenital syphilis.

- *In acquired syphilis*, a *primary* ulcerous lesion, or *chancre*, appears at the site of inoculation about a month after initial infection. This usually heals without treatment but, a month or more after that, the disease enters a *secondary phase* characterized by the appearance of a maculopapular rash and bone and joint changes due to periostitis, osteitis and osteochondritis. After a variable length of time, this phase is followed by a *latent period* which may continue for many years. The term is somewhat deceptive because in about half the cases pathological lesions continue to appear in various organs and 10–30 years later the patient may present again with *tertiary syphilis*. This takes various forms including the appearance of large granulomatous gummata in bones and joints and neuropathic disorders in which the loss of sensibility gives rise to joint breakdown (*Charcot joints*).
- *In congenital syphilis*, the primary infection may be so severe that the fetus is stillborn or the infant dies shortly after birth. The ones who survive manifest pathological changes similar to those described above, though with modified clinical appearances and a contracted timescale (**2.13**).

Clinical features of acquired syphilis

EARLY

The patient usually presents with pain, swelling and tenderness of the bones, especially those with little soft-tissue covering, such as the frontal bones of the skull, the anterior surface of

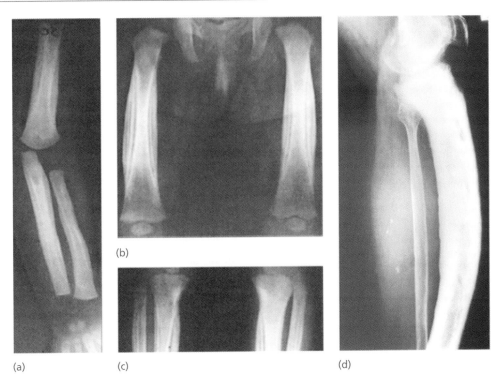

(b)

(a)   (c)   (d)

2.13 Syphilis (a–c) Congenital syphilis, with diffuse periostitis of many bones. **(d)** Acquired syphilitic periostitis of the tibia.

the tibia, the sternum and the ribs. *X-rays* may show typical features of *periostitis* and *thickening of the cortex* in these bones, as well as others that are not necessarily symptomatic. *Osteitis* and *septic arthritis* are less common. Occasionally these patients develop polyarthralgia or polyarthritis.

LATE

The typical late feature, which may appear only after many years, is the syphilitic *gumma*, a dense granulomatous lesion associated with local bone resorption and adjacent areas of sclerosis. This sometimes results in a pathological fracture. *X-rays* may show thick periosteal new bone formation at other sites, especially the tibia.

The other well-recognized feature of tertiary syphilis is a neuropathic arthropathy due to loss of sensibility in the joint, most characteristically the knee.

Other neurological disorders, the early signs of which may only be discovered on careful examination, are tabes dorsalis and 'general paralysis of the insane' (GPI).

Clinical features of congenital syphilis

EARLY

Although the infection is present at birth, bone changes do not usually appear until several weeks afterwards. The baby is sick and irritable and examination may show skin lesions, hepatosplenomegaly and anaemia. Serological tests are usually positive in both mother and child.

The first signs of skeletal involvement may be joint swelling and 'pseudoparalysis' – the child refuses to move a painful limb. Several sites may be involved, often symmetrically, with slight swelling and tenderness at the ends or along the shafts of the tubular bones. The characteristic *X-ray changes* are of two kinds:

- *osteochondritis* (*'metaphysitis'*) – trabecular erosion in the juxta-epiphyseal regions of tubular bones showing first as a lucent band

near the physis and later as frank bone destruction which may result in epiphyseal separation
- less frequently, *periostitis* – diffuse periosteal new bone formation along the diaphysis, usually of mild degree but sometimes producing an 'onion-peel' effect.

LATE

Bone lesions in older children and adolescents resemble those of acquired syphilis and some features occurring 10–15 years after birth may be manifestations of tertiary disease, the result of gumma formation and endarteritis. Gummata appear either as discrete, punched-out radiolucent areas in the medulla or as more extensive destructive lesions in the cortex. The surrounding bone is thick and sclerotic. Sometimes the predominant feature is dense endosteal and periosteal new bone formation affecting almost the entire bone (the classic '*sabre tibia*').

Other abnormalities which have come to be regarded as 'classic' features in older children are dental malformations ('*Hutchinson's teeth*'), erosion of the nasal bones, thickening and expansion of the finger phalanges (*dactylitis*) and painless effusions in the knees or elbows ('*Clutton's joints*').

Treatment

Early lesions will usually respond to intramuscular injections of benzylpenicillin given weekly for three or four doses. Late lesions will require high-dosage intravenous penicillin for a week or 10 days, but some forms of tertiary syphilis will not respond at all. An alternative would be treatment with one of the third-generation cephalosporins.

TUBERCULOSIS

The skeletal manifestations of the disease are seen chiefly in the spine and the large joints, but the infection may appear in any bone or any synovial or bursal sheath. Predisposing conditions include chronic debilitating disorders, diabetes, drug abuse, prolonged corticosteroid medication, AIDS and other disorders resulting in reduced defence mechanisms.

Pathology

Mycobacterium tuberculosis enters the body via the lung or the gut (swallowing infected milk products) or, rarely, through the skin. It causes a granulomatous reaction which is associated with tissue necrosis and caseation.

PRIMARY COMPLEX

The initial lesion in lung, pharynx or gut is a small one with lymphatic spread to regional lymph nodes; this combination is the primary complex. Usually the bacilli are fixed in the nodes and no clinical illness results.

Even though there is often no clinical illness, the initial infection has two important sequels:

- Within nodes which are apparently healed or even calcified, bacilli may survive for many years, so that a reservoir exists.
- The body has been sensitized to the toxin (a positive Mantoux or Heaf test being an index of sensitization) and, if reinfection occurs, the response is quite different, the lesion being a destructive one which spreads by contiguity.

SECONDARY SPREAD

If resistance to the original infection is low, widespread dissemination via the bloodstream may occur, giving rise to miliary tuberculosis, meningitis or multiple tuberculous lesions. More often, blood spread occurs months or years later, perhaps during a period of lowered immunity. Some of these foci develop into destructive lesions to which the term 'tertiary' may be applied.

TERTIARY LESION

Bones or joints are affected in about 5% of patients with tuberculosis. There is a predilection for the vertebral bodies and the large synovial joints. Multiple lesions occur in about one-third of patients.

Bacilli elicit a chronic inflammatory reaction. The characteristic microscopic lesion is the tuberculous granuloma (or 'tubercle'), which is a collection of epithelioid and multinucleated giant cells surrounding an area of necrosis, with round cells (mainly lymphocytes) around the periphery (**2.14**).

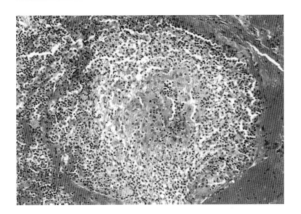

2.14 Tuberculosis – histology A typical tuberculous granuloma, with central necrosis and scattered giant cells surrounded by lymphocytes and histiocytes.

Within the affected area, small patches of caseous necrosis appear. These may coalesce into a larger yellowish mass, or the centre may break down to form an abscess containing pus and fragments of necrotic bone.

Bone lesions tend to spread quite rapidly. Epiphyseal cartilage is no barrier to invasion and soon the infection reaches the joint.

If the synovium is involved, it becomes thick and oedematous, giving rise to a marked effusion. A pannus of granulation tissue may extend from the synovial reflections across the joint; articular cartilage is slowly destroyed, though the rapid and complete destruction elicited by pyogenic organisms does not occur in the absence of secondary infection. At the edges of the joint, along the synovial reflections, there may be active bone erosion. In addition, the increased vascularity causes local osteoporosis.

If unchecked, caseation and infection extend into the surrounding soft tissues to produce a 'cold' abscess ('cold' only in comparison to a pyogenic abscess). This may burst through the skin, forming a sinus or tuberculous ulcer, or it may track along the tissue planes to point at some distant site. Secondary infection by pyogenic organisms is common.

Clinical features

There may be a history of previous infection or recent contact with tuberculosis. The patient complains of pain and joint swelling. In advanced cases there may be attacks of fever, night sweats, lassitude and loss of weight. Relatives tell of 'night cries': the joint, splinted by muscle spasm during the waking hours, relaxes with sleep and the inflamed or damaged tissues are stretched or compressed, causing sudden episodes of intense pain. Muscle wasting is characteristic and synovial thickening is often striking (**2.15**). Regional lymph nodes may be enlarged and tender. Movements are limited in all directions. As articular erosion progresses the joint becomes stiff and deformed.

X-rays

Soft-tissue swelling and periarticular osteoporosis are characteristic. The bone ends take on a 'washed-out' appearance and the articular space

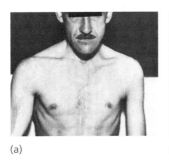
(a)

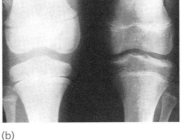
(b)

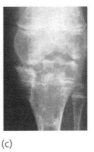
(c)

2.15 Tuberculosis – clinical and X-ray features **(a)** Generalized wasting used to be a common feature of all forms of tuberculosis. Today, skeletal tuberculosis occurs in deceptively healthy-looking individuals. An early feature is periarticular osteoporosis due to synovitis – the left knee in **(b)**. This often resolves with treatment, but if cartilage and bone are destroyed **(c)**, healing occurs by fibrosis and the joint retains a 'jog' of painful movement.

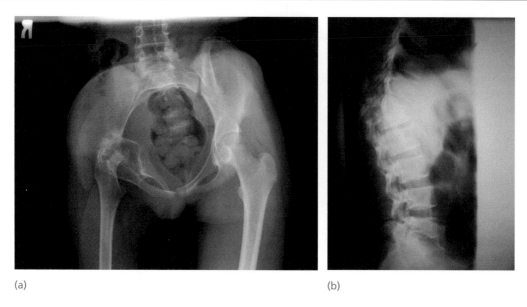

(a)   (b)

2.16 Tuberculosis – bone damage (a) Untreated tuberculosis of the right hip resulting in significant acetabular erosion and avascular necrosis of the femoral head. **(b)** Tuberculosis of the spine with destruction of the T12/L1 intervertebral disc and ankylosis causing a localized kyphosis.

is narrowed. In children, the epiphyses may be enlarged, probably the result of long-continued hyperaemia. Later, there is erosion of the sub-articular bone; characteristically, this is seen *on both sides of the joint*, indicating an inflammatory process starting in the synovium. Cystic lesions may appear in the adjacent bone ends but there is little or no periosteal reaction. In the spine, the characteristic appearance is one of bone erosion and collapse around a diminished intervertebral disc space; the soft-tissue shadows may define a paravertebral abscess (**2.16**).

Investigations

The ESR is usually increased and there may be a relative lymphocytosis. The Mantoux or Heaf test will be positive.

> *Mantoux and Heaf tests* are sensitive but not specific tests; i.e. a negative Mantoux virtually excludes the diagnosis, but a positive test merely indicates tuberculous infection, now or at some time in the past.

If synovial fluid is aspirated, it may be cloudy, the protein concentration is increased and the WBC count is elevated. Acid-fast bacilli are identified in synovial fluid in 10–20% of cases, and cultures are positive in over half. A synovial biopsy is more reliable: sections will show the characteristic histological features and acid-fast bacilli may be identified; cultures are positive in about 80% of patients who have not received antimicrobial treatment. Where facilities allow, polymerase chain reaction (PCR) nucleic acid amplification testing can also be used.

Treatment

CHEMOTHERAPY

The most effective treatment is a combination of antituberculous drugs, which should always include rifampicin and isoniazid. Over the last decade the incidence of drug resistance has increased and this has led to the addition of various 'potentiating' drugs to the list. The following box details one of several recommended regimens.

TUBERCULOSIS: A RECOMMENDED CHEMOTHERAPY REGIMEN

1 Initial *'intensive phase treatment'* consisting of the following antibiotics for 5–6 months:
   • isoniazid 300–400 mg + rifampicin 450–600 mg + fluoroquinolones 400–600 mg per day.
   All replicating sensitive bacteria are likely to be killed by this bactericidal treatment.
2 *'Continuation phase treatment'* lasting 9 months, the purpose of which is to eliminate the 'persisters', slow-growing, intermittently growing, dormant or intracellular mycobacteria:
   • isoniazid + pyrazinamide 1500 mg per day for 4½ months, and then
   • isoniazid + rifampicin for another 4½ months.
3 *'Prophylactic phase'* for a further 3–4 months:
   • isoniazid + ethambutol 1200 mg per day.

OPERATION

Operative drainage or clearance of a tuberculous focus is seldom necessary in high-income countries. However, in LMICs, tuberculosis affecting large joints and the spine remains a significant cause of morbidity. Suspected tuberculosis of the spine requires a biopsy followed by chemotherapy. If there is neurological compromise, decompression is required, often with stabilization to avoid progressive deformity. Neglected tuberculosis of the knee and ankle usually requires arthrodesis, while in the hip, total hip arthroplasty has been successfully used following eradication of the infection. The definitive surgery should be undertaken in conjunction with prophylactic chemotherapy to avoid recurrence.

MYCOTIC INFECTIONS

Mycotic or fungal infection causes an indolent granulomatous reaction, often leading to abscess formation, tissue destruction and ulceration. When the musculoskeletal system is involved, it is usually by direct spread from the adjacent soft tissues. Mycoses are of two basic types: superficial and deep.

• *Superficial mycoses.* These are primarily infections of the skin or mucous surfaces which spread into the adjacent soft tissues and bone. The more common examples are the *maduromycoses* (a group consisting of several species), *Sporothrix* and various species of *Candida*.

The *actinomycoses* are usually included with the superficial fungal infections. The causal organisms, of which *Actinomyces israelii* is the commonest in humans, are not really fungi but anaerobic bacilli with fungus-like appearance and behaviour.

• *Deep mycoses.* This group comprises infections by *Blastomyces*, *Histoplasma*, *Coccidioides*, *Cryptococcus*, *Aspergillus* and other rare fungi. The organisms, which occur in rotting vegetation and bird droppings, gain entry through the lungs and, in humans, may cause an influenza-like illness. Bone or joint infection is uncommon except in patients with compromised host defences.

CANDIDIASIS

Candida albicans is a normal commensal in humans and it often causes superficial infection of the skin or mucous membranes. Deep and systemic infections are rare except under conditions of immunosuppression.

Candida osteomyelitis and arthritis may follow direct contamination during surgery or other invasive procedures such as joint aspiration or arthroscopy. The diagnosis is usually made only after tissue sampling and culture.

Treatment consists of thorough joint irrigation and curettage of discrete bone lesions, together with intravenous amphotericin B.

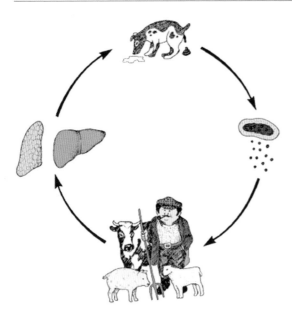

2.17 Hydatid disease The life cycle of the tapeworm that causes hydatid disease.

HYDATID DISEASE

Hydatid disease is caused by the tapeworm *Echinococcus*. Parasitic infestation is common among sheep farmers, but bone lesions are rare.

The organism, a cestode worm, has a complicated life cycle (**2.17**). The definitive host is the dog or some other carnivore that carries the tapeworm in its bowel. Segments of worm and ova pass out in the faeces and are later ingested by one of the intermediate hosts (usually sheep or cattle or man). Here, the larvae are carried via the portal circulation to the liver, and occasionally beyond to other organs, where they produce cysts containing numerous scolices. Infested meat is then eaten by dogs (or humans), giving rise to a new generation of tapeworm.

Scolices carried in the bloodstream occasionally settle in bone and produce hydatid cysts that slowly enlarge with little respect for cortical or epiphyseal boundaries. The bones most commonly affected are the vertebrae, pelvis, femur, scapula and ribs.

Clinical features

The patient may complain of pain and swelling, or may present for the first time with a pathological fracture or compression of the spinal cord. Infestation sometimes starts in childhood but the cysts take so long to enlarge that clinical symptoms and signs may not become apparent for many years. The diagnosis is more likely if the patient comes from a sheep-farming district.

Imaging

X-rays show solitary or multiloculated bone cysts, but only moderate expansion of the cortices (**2.18**). However, cortical thinning may lead to a pathological fracture. In the spine, hydatid disease may involve adjacent vertebrae, with large cysts extending into the paravertebral soft tissues. These features are best seen on *CT* and *MRI*, which should always be performed if operative excision of the lesion is contemplated.

Investigations

Casoni's (complement fixation) test may be positive, especially in long-standing cases.

Diagnosis

Hydatid disease must be included in the differential diagnosis of benign and malignant bone cysts and cyst-like tumours. If the clinical and radiological features are not conclusive, needle biopsy should be considered, though there is a risk of spreading the disease.

Treatment

The antihelminthic drug albendazole is moderately effective in destroying the parasite. It has to be given in repeated courses: a recommended programme is oral administration of 10 mg per kg per day for 3 weeks, repeated at least four times with a 1-week 'rest' between courses. Liver, renal and bone marrow function should be monitored during treatment.

However, the bone cysts do not heal and recurrence is common. The indications for

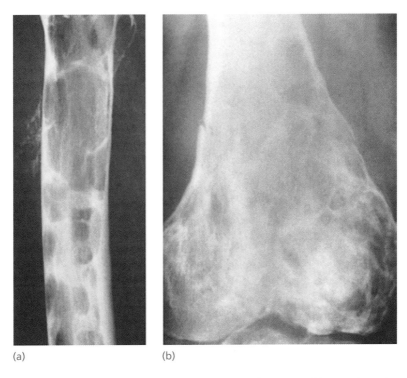

(a)   (b)

2.18 Hydatid disease of bone Two examples of hydatid involvement of bone: there is no expansion of the cortex in **(a)** and very little in **(b)**.

surgery are continuing enlargement or spread of the lesion, a risk of fracture, invasion of soft tissues and pressure on important structures. Curettage and bone grafting will lessen the risk of pathological fracture; at operation the cavity can be 'sterilized' with copious amounts of hypertonic saline, alcohol or formalin to lessen the risk of recurrence.

Radical resection, with the margin at least 2 cm beyond the cyst, is more certain, but also much more challenging.

FINAL COMMENT

Infections are severe clinical entities that need to be considered in many clinical scenarios. When affecting bones or joints, and especially when implants are involved, microorganisms may attach and proliferate until the point of severely damaging the tissue and the general health of the patient and eventually proving fatal. Even if cured, an infection may seriously affect the appropriate function of the bone and joint, and cause long-term or even permanent disability.

Early clinical suspicion, adequate aetiological diagnosis, and properly staged treatment that usually includes surgery, antibiotics and other actions, are crucial to control and eventually heal these complex diseases.

Future management of increasingly complex infections will require a deep knowledge of available diagnostic and therapeutic options and developments. From basic clinical reasoning to sophisticated laboratory tools, from appropriate surgical decisions to specific antibiotic regimes, a multidisciplinary approach is a major asset to successfully orient musculoskeletal infections.

SECTION 1 GENERAL ORTHOPAEDICS

Inflammatory rheumatic disorders

3

- Rheumatoid arthritis   51
- Ankylosing spondylitis   57
- Seronegative spondarthritis   60
- Psoriatic arthritis   60
- Reiter's syndrome and reactive arthritis   61
- Juvenile idiopathic arthritis   62
- Systemic connective-tissue diseases   64
- Fibromyalgia   64

The term 'inflammatory rheumatic disorders' covers a number of diseases that cause chronic pain, stiffness and swelling around joints and tendons. In addition, they are commonly associated with extra-articular features including skin rashes and inflammatory eye disease. Many – perhaps all – are due to a faulty immune reaction resulting from a combination of environmental exposures against a background of genetic predisposition.

RHEUMATOID ARTHRITIS

Rheumatoid arthritis (RA), the commonest cause of inflammatory joint disease, affects about 3% of the population, women three times more often than men. It usually appears in the fourth or fifth decade. It is a systemic disease associated with a decreased life expectancy often due to ischaemic heart disease caused by chronic inflammation.

Cause

The cause of RA is still incompletely understood.

IMPORTANT FACTORS IN THE EVOLUTION OF RA

1 Genetic susceptibility through the human leucocyte antigen HLA-DR4
2 An immunological reaction preferentially focused on synovial tissue
3 An inflammatory reaction in joints and tendon sheaths
4 The appearance of rheumatoid factors (RFs) and anti-citrullinated peptide antibodies (anti-CCPs or ACPAs) in the blood and synovium
5 Perpetuation of the inflammatory process
6 Articular cartilage destruction

Pathology

Although tissues throughout the body are affected, the brunt of the attack falls on synovium. The pathological changes, if unchecked, proceed in four stages (3.1).

Stage 1: Preclinical Well before RA becomes clinically apparent, the immune pathology is

SECTION 1 GENERAL ORTHOPAEDICS

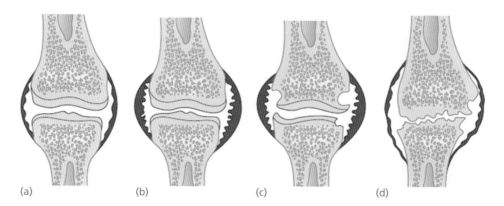

(a)   (b)   (c)   (d)

3.1 Rheumatoid arthritis – pathology (a) The normal joint. **(b)** Stage 1: synovitis and joint swelling. **(c)** Stage 2: early joint destruction with periarticular erosions. **(d)** Stage 3: advanced joint destruction and deformity.

already beginning. Raised erythrocyte sedimentation rate (ESR), C-reactive protein (CRP) and RF may be detectable years before the first diagnosis.

Stage 2: Synovitis The synovial membrane becomes inflamed and thickened, giving rise to a cell-rich effusion. Although painful and swollen, the joints and tendons are still intact and the disorder is potentially reversible.

Stage 3: Destruction Persistent inflammation causes joint and tendon destruction. Articular cartilage is eroded, partly by proteolytic enzymes, partly by vascular tissue in the folds of the synovial reflections, and partly due to direct invasion of the cartilage by a pannus of granulation tissue creeping over the articular surface. At the margins of the joint, bone is eroded by granulation tissue invasion and osteoclastic resorption. Similar changes occur in tendon sheaths, causing tenosynovitis and, eventually, partial or complete rupture of tendons. A synovial effusion, often containing copious amounts of fibrinoid material, produces swelling of the joints, tendons and bursae.

Stage 4: Deformity The combination of articular destruction, capsular stretching and tendon rupture leads to progressive instability and deformity.

EXTRA-ARTICULAR FEATURES

The most characteristic extra-articular lesion is the *rheumatoid nodule*, a small granuloma occurring under the skin (especially over bony

prominences), on tendons, in the sclera and in viscera. Other systemic features are:

- *lymphadenopathy*
- *vasculitis*
- *muscle weakness*
- *visceral disease* affecting the lungs, heart, kidneys, brain and gastrointestinal tract.

It used to be thought that the disease would eventually 'burn itself out', but this does not appear to be the case. Features of different stages can occur simultaneously in different joints and, even when the arthritis is quiescent, systemic pathology may still be active.

Clinical features

The usual pattern is the insidious emergence of a symmetrical polyarthritis affecting mainly the hands and feet (**3.2**), together with early morning stiffness and a lack of well-being. Women are affected more often than men.

EARLY STAGE

The early stage is marked by swelling, stiffness, increased warmth and tenderness of the proximal finger joints and the wrists, as well as of the tendon sheaths around these joints. *X-ray* examination may show soft-tissue swelling and periarticular osteoporosis. Gradually, similar symptoms and signs appear in other joints: the elbows, shoulders, knees, ankles and feet. However, it is important to remember that the condition occasionally begins in one of the larger joints and (at least for a while)

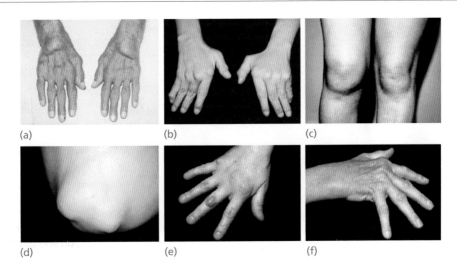

(a)   (b)   (c)

(d)   (e)   (f)

3.2 Rheumatoid arthritis – clinical features **(a)** Early features of swelling and stiffness of the proximal finger joints and the wrists. **(b)** The late hand deformities are so characteristic as to be almost pathognomonic. **(c)** Occasionally, rheumatoid disease starts with synovitis of a single large joint (in this case the right knee). Extra-articular features include subcutaneous nodules **(d,e)** and tendon ruptures **(f)**.

can resemble an inflammatory monarthritis such as gonococcal or tuberculous synovitis.

MID STAGE

As the disease progresses, joint movements become increasingly restricted and isolated tendon ruptures appear at the wrists. Subcutaneous nodules may be felt over the olecranon process; although they occur in only 25% of patients, they are pathognomonic of RA.

LATER STAGES

In the later stages, joint deformity becomes increasingly apparent and the acute pain of synovitis is replaced by the more constant ache of joint destruction. The combination of instability and tendon rupture produces the typical 'rheumatoid' deformities.

TYPICAL 'RHEUMATOID' DEFORMITIES

Ulnar deviation of the fingers
Radial and volar displacement of the wrists
Valgus knees
Valgus feet
Clawed toes

Joint movements are restricted and often very painful. About one-third of all patients develop pain and stiffness in the cervical spine. Function is increasingly disturbed and patients may need help with grooming, dressing and eating

Certain extra-articular features become increasingly apparent in patients with severe disease.

EXTRA-ARTICULAR FEATURES IN SEVERE RA

Muscle wasting
Lymphadenopathy
Nerve entrapment syndromes
Skin atrophy or ulceration
Scleritis
Vasculitis
Peripheral sensory neuropathy

X-rays

Early on, X-rays show only the features of synovitis: soft-tissue swelling and periarticular osteoporosis. The later stages are marked by the appearance of marginal bony erosions and narrowing of the articular space, especially in the proximal joints of the hands and feet. In advanced disease, articular destruction and joint deformity are obvious (**3.3**).

SECTION 1 GENERAL ORTHOPAEDICS

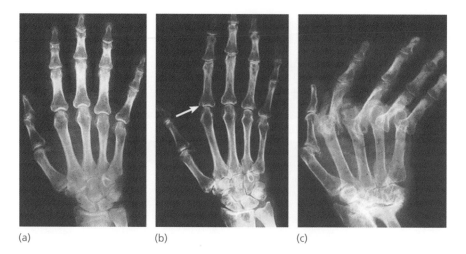

(a)   (b)   (c)

3.3 Rheumatoid arthritis – X-ray changes The progress of disease is well shown in this patient's X-rays. **(a)** First there was only soft-tissue swelling and periarticular osteoporosis; **(b)** later, juxta-articular erosions appeared (arrow); **(c)** ultimately, the joints became unstable and deformed.

Blood investigations

Normocytic, hypochromic anaemia is common and is a reflection of abnormal erythropoiesis. It may be aggravated by chronic gastrointestinal blood loss caused by non-steroidal anti-inflammatory drugs (NSAIDs). In active phases, the ESR and CRP concentrations are usually raised.

Serological tests for RF are positive in about 80% of patients and antinuclear factors are present in 30%. Neither of these tests is specific and neither is required for a diagnosis of RA.

 A positive test for RF in the absence of the above features is not sufficient to diagnose RA, nor does a negative test exclude the diagnosis if all the other features are present.

Diagnosis

The minimal criteria for diagnosing RA are:

- bilateral, symmetrical polyarthritis involving the proximal joints of the hands or feet
- present for at least 6 weeks.

If, in addition, there are subcutaneous nodules or periarticular erosions on X-ray, the diagnosis is certain.

The chief value of the RF tests is in assessing prognosis; high titres herald more serious disease.

In the *differential diagnosis* of polyarthritis, several disorders must be considered (**3.4**).

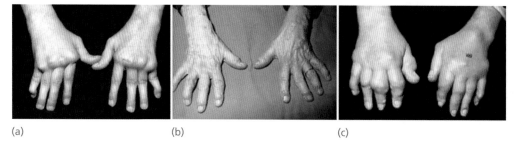

(a)   (b)   (c)

3.4 Rheumatoid arthritis – differential diagnosis All three patients presented with painful swollen fingers. In **(a)** mainly the proximal joints were affected (RA); in **(b)** the distal joints were the worst (Heberden's osteoarthritis); in **(c)** there were asymmetrical nodular swellings around the joints (gouty tophi).

Seronegative polyarthritis   This is a feature of a number of conditions vaguely related to RA:

- psoriatic arthritis
- juvenile chronic arthritis (Still's disease)
- systemic lupus erythematosus and other connective-tissue diseases.

Ankylosing spondylitis (AS)   This may involve the peripheral joints, but it is primarily a disease of the sacroiliac and intervertebral joints, causing back pain and progressive stiffness.

Reiter's disease   This condition affects the large joints and the lumbosacral spine. There is a history of urethritis or colitis and often also conjunctivitis.

Polyarticular gout   This affects large and small joints, and tophi on fingers and toes may be mistaken for rheumatoid nodules.

Polyarticular osteoarthritis (OA)   Affecting the distal interphalangeal joints, this causes nodular swellings with radiologically obvious osteophytes.

Polymyalgia rheumatica   This occurs mostly in middle-aged or elderly women, causing marked stiffness and weakness after inactivity. Pain is most severe around the pectoral and pelvic girdles; tenderness is in muscles rather than joints. The ESR is almost always high. This is a form of giant-cell arteritis and carries the risk of temporal arteritis resulting in blindness. Corticosteroids provide rapid and dramatic relief of all symptoms.

 Swollen finger joints:
- proximal joints = inflammatory arthritis
- distal joints = OA

Complications

Infection   Patients with RA – and even more so those on corticosteroid therapy – are susceptible to infection.

 Sudden clinical deterioration, or increased pain in a single joint, should alert one to the possibility of septic arthritis and the need for joint aspiration.

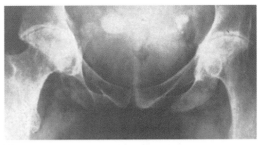

(a)

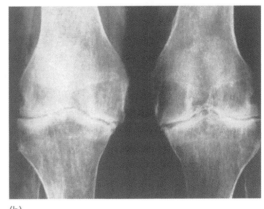

(b)

3.5 Rheumatoid arthritis – aftermath After the acute inflammatory phase has passed, the patient may be left with features of secondary OA, especially in **(a)** the hips and **(b)** the knees.

Tendon rupture   Nodular infiltration may lead to tendon rupture. This is seen most often at the wrist, where it contributes significantly to the development of the characteristic rheumatoid deformities.

Joint rupture   Occasionally, the joint lining ruptures and synovial contents spill into the soft tissues. Treatment is directed at the underlying synovitis – i.e. splintage and injection of the joint, with synovectomy as a second resort.

Secondary OA   Articular cartilage erosion may leave the joint so damaged that, even if the rheumatoid disease subsides or is kept under control, the end stage will be very similar to advanced OA (**3.5**).

Prognosis

RA runs a variable course. When the patient is first seen, it is difficult to predict the outcome;

however, a number of signs indicate a poor prognosis.

POOR PROGNOSTIC SIGNS IN RA

High titres of RF
Periarticular erosions
Rheumatoid nodules
Severe muscle wasting
Joint contractures
Evidence of vasculitis

Women, on the whole, fare somewhat worse than men. Without effective treatment:

- about 10% of patients improve steadily after the first attack of active synovitis
- 60% have intermittent phases of disease activity and remission, but with a slow downhill course over many years
- 20% have severe joint erosion, which is usually evident within the first 5 years
- 10% end up completely disabled.

In addition, a reduction in life expectancy by 5–10 years is common and is often due to premature ischaemic heart disease. However, early aggressive medical treatment appears to reduce the morbidity and mortality.

Treatment

ASSOCIATIONS WITH FASTER PROGRESSION

Female sex
Multiple joint involvement
High ESR and CRP
Positive RF and ACPA
Younger age
The presence of erosions at diagnosis

There is no cure for RA. A multidisciplinary approach is needed from the beginning: ideally, the therapeutic team should include a rheumatologist, orthopaedic surgeon, physiotherapist, occupational therapist, orthotist and social worker. Their deployment and priorities will vary according to the individual and the stage of the disease.

At the onset of the disease, there will be uncertainty about its likely rate of progress, but a number of factors are associated with worse evential outcomes.

PRINCIPLES OF MEDICAL MANAGEMENT

Treatment is aimed at controlling inflammation as rapidly as possible.

Oral corticosteroids These are used for their rapid action (initially an oral dose of 30 mg of prednisolone or 120 mg of methylprednisolone intramuscularly). The dose should be rapidly tapered off to prevent significant side effects.

Disease-modifying antirheumatic drugs (DMARDs) In addition, DMARDs should be started at this time; the first choice is now methotrexate at doses of 10–25 mg/week. This may be used initially alone or in combination with sulfasalazine and hydroxychloroquine. Leflunomide can also be considered if methotrexate is not tolerated. Gold and penicillamine are now rarely used.

NSAIDs These may be needed to control pain and stiffness.

Biological therapies If there is no satisfactory response to DMARDs, it is wise to progress rapidly to biological therapies such as the tumour necrosis factor (TNF) inhibitors infliximab, etanercept and adalimumab. Other biological therapies include inhibitors of T-cell costimulation (abatacept), IL-6 (tocilizumab) and B-cell depleting therapies (rituximab).

Corticosteroid injection Further measures include the injection of long-acting corticosteroid preparations into inflamed joints and tendon sheaths. It is sometimes feared that such injections may themselves cause damage to articular cartilage or tendons. However, there is little evidence that they are harmful, provided they are used sparingly and with full precautions against infection.

PHYSIOTHERAPY AND OCCUPATIONAL THERAPY

Muscle tone and joint mobility are maintained by a balanced programme of exercise, and general advice on coping with the activities of daily living. Preventative splinting and orthotic devices may be helpful; however, it is important to encourage activity.

SURGICAL MANAGEMENT

Operative treatment may be indicated at any stage of the disease if conservative measures alone are not effective. Early on, this consists mainly of soft-tissue procedures (synovectomy, tendon repair or replacement and joint stabilization).

In late rheumatoid disease, severe joint destruction, fixed deformity and loss of function are clear indications for reconstructive surgery. Arthrodesis, osteotomy and arthroplasty all have their place and are considered in the appropriate chapters.

 It should be recognized that patients who are no longer suffering the pain of active synovitis and who are contented with a limited pattern of life may not want or need heroic surgery merely to improve their anatomy. Careful assessment for occupational therapy, the provision of mechanical aids and adjustments to their home environment may be much more useful.

It appears safe to continue methotrexate during elective orthopaedic surgery. However, doses of corticosteroids should be as low as possible and biological therapies such as the TNF inhibitors should be stopped prior to surgery where possible.

ANKYLOSING SPONDYLITIS

Like RA, AS is a generalized chronic inflammatory disease, but its effects are seen mainly in the spine and sacroiliac joints. It is characterized by pain and stiffness of the back, with variable involvement of the hips and shoulders and (more rarely) the peripheral joints. The prevalence is higher in Europeans than other races, at about 0.2%. Males are affected more frequently than females (estimates vary from 2 : 1 to 10 : 1) and the usual age at onset is between 15 and 25 years.

Cause

The disease tends to run in families; close relatives may have either classic AS or one of the other 'spondarthritides' such as Reiter's disease, psoriatic arthritis or enteropathic arthritis. The fact that all these conditions are associated with a particular tissue type, the HLA-B27, suggests a genetic predisposition; the specific clinical syndrome is probably triggered by some recent event – often genitourinary or bowel infection.

Pathology

There are three characteristic lesions.

CHARACTERISTIC AS LESIONS

Synovitis of diarthrodial joints
Inflammation at the fibro-osseous junctions of syndesmotic joints, tendons and ligaments (*enthesopathy*)
Ossification across the periphery of the intervertebral discs

The disease starts as an inflammation of the sacroiliac and vertebral joints and ligaments. Sometimes the hips and shoulders also are affected, and very occasionally the peripheral joints.

Pathological changes follow a constant sequence.

SEQUENCE OF PATHOLOGICAL CHANGES IN AS

1 Inflammation
2 Granulation tissue formation
3 Erosion of articular cartilage or bone
4 Replacement by fibrous tissue
5 Ossification of the fibrous tissue
6 Ankylosis

If many vertebrae are involved, the spine may become absolutely rigid. If the costovertebral joints are involved, respiratory excursion is diminished.

Clinical features

Most patients are young men who complain of persistent backache and stiffness (**3.6**), often worse in the early morning or after inactivity. About 10% have pain in peripheral joints.

The most typical sign is stiffness of the spine. All movements are diminished, but loss of extension is both the earliest and the most severe. The '*wall test*' is useful.

WALL TEST FOR LOSS OF SPINE EXTENSION

If a healthy person stands with their back to a wall, their heels, buttocks, scapulae and occiput could all be made to touch the wall simultaneously, but if extension is seriously diminished, this is impossible. In advanced cases of AS, the entire spine may be rigid ('poker back').

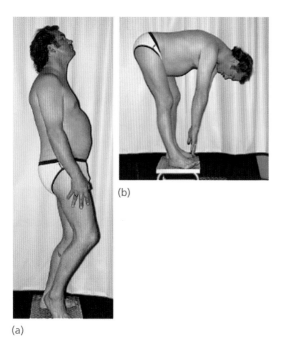

(a)

(b)

3.6 Ankylosing spondylitis – early The cardinal clinical feature is marked stiffness of the spine. **(a)** This patient manages to stand upright by keeping his knees slightly flexed. **(b)** It looks as if he can bend down to touch his toes, but his back is rigid and all the movement takes place at his hips.

Also in advanced cases, chest expansion is decreased to well below the normal 7 cm.

If the hips are involved, they also may go on to complete ankylosis. Occasionally, peripheral joints are swollen and tender. Some patients complain of painful heels and have tenderness at the insertion of the tendo Achillis.

The patient may exhibit a number of extraskeletal manifestations.

EXTRASKELETAL MANIFESTATIONS OF AS

General fatigue and weight loss
Ocular inflammation
Aortic valve disease
Carditis
Pulmonary fibrosis

Imaging

The cardinal X-ray feature is fuzziness or frank erosion of the sacroiliac joints. Later these joints become sclerosed and, eventually, completely ankylosed (**3.7, 3.8**). More subtle changes can be revealed by MRI.

Ossification across the intervertebral discs produces bony bridges (syndesmophytes) spanning the gaps between adjacent vertebral bodies. Bridging at several levels gives the appearance of a 'bamboo spine'.

Peripheral joints may show erosive arthritis resembling that of RA.

Investigations

The ESR is usually elevated during active phases of the disease. HLA-B27 is present in 95% of Caucasian patients and one-half of their first-degree relatives.

Diagnosis

Diagnosis is easy in patients who present with chronic back pain and spinal rigidity. However, in over 10% of cases, the disease starts in a peripheral joint and it may be several years before the true diagnosis reveals itself. Atypical onset is more common in women. A history of AS in a relative is strongly suggestive.

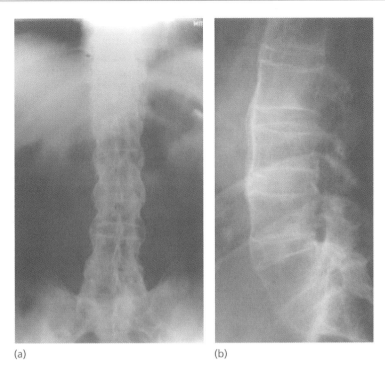

(a)   (b)

3.7 Ankylosing spondylitis – X-ray features (a,b) Bony bridges (syndesmophytes) between the vertebral bodies convert the spine into a rigid column. Note that the sacroiliac joints have fused.

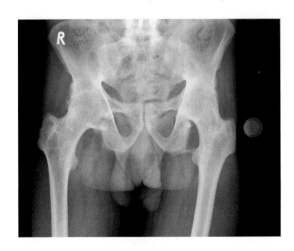

3.8 Ankylosing spondylitis Advanced disease that has resulted in bony ankylosis of the hips, sacroiliac joints and the lumbar–sacral spine.

DIFFUSE IDIOPATHIS HYPEROSTOSIS (FORESTIER'S DISEASE)

This syndrome may be confused with AS. The condition, predominantly of older men, is characterized by widespread ossification of ligaments and tendon insertions. *X-rays* show pronounced but asymmetrical intervertebral spur formation and bridging throughout the dorsolumbar spine. Although it bears a superficial resemblance to AS, it is not an inflammatory disease, spinal pain and stiffness are seldom severe, the sacroiliac joints are not eroded and the ESR is normal.

Treatment

Treatment consists of:

- general measures to maintain satisfactory posture and preserve movement
- anti-inflammatory drugs to counteract pain and stiffness
- the use of TNF inhibitors for severe disease
- operations to correct deformity or restore mobility.

NON-OPERATIVE TREATMENT

General measures Patients are taught how to maintain satisfactory posture and encouraged to remain active and to perform spinal extension exercises every day.

NSAIDs Although these drugs may not retard the progress to ankylosis, they do control pain and counteract soft-tissue stiffness.

TNF inhibitors The introduction of TNF inhibitors has made it possible to treat the underlying inflammatory processes active in AS. This can result in significant improvement in disease activity including remission. TNF inhibitors are generally reserved for patients who cannot be helped by NSAIDs.

OPERATIVE TREATMENT

Significantly damaged hips can be treated by joint replacement, though this seldom provides more than moderate mobility. Deformity of the spine may be severe enough to warrant lumbar or cervical osteotomy. These are difficult and potentially hazardous procedures.

SERONEGATIVE SPONDARTHRITIS

A number of conditions usually associated with seronegative polyarthritis (i.e. without serum RFs) may show changes in the spine and sacro-iliac joints indistinguishable from those of AS. These include:

- *psoriatic arthritis*
- *Reiter's disease*
- the arthritis that sometimes accompanies *ulcerative colitis* or *Crohn's disease*.

SHARED FEATURES OF THE SERONEGATIVE SPONDARTHRITIDES

Characteristic spondylitis and sacroiliitis occur in all of them.
All are associated with HLA-B27.
They show familial aggregation.
There is considerable overlap within families, some members having one disorder and close relatives another.

Together with classic AS, these conditions are often grouped as the '*seronegative spondarthritides*'.

The exact relationship between these disorders is unknown, but they share certain important features.

PSORIATIC ARTHRITIS

About 4% of patients with chronic polyarthritis have psoriasis; not all, however, have psoriatic arthritis, which is a distinct entity and not simply 'RA plus psoriasis' (**3.9**). Unlike RA, psoriatic

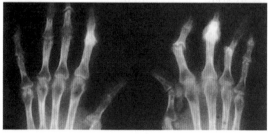

(a)

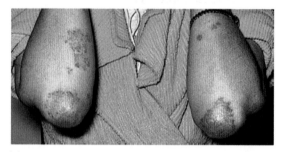

(b)

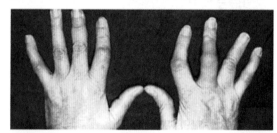

(c)

3.9 Psoriatic arthritis (a) Psoriasis of the elbows and forearms. **(b)** Typical finger deformities. **(c)** X-rays show distal joint involvement - clearly the disease is not simply RA in a patient with psoriasis.

arthritis affects men and women equally and tends to run in families. The arthritis is not as clearly symmetrical as in RA and – in marked contrast to the latter – it occurs mainly in the interphalangeal joints of the fingers and toes. Bone destruction may be so severe that the digits are completely flail or badly deformed ('arthritis mutilans'). About one-quarter of patients develop sacroiliac and vertebral changes like those of AS. HLA-B27 occurs in about 60% of those with overt sacroiliitis.

Treatment

General treatment   This aims at controlling the skin disorder with topical preparations and alleviating joint symptoms with NSAIDs. In resistant forms of arthritis, immunosuppressive agents have proved effective.

Local treatment   Judicious splintage is used to prevent undue deformity, and surgery for unstable joints.

REITER'S SYNDROME AND REACTIVE ARTHRITIS

'Classic' Reiter's disease is a clinical triad of polyarthritis, conjunctivitis and non-specific urethritis (**3.10**). However, the term is now used more loosely for a *reactive arthritis* associated with non-specific urogenital or bowel infection. It is the most common type of large-joint polyarthritis in young men. Familial aggregation, overlap with other forms of seronegative spondarthritis in first-degree relatives, and an increased frequency of HLA-B27 in all these disorders point to a genetic predisposition. *Chlamydia trachomatis* has been implicated as the urogenital infective agent, but arthritis also occurs with bowel infection due to *Shigella*, *Salmonella* or *Yersinia enterocolitica*.

The joints themselves are not infected; the synovitis is the end stage of an abnormal immune response to infection elsewhere or to its products.

Clinical features

ACUTE PHASE

The acute phase of the disease is marked by an asymmetrical inflammatory arthritis of the lower limb joints – usually the knee and ankle but often the tarsal and toe joints as well. The joint may be acutely painful, hot and swollen with a tense effusion, suggesting gout or infection. Tendo Achillis tenderness and plantar fasciitis (evidence of enthesopathy) are common, and the patient may complain of backache even in the early stage.

Typically, there is a history of urethritis, prostatitis, cervicitis or diarrhoea. Ocular lesions include conjunctivitis, episcleritis and uveitis.

The acute disorder usually lasts for a few weeks or months and then subsides, but most patients have either recurrent attacks of arthritis or other features suggesting chronic disease.

CHRONIC PHASE

The chronic phase is more characteristic of a spondyloarthropathy. Over half of patients with Reiter's disease complain of mild, recurrent episodes of polyarthritis (including upper limb

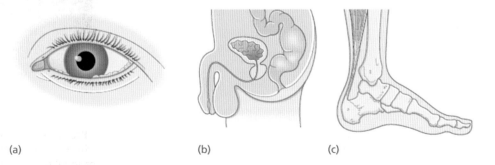

(a)   (b)   (c)

3.10 Reiter's syndrome The classic 'Reiter's triad' consists of conjunctivitis **(a)**, urethritis **(b)** (sometimes colitis) and arthritis. **(c)** Tenderness of the tendo Achillis and the plantar fascia is also common.

SECTION 1 GENERAL ORTHOPAEDICS

joints). Many develop sacroiliitis and spondylitis, with features resembling those of AS.

Special investigations

- *Tests for HLA-B27* are positive in 75% of patients with sacroiliitis.
- The *ESR* may be high in the active phase.
- The causative organism can sometimes be isolated from *urethral fluids or faeces.*
- *Tests for antibodies* may be positive.

Diagnosis

If the condition affects only one or two joints, it is usually mistaken for gout or infective arthritis. Examination of the synovial fluid for organisms and crystals will help to exclude these disorders.

Treatment

General treatment   A short course of antibiotics is usually sufficient for active urogenital or bowel infection, but for *Chlamydia* tetracycline daily for 6 months is recommended.

Symptomatic treatment   This includes the use of analgesia and NSAIDs. If the inflammatory response is aggressive, local injection of corticosteroids or even intramuscular methylprednisolone may be useful. If symptoms and signs do not resolve, DMARDs, as used in the treatment of RA, may be needed. Topical steroids may be used for uveitis.

JUVENILE IDIOPATHIC ARTHRITIS

Juvenile idiopathic arthritis (JIA) is the preferred term for non-infective inflammatory joint disease of more than 3 months' duration in children under 16 years. It embraces a group of disorders in all of which pain, swelling and stiffness of the joints are common features. The prevalence is about 1 per 1000 children, and boys and girls are affected with equal frequency.

The cause is probably similar to that of rheumatoid disease: an abnormal immune response to some antigen in children with a particular genetic predisposition. However, RF is usually absent.

The pathology, too, is like that of RA: a synovial inflammation leading to fibrosis and ankylosis; the joints tend to stiffen in whatever position they are allowed to assume (usually flexion) and growth is retarded.

Clinical features

JIA occurs in several characteristic forms.

- About 15% have a *systemic illness* and arthritis only develops somewhat later.
- The majority (60–70%) have a *pauciarticular arthritis* affecting a few of the larger joints.
- About 10% present with *polyarticular arthritis*, sometimes closely resembling RA.
- The remaining 5–10% develop a *seronegative spondyloarthritis.*

SYSTEMIC JIA

This, the classic Still's disease, is usually seen in children below the age of 3 years. It starts with intermittent fever, rashes and malaise; there may also be lymphadenopathy, splenomegaly and hepatomegaly. Joint swelling occurs some weeks or months after the onset; fortunately, it usually resolves when the systemic illness subsides, but it may go on to a progressive seronegative polyarthritis with permanent deformity of the larger joints and fusion of the cervical apophyseal joints. By puberty, there may also be stunting of growth, often abetted by the use of corticosteroids.

PAUCIARTICULAR JIA

This is by far the commonest form of JIA. It usually occurs below the age of 6 years and is more common in girls. Only a few joints are involved and there is no systemic illness. The child presents with pain and swelling of medium-sized joints (knees, ankles, elbows and wrists) (**3.11**); RF tests are negative. A serious complication is chronic iridocyclitis, which occurs in about 50%. The arthritis often goes into remission after a few years but by then the child is left with asymmetrical deformities and growth defects that may be permanent.

POLYARTICULAR SEROPOSITIVE JIA

This is usually seen in older children, mainly girls. The typical deformities of RA are uncommon

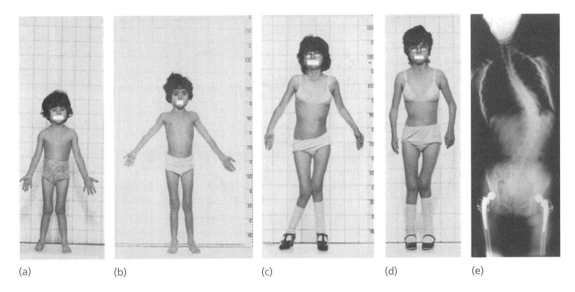

(a)   (b)   (c)   (d)   (e)

3.11 Juvenile idiopathic arthritis This young girl developed JIA when she was 5 years old. Here we see her at 6, 9 and 14 years of age **(a–c)**. The arthritis became inactive, leaving her with a knee deformity which was treated by osteotomy **(d)**. **(e)** X-ray of another girl who required hip replacements at the age of 14 years and, later, surgical correction of her scoliosis.

and RF is usually absent. In some cases, however, the features can be indistinguishable from those of adult RA, with a positive RF test; these probably warrant the designation 'juvenile RA'.

SERONEGATIVE SPONDARTHRITIS

In older children – usually boys – the condition may take the form of sacroiliitis and spondylitis; hips and knees are sometimes also involved. Tests for HLA-B27 are often positive and this should probably be regarded as 'juvenile AS'.

Complications

Stiffness While most patients recover good function, some permanent loss of movement is common.

Growth defects There is general retardation of growth, sometimes aggravated by prolonged corticosteroid therapy.

Iridocyclitis This is most common in pauciarticular disease; untreated it may lead to blindness.

Amyloidosis In children with long-standing active disease, there is a serious risk of amyloidosis, which may be fatal.

Treatment

NON-OPERATIVE TREATMENT

General treatment This is similar to that of RA. Corticosteroids should be used only for severe systemic disease and chronic iridocyclitis unresponsive to topical therapy. Severe inflammatory disease may need to be treated with cytokine inhibitors such as anti-TNF therapies.

Local treatment The aim of this is to prevent stiffness and deformity. Night splints are useful for the wrists, hands, knees and ankles; prone lying for some period each day may prevent flexion contracture of the hips. Between periods of splinting, active exercises are encouraged. Fixed deformities may need correction by serial plasters.

OPERATIVE TREATMENT

When progress is no longer being made, *joint capsulotomy* may help.

Operation is indicated for painful, eroded joints. Useful procedures include custom-designed arthroplasties of the hip and knee (even in children), and arthrodesis of the wrist or ankle. The use of anti-TNF therapy in the worst affected children has greatly reduced the need for early joint replacement.

Outcome

Fortunately, most children with JIA recover from the arthritis and are left with only moderate deformity and limitation of function. However, 5–10% (and especially those with juvenile RA) are severely disabled and require treatment throughout life.

About 3% of children with JIA die as a result of the condition, usually as a result of renal failure due to amyloidosis or following overwhelming infection.

SYSTEMIC CONNECTIVE-TISSUE DISEASES

'Systemic connective-tissue disease' is a collective term for a group of closely related conditions that have features which overlap with those of rheumatoid disease. Like RA, these are 'autoimmune disorders', probably triggered by viral infection in genetically predisposed individuals.

SYSTEMIC LUPUS ERYTHEMATOSUS

Systemic lupus erythematosus (SLE) is the best known systemic connective-tissue disease. It occurs mainly in young females and may be difficult to differentiate from RA. Although joint pain is usual, it is often overshadowed by systemic symptoms such as malaise, anorexia, weight loss and fever.

CHARACTERISTIC CLINICAL FEATURES OF SLE

Skin rashes (especially a 'butterfly rash' on the face)
Raynaud's phenomenon
Peripheral vasculitis
Splenomegaly
Disorders of the kidney, heart, lung, eyes and central nervous system

Anaemia, leucopenia and elevation of the ESR are common. Tests for antinuclear factor are always positive.

Treatment

Corticosteroids are indicated for severe systemic disease and may have to be continued for life. Progressive joint deformity is unusual and the arthritis can almost always be controlled by NSAIDs, physiotherapy and intermittent splintage.

A curious complication of SLE is avascular necrosis (usually of the femoral head). This may be due in part to the corticosteroid treatment, but the disease itself seems to predispose to bone ischaemia.

FIBROMYALGIA

Fibromyalgia is not so much a diagnosis as a descriptive term for a condition in which patients complain of pain and tenderness in the muscles and other soft tissues around the back of the neck and shoulders and across the lower part of the back and the upper parts of the buttocks. What sets the condition apart from other 'rheumatic' diseases is the complete absence of demonstrable pathological changes in the affected tissues. Indeed, it is often difficult to give credence to the patient's complaints, an attitude which is encouraged by the fact that similar symptoms are encountered in some patients who have suffered trivial injuries in a variety of accidents; a significant number also develop psychological depression and anxiety.

The criteria for making the diagnosis were put forward by the American College of Rheumatology in 1990. These included symptoms of widespread pain in all four quadrants of the body, together with at least nine pairs of designated 'tender points' on physical examination. In practice, however, the diagnosis is often made in patients with much more localized symptoms and signs, and it is now quite common to attach this label to myofascial pain where no specific underlying disorder can be identified.

The cause of fibromyalgia remains unknown; no pathology has been found in the 'tender spots'. It has been suggested that this is an abnormality of sensory processing and patients often do display increased sensitivity to pain in other parts of the body. There are also suggestions that the condition is related to stress responses which can be activated by sudden accidents or traumatic life events. This does not mean that such patients will necessarily show other features of psychological dysfunction and the condition cannot be excluded merely by psychological testing.

Treatment

In mild cases, treatment can be limited to keeping up muscle tone and general fitness (hence the advice to have physiotherapy and then continue with daily exercises on their own), perhaps together with injections into the painful areas simply to reduce the level of discomfort. Patients with more persistent and more disturbing symptoms may benefit from various types of psychotherapy.

Crystal deposition disorders

4

■ Gout   67
■ Calcium pyrophosphate dihydrate crystal-associated arthropathy   70
■ Basic calcium phosphate crystal deposition disease   72

Gout and its imitators form a group of conditions characterized by the presence of crystals in and around the joints, bursae and tendons. Three clinical disorders in particular are associated with this phenomenon:

- *gout:* urate crystal deposition disorder
- *pseudogout:* calcium pyrophosphate dihydrate (CPPD) crystal deposition associated arthropathy
- *basic calcium phosphate* (BCP) *deposition disease*.

Characteristically, in each of these conditions, crystal deposition has three distinct consequences.

- The deposit may be inert and asymptomatic.
- It may induce an acute inflammatory reaction.
- It may result in slow destruction of the affected tissues.

GOUT

Gout is caused by deposition of monosodium urate crystals in joints and other tissues, secondary to hyperuricaemia. This leads to cartilage degeneration, renal dysfunction and uric acid kidney stones.

Gout is the most common inflammatory joint disease in men with peak onset in the fifth decade, with an estimated 1–2.5% of adults in developed countries affected. A number of risk factors have been identified.

RISK FACTORS FOR GOUT
Family history (30–40%)
Alcohol (50%)
Renal impairment
Obesity

Atherosclerosis, hyperlipidaemia and hypertension are important associated morbidities. A second group in whom gout is common are older females, invariably on diuretics. In both these groups, under-excretion of urate results in hyperuricaemia.

 Onset of gout in men prior to adulthood or in women before menopause is rare and should raise the possibility of an inherited disorder of urate metabolism resulting in overproduction.

Pathology

Uric acid is produced in the liver as the end product of purine metabolism.

HYPERURICAEMIA

Hyperuricaemia is defined as serum uric acid (SUA) level over 420 µmol/L in men and 360 µmol/L in women. It is predominantly a problem of poor excretion rather than overproduction.

Renal excretion is complex: 90% of filtered urate is actively reabsorbed via urate transporter proteins in the proximal convoluted tubules. Further excretion and reabsorption occur in the distal tubules.

Hyperuricaemia is a prerequisite for formation of urate crystals but pH, temperature and the absence of natural inhibitors are also important – otherwise all hyperuricaemic patients would be constantly forming crystals. Stimulation of the NALP3 inflammasome and other humoral and cellular inflammatory mediators by monosodium urate crystals results in acute gouty arthritis with a neutrophilic synovitis. Chronic cumulative urate crystal formation in tissue fluids leads to deposition of monosodium urate crystals in the synovium, cartilage, tendons and soft tissues, resulting in tophi formation and chronic tophaceous gouty arthritis.

CLINICAL GOUT

Urate crystals are deposited in minute clumps in connective tissue, including articular cartilage; the commonest sites are the small joints of the hands and feet. For months, perhaps years, they remain inert. Then, possibly as a result of local trauma, the needle-like crystals are dispersed into the joint and the surrounding tissues where they excite an acute inflammatory reaction.

With the passage of time, urate deposits may build up in joints, periarticular tissues, tendons and bursae.

COMMONEST SITES FOR URATE DEPOSIT BUILD-UP

Metatarsophalangeal (MTP) joints of the big toes
Achilles tendons
Olecranon bursae
Pinnae of the ears

These clumps of chalky material, or tophi, vary in size from less than 1 mm to several centimetres in diameter. They may ulcerate through the skin or destroy cartilage and periarticular bone.

Urate calculi appear in the urine, and crystal deposition in the kidney parenchyma may cause renal failure.

Classification

CLASSIFICATION OF GOUT

Primary gout (95% of cases) occurs in the absence of any obvious cause and may be due to constitutional under-excretion (the vast majority) or over-production of urate.
Secondary gout (5%) results from prolonged hyperuricaemia due to acquired disorders such as myeloproliferative diseases, administration of diuretics or renal failure.

This division into primary and secondary is somewhat artificial, however: people with an initial tendency to 'primary' hyperuricaemia may develop gout only when secondary factors (e.g. obesity and alcohol abuse, or treatment with diuretics or salicylates which increase tubular reabsorption of uric acid) are introduced.

Clinical features

Asymptomatic hyperuricaemia is ten times more common than gout, and the majority of patients with hyperuricaemia do not develop gout.

Seventy per cent of acute gout affects the first MTP joints (podagra). Other sites include the knee, ankle, midfoot, elbow and wrist. Attacks often begin at night and, within a few hours the affected joint becomes red, hot, swollen and extremely painful. Gout is rarely just 'painful' or 'uncomfortable'; the patient may be unable to walk or bear the touch of bedclothes. Systemic features such as fever and malaise may occur, especially during polyarticular attacks.

The natural history is for the attack to settle after 5–7 days, often with desquamation of the skin over the affected joint. Acute gout may also cause:

- bursitis
- tendinitis
- notably in the elderly, cellulitis of the lower limb.

Untreated, mass collections of urate (tophi) may be deposited in and around joints, notable at the elbows, over the small joints of the hands (**4.1a–c**) and in the ear.

Investigation

Hyperuricaemia remains the cardinal feature of gout, but levels may be normal during acute attacks. *X-rays* are unhelpful in the acute attack, either being normal or showing soft-tissue swelling. In chronic gout, erosions may be seen: classically, these are away from the joint margin, being 'punched-out' with a rounded or oval shape and overhanging edge (**4.1d**).

Acute gout can only be diagnosed with certainty by identifying urate crystals in synovial fluid, bursa or aspirate of tophus. Crystals are needle-shaped and strongly negatively birefringent under polarized light (**4.2**). Absence of the crystals does not rule out the diagnosis. In acute gout, synovial fluid is highly inflammatory, with white blood cell counts of ≥2000 cells/mm³.

Differential diagnosis

Pseudogout Pyrophosphate crystal deposition may cause an acute arthritis indistinguishable from gout – except that it tends to affect large rather than small joints and is somewhat more common in women than in men. *X-rays* may show reticular calcification. Demonstrating the crystals in synovial fluid establishes the diagnosis.

Infection Cellulitis, septic bursitis, an infected bunion or septic arthritis must all be excluded,

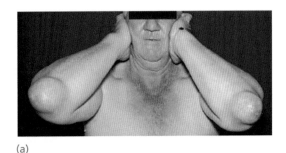

(a)

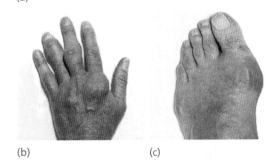

(b)   (c)

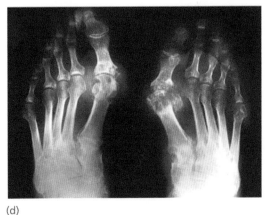

(d)

4.1 Gout (a) This is the stereotypical 'gouty type', with his rubicund face, large olecranon bursae and small subcutaneous tophi over the elbows. **(b,c)** Tophaceous gout affecting the hands and feet; the swollen big toe joint is particularly characteristic. **(d)** X-rays show the typical periarticular excavations (tophi consisting of uric acid deposits) in the big toe MTP joints.

if necessary by immediate joint aspiration and examination of synovial fluid.

Rheumatoid arthritis (RA) Polyarticular gout affecting the fingers may be mistaken for RA, and elbow tophi for rheumatoid nodules. In difficult cases, biopsy will establish the diagnosis.

SECTION 1 GENERAL ORTHOPAEDICS

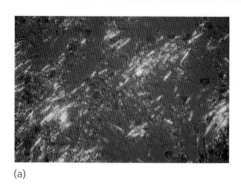
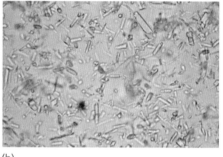

(a)   (b)

4.2 Crystals In polarized light, crystals appear bright on a dark background. If a compensator is added to the optical system, the background appears in shades of mauve and birefringent crystals as yellow or blue. In these two specimens (obtained from crystal deposits in two different joints), *urate crystals (a)* appear needle-like, 5–20 μm long and exhibiting strong negative birefringence, while the *pyrophosphate crystals (b)* are rhomboid-shaped, slightly smaller than urate crystals and show weak positive birefringence. (Courtesy of Professor P.A. Dieppe.)

Treatment

ACUTE GOUT

Non-steroidal anti-inflammatory drugs (NSAIDs) These are the drugs of choice for the treatment of acute gout without comorbid diseases (e.g. indomethacin 50–75 mg bd, naproxen 500 mg bd, etorocoxib 120 mg). A 'decrescendo' regime is employed, using large doses at first, tapering over 5–7 days.

Steroids NSAIDs are unsuitable for many patients with gout due to renal impairment, congestive cardiac failure, peptic ulcer disease or use of anticoagulant treatment. In these cases, steroids are probably the best alternative.

Colchicine This is also helpful, though limited by gastrointestinal side effects such as diarrhoea and nausea.

Non-drug treatment Rest, ice packs and splinting will help, as will powerful analgesia.

CHRONIC GOUT

Patient education This is important in the management of chronic gout. Appropriate lifestyle modification, weight loss and dietary advice such as reduction of alcohol and fructose consumption can be powerful interventions.

Urate-lowering therapy (ULT) ULT aims to keep serum urate below the saturation point for monosodium urate. First-line ULT agents are those that reduce formation of urate by inhibiting xanthine oxidase.

- *Allopurinol* is the drug of choice.

 As it is being introduced, allopurinol can trigger a paradoxical flare of gout. It should therefore not be started until at least 4 weeks after the last acute attack and prophylaxis should be offered (NSAID or low-dose colchicine) until the serum urate is stable in the target range.

- *Febuxostat* is an alternative inhibitor of xanthine oxidase, metabolized and excreted by the liver, so no dose adjustment appears to be necessary in patients with mild-to-moderate renal impairment.

- Other ULT agents are 'uricosuric', increasing excretion of urate at the kidney. In general, they are less effective than allopurinol and are contraindicated in urolithiasis.

CALCIUM PYROPHOSPHATE DIHYDRATE CRYSTAL-ASSOCIATED ARTHROPATHY

Calcium pyrophosphate dihydrate (CPPD) crystal-associated arthropathy is usually the consequence of cartilage changes related to ageing,

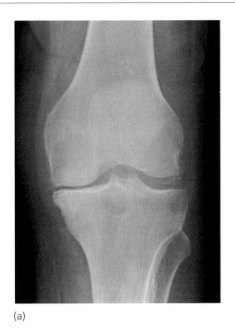 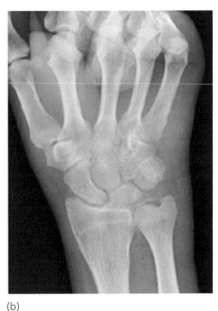

(a)   (b)

4.3 Cartilage calcification CC (also known as chondrocalcinosis) at the knee **(a)** and the wrist **(b)**.

degeneration, enzymatic degradation or trauma which result in deposition of calcium pyrophosphate (CPP) crystals.

Pathology

Pyrophosphate is probably generated in abnormal cartilage by enzyme activity at chondrocyte surfaces, combining with calcium ions in the matrix where crystal nucleation occurs on collagen fibres. The crystals grow to form nests of amorphous material in the cartilage matrix.

Cartilage calcification

Cartilage calcification (CC), also known as *chondrocalcinosis*, refers to the appearance of calcification, usually due to CPP deposition, in cartilage. This is generally seen in fibrocartilage (**4.3**), as cloudy, irregular opacities in the menisci of the knee, triangular fibrocartilage complex of the wrist, pubic symphysis and intervertebral discs. CC is strongly associated with age, prevalence rising from 10–15% in those aged 65–75 to 30–36% in those older than 85 years.

Acute CPP arthritis ('pseudogout')

CPP crystals may trigger an acute inflammatory reaction within the joint. Potential triggers include:

- direct trauma
- intercurrent medical illness
- surgery
- blood transfusion.

This is the commonest cause of acute monoarthritis in the elderly. Any joint may be involved but knee, wrist, shoulder and ankle are most common. Typical onset is with swelling and pain, which becomes severe over 6–24 hours. Fever is common and elderly patients in particular may appear systemically unwell.

Differentiation from gout can be very difficult. Crystal identification (positively birefringent rhomboid-shaped crystals) is required (**4.4**).

Treatment options include:

- rest
- analgesia
- aspiration

SECTION 1 GENERAL ORTHOPAEDICS

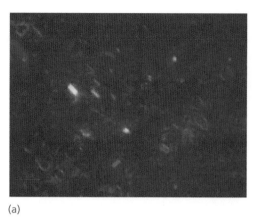

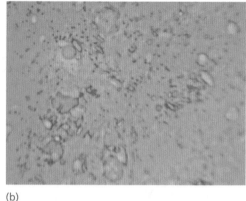

(a)   (b)

4.4 Pyrophosphate crystals CPPD crystals are seen as several different shapes (rods, barrels, rhomboid and ovoid). Only the larger ones are visible under normal light **(a)**. In compensated polarized light they are weakly positively birefringent **(b)**. (Images courtesy of Andrew Bird, Senior Biomedical Scientist, Cytology, North Bristol NHS Trust.)

- injection with steroid
- NSAIDs.

Colchicine may also be effective – a good response to this drug does not differentiate gout and acute CPP.

OSTEOARTHRITIS WITH CPPD

The presence of CPP crystals appears to modulate the development of osteoarthritis (OA). Characteristically, there is a hypertrophic reaction with marked osteophyte formation. There are the usual features of pain, stiffness, swelling, joint crepitus and loss of movement. The subgroup is commonest in older women, with polyarticular OA affecting knees in particular, but also more unusual joints, such as the metacarpophalangeal (MCP), radiocarpal, midcarpal, glenohumeral, ankle and midfoot.

The characteristic *X-ray* features arise from a combination of intra-articular and periarticular calcification and OA. OA appearances are similar to those of non-CPPD disease apart from unusual distribution.

Haemochromatosis

Haemochromatosis is an uncommon disorder of middle-aged people (usually men), resulting from chronic iron overload. The clinical features are those of cirrhosis and diabetes, with a typical bronze pigmentation of the skin. About half of patients develop joint symptoms (particularly in the hands and fingers). It is associated with CC but may also result in a form of OA, though unusual in that MCP joints are affected. The plasma iron and iron-binding capacity are raised.

CHRONIC CPP CRYSTAL INFLAMMATORY ARTHRITIS

This presents as a chronic oligo- or polyarthritis with inflammatory symptoms and signs and often an acute phase response with elevated erythrocyte sedimentation rate (ESR) or C-reactive protein (CRP). It thus forms part of the differential diagnosis of RA. There may be typical acute attacks of acute CPP arthritis. The commonest affected joints are knee, radiocarpal and glenohumeral.

BASIC CALCIUM PHOSPHATE CRYSTAL DEPOSITION DISEASE

Basic calcium phosphate (BCP) is a normal component of bone, as calcium hydroxyapatite crystals. BCP crystal deposition may occur in and

SECTION 1 GENERAL ORTHOPAEDICS

around joints as a result of local tissue damage. Such deposition is common, especially with increasing age. It is usually asymptomatic but may give rise to acute periarthritis or tendinitis.

Pathology

BCP crystals are deposited in relatively avascular or damaged parts of tendons and ligaments – most notably around the shoulder and knee – and also around chondrocytes in articular cartilage. The deposits grow by crystal accretion and eventually may be seen on X-ray. Macroscopically, the BCP deposit has a chalky appearance. The deposit may be completely inert but, for reasons that are often unclear, may suddenly provoke an acute vascular reaction and inflammation. Crystal shedding into joints may give rise to synovitis.

Clinical features

Two clinical syndromes are associated with BCP crystal deposition:

- an acute periarthritis
- a chronic rapidly destructive arthritis.

ACUTE PERIARTHRITIS

This is by far the commonest form of BCP crystal deposition disorder affecting joints and it usually affects the rotator cuff. The patient, usually a

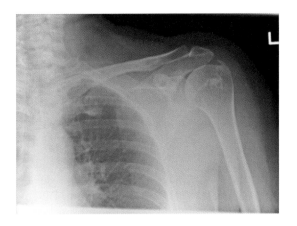

4.5 Calcification in supraspinatus.

female between 30 and 50 years of age, complains of pain around the shoulder. Symptoms may start suddenly and rise to a crescendo during which the tissues around the joint are swollen, warm and exquisitely tender. Surgical intervention may disclose a tense globule of creamy material oozing from between the frayed fibres of tendon or ligament.

Diagnosis is usually presumptive from the history. Radiographs may show calcification around the shoulder (**4.5**). Detection of BCP crystals is not practical in routine service: individual crystals are less than 0.1 μm long and cannot be seen on light microscopy.

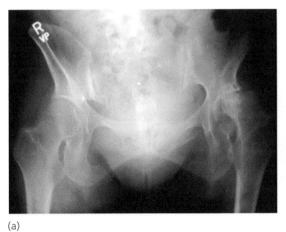

(a)

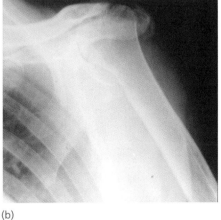

(b)

4.6 Apatite-associated destructive arthropathy (rapidly destructive OA) Radiographs of the hip (a) and shoulder (b). Common features are rapid progression to joint disruption, crumbling of the subarticular bone and periarticular ossification.

Treatment of acute periarthritis includes rest and NSAIDs. Resistant cases may respond to local injection of corticosteroids during the acute attack. Persistent pain and tenderness may call for operative removal of the calcific deposit or 'decompression' of the affected tendon or ligament.

CHRONIC DESTRUCTIVE ARTHRITIS

A destructive form of OA affecting the shoulder or hip (rarely, knee) has been described in elderly individuals, associated with rotator cuff defects and aggregates of BCP in the fluid. Patients are usually female and aged over 70, presenting with pain, swelling and loss of function of the affected shoulder. Night pain is often present.

On examination, a large effusion is typically seen: occasionally rupture of the capsule leads to extravasation of blood and synovial fluid into surrounding tissues. The glenohumeral joint has reduced movement in all planes. Aspiration of the joint is frequently blood-stained.

X-rays (**4.6**) show loss of the articular space, with little or no sclerosis or osteophyte formation. Rapid erosion and destruction of subchondral bone may occur, resulting in instability and dislocation.

Management is often difficult: aspiration and steroid injection may be tried but effusions usually recur and the inevitable associated massive rotator cuff tears make surgery difficult.

Osteoarthritis

5

- Introduction 75
- Prevalence and distribution 76
- Aetiology and risk factors 76
- Pathology 78
- Natural history and outcomes 78
- Assessment 82
- Management 83

INTRODUCTION

Osteoarthritis (OA) is the most common form of joint disease throughout the world. It is strongly associated with age, and extremely common in older people; some studies estimate that over 80% of people over 55 years of age have OA of at least one joint. It mainly affects the hips, knees, spine, hands and feet.

The disease processes leading to OA result in a final common pathway of joint failure. Clinically, OA is a very heterogeneous condition, but it is the end result of biochemical and mechanical insult that exceeds the joint's ability to repair itself.

All of the structures that compose synovial joints can fail and lead to the final common outcome of OA. Once one structure begins to fail, the surrounding structures are affected adversely and then also fail. Normally, the insult, whether biological or mechanical, affects a number of structures simultaneously and the remaining structures secondarily. For example, a traumatic knee injury could lead to a tear of the meniscus, fracture of subchondral bone, disruption of the hyaline cartilage and stretching of entheses, all occurring simultaneously.

Subchondral bone supports the overlying hyaline cartilage. It is susceptible to fracture when subjected to great compressive force or to avascular necrosis when subjected to shear forces. Collapse of the subchondral bone leads to splitting of the overlying hyaline cartilage. Synovium can become inflamed due to chemical irritants such as crystals, or infection; additionally, the synovium is prone to inflammation resulting from systemic immune-related problems, as in rheumatoid arthritis (RA). Synovitis of any cause results in the release of inflammatory mediators such as cytokines, and affects the production of hyaluronic acid, thereby altering the viscosity of the synovial fluid. The cytokines in the synovial fluid affect the catabolic and anabolic activities of the chondrocytes and osteocytes in the nearby cartilage and bone, as well as the capsule, leading to alterations in the normal integrity of these tissues, rendering them more susceptible to mechanical insults. The entheses are commonly stretched by injuries producing inflammation and oedema in the adjacent bone. The menisci or the labrum are susceptible to tearing under excessive shear forces. Once their function is compromised, the hyaline cartilage can become exposed to abnormal load and can fail.

Failure of hyaline cartilage results in the subchondral bone being subjected to both increased load and direct pressure from synovial fluid.

FINAL COMMON PATHWAY TO OA

1 Damage to hyaline cartilage
2 Increased load on the underlying bone
3 Cyst formation due to penetration of the subchondral bone by synovial fluid under pressure
4 New bone formation on the joint margins (osteophytes)

PREVALENCE AND DISTRIBUTION

OA affects focal areas within joints: early in the disease only a localized area is affected, although later it may spread to affect the whole joint. The sites most commonly affected are:

- *in the knee*: the anteromedial compartment of the tibiofemoral joint and the lateral facet of the patellofemoral joint
- *in the hip*: the superolateral aspect
- *in the hands and feet*: the terminal (distal) interphalangeal joints, as well as the first metatarsophalangeal (MTP) and thumb base.

Increasing age is a strong risk factor, and there are differences in prevalence and distribution in men and women (e.g. **5.1**). Some racial/ethnic differences also exist. For example, superolateral hip OA, which is very common in Caucasians, is relatively uncommon in people of Chinese origin. This may be due to subtle differences in skeletal shape.

AETIOLOGY AND RISK FACTORS

OA has no single cause; rather, it is due to a variable combination of both systemic predisposition and local biomechanical risk factors affecting different individuals and different joint sites, which explains its heterogeneity (**5.2**).

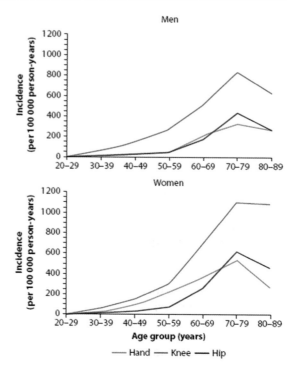

5.1 Incidence of symptomatic OA of the hand, knee and hip as a function of age (Data from Fallon Community Health Plan (Oliveria et al., 1995) reproduced from Nelson & Jordan, 2015.)

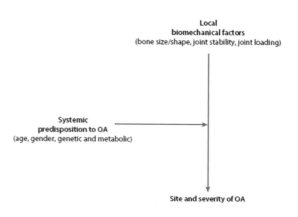

5.2 Osteoarthritis Systemic predisposition and local biomechanical risk factors.

MAJOR RISK FACTORS FOR OA

Systemic predisposition

- Genetics
- Age
- Gender
- Diet and obesity

Local biomechanical factors

- Abnormal joint shape and size
- Previous injury
- Neuromuscular problems
- Obesity
- Loading/occupational factors

Bone mineral density

(It is unclear whether this is a local or a systemic factor)

Systemic predisposition

GENETIC PREDISPOSITION

Twin studies and other data indicate that about 40% of the predisposition to OA may be genetic. However, there is no 'OA gene'; rather, several different sites within the genome each confer a small increased risk. Many of these sites relate to genes important for skeletal development, adding to other evidence that suggests that bone size and shape are important determinants of the likelihood of getting OA.

AGE

OA is strongly associated with increasing age although there are major differences in the 'pathology' of ageing joints from those of OA, and it has been suggested that we would need to live for over 200 years before the age-related changes in the joints alone (such as thinning of the cartilage) would cause OA! The association with age may have more to do with joint stability and muscles than joints. As we age, our cartilage gets thinner and our muscles get weaker, and the stability of major joints such as the knee may be affected in subtle but important ways by these changes.

GENDER

As shown in 5.1, there are differences in prevalence of OA between men and women. Changes related to the female menopause appear to be particularly important, as knee OA prevalence in women rises sharply after the menopause, and inflammatory OA of the hands often starts during the menopause.

DIET AND OBESITY

Obesity is a strong risk factor, particularly for knee OA. It is also a risk factor for increased incidence of hand OA, suggesting that it may have some systemic influence, perhaps through changes in obesity-related biochemical factors such as leptin levels. Studies suggest that deficiencies in some vitamin deficiencies, including C, D and K, may be important in the development of OA.

Local biomechanical factors

ABNORMAL JOINT SHAPE AND SIZE

Joint shape is an important risk factor, particularly for hip OA. Hip dysplasia predisposes to hip OA in later life, and more subtle abnormalities of the size or shape of the head of the femur or acetabulum (such as the shape changes that cause femoroacetabular impingement) may be responsible for much of the common hip OA seen. The differences in shape of hips in Chinese from that in Caucasians may explain the low prevalence of hip OA in Chinese people.

PREVIOUS INJURY

Injuries that affect the shape or stability of a joint predispose to OA. At the knee joint, meniscal and ligament injuries, particularly ACL rupture, are important predisposing factors.

NEUROMUSCULAR PROBLEMS

Severe neurological problems of specific types can lead to the important variant of OA called 'Charcot's joints'. Muscle weakness, loss of proprioception and joint laxity predispose to OA. Conversely, spasticity results in very tight joints accompanied by abnormal joint loading leading to joint damage and secondary OA. OA of the hip is particularly common in persons suffering from spastic cerebral palsy.

JOINT LOADING, OCCUPATION AND OBESITY

The extent to which normal or excessive joint use, including exercise, are risk factors for OA or alternatively protective to the condition is a contentious issue, and we do not yet understand exactly what aspects of joint loading matter most to joint health. However, certain specific occupations involving repetitive 'overuse' of joints can predispose to OA.

Bone density

People who come to hip replacement because of fractures caused by osteoporosis are unlikely to have hip OA. Studies have confirmed that, at both the knee and the hip, high bone mineral density is a risk factor for OA, and low bone mineral density is protective.

PATHOLOGY

The key *pathological features* of OA and their radiographic correlates are shown in **Table 5.1**.

The cartilage changes are accompanied by extensive changes in the tidemark between bone and cartilage, with vascular invasion and extension of the calcified zone as well as thickening of the subchondral bone. At the margins of the joint, periosteal cells proliferate and change their phenotype to form bone (osteophytes) (**5.3**). In addition, there is usually some

Table 5.1 Key pathological features of OA

Pathology	Radiographic correlates
Focal areas of loss of articular cartilage	Joint space narrowing (if loss is extensive)
Bone growth at the joint margins	Osteophytes
Sclerosis of underlying bone	Sclerosis of subchondral bone
Cyst formation in underlying bone	Bone cysts
Loss of bone	Bone attrition
Varying degrees of synovial inflammation	Effusions may be apparent
Fibrosis and thickening of the joint capsule	Not visible on radiographs

synovial inflammation (which may result in joint effusions) as well as thickening and fibrosis of the joint capsule (which may be extensive). In advanced cases, the damage to the subchondral bone can lead to the formation of cysts (**5.4**) and loss of bone volume.

NATURAL HISTORY AND OUTCOMES

OA is not a degenerative process; the changes that are going on in cartilage and other tissues are very active ones. Similarly, OA is not necessarily progressive. Natural history and physiological

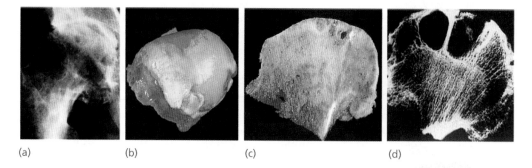

(a)   (b)   (c)   (d)

5.3 Osteoarthritis – pathology (a) The X-ray shows loss of articular cartilage at the superior pole and cysts in the underlying bone; the specimen **(b)** shows that the top of the femoral head was completely denuded of cartilage and there are large osteophytes around the periphery. In the coronal section **(c)** the subarticular cysts are clearly revealed. **(d)** A fine-detail X-ray shows the extent of the subarticular bone destruction.

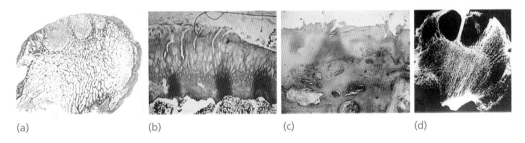

(a)　　　　(b)　　　　(c)　　　　(d)

5.4 Osteoarthritis – histology (a) Destructive changes (loss of articular cartilage and cyst formation) are most marked where stress is greatest; reparative changes are represented by sclerosis around the cysts and new bone formation (osteophytes) in less stressed areas. **(b)** In this high-power view, the articular cartilage shows loss of metachromasia and deep clefts in the surface (fibrillation). Attempts at repair result in **(c)** subarticular sclerosis and buds of fibrocartilage mushrooming where the articular surface is destroyed **(d)**.

imaging studies (such as bone scintigraphy) suggest that it goes through periods of activity and quiescence. Thus, a joint may be mechanically compromised in a susceptible person, and respond by activation of the OA process, leading to some changes to cartilage and bone and to the characteristic radiographic changes (**5.5**). This may result in the process then becoming quiescent for long periods, although physical examination and radiographs of the joint will still reveal the changes of OA.

Clinically, it is also clear that patients can have periods of more severe symptoms, followed by quiescent periods. In a significant proportion of cases (probably about 30%), time results in clinical improvement rather than deterioration.

Repair of the pathological changes is less common but can occur: spontaneous improvement in hip OA is well described, as is joint repair in response to major mechanical treatment interventions (e.g. osteotomy at the knee) or mechanical unloading (e.g. by use of Ilizarov frames for

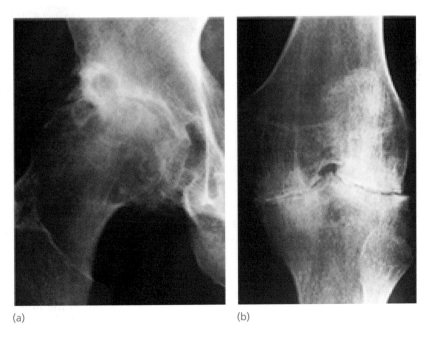

(a)　　　　(b)

5.5 Osteoarthritis – X-rays The cardinal features of OA are remarkably constant whether in **(a)** the hip or **(b)** the knee.

SECTION 1 GENERAL ORTHOPAEDICS

ankle OA). However, the repaired OA joint is not normal, as the hyaline articular cartilage is replaced by fibrocartilage.

Symptoms and signs

Pain is the main clinical problem, but there is poor correlation between the radiographic evidence of OA in joints and the prevalence of the clinical symptoms such as pain (**5.6**).

MAJOR SYMPTOMS AND SIGNS OF CLINICAL OA

Symptoms
- Pain (the nature and severity of which is very variable)
- Joint stiffness (particularly short-lasting stiffness after a period of inactivity)
- Fatigue
- Sleep disturbance
- Anxiety/depression
- Reduced functional ability and activities

Signs
- Tenderness of the joint
- Bony swelling
- Reduced range of movement with pain at the end of the range
- Crepitus on movement of the joint
- Weakness and wasting of muscles acting on the joint
- Signs of inflammation (usually fairly mild)
- Deformity and instability in severe/advanced cases

PAIN

Most patients with clinical OA report discomfort or pain in or around the joints affected. They often refer to the sensation as a deep-seated discomfort similar to a toothache emanating from within the joint. Experiences vary:

- a dull ache after exercise
- (more common) moderate activity-related pain
- excruciating continuous pain and pain at night.

Severe pain that wakes the patient nightly is a particularly debilitating symptom of severe arthritis and leads to sleep deprivation.

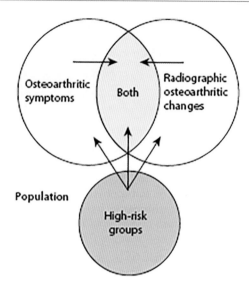

5.6 The relationship between osteoarthritic symptoms and radiological features of OA (From Dieppe & Lohmander, 2005.)

Many people report that no two days are the same, the pain experience being variable and seemingly inexplicable.

OTHER SYMPTOMS

Stiffness, or gelling of the joint after inactivity, is a classic feature of OA, resulting in people having difficulty getting moving after resting. It is particularly common in the morning after first awakening. Less well-appreciated symptoms of OA include *fatigue, sleep disturbance* caused by pain, and *anxiety/depression*. Each of these is very common, can have a significant impact on individuals and may need management separately from any attempt to deal with joint damage or pain.

SIGNS

Look for the signs of OA on examination, palpation and movement.

On examination

- The joints affected may appear swollen.
- There may be evidence of wasting (e.g. in quadriceps muscle wasting at the knee).
- Surrounding muscles may be weak (e.g. the Trendelenburg sign at the hip, which signifies weakness of hip abductors)
- In advanced OA, there may be joint deformity.

On palpation

- There may be bony swelling at the margin of the joint.
- There may be signs of mild inflammation (e.g. heat over the joint line).
- An effusion may be felt.

On movement

- There is usually a reduced range, with pain at the end of the range.
- Crepitus may be felt as the joint is moved.
- In advanced disease, instability may be detected.

SYMPTOMS AND SIGNS AT DIFFERENT JOINT SITES

Hips Pain usually is felt in the groin and laterally over the hip and radiates down the anterolateral aspect of the thigh to the knee. Occasionally, the pain can radiate beyond the knee.

 Referred pain felt only in the knee is not uncommon, and clinicians should always consider hip OA as a cause of isolated knee pain.

Pain is worse on exercise and walking distance is reduced. Pain at rest and night pain can be particularly troublesome. Stiffness is usually experienced first thing in the morning and after having sat still for a while, but it quickly resolves on movement to be replaced by pain. Complex movements, such as getting in and out of a car or putting on socks, which involve deep flexion combined with rotation, are often difficult or impossible. Patients struggle with stairs and, in the absence of a banister, may only manage stairs on all fours.

Examination reveals:

- an antalgic gait, characterized by an uneven cadence, in which less time is spent in the stance phase of the painful limb
- globally reduced range of movement with internal rotation often restricted early in the disease progression
- joint movement that is limited by pain at the extremes of movement.

Knees Knee OA occurs most commonly in the medial tibiofemoral joint but can occur in all three compartments and is often tricompartmental. Isolated patellofemoral OA is probably due to altered biomechanics of the extensor mechanism. Pain is felt globally over the knee and the proximal tibia. In isolated patellofemoral OA, the pain is felt anteriorly over the knee and is often worst when ascending or descending stairs as the patella is compressed against the femur. As in the hip, the pain is a deep-seated aching sensation related to exercise. Rest pain and night pain develop in the later stages of the disease. Patients sometimes report audible crepitus (crackling or grating sounds) coming from the knee as well as symptoms of instability (a feeling that the knee is going to give way). They may notice gradual deformity of the knee, in particular varus deformity (**5.7**), but less commonly valgus deformity.

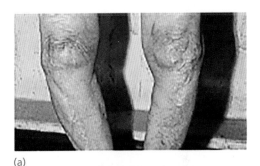

(a)

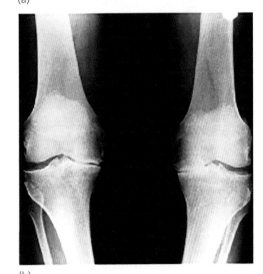

(b)

5.7 Polyarticular (generalized) OA of the knees.

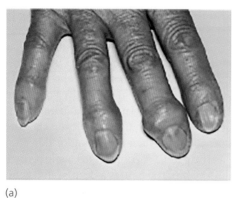

(a)

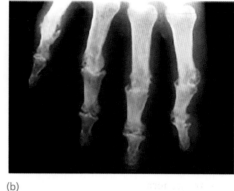

(b)

5.8 Polyarticular (generalized) OA of the hands (a,b) An almost invariable feature of the polyarticular OA is involvement of the terminal finger joints – Heberden's nodes.

Fixed flexion deformity means that the knees cannot lock in full extension and thus patients cannot stand comfortably for prolonged periods due to muscle fatigue. Loss of flexion beyond 90 degrees makes standing from a sitting position difficult as patients cannot move their centre of gravity anterior to their mid-coronal plane. Swelling and stiffness are common features.

Examination reveals:

- an antalgic gait
- wasting of quadriceps muscles
- joint effusion
- joint deformity
- crepitus palpable and sometimes audible on movement.

The joint deformity may be passively correctable. Deformity is towards the compartment most severely affected, usually varus deformity with predominantly medial compartment OA. There is sometimes tenderness along the joint line and palpable osteophytes that can be tender.

Hands The joint sites commonly affected in the hand are the distal interphalangeal joints and the thumb base (**5.8**).

OA of the hand is strongly associated with OA at other joint sites and is far more common in women than in men. It often starts relatively abruptly around the time of the menopause. Distal interphalangeal joint OA is not generally a major problem in terms of function, but thumb base OA can be, as it leads to instability and difficulty with pinch grip.

Other joints Almost any joint can be affected by OA, particularly if it is damaged by severe trauma. However, there are peculiarities to the phenotype of the condition at different sites.

- *Elbow OA* is almost always asymptomatic (just causing loss of full extension of the elbow).
- *Shoulder OA* is more likely to result in severe bone destruction (a condition sometimes called 'Milwaukee shoulder').

ASSESSMENT

Pain is a subjective experience which cannot easily be measured or assessed. Similarly, it is not easy to ascertain the severity of the functional problems that any individual patient may be experiencing. One is largely reliant on what the patient says, supplemented by the observation of gait, any difficulties the patient has undressing, dressing or getting onto or off the examination couch and clinical examination.

A number of instruments are available to assess the severity and impact of OA. Patient self-assessment questionnaires such as the 'WOMAC', Oxford hip, knee and shoulder scores are often used. In addition, semi-objective tests of function, such as walking speed, can be measured to assess disability. Plain radiographs are so characteristic as to make other imaging studies unnecessary. There are four cardinal signs.

SECTION 1 GENERAL ORTHOPAEDICS

THE FOUR CARDINAL SIGNS OF OA
Osteophyte formation
Joint space narrowing
Sclerosis of the underlying bone
Subchondral bone cysts

MANAGEMENT

Interventions are generally divided into symptomatic therapies and disease-modifying therapies. As yet, there are no drugs with proven ability to modify the disease process. Disease modification can occur in response to mechanical interventions, such as joint distraction and osteotomy. All other interventions are symptomatic.

The main symptoms of OA (pain, stiffness, fatigue and anxiety/depression) are very susceptible to so-called 'placebo' and 'nocebo' effects. Placebo is generally thought of as a sham or dummy intervention, and we know that sham surgery can work well in OA, but what placebo research teaches us is that symptoms of conditions such as OA are highly responsive to the whole context in which any therapy is administered. If patients and clinicians feel safe and trusting of each other, and if the clinician is able to validate the patient's experiences (i.e. the patient feels fully understood), then outcomes will be good, whatever the intervention.

Symptomatic therapy

The basic principles of the symptomatic management of OA can be illustrated as a pyramid (**5.9**).

The UK National Institute for Health and Care Excellence (NICE) 2014 guideline *CG177: Osteoarthritis: Care and Management* recommends that clinicians follow the four steps described below.

STEP 1: *Take a holistic approach and encourage self-management*
This means assessing the impact of the OA on the individual's quality of life, function, mood, relationships and activities, thinking about their

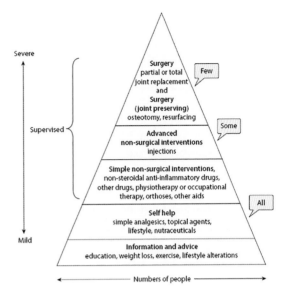

5.9 The pyramid of treatment for symptomatic OA (From Dieppe & Lohmander, 2005.)

context and any comorbidities (including depression) and about the potential risks and benefits of any intervention.

Self-management strategies include:

- considering alterations of diet (particularly to lose weight)
- alteration in activities
- changing footwear
- taking a more positive approach to the condition
- exercising more.

STEP 2: *Introduce the 'core treatments' appropriate for most people with OA*
These core treatments include:

- the provision of information about the condition and its management
- helping people to increase their exercise level and to do specific exercises to strengthen muscles around affected joints
- footwear advice
- help with weight loss for those who are obese.

STEP 3: *Introduce specific non-surgical interventions*
These may be pharmacological or non-pharmacological.

Non-pharmacological The non-pharmacological interventions of proven value include:

- supervised courses of physical therapy
- use of aids and devices to reduce instability of to help with functional problems
- walking aids, e.g. sticks or crutches
- some electrotherapy techniques, e.g. TENS machines for pain control
- some manipulations, particularly in the case of hip OA with a reduced range of motion of the hip.

Pharmacological Options include the following.

- Regular or on-demand paracetamol and topical non-steroidal anti-inflammatory drugs (NSAIDs) are considered to be the first choices for pain. Recent evidence has suggested that paracetamol is no better than placebo, but both have been demonstrated to reduce pain.
- If they are insufficient, NSAIDs, COX-2 inhibitors and opioid analgesics can be considered.
- Intra-articular local anaesthetic and corticosteroid injections can be considered as an adjunct to other treatments, but hyaluronan injections are not recommended because of lack of evidence.

The very widely used 'nutriceuticals' such as glucosamine and chondroitin are not recommended because of the lack of robust evidence to support their use.

STEP 4: *Consider surgical options*

There are many different surgical options available, as discussed in more detail in other chapters. Surgery is broadly divided into:

- joint realignment
- joint fusion
- joint excision
- joint replacement (arthroplasty), which may be total or partial (e.g. unicompartmental knee replacement).

Joint debridement such as arthroscopic knee debridement has largely been discredited by randomized controlled trials of sham surgery versus debridement, which showed no treatment benefit.

Surgery is usually confined to end-stage disease once pain has become refractory to other treatment options. *Hip and knee replacements* are particularly successful treatments for advanced OA, often resulting in complete resolution of pain and a dramatic improvement in function and quality of life. However, a small but important minority of patients do not benefit from joint replacement (5–15%, lack of response more common for knee replacement than hip replacement) and have persistent severe pain in the long-term post surgery despite no evidence of technical issues with the surgery performed.

Principles of management

The natural history, presentation, impact and prognosis are different for each of the major joint sites affected, and management needs to be based on prognosis and impact in particular.

 Most people with OA do not progress to a severe enough state to warrant surgical intervention and the prognosis is generally relatively good. Interventions should therefore be kept as simple and as safe as possible.

HIP OA

OA of the hip often progresses relatively rapidly: patients may report a relatively long period of mild problems, such as exercise-related aching in the groin, followed by the development of severe pain over a period of a few weeks or months.

Spontaneous recovery from severe hip OA occasionally occurs, particularly in those who stay active, but this cannot be predicted or relied upon.

Hip OA responds relatively well to physical therapy. It is important to assess leg length and think about corrective footwear, and shock-absorbing shoes can help.

MAINSTAYS OF TREATMENT FOR HIP OA

Weight loss

Walking aids – the use of a stick in the contralateral hand to reduce loading while walking is helpful

Physiotherapy aimed at increasing the range of motion and improving muscle strength and pelvic stability

Simple analgesics combined with NSAIDs

When these treatment modalities no longer control symptoms and pain becomes very severe, interfering with activities and sleep, total hip replacement is likely to be the best option and is usually very effective.

KNEE OA

OA of the knee often responds well to simple non-surgical interventions, and it often remains relatively stable and mild for many years, during which people can adjust to it, and find ways of making sure it interferes with life minimally.

There are many surgical options if the condition becomes severe. These include osteotomies of various types, and unicompartmental or total joint replacements. Arthroscopic joint lavage is not recommended because of insufficient evidence for efficacy over and above its significant placebo effect.

MAINSTAYS OF TREATMENT FOR KNEE OA

Weight loss – knee OA is strongly related to obesity and even modest weight loss can result in marked reduction in symptoms, so this should be prioritized.

Keeping the quadriceps muscles strong is important, as they are key to knee stability.

Topical NSAIDs are useful.

Shoes or appliances that reduce impact loading (shock-absorbing) and/or adjustments to unload the most affected compartments (usually the medial tibiofemoral compartment) are helpful.

Patella strapping is useful for patellofemoral OA.

Corticosteroid injections can result in good pain relief for relatively short periods of time.

HAND OA

OA in the hand often has a relatively good long-term prognosis, unless there is severe thumb base disease. Management therefore usually involves strategies that reduce pain without putting the patient at risk. Topical NSAIDs and capsaicin are of proven value for interphalangeal joint disease. There are good surgical options for advanced thumb base OA.

Osteonecrosis and osteochondritis

6

- Osteonecrosis   87
- Systemic disorders associated with osteonecrosis   92
- Osteochondrosis ('osteochondritis')   94

OSTEONECROSIS

The prototypical example of avascular necrosis (AVN) is aseptic death of a large segment of the femoral head following fracture of the femoral neck and severance of the local blood supply. It is now recognized that aseptic osteonecrosis occurs at a number of other sites, due either to local injury or to non-traumatic conditions (including Legg-Calvé-Perthes disease, high-dosage corticosteroid administration and alcohol abuse) which result in ischaemia of a substantial segment of bone.

MAIN CONDITIONS ASSOCIATED WITH NON-TRAUMATIC OSTEONECROSIS

Bone infections
Septic arthritis
Legg-Calvé-Perthes disease
Cortisone administration
Alcohol abuse
Sickle-cell disease
Gaucher's disease
Haemoglobinopathies
Caisson disease
Ionizing radiation

The sites most susceptible are:

- the femoral head (most common)
- the femoral condyles
- the head of humerus
- the proximal poles of scaphoid and talus (**6.1**).

What they have in common is that they lie at the outskirts of the bone's main vascular supply and they are largely enclosed by articular cartilage, which is itself avascular and which restricts the area for entry of local blood vessels. Furthermore, at some of these sites, the subarticular trabeculae are sustained largely by endarterioles with limited arterial connections.

Another factor which needs to be taken into account is that the vascular sinusoids which nourish the marrow and bone cells, unlike arterial capillaries, have no adventitial layer and their patency is determined by the volume and pressure of the surrounding marrow tissue, which itself is encased in unyielding bone. The system functions essentially as a closed compartment within which one element can expand only at the expense of the others. Local changes such as vascular stasis, haemorrhage or marrow swelling can, therefore, rapidly spiral to a vicious cycle of ischaemia, reactive oedema or inflammation, further marrow swelling, increased intraosseous pressure and further ischaemia.

SECTION 1 GENERAL ORTHOPAEDICS

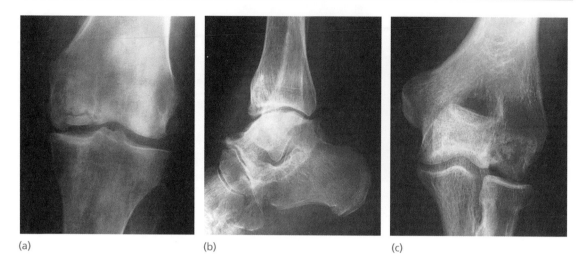

(a)   (b)   (c)

6.1 Osteonecrosis – distribution The most common site for osteonecrosis is the head of the femur but, as shown here, other sites can also be affected: examples are **(a)** the medial condyle of the femur, **(b)** the talus and **(c)** the capitulum. All these areas are located beneath convex articular surfaces; osteonecrosis is very seldom seen beneath a concave articular surface.

The process described above can be initiated in at least four different ways.

FACTORS CAUSING INITIATION OF OSTEONECROSIS

Severance of the local blood supply
Venous stasis and retrograde arteriolar
    stoppage
Intravascular thrombosis
Compression of capillaries and sinusoids
    by marrow swelling

 Ischaemia, in the majority of cases, is due to a combination of several initiating factors.

Traumatic osteonecrosis

In fractures and dislocations of the hip the retinacular vessels supplying the femoral head are easily torn; if, in addition, there is damage to or thrombosis of the ligamentum teres, osteonecrosis is inevitable. Other injuries which are prone to osteonecrosis are fractures of the scaphoid and talus; significantly, in these cases it is always the proximal fragment which suffers because the principal vessels enter the bones near their distal ends and course through the bone from distal to proximal.

Impact injuries and osteoarticular fractures at any of the convex articular surfaces behave in the same way and may cause localized ischaemic changes affecting a small segment of bone just below the articular surface. These small lesions are usually referred to as '*osteochondroses*' and many of them have acquired eponyms which are now firmly embedded in orthopaedic history.

Non-traumatic osteonecrosis

The mechanisms here are more complex and may involve several pathways to intravascular stasis or thrombosis, as well as extravascular swelling and capillary compression. These changes, acting either independently or in combination, are believed to cause the critical bone ischaemia in osteonecrotic lesions associated with Legg-Calvé-Perthes disease, caisson disease, sickle-cell disease, Gaucher's disease, high-dosage corticosteroid medication and alcohol abuse.

Pathology

Dead bone is structurally and radiographically indistinguishable from live bone. However, lacking a blood supply, it does not undergo renewal, and after a limited period of repetitive stress it collapses (**6.2**). The changes develop in four overlapping stages.

STAGE 1: *BONE DEATH WITHOUT STRUCTURAL CHANGE*

Within 48 hours after infarction there is marrow necrosis and cell death. However, for weeks or even months the bone may show no alteration in macroscopic appearance.

STAGE 2: *REPAIR AND EARLY STRUCTURAL FAILURE*

Some days or weeks after infarction the surrounding, living bone shows a vascular reaction; new bone is laid down upon the dead trabeculae and the increase in bone mass shows on the X-ray as exaggerated density.

STAGE 3: *MAJOR STRUCTURAL FAILURE*

Small fractures begin to appear in the dead bone. The necrotic portion starts to crumble and the bone outline becomes distorted.

STAGE 4: *ARTICULAR DESTRUCTION*

Cartilage, being nourished mainly by synovial fluid, is preserved even in advanced osteonecrosis. However, severe distortion of the surface eventually leads to cartilage breakdown and secondary osteoarthritis.

Clinical features

By the time the patient presents, the lesion is often well advanced.

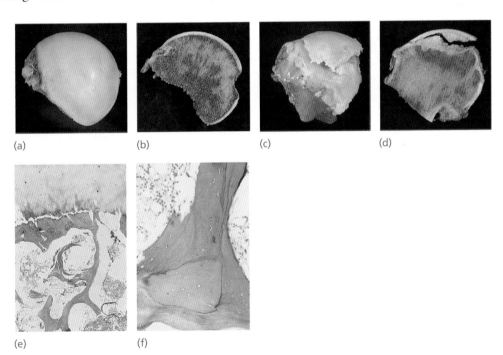

(a) (b) (c) (d)

(e) (f)

6.2 Osteonecrosis – pathology (a,b) Normal femoral head and cut section. The articular cartilage is obviously intact and the subchondral bone is well vascularized. **(c,d)** In this femoral head with osteonecrosis, the articular cartilage is lifted off the bone; the coronal section in **(d)** shows that this is due to a subarticular fracture through the necrotic segment in the dome of the femoral head. **(e)** Histological section across the junction between articular cartilage and bone showing living cartilage cells but necrotic subchondral marrow and bone. **(f)** High-power view showing islands of dead bone with empty osteocytic lacunae enfolded by new, living bone.

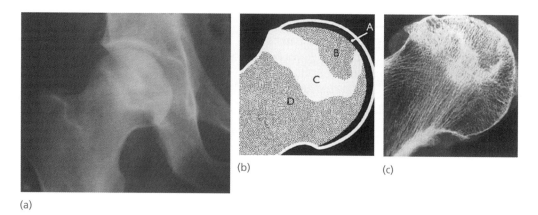

(a)

(b)

(c)

6.3 Osteonecrosis – X-ray (a) The cardinal X-ray feature is increased radiographic density in the weight-bearing part of the subarticular bone. The 'density' is due to new bone formation spreading into the necrotic segment. This is shown in the diagram **(b)** and the corresponding fine-detail X-ray of the femoral head specimen **(c)**. (A, articular cartilage; B, dead bone; C, new bone formation; D, normal bone.)

- *Pain* is the usual complaint; it is felt near a joint and is accompanied by *stiffness*.
- Local *tenderness* may be present with *swelling* of the nearby joint.
- *Restricted movement* is usual.

Imaging

X-RAYS

The distinctive X-ray feature of AVN is a subarticular segment of increased bone density (**6.3**). This is not because dead bone is more radio-opaque than living bone; it is due to reactive new bone formation in the surrounding living tissue which increases the total mass of calcified bone. Later changes are fracturing and collapse of the necrotic segment. A cardinal feature that distinguishes these progressive changes from those of osteoarthritis is that the radiographic 'joint space' retains its normal width because the articular cartilage is not destroyed until very late.

RADIOSCINTIGRAPHY

Radionuclide scanning with ^{99m}technetium hydroxymethylene diphosphonate (^{99m}Tc-HDP) may reveal an avascular segment (a 'cold' area signifying diminished activity) (e.g. after fracture of the femoral neck). More often, however, the picture is dominated by increased activity, reflecting hyperaemia and new bone formation in the area around the infarct.

MAGNETIC RESONANCE IMAGING

Magnetic resonance imaging (MRI) is the only reliable method of picking up the early signs of osteonecrosis. The first sign is a band-like low-intensity signal on the T1-weighted spin echo (SE) image and a similar but high-intensity signal on the short-tau inversion recovery (STIR) image (**6.4**).

MODIFIED ARCO STAGING OF OSTEONECROSIS

Stage 0 Patient asymptomatic and all clinical investigations 'normal'; biopsy shows osteonecrosis

Stage 1 X-rays normal; MRI or radionuclide scan shows osteonecrosis

Stage 2 X-rays and/or MRI show early signs of osteonecrosis but no distortion of bone shape or subchondral intraosseous fracture ('crescent sign')

Stage 3 X-ray shows early abnormality but femoral head still spherical

Stage 4 Signs of flattening or collapse of femoral head

Stage 5 Changes as above plus loss of 'joint space'

Stage 6 Changes as above plus marked destruction of articular surfaces

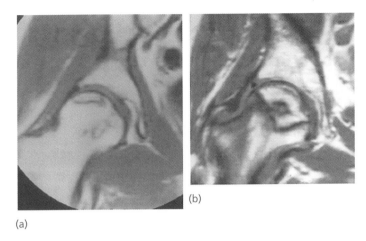

(b)

(a)

6.4 Osteonecrosis – MRI (a) Before any change is discernible on the plain X-ray, MRI will show a typical hypointense band in the T1-weighted image, outlining the ischaemic segment beneath the articular surface. **(b)** In this case the size of the ischaemic segment is much larger – and the likelihood of bone crumbling much greater.

Staging the lesion

It has long been recognized that the prognosis and planning of treatment for osteonecrosis depend largely on the stage at which the disorder is encountered. The most widely used system of staging is the one promoted by the International Association of Bone Circulation and Bone Necrosis (*Association Research Circulation Osseous — ARCO*), which applies mainly to femoral head necrosis.

Diagnosis of the underlying disorder

In many cases of osteonecrosis, an underlying disorder will be obvious from the history. Examples include:

- a known episode of trauma
- an occupation such as deep-sea diving or working under compressed air
- a family background of Gaucher's disease or sickle-cell disease
- a history of long-standing alcohol abuse
- a record of high-dosage corticosteroid administration (e.g. after organ transplantation where the drug is used for immunosuppression).

 Smaller doses of corticosteroid administration (e.g. as short-term treatment for asthma or as an adjunct in neurosurgical emergencies) can also be dangerous in patients with other risk factors.

Treatment

If possible, the cause should be eliminated.

- *In ARCO stages 1 and 2*, bone collapse can sometimes be prevented by a combination of weight-relief, splintage and (in some cases, associated with venous stasis and marrow oedema) surgical decompression of the bone.
- Once bone collapse has occurred, and provided the area of involvement is less than 30% or in a non-load-bearing position (*stage 3*), a realignment osteotomy, by transferring stress to an undamaged area, may relieve pain and prevent further bone distortion.
- *In stages 4–6*, the treatment is essentially the same as for osteoarthritis.

TREATMENT FOR STAGE 4–6 OSTEONECROSIS

1. Pain control and modification of daily activities
2. Arthrodesis of the joint if mobility is not a major issue (e.g. the ankle or wrist)
3. Partial or total joint replacement, the preferred option for the shoulder, hip and knee

SECTION 1 GENERAL ORTHOPAEDICS

SYSTEMIC DISORDERS ASSOCIATED WITH OSTEONECROSIS

SICKLE-CELL DISEASE

This is a genetic disorder, limited to people of black Central and West African descent. Red cells containing abnormal haemoglobin (HbS) become distorted and sickle-shaped; this is especially likely to occur with hypoxia (e.g. under anaesthesia or in extreme cold). Clumping of the sickle-shaped cells causes diminished capillary flow and repeated episodes of pain ('bone crises') or, if more severe, ischaemic necrosis. Almost any bone may be involved and there is a tendency for the infarcts to become infected, sometimes with unusual organisms such as *Salmonella*.

Imaging

X-rays of the tubular bones (including the phalanges) may show irregular endosteal destruction and medullary sclerosis, together with periosteal new bone formation (**6.5**). Not only does this resemble osteitis, but true infection is often superimposed on the infarct. In children, femoral head necrosis could be mistaken for Legg-Calvé-Perthes disease.

Treatment

Acute episodes are treated by rest and analgesics, followed by physiotherapy to minimize stiffness. Established necrosis is treated according to the principles described above, but with the emphasis on conservatism. Anaesthesia carries serious risks and may even precipitate vascular occlusion in the central nervous system, lungs or kidneys. The chances of postoperative infection are high.

CAISSON DISEASE

Decompression sickness (caisson disease) and osteonecrosis are important causes of disability in deep-sea divers and compressed-air workers building tunnels or underwater structures. Under increased

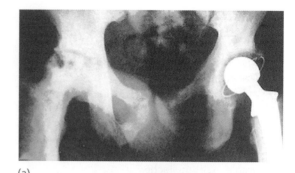

(a)

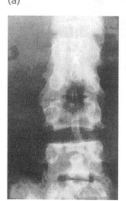

(b)

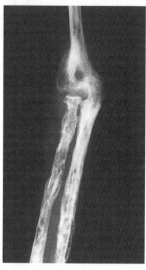

(c)

6.5 Sickle-cell disease (a) Typical changes in the femur due to marrow hyperplasia, with bone infarction and necrosis of the femoral head. **(b)** The spine also may be involved. **(c)** In severe cases, infarctions of tubular bones may resemble osteomyelitis.

air pressure, the blood and other tissues (especially fat) become supersaturated with nitrogen; if decompression is too rapid, the gas is released as bubbles, which cause local tissue damage and generalized embolic phenomena. The symptoms of decompression sickness are pain near the joints ('the bends'), breathing difficulty and vertigo ('the staggers'). In the most acute cases, there can be circulatory and respiratory collapse, severe neurological changes, coma and death. Bone necrosis may be due to capillary obstruction by gas bubbles and changes in marrow fat.

The patient complains of pain and loss of joint movement, but many lesions remain silent and are found only on routine X-ray examination.

Management

The aim is prevention; the incidence of osteonecrosis is proportional to the working pressure, the length of exposure, the rate of decompression and the number of exposures. Strict enforcement of suitable working schedules has reduced the risks considerably. The treatment of established lesions follows the principles already outlined.

GAUCHER'S DISEASE

Gaucher's disease is a familial metabolic disorder caused by inherited deficiency of lysosomal enzyme glucocerebrosidase and characterized by accumulation of glucosylceramide in the lysosomes of reticuloendothelial cells to produce Gaucher's cells. The effects are seen chiefly in the liver, spleen and bone marrow. Accumulation of Gaucher's cells in the bone marrow triggers a series of events that lead to skeletal pathology, of which osteonecrosis is the worst. The sites affected are:

- the hip (most frequently affected)
- the distal femur
- the talus
- the head of the humerus.

Bone ischaemia is usually attributed to the increase in medullary cell volume and sinusoidal compression.

Symptoms may occur at any age; the patient complains of pain around one of the larger joints and movements may be restricted. There is a tendency for the Gaucher deposits to become infected and the patient may present with septicaemia. A diagnostic, though inconstant, finding is a raised serum acid phosphatase level.

A special feature of *X-rays* is expansion of the tubular bones, especially the distal femur, producing a flask-like appearance due to replacement of myeloid tissue by Gaucher cells (**6.6**). Osteonecrosis of the femoral head is common.

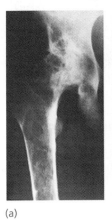
(a)

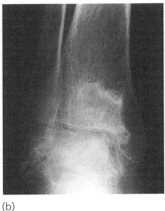
(b)

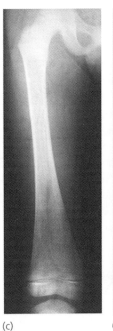
(c)

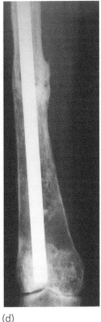
(d)

6.6 Gaucher's disease (a) Gaucher deposits are seen throughout the femur. The cortices are thin and there is osteonecrosis of the femoral head. **(b)** Bone infarction is seen in the distal end of the tibia and the talus. **(c)** The typical Erlenmeyer flask appearance is seen in the X-ray of this teenager. **(d)** Ten years later, the bone changes are much more marked, the cortices are extremely thin and the patient has obviously suffered a pathological fracture.

Treatment

The general disorder can now be treated by enzyme replacement. Management of the osteonecrosis follows the principles outlined in Chapter 8. If joint replacement is contemplated, antibiotic cover is essential.

DRUG-INDUCED NECROSIS

Corticosteroids in high dosage may give rise to 'spontaneous' osteonecrosis; thus, the condition is fairly common in renal transplant patients on immunosuppressive corticosteroids. Alcohol abuse is another potent cause. Both conditions result in widespread fatty changes and marrow infarction, which may be the cause of the bone necrosis. The sites usually affected are:

- the femoral head
- the femoral condyles
- the head of the humerus.

Pain may be present for many months before X-rays show any abnormality. *MRI* is the only reliable way of making an early diagnosis; typical changes are often discovered in asymptomatic joints.

Treatment

Early changes, if not actually reversible, can be prevented from extending by stopping the cortisone or alcohol. Analgesics, weight-relief and physiotherapy are often all that is required. Decompression of the affected bone by drilling may relieve symptoms and even prevent progressive changes in very early cases. If the joint surface has collapsed, reconstructive surgery is required.

OSTEOCHONDROSIS ('OSTEOCHONDRITIS')

The term '*osteochondrosis*' or '*osteochondritis*' is applied to a group of conditions in which there is compression, fragmentation or separation of a small segment of bone, usually at the bone end and involving the attached articular surface. The affected portion of bone shows many of the features of ischaemic necrosis, including increased vascularity and reactive sclerosis in the surrounding bone. These conditions occur in children and adolescents, often during phases of rapid growth and increased physical activity.

The pathogenesis of these lesions is still not completely understood. Impact injuries can cause oedema or bleeding in the subarticular bone, resulting in capillary compression or thrombosis and localized ischaemia. The critical event may well be a small osteochondral fracture, too faint to show up on plain X-ray examination but often visible on MRI. If the crack fails to unite, the isolated fragment may lose its blood supply and become necrotic.

Clinical features

The condition usually occurs in adolescents and young adults and the classic example is *osteochondritis dissecans* of the lateral part of the medial femoral condyle at the knee (6.7). Similar lesions are seen at other sites:

- the anteromedial corner of the talus
- the superomedial part of the femoral head
- the humeral capitulum (*Panner's disease*)
- the head of the second metatarsal (*Freiberg's disease*)
- the carpal lunate (*Kienböck's disease*).

The patient usually complains of intermittent pain; there is sometimes swelling and a small effusion in the joint. If the necrotic fragment becomes completely detached (not uncommon in osteochondritis dissecans), it may cause locking of the joint or episodes of 'giving way' in the knee or ankle.

Imaging

The early changes (i.e. before demarcation of the ischaemic fragment) are best shown by *MRI*: there is decreased signal intensity in the area around the affected osteochondral segment. *Radionuclide scanning* with ^{99m}Tc-HDP shows markedly increased activity in the same area.

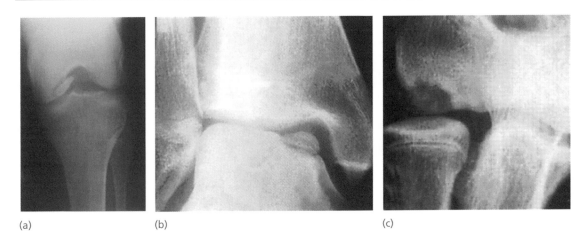

(a) (b) (c)

6.7 Osteochondrosis At the knee **(a)**, the osteochondral fragment separates on the lateral side of the medial femoral condyle. Other sites where this occurs are **(b)** the medial corner of the talus and **(c)** the capitulum at the elbow.

X-ray changes come later. The ischaemic or dissecting fragment is defined by a radiolucent line of demarcation. When it separates, the resulting 'crater' may be obvious.

Treatment

Treatment in the early stage consists of load reduction and restriction of activity. In young people, complete healing may occur, though it can take up to 2 years. For a large joint like the knee, it is generally recommended that partially detached fragments be pinned back in position after roughening of the base, while completely detached fragments should be pinned back only if they are completely preserved.

Treatment of osteochondrosis at the elbow, wrist and metatarsal head is discussed in the relevant chapters.

Metabolic and endocrine bone disorders

7

Bone and Bones	**97**	■ Hypocalcaemia	116
■ Bone composition and structure	98	■ Rickets and osteomalacia	117
■ Bone development and growth	102	■ Chronic kidney disease mineral bone	
■ Bone maintenance	104	disorder	122
■ Mineral exchange	105	■ Hypercalcaemia	123
■ Other influences on bone metabolism	106	■ Hyperparathyroidism	124
Metabolic bone disorders	**107**	■ Hypercalcaemia of malignancy	125
■ Assessment	107	■ Paget's disease of bone	126
■ Osteoporosis	111		

BONE AND BONES

Understanding of disorders of the musculoskeletal system begins with a basic knowledge of the anatomical structure and physiology of the bones and joints – the framework that supports the body, protects the soft tissues, transmits load and power from one part of the body to another and mediates movement and locomotion.

The illustration in 7.1 summarizes the stages of bone development. Embryonic development of the limbs begins with the appearance of the arm buds at about 4 weeks from ovulation and the leg buds shortly afterwards. At first, these have the appearance of miniature paddles, but by around 5 weeks the finger and toe rays become differentiated. By then, primitive skeletal elements and pre-muscle masses have begun to differentiate in the limbs. From about 6 weeks after ovulation the primitive cartilaginous bone-models start to become vascularized and primary ossification centres appear in the chondroid anlage. By now, spinal nerves are growing into the limbs. At 7–8 weeks, cavitation occurs where the joints will appear, and during the next few weeks the cartilaginous epiphyseal precursors become vacularized. Between 8 and 12 weeks the primitive joints and synovium become defined.

From then, further development goes hand in hand with growth. Bone formation in the cartilaginous model progresses along the diaphysis but the epiphyseal ends remain unossified until after birth.

Soon after birth secondary ossification centres begin to appear in the still cartilaginous ends of the tubular bones, a process that will occur during childhood in all the *endochondral bones* (bones formed in cartilage). By then, each bone end is defined as an *epiphysis*, the growth plate between the epiphysis and the rest of the bone as the *physis*, the adjacent end of the long bone the *metaphysis*, and the shaft as the *diaphysis*.

Longitudinal growth continues up until late adolescence, by a process of *endochondral bone*

SECTION 1 GENERAL ORTHOPAEDICS

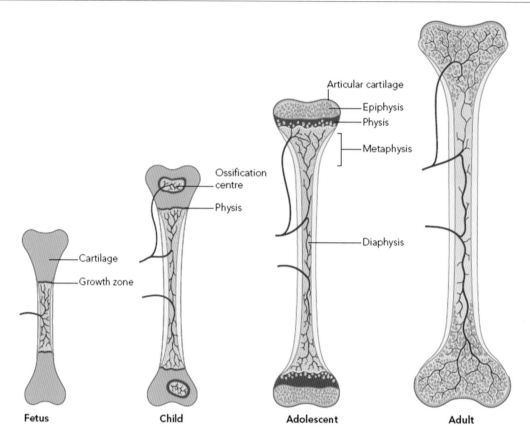

7.1 Stages in bone development Schematic representation of the stages in the development of a tubular bone showing the progress from diaphyseal ossification, through endochondral growth at the physis and increase in width of the diaphysis by sub-periosteal appositional bone formation.

formation, whereby cartilage formed beneath the growth plate becomes calcified to produce the primary spongiosa, which is then replaced by the secondary spongiosa following vascular invasion. Cessation of longitudinal growth is heralded by the growth plate becoming ossified, resulting in fusion of the epiphysis to the metaphysis.

An increase in bone circumference occurs by a different process: *periosteal bone formation*. This involves small generative cuboidal cells in the deepest layer of the periosteum. In contrast to longitudinal growth, periosteal bone formation does not involve the intermediary formation of cartilage. Whereas longitudinal growth ceases once growth plates have fused, periosteal bone formation may continue through life, depending on the anatomical site.

Where bones connect with each other, i.e. at the joints, the contact surfaces remain cartilaginous. *Diarthrodial joints* (freely movable, synovial joints) comprise *hyaline cartilage*, which is ideally suited to permit low-friction movement and to accommodate both compressive and tensile forces. In *synarthroses*, where greater resistance to shearing forces is needed, the interface usually consists of tough *fibrocartilage* (e.g. the pubic symphysis).

BONE COMPOSITION AND STRUCTURE

Bones as structural organs have three main functions:

- *support*
- *protection*
- *leverage*.

Bone as tissue has an equally important role as a mineral reservoir which helps to regulate the composition – and in particular the calcium ion concentration – of the extracellular fluid. For all its solidity, it is in a continuous state of flux, its internal shape and structure changing continuously.

All modulations in bone structure and composition are brought about by cellular activity, which is regulated by hormones and local factors; these agents, in turn, are controlled by alterations in mineral ion concentrations. Disruption of this complex interactive system results in systemic changes in mineral metabolism and generalized skeletal abnormalities.

BONE COMPOSITION

Bone consists of a largely collagenous *matrix* which is impregnated with mineral salts and populated by cells (*osteoblasts* and *osteoclasts*).

The matrix

Type I collagen fibres make up over 80% of the unmineralized matrix. They consist of collagen fibrils comprising a triple helix, with the overall structure stabilized by cross-linking between adjacent fibrils. Collagen is responsible for the skeleton's tensile strength. It also serves as a scaffold on which the mineral component is deposited.

Other non-collagenous proteins exist in small amounts in the mineralized matrix – mainly *osteopontin, osteonectin, osteocalcin* and *alkaline phosphatases* (*ALPs*). Their functions have not been fully elucidated but they appear to be involved in the regulation of bone cells and matrix mineralization.

Bone mineral

Almost half the bone volume is mineral matter, predominantly hydroxyapatite.

While the collagenous component lends tensile strength to bone, the crystalline mineral enhances its ability to resist compression.

Unmineralized matrix is known as *osteoid*; normally, it is seen only as a thin layer on surfaces where active new bone formation is taking place, but the proportion of osteoid to mineralized bone increases significantly in rickets and osteomalacia.

Bone cells

There are of three types of bone cell:

- *osteoblasts*
- *osteocytes*
- *osteoclasts.*

OSTEOBLASTS

Osteoblasts are concerned with bone formation and osteoclast activation.

Mature osteoblasts form rows of small (20 μm) mononuclear cells along the free surfaces of trabeculae and haversian systems where *osteoid* is laid down prior to calcification (**7.2**). They are rich in ALP and are responsible for the production of type I collagen as well as the non-collagenous bone proteins and for the mineralization of bone matrix. Stimulated by parathyroid hormone (PTH), they play a critical role in the initiation and control of osteoclastic activity.

OSTEOCYTES

Osteocytes are osteoblasts that become entombed in their own matrix. Lying in their bony lacunae, they communicate with each other and with the surface lining cells by slender cytoplasmic processes. They are sensitive to mechanical stimuli and communicate information and changes in stress and strain to the active osteoblasts which can then modify their osteogenic activity accordingly.

OSTEOCLASTS

These large multinucleated cells are the principal mediators of bone resorption.

Mature osteoclasts have a foamy appearance, due to the presence of numerous vesicles in the cytoplasm. In response to appropriate stimuli, the osteoclast forms a sealed attachment to a bone surface, where the cell membrane develops a ruffled border within which bone resorption takes place.

Following resorption of the bone matrix, the osteoclasts are left in shallow excavations – *Howship's lacunae* – along free bone surfaces (**7.2**).

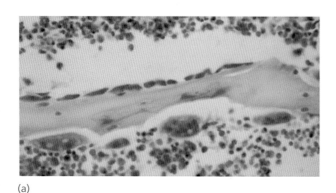

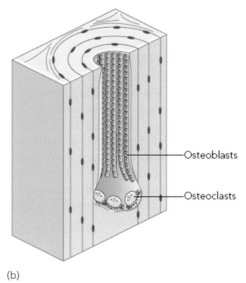

(a)   (b)

7.2 Bone cells **(a)** Histological section showing a trabecula lined on one surface by excavating osteoclasts and on the other surface by a string of much smaller osteoblasts. These two types of cell, working in concert, continuously remodel the internal bone structure. **(b)** In compact bone the osteoclasts burrow deeply into the existing bone, with the osteoblasts following close behind to re-line the cavity with new bone.

BONE STRUCTURE

Bone is laid down either in a haphazard manner known as *woven bone*, or in parallel sheets known as *lamellar bone*. Woven bone occurs where bone tissue is formed in its immature state, as in the early stages of fracture healing, where it acts as a temporary weld before being replaced by mature bone, or when formed in pathological states such as infection or Paget's disease.

In lamellar bone, collagen fibres are arranged parallel to each other to form multiple layers (or laminae) with the osteocytes lying between the lamellae. Unlike woven bone, which is laid down in fibrous tissue, lamellar bone forms only on existing bone surfaces.

Lamellar bone exists in two structurally different forms:

- *compact (cortical) bone*
- *cancellous (trabecular) bone*.

Compact bone

Compact bone is dense to the naked eye. It is found where support matters most: the outer walls of all bones but especially the shafts of tubular bones, and the subchondral plates supporting articular cartilage. It is made up of compact units – haversian systems or osteons – each of which consists of a central canal (the haversian canal) containing blood vessels, lymphatics and nerves and enclosed by closely packed, more or less concentric lamellae of bone. Between the lamellae lie osteocytes, bedded in lacunae which appear to be discrete but which are in fact connected by a network of fine canaliculae.

Cancellous bone

Cancellous (trabecular) bone has a honeycomb appearance; it makes up the interior meshwork of all bones and is particularly well developed in the ends of the tubular bones and the vertebral bodies. The structural units of trabecular bone are flattened sheets or spars. Three-dimensionally, the trabecular sheets are interconnected (like a honeycomb) and arranged according to the mechanical needs of the structure, the thickest and strongest along trajectories of compressive stress and the thinnest in the planes of tensile stress. The spaces between trabeculae – the 'opened-out' vascular spaces – contain the marrow and fine sinusoidal vessels that course through the tissue, nourishing both marrow and bone.

Haversian system

Bones vary greatly in size and shape. At the most basic level, however, they are similar: compact on the outside and spongy on the inside. Their outer surfaces (except at the articular ends) are covered by a tough *periosteal membrane*, the deepest layer of which consists of potentially bone-forming cells. The inner, endosteal, surfaces are irregular and lined by a fine *endosteal membrane* in close contact with the marrow spaces.

The osteonal pattern in the cortex is usually depicted from 2D histological sections. A 3D reconstruction would show that the *haversian canals* are long, branching channels running in the longitudinal axis of the bone (7.3). These connect extensively with each other and with the endosteal and periosteal surfaces by smaller channels (*Volkmann canals*). In this way the vessels in the haversian canals form a rich anastomotic network between the medullary and periosteal blood supply (7.4). Blood flow in this capillary network is normally centrifugal – from the medullary cavity, which is fed by a nutrient artery, outwards. The outermost layers of the cortex are normally also supplied by periosteal vessels; if the medullary vessels are blocked or destroyed, the periosteal circulation can take over entirely and the direction of blood flow is reversed.

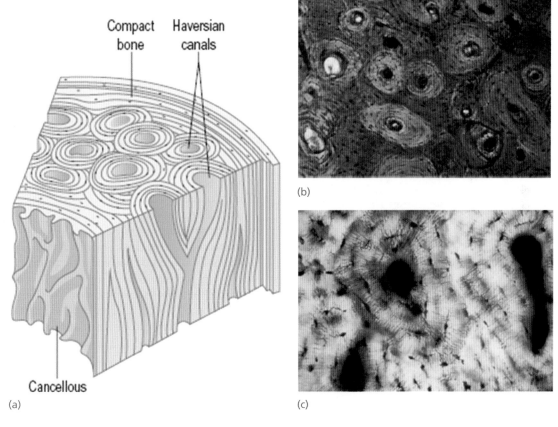

7.3 The haversian systems (a) A schematic diagram representing a wedge taken from the cortex of a long bone. It shows the basic elements of compact bone: densely packed osteons, each made up of concentric layers of bone and osteocytes around a central haversian canal which contains the blood vessels; outer laminae of sub-periosteal bone; and similar laminae on the interior surface (endosteum) merging into a lattice of cancellous bone. **(b,c)** Low- and high-power views showing the osteons in various stages of formation and resorption.

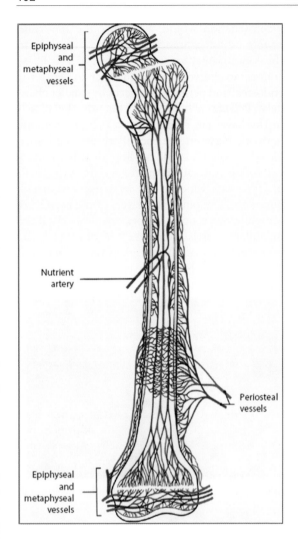

7.4 Blood supply to bone Schematic presentation of the blood supply in tubular bones. (Reproduced from Bullough P.G. *Atlas of Orthopaedic Pathology: With Clinical and Radiological Correlations*, 2nd edn. Baltimore: University Park Press, 1985. By kind permission of Dr Peter G. Bullough and Elsevier.)

BONE DEVELOPMENT AND GROWTH

Bones develop in two different ways:

- by ossification of a prior cartilage model or framework *(endochondral ossification)*
- by direct *intramembranous ossification*.

ENDOCHONDRAL OSSIFICATION

This is the usual manner in which tubular bones develop, and it is also the process involved in longitudinal growth of bones. At birth the cartilage model is complete and ossification has already begun at the centre of the diaphysis. After secondary ossification of the epiphyseal ends has begun, further growth in length takes place in the still-cartilaginous zone between the extending area of diaphyseal bone and the epiphysis. In this way the still-cartilaginous zone between the ossifying diaphysis and the epiphysis gradually narrows down but does not disappear until late adolescence. This actively growing cartilage disc is called the *physis* (growth plate), situated between the epiphysis and the diaphysis.

The growth plate consists of four distinct zones (7.5):

- Co-extensive with the epiphysis is a *zone of resting chondrocytes* in haphazard array.
- This merges into a *proliferative zone* in which the chondrocytes are lined up longitudinally; being capable of interstitial growth, they add progressively to the overall length of the bone.
- The older cells in this zone (those 'left behind' nearest the advancing new bone of the diaphysis) gradually enlarge and constitute a *hypertrophic zone*.
- Close to the interface between cartilage and bone the cartilage becomes calcified (probably with the involvement of ALP produced by the hypertrophic cells); this *zone of calcified cartilage* finally undergoes osteoclastic resorption and, with the ingrowth of new blood vessels from the metaphysis, ossification. Woven bone is laid down on the calcified scaffolding and this in turn is replaced by lamellar bone which forms the newest part of the bone shaft, now called the *metaphysis*.

It should be noted that a similar process takes place in the late stage of fracture repair.

INTRAMEMBRANOUS OSSIFICATION

With the growth in length, the bone also has to increase in circumference and, since a tubular

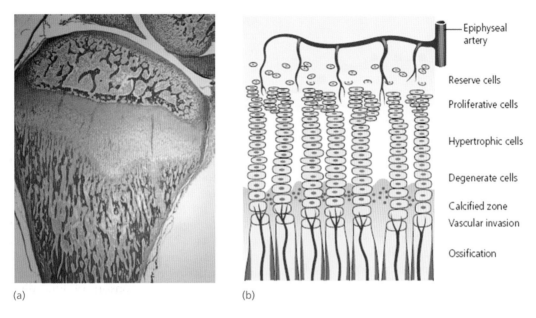

(a)   (b)

7.5 Endochondral ossification Histological section of a growing endochondral bone with a schematic figure showing the layers of the growth disc (physis). (Reproduced from Bullough P.G. *Atlas of Orthopaedic Pathology: With Clinical and Radiological Correlations*, 2nd edn. Baltimore: University Park Press, 1985. Part **(b)** by kind permission of Dr Peter G. Bullough and Elsevier.)

bone is an open cylinder, this inevitably demands that the medullary cavity increase in size proportionately. New bone is added to the outside by direct ossification at the deepest layer of the periosteum where mesenchymal cells differentiate into osteoblasts *(intramembranous, or 'appositional', bone formation)* and old bone is removed from the inside of the cylinder by osteoclastic *endosteal resorption.*

Intramembranous periosteal new bone formation also occurs as a response to periosteal stripping due to trauma, infection or tumour growth, and its appearance is a useful radiographic pointer.

BONE MODELLING

Bone modelling describes the process by which changes in the overall size and shape of bone are accomplished. Though primarily occurring during longitudinal growth, outward growth via intramembranous bone formation may continue long after the former has ceased through closure of growth plates. Whereas the outer dimension

of long bones continues to expand during the third decade as part of the process of peak bone mass achievement, at certain sites such as the femoral neck, expansion may continue lifelong. In contrast to bone modelling, which is driven by bone formation, bone resorption occurs as a secondary process intended to maintain overall shape, as in the maintenance of the flared ends of bone during longitudinal growth.

PEAK BONE MASS

Dual-energy X-ray absorptiometry (DEXA) scans are used to measure the amount of skeletal tissue by evaluation of calcium content, termed bone mass (see 'Measurement of bone mass' below). Bone mass increases during childhood, in keeping with the increase in bone size which is characterized by acceleration around puberty, followed by a less rapid gain until the cessation of linear growth. Once longitudinal growth has ceased, further skeletal consolidation continues, with peak bone mass reached in the late twenties (7.6). Peak bone mass remains stable into

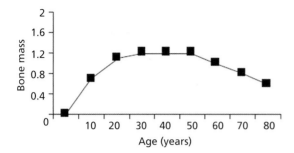

7.6 Bone mineral density over the life course
Graph showing change in bone mass in women from birth to mid-eighties.

later adulthood, until processes contributing to bone loss take effect, particularly oestrogen deficiency after the menopause in women (see Postmenopausal osteoporosis). Skeletal consolidation involves a number of factors including periosteal expansion and modelling, secondary mineralization of newly formed bone, and in-filling of haversian canals due to reduced bone remodelling after longitudinal growth has ceased.

By the end of bone growth, mean bone mass is about 5–10% greater in young men than in young women, due mainly to increased appositional bone formation when androgen levels rise after puberty. The level of peak bone mass attained is thought to be important in terms of risk of fractures and osteoporosis in later life. Of the many genetic factors that have been identified as influencing bone mineral density (BMD) and fracture risk, several of these are likely to act by influencing peak bone mass. Environmental factors are probably also important, such as physical activity and diet. Disorders affecting peak bone mass acquisition have important effects in terms of subsequent fracture risk, including anorexia nervosa, primary amenorrhea, and inflammatory paediatric disorders such as inflammatory bowel disease.

BONE MAINTENANCE

As well as contributing to bone growth and modelling, bone formation and resorption continue as a lifelong process. These two processes are carefully coordinated as part of the remodelling cycle that serves to maintain bone integrity. They are also activated during repair following injury (e.g. after a fracture).

BONE RESORPTION

Bone resorption is carried out by the *osteoclasts* under the influence of stromal cells (including *osteoblasts*) and both local and systemic activators. Though it has long been known that PTH promotes bone resorption, osteoclasts have no receptor for PTH. The hormone acts indirectly through its effect on $1,25\text{-}(OH)_2D_3$ and osteoblasts.

Before mature osteoclasts start to resorb bone, osteoblasts are thought first to 'prepare' the resorption site by removing osteoid from the bone surface while other matrix constituents act as osteoclast attractors. During resorption, each osteoclast forms a sealed attachment to the bone surface where the cell membrane folds into a characteristic ruffled border within which hydrochloric acid and proteolytic enzymes are secreted. At this low pH, minerals in the matrix are dissolved and the organic components are destroyed by lysosomal enzymes.

BONE FORMATION

Bone formation is carried out by teams of osteoblasts, which are recruited to a bone surface or haversian system and proceed to secrete osteoid, composed of type I collagen fibrils, which becomes deposited on the adjacent bone surface. Bone mineral, in the form of hydroxyapatite crystals, subsequently becomes deposited in spaces between collagen fibrils.

Whereas osteoid is rapidly mineralized following its synthesis, a process of secondary mineralization takes place after bone formation is complete.

Like bone resorption, bone formation is regulated by a combination of systemic and locally produced factors acting to promote osteoblast differentiation. Arguably the most important local factors in regulating osteoblast differentiation are the bone morphogenetic proteins

(BMPs) and the Wnt signalling system, both of which comprise complex systems of multiple ligands, cell surface receptors, intracellular signalling pathways and endogenous inhibitors.

BONE REMODELLING

Osteoblast and osteoclast activity are coordinated during bone remodelling, which describes a process by which previously formed bone is removed and then replaced in a specific sequence comprising the bone remodelling cycle. This process, which determines the internal architecture of bone, occurs not only during growth but throughout life. Bone remodelling serves several crucial purposes:

- 'Old bone' is continually replaced by 'new bone' and in this way the skeleton is protected from the excess accumulation of fatigue damage and the risk of stress failure.
- Bone turnover is sensitive to the demands of function, and trabeculae are fashioned in accordance with the stresses imposed upon the bone.

At each *remodelling site*, work proceeds in an orderly sequence.

SEQUENCE OF BONE REMODELLING

1 Prompted by the osteoblasts, osteoclasts gather on a free bone surface and proceed to excavate a cavity.
2 After 2–4 weeks, resorption ceases; the osteoclasts undergo apoptosis and are phagocytosed.
3 There is a short quiescent period, then the excavated surface is covered with osteoblasts and for the next 3 months osteoid is laid down and mineralized to leave a new 'packet' of bone (or *osteon*).

The entire *remodelling cycle* takes 4–6 months and at the end the boundary between 'old' and 'new' bone is marked by a histologically identifiable 'cement line'.

The annual rate of bone turnover in healthy adults has been estimated as 4% for cortical bone and 25% for trabecular bone. During the first half of life, formation slightly exceeds resorption and bone mass increases; in later years, resorption exceeds formation and bone mass steadily diminishes.

MINERAL EXCHANGE

Calcium and phosphorus have an essential role in a wide range of physiological processes. More than 98% of the body's calcium and 85% of its phosphorus are tightly packed as hydroxyapatite crystals in bone and capable of only very slow exchange. A small amount exists in a rapidly exchangeable form, either in partially formed crystals or in the extracellular fluid and blood.

A number of essential metabolic processes require extracellular calcium levels to be maintained within a very narrow range, which is achieved through the action of PTH. Transient alterations in blood levels are rapidly compensated for by changes in renal tubular absorption. A more persistent fall in extracellular calcium concentration can be accommodated by increasing bone resorption.

Calcium

Calcium is essential for normal cell function and physiological processes such as blood coagulation, nerve conduction and muscle contraction. An uncompensated fall in extracellular calcium concentration (hypocalcaemia) may cause tetany; an excessive rise (hypercalcaemia) can lead to depressed neuromuscular transmission.

The main sources of calcium are dairy products, green vegetables and soya. Absorption is inhibited by excessive intake of phosphates (common in soft drinks), oxalates (found in tea and coffee), phytates (chapati flour) and fats, by the administration of certain drugs (including corticosteroids) and in malabsorption disorders of the bowel.

If the plasma ionized calcium concentration falls, PTH is released and causes:

- increased renal tubular reabsorption of calcium and reduced renal tubular reabsorption of phosphate

- a switch to increased 1,25-(OH)$_2$ vitamin D production and enhanced intestinal calcium absorption.

If the calcium concentration remains low, calcium is drawn from the skeleton by increased bone resorption through the influence of PTH.

Phosphorus

Apart from its role in the composition of hydroxyapatite crystals in bone, phosphorus is needed for energy transport and intracellular cell signalling. It is abundantly available in the diet and is absorbed in the small intestine, more or less in proportion to the amount ingested; however, absorption is reduced in the presence of antacids such as aluminium hydroxide, which binds phosphorus in the gut. Phosphate excretion is extremely efficient, but 90% is reabsorbed in the proximal tubules.

The solubility product of calcium and phosphate is held at a fairly constant level; any increase in one will cause the other to fall. If Pi rises abnormally, a reciprocal fall in calcium concentration will stimulate PTH secretion, which in turn will suppress urinary tubular reabsorption of Pi, resulting in increased Pi excretion and a fall in plasma Pi. High Pi levels also result in diminished 1,25-(OH)$_2$D production, causing reduced intestinal absorption of phosphorus.

Vitamin D

Vitamin D, through its active metabolites, is principally concerned with calcium absorption and transport and (acting together with PTH) bone remodelling. Target organs are the small intestine and bone.

Vitamin D itself is inactive. Conversion to active metabolites takes place first in the liver by 25-hydroxylation to form 25-hydroxycholecalciferol [25-OHD], and then in the kidneys by further hydroxylation to 1,25-dihydroxycholecalciferol [1,25-(OH)$_2$D] (calcitriol) (7.7).

PTH

PTH is the major regulator of extracellular calcium concentration, acting on the renal tubules, the renal parenchyma, the intestine and bone (Table 7.1).

OTHER INFLUENCES ON BONE METABOLISM

Gonadal hormones

Sex steroids have a major role in the attainment of peak bone mass as a consequence of their role in puberty, which is associated with not only rapid growth but also a rapid gain in bone mass.

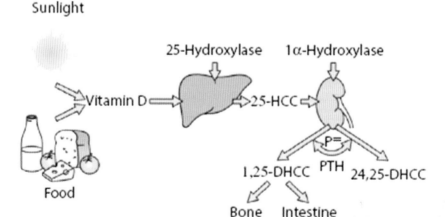

7.7 Vitamin D metabolism The active vitamin D metabolites are derived either from the diet or by conversion of precursors when the skin is exposed to sunlight. The inactive 'vitamin' is hydroxylated, first in the liver and then in the kidney, to form the active metabolites 25-HCC and 1,25-DHCC.

Table 7.1 Role of PTH

Site of action	Action of PTH
Renal tubules	Increases phosphate excretion by restricting its reabsorption Conserves calcium by increasing its reabsorption
Kidney parenchyma	Controls hydroxylation of the vitamin D metabolite 25-OHD: • a rise in PTH concentration stimulates conversion to the active metabolite 1,25-$(OH)_2$D • a fall causes a switch towards the inactive metabolite 24,25-$(OH)_2$D
Intestine	Has the indirect effect of stimulating calcium absorption by promoting the conversion of 25-OHD to 1,25-$(OH)_2$D in the kidney
Bones	Acts to promote osteoclastic resorption Increases the release of calcium and phosphate into the blood

Sex steroids are also important for maintaining bone mass subsequently, with loss of sex steroids in later life leading to significant bone loss.

Oestrogen This acts to suppress longitudinal growth and periosteal expansion, and its rise around puberty contributes to growth plate closure. The major impact of oestrogen deficiency on the skeleton in cases of primary amenorrhoea is a reduction in bone mineral density. Oestrogen also acts to preserve bone mass, with its loss at the menopause leading to an increase in bone turnover, a decline in bone mineral density, a deterioration in bone architecture and a consequential increase in fracture risk.

Androgens These stimulate bone growth, and act to maintain bone mass, through a combination of suppression of bone resorption and stimulation of bone formation.

Other hormones

Glucocorticoid Excess glucocorticoid in Cushing's disease is associated with adverse effects on bone metabolism characterized by suppressed bone formation, leading to a decrease in BMD and increased risk of osteoporosis.

Thyroxine Excess thyroxine in thyrotoxicosis, or over-replacement with thyroxine in hypothyroidism, is associated with increased bone turnover and is a recognized risk factor for low BMD and osteoporosis.

Growth hormone (GH) GH is thought to influence bone remodelling, as well as playing an important role in skeletal growth.

Calcitonin Produced by C cells of the thyroid, calcitonin acts to reduce osteoclast activity.

Mechanical stress

One of the primary roles of the skeleton is to provide an endoskeleton, transmitting forces applied by muscles acting as external levers for the purposes of locomotion and other activities. The skeleton is designed to withstand different types of forces such as compression, tension, shear and torsion. However, at any one site, a specific type of force tends to predominate; for example, compression is the predominant force acting on lumbar vertebrae while tensile forces predominate at the superior surface of the femoral neck. The direction and thickness of trabeculae in cancellous bone are related to regional stress trajectories. This is recognized in Wolff's law (1896), which states that the architecture and mass of the skeleton are adjusted to withstand the prevailing forces imposed by functional need or deformity (7.8). This has led to the concept of the mechanostat, whereby bone remodelling and bone mass are regulated to ensure that bone strain (defined as deformation in response to an externally applied load per unit length) is kept within a target range.

METABOLIC BONE DISORDERS

ASSESSMENT

Patients with metabolic bone disorders usually present to the orthopaedic surgeon in one of several guises.

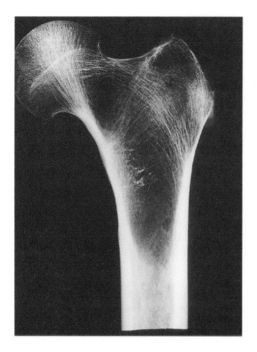

7.8 Wolff's law Wolff's law is beautifully demonstrated in the trabecular pattern at the upper end of the femur. The thickest trabeculae are arranged along the trajectories of greatest stress.

MOST COMMON PRESENTATION OF METABOLIC BONE DISORDERS

Child with bone deformities (*rickets*)

Elderly person with a fracture of the femoral neck or a vertebral body following comparatively minor trauma (*postmenopausal osteoporosis*)

Elderly patient with bone pain and multiple compression fractures of the spine (*osteomalacia*)

Middle-aged person with hypercalcaemia and pseudogout (*hyperparathyroidism*)

Person with multiple fractures and a history of prolonged *corticosteroid treatment*

X-rays may show:

- *stress fractures*
- *vertebral fractures*
- *cortical thinning*
- *loss of trabecular structure*

- an ill-defined loss of radiographic density – *radiographic osteopenia* – which can signify either osteomalacia or osteoporosis.

History

Children are likely to be brought for examination because of failure to thrive, below-normal growth or deformity of the lower limbs. Adults may complain of back pain, the sudden onset of bone pain near one of the large joints or symptoms suggesting a full-blown fracture following some comparatively modest injury. Generalized muscle weakness is common in osteomalacia.

Details such as the patient's sex, age, race, onset of menopause, nutritional background, level of physical activity, previous illnesses, medication and operations are important. The onset and duration of symptoms and their relationship to previous disease or trauma should be carefully considered, especially in older people who may have suffered insufficiency fractures. Other causal associations are retarded growth, malnutrition, dietary fads, intestinal malabsorption, alcohol abuse and cigarette smoking.

Examination

The patient's appearance may be suggestive of an endocrine or metabolic disorder.

APPEARANCE SUGGESTIVE OF ENDOCRINE/ METABOLIC DISORDER

Moon face and Cushingoid build (*hypercortisonism*)

Smooth, hairless skin (*testicular atrophy*)

Physical underdevelopment and bone deformities (*rickets*)

Thoracic kyphosis (a non-specific feature of *vertebral osteoporosis*)

X-rays

Decreased skeletal radiodensity is a late and unreliable sign of bone loss; it becomes apparent only after a 30% reduction in mineral or skeletal mass and, even then, one cannot tell whether this is due to *osteoporosis* (a decrease in bone mass) or *osteomalacia* (insufficient mineralization of bone) or a combination of both.

A more reliable sign of osteoporosis is the presence of fractures – new and old – especially in the spine, ribs, pubic rami or corticocancellous junctions of the long bones.

In addition to these general signs of reduced bone mass or defective mineralization, there may be specific features of bone disorders such as rickets, hyperparathyroidism, metastatic bone disease or myelomatosis.

Measurement of bone mass

The gold standard investigation for measurement of bone mass is the DEXA scan. Additional techniques are available but are reserved for research purposes. These research tools include peripheral quantitative computer tomography (pQCT) and calcaneal ultrasound (US).

DEXA

This is now the method of choice. Precision and accuracy are excellent, radiation exposure is not excessive and it is low-cost. Measurements are usually taken from the lumbar spine and hip. Bone mass values from DEXA scans are 2D estimates of bone density presented as the number of standard deviations below the young adult mean (T score) and the number of standard deviations below the age-matched mean (Z score) (**7.9**).

WORLD HEALTH ORGANIZATION DEFINITIONS OF BONE MASS	
Osteoporosis	T score below –2.5
Osteopenia	T score between –1.0 and –2.5
Normal bone mass	T score above –1.0

QUANTITATIVE COMPUTED TOMOGRAPHY

Quantitative computed tomography (QCT) permits measurement of mineral content per unit volume of bone, which is a true 3D measurement of bone density. It also provides separate values for cortical and cancellous bone.

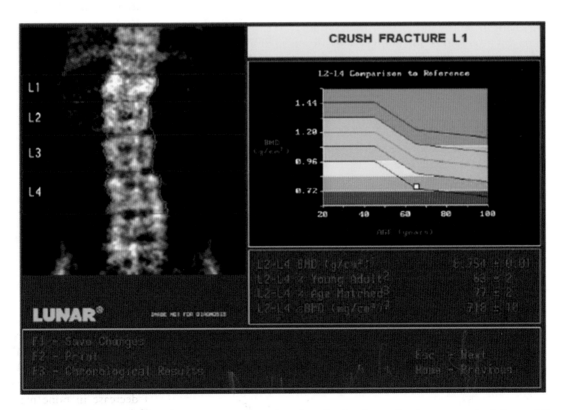

7.9 DEXA output The output from a DEXA scan showing the lumbar spine image on the left, and the measured BMD compared to the reference range on the right.

Indications for bone densitometry

> **MAIN INDICATIONS FOR BONE DENSITOMETRY**
>
> Adults over the age of 50 who have experienced a low trauma fracture
>
> All women over the age of 65 and all men over the age of 75 to assess risk of future fracture
>
> To assess the degree and progress of bone loss in patients with clinically diagnosed metabolic bone disease or conditions such as hyperparathyroidism, corticosteroid-induced osteoporosis, gonadal deficiency or other endocrine disorders
>
> To monitor the effect of treatment for osteoporosis
>
> Patients on medications known to adversely affect bone health (e.g. corticosteroids, aromatase inhibitors)

Biochemical tests

- *Serum calcium and phosphate concentrations* should be measured in the fasting state, and it is the ionized calcium fraction that is important.
- *Serum bone ALP* concentration is an index of osteoblastic activity; it is raised in osteomalacia and in disorders associated with high bone turnover (hyperparathyroidism, Paget's disease, bone metastases).
- *PTH activity* can be estimated from serum assays of the carboxylic acid (COOH) terminal fragment. However, in renal failure, the test is unreliable because there is reduced clearance of the COOH fragment.
- *Vitamin D activity* is assessed by measuring the serum 25-OHD concentration. Serum $1,25\text{-}(OH)_2D$ levels do not necessarily reflect vitamin uptake but are reduced in advanced renal disease.
- *Urinary calcium and phosphate* excretion can be measured. Significant alterations are found in malabsorption disorders, hyperparathyroidism and other conditions associated with hypercalcaemia.

- *Bone turnover markers* can be measured if identification of high or low bone turnover states will be useful. The most common markers are the bone formation marker, serum type I collagen extension propeptide (P1NP), and the bone resorption marker, serum C-terminal cross-linking telopeptide of type I collagen (CTX).

> ⚠ *Laboratory reports* should always state the normal range for each test, which may be different for infants, children and adults.

Bone biopsy

Standardized bone samples are obtained from the iliac crest and can be examined (without prior decalcification) for histological bone volume, osteoid formation and the relative distribution of formation and resorption surfaces (**7.10**). The rate of bone remodelling can also be gauged by labelling the bone with tetracycline on two occasions (2 weeks apart) before obtaining the biopsy. Tetracycline is taken up in new bone and produces a fluorescent strip on ultraviolet light microscopy. By measuring the distance between the two labels, the rate of new bone formation can be calculated. Characteristically in osteomalacia there is a decrease in the rate of bone turnover and an increase in the amount of uncalcified osteoid.

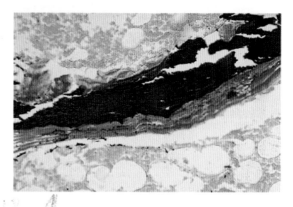

7.10 Bone biopsy Von Kossa stain showing the unusually wide osteoid layer (in red) in a patient with osteomalacia.

OSTEOPOROSIS

Osteoporosis as a clinical disorder is character-ized by an abnormally low bone mass and defects in bone structure, a combination which renders the bone unusually fragile and at greater than normal risk of fracture in a person of that age, sex and race. Although the cancellous regions are more porous and the cortices thinner than nor-mal, the existing bone is fully mineralized (**7.11**).

Bone depletion may be brought about by pre-dominant bone resorption, decreased bone for-mation or a combination of the two.

- *From the onset of the menopause and for the next 10 years* the rate of bone loss in women accelerates to about 3% per year, occurring predominantly in trabecular bone. This steady depletion is due mainly to excessive resorption – osteoclastic activity seeming to be released from the restraining influence

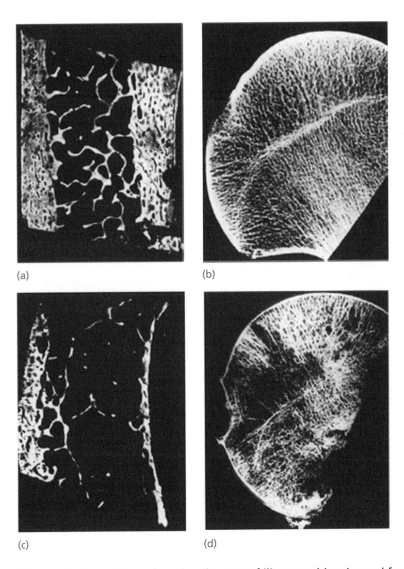

(a)

(b)

(c)

(d)

7.11 Age-related changes in bone These fine-detail X-rays of iliac crest biopsies and femoral head slices show the marked contrast between trabecular density in a healthy 40-year-old woman (**a,b**) and one of 75 years (**c,d**).

of gonadal hormone. About 30% of white women will lose bone to the extent of developing postmenopausal osteoporosis.

- *From the age of 65–70 years* the rate of bone loss in women gradually tails off and by the age of 75 years it is about 0.5% per year. This later phase of depletion is due mainly to diminishing osteoblastic activity.

Men are affected in a similar manner, but the phase of rapid bone loss occurs 15–20 years later than in women.

Bone mass and bone strength

It is important to recognize that throughout life, and regardless of whether *bone mass* increases or decreases, the degree of *mineralization* in normal people varies very little from age to age or from one person to another.

With advancing years, the loss of bone mass is accompanied by a *disproportionate loss of bone strength*, which is explained in a number of ways.

- The absolute diminution in bone mass is the most important factor.
- With increased postmenopausal bone resorption, perforations and gaps appear in the plates and cross-spars of trabecular bone.
- In old age, the decrease in bone cell activity makes for a slower remodelling rate.

This tendency to increased bone fragility with age is counteracted to some extent in tubular bones by the fact that they actually increase in diameter as their cortices become thinner. During each remodelling cycle, resorption exceeds formation on the endosteal surface while formation slightly exceeds resorption on the periosteal surface. Simple mechanics can show that, of two cylinders with equal mass, the one with a greater diameter and thin walls is stronger than one with thicker walls but lesser diameter. Nonetheless, the age-related decrease in bone mass leads to a clear increase in fracture risk with increasing age (**7.12**).

The boundary between 'normal' age-related bone loss and a clinical disorder (*osteoporosis*) is poorly defined. Factors that have an adverse influence on bone mass are shown in the box. Ageing individuals also often have some degree

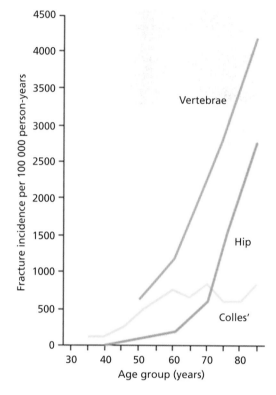

7.12 Fracture incidence The incidence of fractures of the vertebrae, hip and wrist rises progressively after the menopause.

of *osteomalacia* due to lack of dietary vitamin D and poor exposure to sunlight. This, added to the normal age-related bone depletion, makes them more vulnerable than usual to insufficiency fractures.

RISK FACTORS FOR OSTEOPOROSIS

Age
Female
Previous fragility fracture
Current use or frequent recent use of oral or systemic glucocorticoids
Family history of hip fracture
Low body mass index (BMI) (less than 18.5 kg/m²)
Smoking
Alcohol intake of more than 14 units per week for women and more than 21 units per week for men

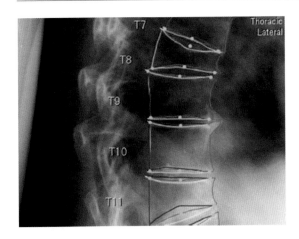

7.13 Vertebral fractures and their grading A lateral spinal image showing the quantitative morphometry method of grading of osteoporotic vertebral fractures by utilising six points on each vertebral body. There is a severe fracture at T8 and a moderate fracture at T11.

X-rays

Osteoporosis cannot be diagnosed from plain radiographs. 'Radiological osteopenia' is a term sometimes used to describe bone which appears to be less 'dense' than normal on X-ray. Typical signs of radiological osteopenia are loss of trabecular definition, thinning of the cortices and insufficiency fractures. Compression fractures of the vertebral bodies, sometimes described as wedging or compression of the vertebral end plates, are typical of severe postmenopausal osteoporosis (7.13).

Assessment of fracture risk

Increasingly, physicians are moving away from simple identification and treatment of low bone density from DEXA scans to individualized assessment of fracture risk. This is because bone density is only one risk factor for fracture. There are now many tools available to calculate a patient's probability of fracture over the next few years based on a combination of clinical risk factors plus bone density. Examples of these tools include FRAX (www.shef.ac.uk/frax/) and QFracture (www.Qfracture.org).

POSTMENOPAUSAL OSTEOPOROSIS

Postmenopausal osteoporosis is an exaggerated form of the physiological bone depletion that normally accompanies ageing and loss of gonadal activity. Around the menopause, and for the next 10 years, bone loss normally accelerates to about 3% per year compared with 0.3% during the preceding two decades. This is due mainly to increased bone resorption, the withdrawal of oestrogen having removed one of the normal restraints on osteoclastic activity. Genetic influences play an important part in determining when and how this process becomes exaggerated, but a number of other risk factors have been identified (see risk factors box on previous page).

Clinical features and investigations

Osteoporosis is asymptomatic unless fractures occur. The fractures are classically low trauma defined as a fall from standing height or less. Fracture of the distal radius (Colles' fracture) is usually the first fracture to occur, followed by vertebrae and hip unless treatment is initiated. Osteoporotic vertebral fractures are particularly difficult to diagnose as they may be clinically silent. Less than a third of vertebral fractures are diagnosed. In severe cases, significant height loss (often exceeding 4 cm) and thoracic kyphosis can occur due to multiple vertebral fractures (7.14).

ADVICE TO WOMEN FOR MAINTENANCE OF HEALTHY BONES

Eat a diet rich in calcium and vitamin D.
Do weight-bearing physical activity.
Avoid smoking.
Avoid excessive consumption of alcohol.
If necessary, take calcium and vitamin D supplements to ensure the recommended daily requirements are met. These measures have been shown to reduce the risk of low-energy fractures in elderly women.

Prevention

Adults over the age of 50 who have a low-energy fracture should have their fracture risk assessed by one of the clinical tools such as FRAX as well as bone density assessment by DEXA. Those above the local treatment thresholds should be offered medications to reduce their fracture risk. All women should be advised on lifestyle choices to maintain healthy bones.

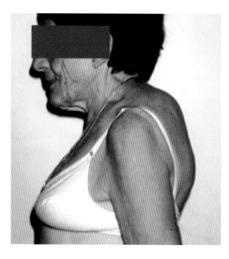

7.14 Dowager's hump Kyphotic deformity of the thoracic spine in a patient with osteoporosis.

Treatment

REDUCTION OF FRACTURE RISK

The current goal of treatment is to reduce risk of future fracture. There is also increasing interest in a 'treat to target' approach, but this is not yet widespread. Medications are now recommended for a period of time, typically 3–5 years, at which point the need for ongoing treatment should be reconsidered by further assessment of fracture risk.

Bisphosphonates   Taken orally, these are now regarded as the first-line medication for reduction of fracture risk in postmenopausal women, although intravenous (IV) formulations are also available. They act by reducing osteoclastic bone resorption and the general rate of bone turnover. They have been shown to prevent bone loss and to reduce the risk of vertebral and hip fractures. Gastrointestinal side effects are the most common adverse event with oral preparations. Rarer, more serious adverse events mainly associated with the IV preparations include atypical femoral fractures and osteonecrosis of the jaw (ONJ).

Denosumab   This is an antibody to RANKL, essential for promoting osteoclastogenesis. Uniquely, it has quite a rapid 'off-set' on stopping the medication, with rapid reversal of bone turnover. Potential adverse events also include atypical femoral fractures and ONJ.

PTH   Preotact and Teriparatide are anabolic agents, given intermittently at low doses, which stimulate bone formation to a greater and earlier extent than bone resorption.

Selective oestrogen receptor modulators (SERMs)   Raloxifene is licensed for fracture risk reduction in women and has been shown to reduce the risk of vertebral fractures. The main side effect is hot flushes, but use can also increase the risk of venous thromboembolism.

Strontium ranelate   This is thought to increase bone formation and reduce bone resorption *in vitro*. Clinical trials show a reduction in the risk of vertebral fractures and non-vertebral fractures.

The use of strontium is limited by the following contraindications:

- current or previous venous thromboembolism
- ischaemic heart disease
- peripheral arterial disease
- cerebrovascular disease.

MANAGEMENT OF FRACTURES

Femoral neck and other long-bone fractures may need operative treatment.

Vertebral fractures can be painful and patients will need analgesic treatment. Physiotherapy should initially be aimed at maintaining muscle tone; if pain is adequately controlled, patients should be encouraged to walk and, when symptoms allow, they can be introduced to postural training. Spinal orthoses may be needed for support and pain relief, but they cannot be expected to correct any structural deformity. Vertebral augmentation such as kyphoplasty or vertebroplasty are occasionally called for to treat extremely painful vertebral fractures that have caused symptoms for more than 6–8 weeks.

OSTEOPOROSIS IN MEN

With the gradual depletion in androgenic hormones, men eventually suffer the same bone changes as postmenopausal women, only this occurs about 15 years later unless there is some specific cause for testicular failure.

 Osteoporotic fractures in men under 60 years of age should arouse the suspicion of some underlying disorder – notably hypogonadism, metastatic bone disease, multiple myeloma, liver disease, renal hypercalciuria, alcohol abuse, malabsorption disorder, malnutrition, glucocorticoid medication or anti-gonadal hormone treatment for prostate cancer.

SECONDARY OSTEOPOROSIS

Secondary osteoporosis can be caused by a number of different conditions.

SECONDARY CAUSES OF OSTEOPOROSIS

Endocrine

- Hypogonadism in either sex including untreated premature menopause, treatment with aromatase inhibitors or androgen deprivation therapy
- Hyperthyroidism
- Hyperparathyroidism
- Hyperprolactinaemia
- Cushing's disease
- Diabetes

Respiratory

- Cystic fibrosis
- Smoking-related lung disease

Metabolic

- Homocystinuria

Chronic renal disease
Gastrointestinal

- Coeliac disease
- Inflammatory bowel disease
- Chronic liver disease
- Chronic pancreatitis
- Other causes of malabsorption

Rheumatological

- Rheumatoid arthritis
- Other inflammatory arthropathies

Haematological

- Multiple myeloma
- Haemoglobinopathies
- Systemic mastocytosis

Immobility

- Neurological injury
- Neurological disease

(Based on NICE (2012) CG146: *Osteoporosis: Assessing the risk of fragility fracture.*)

Glucocorticoid-induced osteoporosis

Glucocorticoid overload occurs in endogenous Cushing's disease or after prolonged treatment with corticosteroids. This often results in severe osteoporosis, especially if the condition for which the drug is administered is itself associated with bone loss (e.g. rheumatoid arthritis).

Glucocorticoids have a complex mode of action. The deleterious effect on bone is mainly by suppression of osteoblast function, but it also causes reduced calcium absorption, increased calcium excretion and stimulation of PTH secretion.

Gonadal hormone insufficiency

Oestrogen lack is an important factor in postmenopausal osteoporosis. It also accounts for osteoporosis in younger women who have undergone oophorectomy, and in pubertal girls with ovarian agenesis and primary amenorrhoea

SECTION 1 GENERAL ORTHOPAEDICS

(Turner's syndrome). Treatment is the same as for postmenopausal osteoporosis.

A decline in testicular function probably contributes to the continuing bone loss and rising fracture rate in men over 70 years of age. A more obvious relationship is found in young men with overt hypogonadism; this may require long-term treatment with testosterone.

Hyperthyroidism

Thyroxine speeds up the rate of bone turnover, but resorption exceeds formation. Osteoporosis is quite common in untreated hyperthyroidism, but fractures usually occur only in older people who suffer the cumulative effects of the menopause and thyroid overload. In the worst cases osteoporosis may be severe with spontaneous fractures, a marked rise in serum ALP, hypercalcaemia and hypercalciuria.

Multiple myeloma and carcinomatosis

Generalized osteoporosis, anaemia and a high ESR are characteristic features of myelomatosis and metastatic bone disease. Bone loss is due to overproduction of local osteoclast-activating factors. Treatment with bisphosphonates may reduce the risk of fracture.

Alcohol excess

This is a common and often neglected cause of osteoporosis at all ages, with the added factor of an increased tendency to falls and other injuries. Bone changes are due to a combination of decreased calcium absorption, liver failure and a toxic effect on osteoblast function. Alcohol also has a mild glucocorticoid effect.

Immobilization

The worst effects of stress reduction are seen in states of weightlessness; bone resorption, unbalanced by formation, leads to hypercalcaemia, hypercalciuria and severe osteoporosis. Lesser degrees of osteoporosis are seen in bedridden patients, and regional osteoporosis is common after immobilization of a limb. The effects can be mitigated by encouraging mobility, exercise and weight-bearing.

Diabetes

People with type 1 diabetes have a reduced bone mass and increased risk of fragility fractures compared to people without diabetes. However, despite having normal or above-normal bone density, people with type 2 diabetes are susceptible to low-trauma fractures, even after adjusting for age, physical activity and body weight. 'Diabetic bone disease' is a term being used to describe the bone health of people with type 2 diabetes, and it is thought to be related to poor bone quality, perhaps due to the influence of hyperglycaemia, diabetic complications or other lifestyle factors.

HYPOCALCAEMIA

Regulatory pathways described above, particularly PTH, are generally very effective at maintaining normocalcaemia, which is required for a number of essential cellular processes. Symptomatic hypocalcaemia is therefore rare, but when it is present it needs to be treated promptly. Causes of hypocalcaemia are listed in the box. The most important are hypoparathyroidism, severe vitamin D deficiency and chronic kidney disease.

CAUSES OF HYPOCALCAEMIA

Vitamin D deficiency

- *Acquired:* dietary deficiency, malabsorption
- *Congenital:* 1 alpha-hydroxylase mutation, vitamin D receptor mutation

Chronic renal failure
Hypoparathyroidism

- *Congenital:* DiGeorge syndrome, calciumsensing receptor (activating) mutations, pseudohypoparathyroidism
- *Acquired:* autoimmune, post-parathyroidectomy

> Hypomagnesaemia
> Pancreatitis
> Hyperphosphataemia
> Drug-induced (denosumab, zoledronate, cinacalcet)

HYPOPARATHYROIDISM

This is an important cause of hypocalcaemia immediately following parathyroidectomy, during which calcium levels need to be carefully monitored. Rarely, hypoparathyroidism can develop as part of an autoimmune disease, due to iron overload resulting from haemochromatosis, or due to magnesium deficiency which interferes with PTH release. Congenital hypoparathyroidism may result from failure to develop parathyroid glands (DiGeorge syndrome), and from rare genetic disorders associated with activating mutations of the calcium-sensing receptor.

Diagnosis of hypoparathyroidism is supported by finding of a low serum calcium and elevated serum phosphate and low or absent PTH. In cases of activating mutations of the calcium-sensing receptor, PTH levels may be close to the normal range, but they are nonetheless inappropriately low given the low calcium level.

Clinical features

Mild hypocalcaemia itself is often asymptomatic. Occasionally, severe hypocalcaemia develops acutely and can potentially be fatal. Typical features include tetany, numbness/paraesthesias and muscle spasms. More severe features include convulsions, cardiac arrhythmias and laryngeal spasm. Typical signs are the Trousseau sign (tetany caused by inflating a blood-pressure cuff), Chvostek's sign (facial spasms caused by tapping over the facial nerve), and prolongation of the QT interval on ECG.

Treatment

 Acute hypocalcaemia is a medical emergency and needs to be treated promptly with IV calcium, usually in the form of calcium gluconate.

Chronic hypocalcaemia is often managed with vitamin D metabolites such as calcitriol, however caution needs to be used as calcitriol treatment can lead to significant hypercalciuria, especially in hypoparathyroidism. This increases the risk of renal complications such as nephrocalcinosis and nephrolithiasis. In patients with chronic hypoparathyroidism, replacement treatment with teriparatide may be helpful. In cases of activating mutations of the calcium-sensing receptor, newly developed inhibitors may play a role in future.

RICKETS AND OSTEOMALACIA

Rickets and osteomalacia are different expressions of the same disease: inadequate mineralization of bone in children is called rickets; in adults, it is known as osteomalacia. They are distinct from osteoporosis (**Table 7.2**).

Osteoid throughout the skeleton is incompletely calcified, and the bone is therefore 'softened' (*osteomalacia*). This leads to an increase in bone fragility and fracture risk. In children, the growth plate is also disrupted and, in combination with softening of bone, leads to characteristic deformities (*rickets*).

Reduced serum 1,25-OHD is by far the most common cause of rickets/osteomalacia, usually due to a lack of 25-OHD substrate, resulting from a combination of nutritional deficiency and lack of sunlight exposure. Several risk factors are

Table 7.2 Osteomalacia and osteoporosis compared

	Osteomalacia	Osteoporosis
Similarities	Common in ageing women Prone to pathological fracture Decreased bone density	
Individual	Unwell	Well
Pain	Generalized chronic ache	Pain only after fracture
Muscles	Weak	Normal
Looser's zones	YES	NO
ALP	Increased	Normal
Serum phosphorus	Decreased	Normal
Ca × P	<2.4 mmol/L	>2.4 mmol/L

recognized including childhood and pregnancy when vitamin D requirements are higher, strict veganism, dress codes which limit sun exposure, and nursing-home residence where poor diet is compounded by reduced sunlight exposure. Other causes include intestinal malabsorption of which coeliac disease is the most common, and defective vitamin D activation; decreased 25-hydroxylation is seen in liver disease and treatment with anticonvulsants; reduced 1α-hydroxylation is present in renal disease, nephrectomy and genetic 1α-hydroxylase deficiency.

In contrast, *vitamin D-resistant rickets/osteomalacia* is caused by phosphate deficiency and has distinct clinical features (see Clinical features).

Pathology

Rickets is associated with the inability to calcify the intercellular matrix in the growth plate, causing chondrocytes to pile up irregularly, increase in the width of the growth plate, poor mineralization of the zone of calcification and sparse bone formation in the zone of ossification. The new trabeculae are thin and weak, and the metaphysis becomes broad and cupshaped. *Osteomalacia* is characterized by widened osteoid seams and thinner cortices.

Clinical features

IN CHILDREN

The infant with *rickets* may present with tetany or convulsions due to hypocalcaemia. Later the parents may notice that there is a failure to thrive, listlessness and muscular flaccidity. Early bone changes are deformity of the skull (craniotabes) and thickening of the knees, ankles and wrists from growth plate overgrowth. Enlargement of the costochondral junctions ('rickety rosary') and lateral indentation of the chest (Harrison's sulcus) may also be present. Lower limb deformities such as coxa vara and bowing of the femora and tibiae may develop after weight-bearing, while overall growth may be stunted (**7.15**).

IN ADULTS

Osteomalacia may have an insidious course and patients may complain of relatively non-specific symptoms such as widespread bone pain and

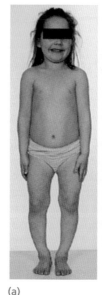
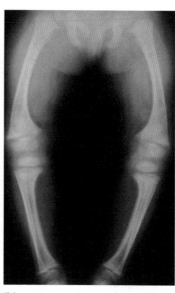

(a)   (b)

7.15 Rickets Nutritional rickets is now uncommon in countries with advanced health systems. **(a)** This 5-year-old girl, after investigation, was found to have familial hypophosphataemic rickets. In addition to the obvious varus deformities on her legs, her lower limbs are disproportionately short compared to her upper body. **(b)** X-ray of another child with classical nutritional rickets, showing the well-marked physes, the flared metaphyses and the bowing deformities of the lower limb bones.

muscle weakness. Unexplained pain in the hip or one of the long bones may presage a stress fracture. *Osteomalacia* increases the risk of fractures throughout the skeleton. When present, muscle weakness is of a proximal distribution, causing a 'waddling' gait.

X-rays

CHILDREN

In active *rickets* there is thickening and widening of the growth plate, cupping of the metaphysis and, sometimes, bowing of the diaphysis (**7.16–7.18**). The metaphysis may remain abnormally wide even after healing has occurred. If the serum calcium remains persistently low, there may be signs of *secondary hyperparathyroidism*: subperiosteal erosions are at the sites of maximal remodelling such

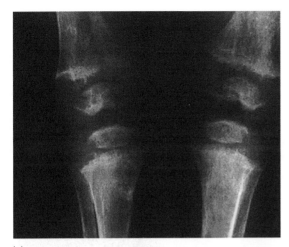

(a)

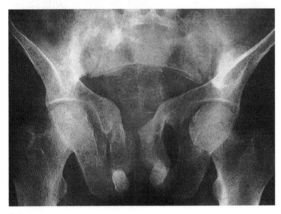

(b)

7.16 Rickets X-rays obtained at two points during growth in a child with nutritional rickets. The typical features such as widening of the physis and flaring of the metaphysis are well marked **(a)**. After treatment, the bones have begun to heal but the bone deformities are still noticeable **(b)**.

as the radial aspects of the proximal and middle phalanges of the middle and index fingers, medial borders of the proximal humerus, femoral neck, distal femur and proximal tibia.

ADULTS

The classic lesion of *osteomalacia* is the Looser's zone, a thin transverse band of rarefaction in an otherwise normal-looking bone (**7.19**). These zones, seen especially in the pubic rami, medial proximal femur and axillary edge of the scapula, are due to incomplete stress fractures which heal with callus lacking in calcium. Vertebral fractures may show either a characteristic biconcave appearance or wedge-shaped deformities indistinguishable from osteoporotic fractures. There may also be signs of *secondary hyperparathyroidism*.

Biochemistry

Overt hypocalcaemia is relatively uncommon in adults presenting with osteomalacia. More commonly, serum calcium is maintained at the lower part of the normal range as a result of secondary hyperparathyroidism, the latter causing raised levels of PTH and ALP (ALP may increase further following a fracture, or during bone healing after initiation of vitamin D replacement), and reduced serum phosphate. Low vitamin D status is indicated by a very low 25-OHD level (typically <10 nmol/L).

Treatment

In high-risk populations, osteomalacia is generally preventable by dietary modification or use of vitamin D supplements.

HYPOPHOSPHATAEMIC RICKETS AND OSTEOMALACIA

Rarely, osteomalacia occurs secondary to renal phosphate wasting as a consequence of impaired renal tubular reabsorption of phosphate.

FAMILIAL HYPOPHOSPHATAEMIC RICKETS

This is the commonest heritable phosphate wasting genetic disorder. It is an X-linked genetic disorder with dominant inheritance. The condition starts in infancy or soon after and causes bony deformity of the lower limbs if it is not recognized and treated (**7.20**). During infancy, the children look normal but deformities of the lower limbs such as genu valgum or varum develop when they begin to walk and growth is below normal. There is no myopathy.

During adulthood, there is a tendency to develop heterotopic bone formation around some

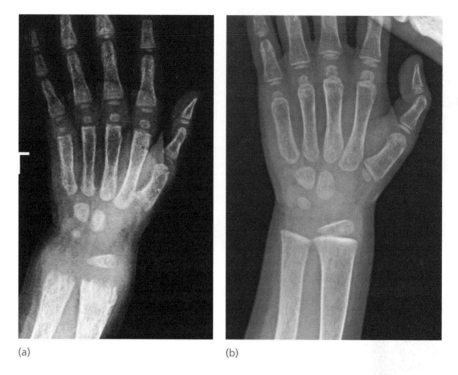

(a)   (b)

7.17 Rickets X-rays of the wrist of a 3-year-old patient with florid vitamin D-deficieny rickets.
(a) Note the profound osteopenia and widened physis. **(b)** The same patient 6 months later,
after vitamin D and calcium supplementation.

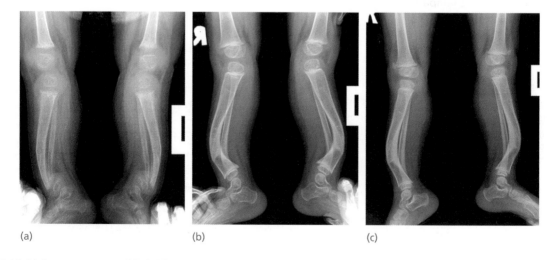

(a)   (b)   (c)

7.18 Rickets A 4-year-old child with vitamin D-deficiency rickets. Considerable modelling can be
seen from the initial radiograph **(a)** to those **(b)** 6 months and **(c)** 18 months following vitamin D and
calcium supplementation. Surgical management for deformity correction should be delayed until the
physes have recovered and remodelling has plateaued.

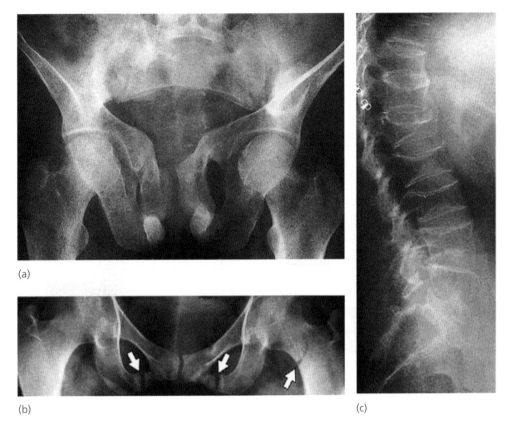

(a)

(b)

(c)

7.19 Osteomalacia Characteristic features of osteomalacia: **(a)** indentation of the acetabula producing the trefoil or champagne glass pelvis; **(b)** Looser's zones in the pubic rami and left femoral neck; **(c)** biconcave vertebrae.

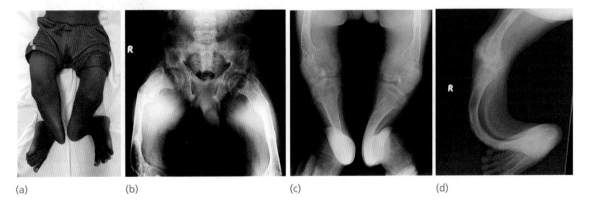

(a)   (b)   (c)   (d)

7.20 X-linked hypophosphataemic rickets The untreated condition in a 13-year-old male patient. Initial management requires high-dose phosphate to correct the metabolic imbalance and improve bone quality prior to multiple corrective osteotomies and intramedullary rodding of both tibiae and femora.

of the larger joints and in the longitudinal ligaments of the spinal canal, which may give rise to enthesopathies and neurological symptoms. As in other forms of osteomalacia, these patients are at increased risk of fractures including stress fractures, but in contrast to other forms of osteomalacia, bones can appear sclerotic. Biochemically these patients have low levels of phosphate, but serum calcium and PTH levels are usually normal.

Treatment requires the use of phosphate (up to 3 g per day, to replace that which is lost in the urine) and large doses of vitamin D. Bony deformities may require bracing or osteotomy. If the child needs to be immobilized, vitamin D must be stopped temporarily to prevent hypercalcaemia from the combined effects of treatment and disuse bone resorption.

CHRONIC KIDNEY DISEASE MINERAL BONE DISORDER

Chronic kidney disease is associated with skeletal and soft-tissue abnormalities termed chronic kidney disease mineral bone disorder (CKD-MBD); the specific skeletal manifestations are termed renal osteodystrophy. Although CKD-MBD may coexist with osteoporosis, it should always be considered as a separate diagnosis in patients with CKD stage 4/5 (i.e. estimated glomerular filtration rate (eGFR) <30 mL/min) presenting with a low trauma fracture.

Pathology

In CKD-MBD, osteoblast function is impaired due to systemic consequences of CKD including acidosis and increased sclerostin levels. High bone turnover is also a consequence of raised PTH levels known as secondary hyperparathyroidism.

Three distinct abnormalities are seen pathologically:

- *High turnover disease* is observed most commonly. As well as evidence of increased bone turnover in the form of increased numbers of osteoblasts and osteoclasts, there may be typical features of hyperparathyroidism including osteitis fibrosa and woven bone.

- *Adynamic bone disease* is observed in a small proportion, with evidence of reduced bone turnover including reduced levels of bone resorption and particularly bone formation.
- *Mineralization* defects may also be present, as indicated by widened osteoid seams and defective mineralization on tetracycline labelling.

Clinical features

CKD-MBD is associated with an increased fracture risk, even at relatively mild levels of renal impairment. This may be exacerbated by concurrent risk factors for osteoporosis such as hypogonadism and glucocorticoid therapy. In more advanced CKD-MBD, when features of renal osteodystrophy are present, bone pain may occur, combined with fractures. In children, growth retardation occurs combined with deformities seen in rickets. Slipped epiphyses may also occur, particularly at the hips when it can cause limping. A major clinical manifestation of CKD-MBD is vascular calcification.

X-rays

There are few specific skeletal manifestations of CKD-MBD radiologically. A rare manifestation is the 'rugger jersey spine' caused by osteosclerosis of the superior and inferior vertebral end plates. There may be evidence of increased soft-tissue calcification, particularly vascular calcification. DEXA scans may not be helpful as fracture risk may be elevated in the presence of a relatively normal BMD.

Biochemistry

Raised PTH is a cardinal feature of CKD stage 5, often increasing to many times the upper normal limit; PTH levels less than two times the upper normal limit may be indicative of adynamic bone disease. Although calcium levels tend to fall as a consequence of reduced calcitriol, they are generally maintained within the normal range by secondary hyperparathyroidism. Extremely high PTH levels and hypercalcaemia may develop due to tertiary hyperparathyroidism as a result of autonomous unregulated PTH secretion, following prolonged secondary hyperparathyroidism.

Treatment

Hyperphosphataemia and secondary hyperpara-thyroidism can be treated by restricting the intake of phosphorus and taking phosphate binders, and by administering a vitamin D analogue, most commonly alfacalcidol. Calcium-sensing receptor agonists such as cinacalcet may also be used to inhibit PTH secretion. However, the biochemical changes are complex and treatment should always be managed by a renal specialist.

HYPERCALCAEMIA

As previously mentioned, regulatory pathways described above, particularly PTH, are generally very effective at maintaining normocalcaemia, which is required for a number of essential cellular processes. Underlying causes of hypercalcaemia need to be identified and managed promptly. The most important are primary hyperparathyroidism and malignancy.

CAUSES OF HYPERCALCAEMIA

Increased calcium/vitamin D resorption
Increased bone resorption

- Primary and tertiary hyperparathyroidism
- Malignancy
- Hyperthyroidism

Granulomatous disorders

- Sarcoidosis
- Tuberculosis
- Histoplasmosis

Drugs

- Lithium
- Thiazides
- Theophylline toxicity
- Vitamin A toxicity
- Vitamin D excess

Familial

- MEN I and II
- Familial hypocalciuric hypercalcaemia

Other

- Addison's disease
- Phaeochromocytoma
- Solid tumours
- Prolonged immobilization

Clinical features

Clinical features vary with the degree of hyper-calcaemia: a mild elevation of serum calcium concentration may cause no more than general lassitude, polyuria and polydipsia. With plasma levels of 3.0–3.5 mmol/L, patients may complain of anorexia, nausea, muscle weakness and fatigue. Those with severe hypercalcaemia (<3.5 mmol/L) have a plethora of symptoms including abdominal pain, nausea, vomiting, severe fatigue and depression. In long-standing cases, patients may develop kidney stones or nephrocalcinosis due to chronic hypercalciuria; some complain of joint symptoms, due to chondrocalcinosis. The clinical picture is summarized in the adage 'moans, groans, bones and stones'.

There may also be symptoms and signs of the underlying cause, which should always be sought.

Hyperparathyroidism This is an important cause of hypercalcaemia.

- *Primary hyperparathyroidism* is usually due to an adenoma or hyperplasia.
- *Tertiary hyperparathyroidism* is when secondary hyperplasia leads to autonomous overactivity.

Both of these cause hypercalcaemia. Primary is more common and the diagnosis of this is supported by finding hypercalcaemia, hypophosphataemia and a raised serum PTH.

Malignancy Malignancy is another important cause of hypercalcaemia and may be due to locally increased bone resorption resulting from secondary bony metastases or multiple myeloma, or more generalized increased bone resorption mediated by parathyroid hormone-related peptide (PTHrP) secreted by solid tumours. Multiple endocrine neoplasia (MEN) syndromes can also cause hypercalcaemia.

Familial hypocalciuric hypercalcaemia (FHH)

FHH caused by inactivating mutations in the gene for the calcium-sensing receptor has a clinical spectrum of hypercalcaemia ranging from life-threatening disorders in the case of neonatal FHH to an asymptomatic biochemical abnormality found on a routine blood testing.

Investigations

Radiographs may show a variety of appearances depending on the underlying cause, including evidence of a primary lung tumour on chest radiography, or evidence of granulomatous diseases such as tuberculosis or sarcoidosis. Finding of a high serum calcium should be followed up by measurement of PTH. If this is normal or high, 24-hour urinary calcium excretion should be measured. The combination of normal/high PTH plus normal or high urinary calcium excretion confirms primary or tertiary hyperparathyroidism. The combination of normal/high PTH plus low urinary calcium excretion suggests familial hypocalciuric hypercalcaemia. Suppressed levels of PTH in the context of hypercalcaemia require symptom-guided investigations for malignancy and tests for other endocrinopathies such as hyperthyroidism (measure thyroid-stimulating hormone, TSH) or adrenal insufficiency (measure cortisol).

Treatment

 Acute severe hypercalcaemia is a medical emergency and needs to be treated promptly with IV fluids. IV bisphosphonates and glucocorticoids can also be used as second line.

Long-term management needs to be guided towards the underlying cause. Primary hyperparathyroidism is often treated with surgery.

HYPERPARATHYROIDISM

Hyperparathyroidism (excessive secretion of PTH) may be:

- *primary* – usually due to an adenoma or hyperplasia
- *secondary* – due to persistent hypocalcaemia

- *tertiary* – when secondary hyperplasia leads to autonomous overactivity.

Pathology

Overproduction of PTH enhances calcium conservation by stimulating tubular absorption, intestinal absorption and bone resorption. The resulting hypercalcaemia increases glomerular filtration of calcium to such an extent that there is hypercalciuria despite the augmented tubular reabsorption. Urinary phosphate is also increased, due to suppressed tubular reabsorption. The main effects of these changes are seen in the kidney: calcinosis, stone formation, recurrent infection and impaired function. There may also be calcification of soft tissues.

There is a general loss of bone substance. In severe cases, osteoclastic hyperactivity produces subperiosteal erosions, endosteal cavitation and replacement of the marrow spaces by vascular granulations and fibrous tissue (osteitis fibrosa cystica). Haemorrhage and giant-cell reaction within the fibrous stroma may give rise to brownish, tumour-like masses, whose liquefaction leads to fluid-filled cysts.

PRIMARY HYPERPARATHYROIDISM

Primary hyperparathyroidism is usually caused by a solitary adenoma in one of the small glands. Patients are middle-aged (40–65 years) and women are affected twice as often as men. Many remain asymptomatic and are diagnosed only because routine biochemistry tests unexpectedly reveal a raised serum calcium level.

Clinical features

Symptoms and signs are mainly due to *hypercalcaemia*:

- anorexia
- nausea
- abdominal pain
- depression
- fatigue
- muscle weakness.

Patients may develop polyuria, kidney stones or nephrocalcinosis due to chronic hypercalciuria.

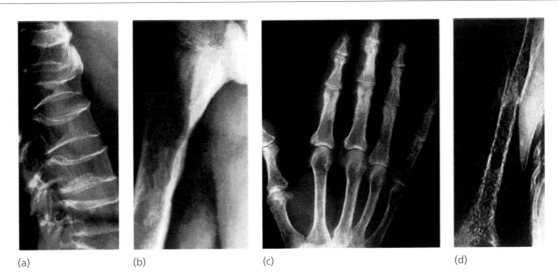

(a)   (b)   (c)   (d)

7.21 Hyperparathyroidism (a) This hyperparathyroid patient with spinal osteoporosis later developed pain in the right arm; **(b)** an X-ray showed cortical erosion of the humerus; **(c)** he also showed typical erosions of the phalanges. **(d)** Another case, showing 'brown tumours' of the humerus and a pathological fracture.

Some complain of joint symptoms, due to chondrocalcinosis. Only a minority (probably less than 10%) present with bone disease; this is usually generalized osteoporosis rather than the classic features of osteitis fibrosa, bone cysts and pathological fractures.

X-rays

Typical radiographic features are osteoporosis (sometimes including vertebral collapse) and areas of cortical erosion (**7.21**). Hyperparathyroid 'brown tumours' should be considered in the differential diagnosis of atypical cyst-like lesions of long bones. The classic – and almost pathognomonic – feature, which should always be sought, is subperiosteal cortical resorption of the middle phalanges. Nonspecific features of hypercalcaemia are renal calculi, nephrocalcinosis and chondrocalcinosis.

Biochemical tests

There may be hypercalcaemia, hypophosphataemia and a raised serum PTH concentration. Serum ALP is raised with osteitis fibrosa.

Diagnosis

It is necessary to exclude other causes of hypercalcaemia (*multiple myeloma, metastatic disease,*

sarcoidosis) in which PTH levels are usually depressed. Hyperparathyroidism also comes into the differential diagnosis of all types of *osteoporosis* and *osteomalacia.*

Treatment

Treatment is usually conservative and includes adequate hydration and decreased calcium intake. The indications for parathyroidectomy are marked and unremitting hypercalcaemia, recurrent renal calculi, progressive nephrocalcinosis and severe osteoporosis.

 Postoperatively, there is a danger of severe hypocalcaemia due to brisk formation of new bone (the 'hungry bone syndrome'). This must be treated promptly, with one of the fast-acting vitamin D metabolites.

HYPERCALCAEMIA OF MALIGNANCY

Pathology

Hypercalcaemia of malignancy is due to either local or generalized increase in bone resorption. Secondary bony metastases (usually from prostate, breast, lung, kidney or thyroid primaries) or multiple myeloma cause local bone resorption due to cytokine induced bone lysis. Hodgkin's lymphoma causes hypercalcaemia through increased production of calcitriol. MEN syndromes (benign or malignant tumours of endocrine tissues inherited in an autosomal dominant pattern) can also cause hypercalcaemia. In MEN type 1, hyperfunction of the parathyroid glands cause hypercalcaemia. In MEN type 2, the hypercalcaemia is associated with medullary thyroid carcinoma.

Investigations

Investigations for hypercalcaemia of malignancy need to be directed towards finding the primary tumour and should be based on symptoms, signs and basic blood tests. A history of smoking, cough, haemoptysis or shortness of breath should direct investigations towards the lungs, but there should be a low threshold for imaging (usually CT scanning) of the entire chest, abdomen and pelvis. A skeletal survey or nuclear medicine bone scan can be useful to identify all bone metastases (7.22). A myeloma screen (serum and urine electrophoresis) should be performed.

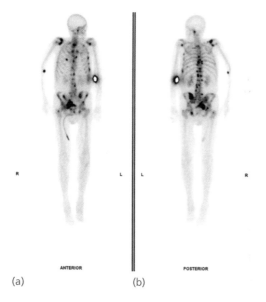

(a)   (b)

7.22 Nuclear medicine bone scans Multiple bony metastases can be seen clearly. (Image provided with kind permission from Dr Paul McCoubrie, Consultant Radiologist, North Bristol NHS Trust.)

Treatment

Treatment of acute severe hypercalcaemia of malignancy should be with IV fluids. IV bisphosphonates and glucocorticoids can also be used as second line. Management of the underlying malignancy can resolve the hypercalcaemia. Local radiotherapy to bone metastases can provide temporary relief of pain and hypercalcaemia caused by local bone resorption.

PAGET'S DISEASE OF BONE

Paget's disease of bone (PDB) is characterized by localized sites of increased bone turnover followed by enlargement and thickening of the bone, but the internal architecture is abnormal and the bone is unusually brittle.

Pathology

PDB may appear in one or several sites; in the long bones it starts at the metaphysis and progresses slowly towards the diaphysis, leaving altered architecture behind. The characteristic cellular change is a marked increase in osteoclastic and osteoblastic activity. Bone turnover is accelerated and plasma ALP is raised.

In the osteolytic (or 'vascular') stage there is avid resorption of existing bone by large osteoclasts, the excavations being filled with vascular fibrous tissue. In adjacent areas, osteoblastic activity produces new woven and lamellar bone, which in turn is removed by osteoclasts. This alternating activity extends to both endosteal and periosteal surfaces, so the bone increases in thickness but is structurally weak and prone to deformation. In the late, osteoblastic, stage, the thickened bone becomes increasingly sclerotic and brittle.

Clinical features

PDB affects men and women equally. Only occasionally does it present in patients under 50 years of age, but from that age onwards it becomes increasingly common. The disease may for many years remain localized to part or the whole of one bone, with the pelvis and tibia being the commonest sites, and the femur, skull, spine and clavicle the next commonest.

Most people with PDB are asymptomatic, the disorder being diagnosed when an X-ray is taken for some unrelated condition or after the incidental discovery of a raised serum ALP level. When patients do present, it is usually because of pain or deformity, or some complication of the disease.

The pain is a dull constant ache, worse in bed when the patient warms up, but rarely severe unless a fracture occurs or sarcoma supervenes.

Steal syndromes, in which blood is diverted from internal organs to the surrounding skeletal circulation, may cause cerebral impairment and spinal cord ischaemia. If there is also spinal stenosis, the patient develops typical symptoms of 'spinal claudication' and lower limb weakness.

Imaging

X-RAYS

X-ray appearances are characteristic. During the resorptive phase, there may be localized areas of osteolysis; most typical is the flame-shaped lesion extending along the shaft of the bone (7.23b). Later, the bone becomes thick and sclerotic, with coarse trabeculation (7.23c,d). The femur or

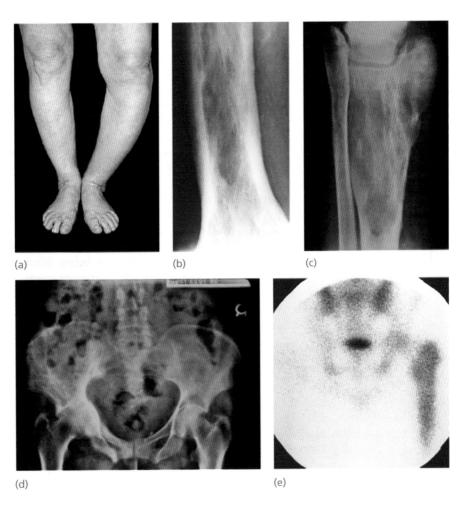

(a) (b) (c)

(d) (e)

7.23 Paget's disease of bone (a) Deformity of the tibia due to Paget's disease. **(b)** Flame-shaped area of osteopenia. **(c,d)** Anteroposterior radiographs showing coarse trabecular patterning of the upper tibia and fibula **(c)**, and right hemipelvis **(d)**. **(e)** Radionuclide scan showing increased activity in the left femur.

tibia sometimes develops fine cracks on the convex surface. These are stress fractures that heal with increasing deformity of the bone.

RADIONUCLIDE SCANS

These can be helpful in showing the distribution of active lesions; the distribution of increased uptake within an affected bone is relatively extensive, which can be helpful in distinguishing from other causes such as malignant secondary deposits (7.23e).

Complications

Fractures   These are common, especially in the weight-bearing long bones. In the femoral neck, they are often vertical; elsewhere, the fracture line is usually partly transverse and partly oblique. In the femur, there is a high rate of non-union; for femoral neck fractures prosthetic replacement and for shaft fractures early internal fixation is recommended. Small stress fractures may be very painful; they resemble Looser's zones on X-ray, except that they occur on convex surfaces.

Osteoarthritis   OA of the hip or knee is not merely a consequence of abnormal loading due to bone deformity; in the hip it seldom occurs unless the innominate bone is involved. The X-ray appearances suggest an atrophic arthritis with sparse remodelling, and at operation joint vascularity is increased.

Nerve compression and spinal stenosis Occasionally the first abnormalities to be detected, these may call for definitive surgical treatment. Local bone hypertrophy may cause hearing loss.

Bone sarcoma   Osteosarcoma arising in an elderly patient is almost always due to malignant transformation in Paget's disease. The frequency of malignant change is probably around 1%. It should always be suspected if a previously diseased bone becomes more painful, swollen and tender. Occasionally it presents as the first evidence of PDB. The prognosis is extremely grave.

High-output cardiac failure   This is a rare but important general complication. It is due to prolonged, increased bone blood flow.

Hypercalcaemia   If the patient is immobilized for prolonged periods, hypercalcaemia may occur.

Intraoperative bleeding   Bleeding from cut bony surfaces is common.

Treatment

IV ZOLEDRONATE

IV zoledronate given as a single infusion (dose 4–5 mg) is very effective at treating active PDB; as well as inducing remission in the great majority of patients, patients often remain in remission for several years thereafter. Whereas remission as reflected by a reduction in bone pain and ALP (which is often normalized) generally occurs, whether long-term sequelae (e.g. deafness and deformity) are prevented is currently unclear. Other than renal impairment (eGFR <30 mL/min), IV zoledronate has no major contraindications or cautions, and it is well tolerated apart from a risk of flu-like symptoms for 24 hours after the first infusion.

IV zoledronate should be considered in the following groups:

- patients with symptoms related to PDB, even if there is some uncertainty (e.g. patients with pelvic involvement and hip pain in whom some of the symptoms may be attributable to hip OA)
- patients who are considered at imminent risk of fracture (e.g. the presence of flame-shaped lytic lesions of the femur or tibia on radiographs).

SURGERY

The main indication for operation is a pathological fracture, which (in a long bone) usually requires internal fixation. When the fracture is treated, the opportunity should be taken to straighten the bone. Other indications for surgery are painful osteoarthritis (total joint replacement), nerve entrapment (decompression) and severe spinal stenosis (decompression). Some sources advocate pretreatment with IV zoledronate to limit blood loss, which may be excessive in these cases.

Genetic disorders, dysplasias and malformations

8

■ The human genome 129
■ Patterns of inheritance 131
■ Diagnosis 132
■ Principles of management 133
■ Classification of skeletal dysplasia 134
Chondro-osteodystrophies **134**
■ Dysplasias with predominantly epiphyseal changes 135
■ Dysplasias with predominantly physeal and metaphyseal changes 137

■ Dysplasias with predominantly diaphyseal changes 139
Connective-tissue disorders **140**
Storage disorders **145**
■ Mucopolysaccharidoses 145
Chromosome disorders **150**
Localized malformations **152**
■ Vertebral anomalies 152
■ Limb anomalies 153

Abnormal development of the musculoskeletal system may give rise to a variety of physical defects which are described as *skeletal dysplasias* (abnormal bone growth and/or modelling), *malformations* (e.g. absence or duplication of certain parts) or structural *defects of connective tissue*; in some, a specific *metabolic abnormality* has been identified.

In many cases the main determinant of the abnormality is a genetic defect. Such conditions can be broadly divided into three categories:

• *chromosome disorders*
• *single gene disorders*
• *polygenic* or *multifactorial disorders.*

Some anomalies may also result from injury to the formed embryo.

THE HUMAN GENOME

Each cell (apart from germ cells) in the human body contains within its nucleus 46 *chromosomes*, each of which consists of a single molecule of *deoxyribonucleic acid* (DNA); unravelled, this life-imparting molecule would be several centimetres long, a double-stranded chain along which thousands of segments are defined and demarcated as *genes*. These are the basic units of inherited biological information, each gene coding for the synthesis of a specific protein. Working as a set (or *genome*) they tell the cells how to develop, differentiate and function in specialized ways.

Chromosomes can be identified and numbered by microscopic examination of suitably prepared blood cells or tissue samples; the *cell karyotype* defines its chromosomal complement. *Somatic (diploid) cells* should have 46 chromosomes: 44 (numbers 1–22), called *autosomes,* are disposed in 22 homologous pairs, one of each pair being derived from the mother and one from the father and both carrying the same type of genetic information; the remaining two chromosomes are the *sex chromosomes*, females having two X chromosomes (one from each parent) and males having one X chromosome from the mother and one Y chromosome from the father. Thus, *germ-line cells* (eggs and sperm) have a *haploid* number of chromosomes (22 plus either an X or a Y).

Genes are distributed along the DNA chains, each gene at a specific point, or *locus*, on a specific chromosome. The chromosomes being paired, there will be two forms, or *alleles,* of each gene (one maternal, one paternal) at each locus; if the two alleles coding for a particular trait are identical, the person is said to be *homozygous* for that trait; if they are not identical, the individual is *heterozygous.*

The full genetic make-up of an individual is called the *genotype.* The finished person – a product of inherited traits and environmental influences – is the *phenotype.*

An important part of the unique human genotype is the *major histocompatibility complex* (MHC), also known as the *HLA system* (after human leucocyte antigen). This is a cluster of genes on chromosome 6 that is responsible for immunological specificity.

Genetic mutation

Mutation is any permanent change in DNA sequencing or structure. Such changes in a somatic cell are characteristic of malignancy. In a germ-line cell, mutations contribute to generational diversity.

Point mutations The substitution of one nucleotide for another is the most common type of mutation. The effect varies from production of a more useful protein to a new but functionless protein, or an inability to form any protein at all; the result may be compatible with an essentially normal life or it may be lethal.

Deletions/insertions Deletion or insertion of a segment in the gene chain can result in an unusual protein being synthesized, perhaps a more advantageous one but maybe one that is non-functional or one that has a dire effect on tissue structure and function.

Single gene disorders

Gene mutation may occur by insertion, deletion, substitution or fusion of amino acids or nucleotides in the DNA chain. This can have profound consequences for cartilage growth, collagen structure, matrix patterning and marrow cell metabolism. The abnormality is then passed on to future generations according to simple Mendelian rules (see Connective Tissue Disorders). There are thousands of single gene disorders, accounting for over 5% of child deaths, yet it is rare to see any of them in an orthopaedic practice.

Chromosome disorders

Additions, deletions or changes in chromosomal structure usually have serious consequences, the affected fetuses being either stillborn or developing with severe physical and mental abnormalities. Examples are:

- *Down's syndrome,* in which there is one extra chromosome 21 (trisomy 21)
- *Turner's syndrome,* in which one of the X chromosomes is lacking (monosomy X)
- *Klinefelter's syndrome,* in which there is one Y but several X chromosomes.

Polygenic and multifactorial disorders

Many normal traits (e.g. body build) derive from the interaction of multiple genetic and environmental influences. Likewise, certain diseases have a polygenic background, and some occur only when a genetic predisposition combines with an appropriate environmental 'trigger'. Gout, for example, is more common than usual in families with hyperuricaemia: the uric acid level is a polygenic trait, reflecting the interplay of multiple genes; it is also influenced by diet and may be more than usually elevated after a period of over-indulgence; finally, a slight bump on the toe acts as the proximate trigger for an acute attack of gout.

Non-genetic developmental disorders

Many fetal abnormalities result from injury to the developing embryo. Most are of unknown aetiology but some are due to specific teratogenic agents which damage the embryo or the placenta during the first few months of gestation. Suspected or known teratogens include viral infections (e.g. rubella), certain drugs (e.g. tha-lidomide) and ionizing radiation. The resulting defects are usually asymmetrical and localized, ranging from mild anatomical faults to severe malformations such as non-development of an entire limb (phocomelia).

PATTERNS OF INHERITANCE

The single gene disorders have characteristic patterns of inheritance, which may be *autosomal* or *X-linked*, and *dominant* or *recessive*.

AUTOSOMAL DOMINANT TRANSMISSION

Autosomal dominant transmission means that the abnormality is inherited even if only one allele of a pair on a non-sex chromosome is abnormal, i.e. only one parent need have been affected and the condition is said to be *heterozygous* (e.g. hereditary multiple exostoses). In that case, one-half of the children of either sex are likely to develop the disease, though it may appear in varying degrees of severity (*variable expressivity*). The pedigree shows a 'vertical' pattern of inheritance, with several affected siblings in successive generations.

AUTOSOMAL RECESSIVE TRANSMISSION

Autosomal recessive transmission means that both alleles of a pair have to be abnormal for the child to be affected, i.e. the condition is *homozygous*. Each parent contributes a faulty gene, though if both are heterozygous, they themselves will be clinically normal. Theoretically one in four of the children will be homozygous and will therefore develop the disease; two out of four will be *heterozygous carriers* of the faulty gene. The typical pedigree shows a 'horizontal' pattern of inheritance: several siblings in one generation are affected but neither their parents nor their children have the disease.

X-LINKED DISORDERS

X-linked disorders are caused by a faulty gene in the X chromosome. Characteristically, therefore, they never pass directly from father to son because the father's X chromosome inevitably goes to the daughter and the Y chromosome to the son.

X-linked dominant disorders   These disorders (e.g. hypophosphataemic rickets) pass from an affected mother to one-half of her daughters and one-half of her sons, or from an affected father to all of his daughters but none of his sons. (Not surprisingly, these conditions are twice as common in girls as in boys.)

X-linked recessive disorders   These disorders – of which the most notorious is haemophilia – have a highly distinctive pattern of inheritance: an affected male will pass the gene only to his daughters, who will become unaffected heterozygous carriers; they, in turn, will transmit it to one-half of their daughters (who will likewise be carriers) and one-half of their sons (who will be affected).

Inbreeding

All types of genetic disease are more likely to occur in the children of consanguineous marriages or in closed communities where many people are related to each other. The rare recessive disorders, in particular, are seen in these circumstances, where there is an increased risk of a homozygous pairing between two mutant genes.

Genetic heterogeneity

The same phenotype (i.e. a patient with a characteristic set of clinical features) can result from widely different gene mutations. For example, there are four different types of osteogenesis imperfecta (brittle bone disease), some showing autosomal dominant and some autosomal recessive inheritance. Where this occurs, the recessive form is usually the more severe. This must be borne in mind when counselling parents.

Genetic markers

Many common disorders show an unusually close association with certain blood groups, tissue types or other serum proteins that occur with higher-than-expected frequency in the patients and their relatives. These are referred to as genetic markers. A good example is ankylosing spondylitis: over 90% of patients and 60% of their first-degree relatives are positive for HLA-B27.

Gene mapping

With advancing recombinant DNA technology, the genetic disorders are gradually being mapped to specific loci. In some cases (e.g. Duchenne muscular dystrophy) the mutant gene itself has been cloned, holding out the possibility of effective treatment in the future.

DIAGNOSIS

Prenatal diagnosis

Many genetic disorders can be diagnosed before birth, thus giving the parents the choice of selective abortion. *High-resolution ultrasound imaging* is harmless and is now carried out almost routinely. Tests that involve *amniocentesis* or *chorionic villus sampling*, however, carry a risk of injury to the fetus and are therefore used only when there is an increased likelihood of some abnormality.

INDICATIONS FOR AMNIOCENTESIS OR CHORIONIC VILLUS SAMPLING
Maternal age over 35 years (increased risk of Down's syndrome) or an unduly high paternal age (increased risk of achondroplasia)
Previous history of chromosomal abnormalities (e.g. Down's syndrome) or genetic abnormalities amenable to biochemical diagnosis (neural-tube defects or inborn errors of metabolism) which will benefit from prompt neonatal treatment
To confirm non-invasive tests suggesting an abnormality

Diagnosis in childhood

Physical abnormalities may be obvious *at birth* (e.g. disproportionately short limbs suggesting achondroplasia). *During infancy,* the reasons for presentation are failure to grow normally, disproportionate shortness of the limbs, a delay in walking or repeated fractures.

Older children are more obviously abnormal. Features suggestive of skeletal dysplasia are retarded growth, deformities of the spine and/or limbs, unusual facial characteristics and a history of repeated fractures. There is a remarkable consistency about the deformities, which makes for a similarity of appearance in members of a particular group.

X-ray examination is important even if the physical features look familiar.

INITIAL RADIOGRAPHIC SURVEY
Posteroanterior view of the chest
Anteroposterior views of the pelvis knees and hands
Additional views of one arm and one leg
Lateral view of the thoracolumbar spine
Standard views of the skull

Fractures, bent bones, exostoses, epiphyseal dysplasia and spinal deformities may be obvious, especially in the older child. Sometimes a complete survey is needed and it is important to note which portion of the long bones (epiphysis, metaphysis or diaphysis) is affected.

 If there are *multiple fractures in different stages of healing,* or features of *several old healed fractures,* consider the possibility of *non-accidental injury* ('battered baby' syndrome).

The family history may reveal a characteristic pattern of inheritance. However, even an apparently normal parent may be very mildly affected, a fact which will not come to light if one relies entirely on the 'history', without the benefit of direct observation. *Racial background* is sometimes important: some diseases are particularly common in specific communities (e.g. sickle-cell disease in some black peoples and Gaucher's disease in Ashkenazi Jews).

Special investigations may be indicated to identify specific enzyme or metabolic abnormalities. *Direct testing for gene mutations* is already available for a number of conditions and is rapidly being extended to others.

Diagnosis in adults

Dysmorphic individuals who reach adulthood may lead fulfilling lives and have children of their own. Nevertheless, they often seek medical advice for problems such as abnormally short stature, local bone deformities, spinal stenosis, repeated fractures, secondary osteoarthritis (OA) or joint instability. As in children, family history and special investigations for enzyme or metabolic abnormalities are important.

PRINCIPLES OF MANAGEMENT

Communication

Once the diagnosis has been made, the next step is to explain as much as possible about the disorder to the patient and family without causing unnecessary distress. Nowadays, with quick and easy access to the internet, it is relatively easy to obtain useful information about almost any condition, which the clinician can pass on in simple language. Rare developmental disorders are best treated in a centre that offers a 'special interest' team consisting of a paediatrician, medical geneticist, orthopaedic surgeon, psychologist, social worker, occupational therapist, orthotist and prosthetist.

Counselling

It is important to make expert counselling available to patients and families when a genetic disorder is diagnosed. Where there are severe deformities or mental disability, the entire family will need counselling.

IMPORTANT TOPICS IN GENETIC COUNSELLING

The likely outcome of the disorders
What will be required of the family
The risk of siblings or children being affected

Intrauterine surgery

The concept of operating on the unborn fetus is already a reality; however, it is too early to say whether the advantages (e.g. prenatal skin closure for dysraphism) will outweigh the risks.

Specific medication

The ideal form of treatment would be modification or replacement of the abnormal gene. For the present, however, treatment is directed mainly at identifying the faulty protein or enzyme and then, where possible, administering the essential ingredient that will restore physiological function or counteract the pathological effects of the abnormality. One example is the treatment of Gaucher's disease by administering the missing enzyme, alglucerase.

Gene therapy is still at the experimental stage. A carrier molecule or vector (often a virus that has been genetically modified to carry some normal human genetic material) is used to deliver the therapeutic material into the abnormal target cells where the DNA is 'uploaded' allowing, for example, functional protein production to be resumed.

Prevention and correction of deformities

Realignment of the limb, correction of ligamentous laxity and joint reconstruction can improve joint stability and gait. Anomalies such as coxa vara, genu valgum, club foot, radial club hand or scoliosis (and many others outside the field of orthopaedics) are amenable to corrective surgery. Short-limbed patients may benefit from lengthening operations; however, the risks should be carefully explained. One should bear in mind that cosmetic improvement is not always accompanied by any significant functional change. Conservative measures such as physiotherapy and splinting still have an important role to play.

Several developmental disorders are associated with potentially dangerous spinal anomalies (e.g. spinal stenosis and cord compression in achondroplasia and severe kyphoscoliosis in various types of vertebral dysplasia). Cord decompression or occipitocervical fusion are feasible, but spinal operations carry considerable risks and should be undertaken only in specialized units.

> ⚠ Patients with spinal dysplasia undergoing any procedure under anaesthesia should be examined beforehand for odontoid hypoplasia and atlantoaxial instability.

CLASSIFICATION OF SKELETAL DYSPLASIA

There is no completely satisfactory classification of developmental disorders. The same genetic abnormality may be expressed in different ways, while a variety of gene defects may cause almost identical clinical syndromes. The grouping presented in **Table 8.1** is no more than a convenient way of cataloguing the least rare of the clinical syndromes. Only a few representative conditions will be described in this chapter.

CHONDRO-OSTEODYSTROPHIES

The chondro-osteodystrophies, or skeletal dysplasias, are a large group of disorders characterized by abnormal cartilage and bone growth. Only a few of the least rare conditions are discussed here. They are presented in clinical rather than aetiological groups of dysplasias with:

- predominantly epiphyseal changes
- predominantly physeal and metaphyseal changes
- mainly diaphyseal changes
- a mixture of abnormalities.

Table 8.1 A practical grouping of generalized developmental disorders

Grouping		Disorder(s)
Genetic disorders of cartilage and bone growth (chondro-osteodystrophies)	Dysplasias with predominantly epiphyseal changes	Multiple epiphyseal dysplasia Spondyloepiphyseal dysplasia
	Dysplasias with predominantly physeal and metaphyseal changes	Hereditary multiple exostosis Achondroplasia Metaphyseal chondrodysplasia Dyschondroplasia (enchodromatosis, Ollier's disease)
	Dysplasias with predominantly diaphyseal changes	Osteopetrosis (marble bones, Albers–Schönberg disease) Diaphyseal dysplasia (Engelmann's disease, Camurati's disease)
Collagen disorders	Osteogenesis imperfecta (brittle bones) Generalized joint laxity Ehlers–Danlos syndrome	
Enzyme defects and metabolic disorders	Mucopolysaccharidoses Gaucher's disease	Hurler's syndrome (MPS I) Hunter's syndrome (MPS II) Morquio–Brailsford syndrome (MPS IV)
Chromosome disorders	Down's syndrome	

DYSPLASIAS WITH PREDOMINANTLY EPIPHYSEAL CHANGES

MULTIPLE EPIPHYSEAL DYSPLASIA

Multiple epiphyseal dysplasia (MED) varies in severity from a trouble-free disorder with mild anatomical abnormalities to a severe crippling condition. There is widespread involvement of the epiphyses but the vertebrae are not at all, or only mildly, affected.

Clinical features

MED is a familial disorder (autosomal dominant in most cases) in which the long-bone epiphyses develop abnormally. Children may present with stunted growth or with joint pain and progressive deformity. The face, skull and spine are normal. In adult life, residual bone defects may lead to joint incongruity and secondary OA.

X-rays

Common *radiographic features* of dominant MED include delayed epiphyseal ossification. When the epiphysis appears, the shape is abnormal, but this may be subtle. There is a gradual deterioration of epiphyseal shape, with progressive flattening leading to articular incongruity at skeletal maturity (**8.1, 8.2**).

Management

Management is generally symptomatic, with advice on activity modification, avoiding repetitive loading, physiotherapy and analgesic and anti-inflammatory medication. Weight control is also very important and this in isolation is an efficient method of reducing pain and possibly prolonging native joint function.

As patients near skeletal maturity, those with more severe forms of the condition may be considered for osteotomies to correct deformity and improve the mechanical environment. Consideration for realignment osteotomies of the hip should be approached cautiously, as pain relief is unpredictable and joint stiffness is common. Arthroplasty is the conventional method for managing deteriorating joint pain and may be required at a young age in severely affected individuals.

SPONDYLOEPIPHYSEAL DYSPLASIA

Spondyloepiphyseal dysplasia (SED) is an uncommon condition with an approximate incidence of 1 : 100 000. Affected individuals have significant shortening of the neck, spine and limbs.

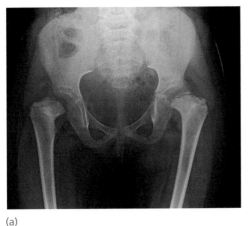

(a)

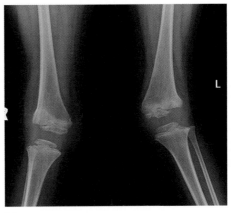

(b)

8.1 Multiple epiphyseal dysplasia Note the symmetrical condition in this child with flattened epiphyses, hip subluxation **(a)** and genu valgum **(b)**. Corrective osteotomies around the knee are indicated to improve the mechanical axis and joint longevity.

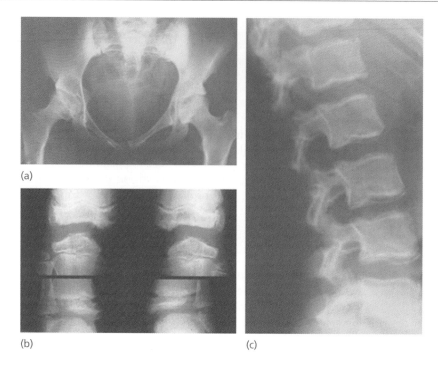

8.2 Multiple epiphyseal dysplasia (a,b) X-rays show epiphyseal distortion and flattening at multiple sites, in this case the hips, knees and ankles. **(c)** The ring epiphyses of the vertebral bodies also may be affected and in spondyloepiphyseal dysplasia this is the dominant feature.

The condition presents with two distinct phenotypes, due to a mutation in *COL2A1* leading to impaired synthesis of type II collagen.

- *SED congenita* is the more severe form, characterized by an autosomal dominant inheritance pattern.
- *SED tarda* is characterized by an X-linked recessive inheritance pattern and is associated with milder phenotypic changes.

Maxillary flattening, facial abnormalities and cleft palate are common associations diagnosed in the postnatal period. Severe myopia, vitreous abnormalities and retinal detachment cause visual impairment, and hearing loss becomes obvious in early childhood.

> ⚠ Atlantoaxial instability is a very significant association in patients with SED congenita.

Patients may require cervico-occipital fusion in the presence of significant instability to prevent cervical myelopathy. Thoracolumbar kyphoscoliosis, chest wall abnormalities with respiratory insufficiency and lumbar lordosis are commonly seen (**e8.1**).

Radiographic findings include:

- platyspondyly
- odontoid hypoplasia
- narrowed intervertebral discs
- pubic bones unossifed at birth with coxa vara and delayed ossification of the femoral head in later childhood.

The eventual consequence of abnormal collagen and an unfavourable mechanical environment is the premature onset of OA. Joint deformity can be managed with multilevel corrective osteotomies and the small size and complex anatomy introduces a dimension of complexity that requires advanced arthroplasty solutions.

SED tarda is less severe. Males are more commonly affected than females and present with chest wall and spinal abnormalities or concerns about stature. The radiographic features are similar to SED congenita.

The initial approach is symptomatic improvement, using physiotherapy, core strengthening, analgesic and anti-inflammatory medication and activity modification for back pain. Joint deformities may require corrective osteotomies, and arthritis of the hips or knees is managed with arthroplasty.

DYSPLASIAS WITH PREDOMINANTLY PHYSEAL AND METAPHYSEAL CHANGES

HEREDITARY MULTIPLE EXOSTOSIS (DIAPHYSEAL ACLASIS)

This is a congenital disorder in which multiple exostoses appear at the long-bone metaphyses and the apophyseal borders of the scapula and pelvis. It is inherited by autosomal dominant transmission and starts with unrestrained lateral growth of the cartilaginous physis and defective modelling at the physeal/metaphyseal junction. Each exostosis is covered by a cartilage cap and can go on growing as long as endochondral growth proceeds normally.

> ⚠ Any enlargement after endochondral growth ceases may herald malignant change to a chondrosarcoma.

The failure of modelling results in deformities of the long bones (e8.2).

Clinical features

The condition is usually discovered in childhood; hard lumps appear near the ends of the long bones (8.3, 8.4) and along the edges of the scapula and pelvis. The child may be slightly short, with bowing of the forearms and often a lower limb growth disturbance with genu valgum, genu varum or leg length discrepancy. Occasionally, one of the lumps becomes tender or causes trouble due to pressure on a tendon. Large exostoses at the fibula neck can irritate the common peroneal nerve.

X-rays show the pathognomonic exostoses as well as broadening and imperfect modelling of the metaphyses.

Management

If an exostosis is troublesome (and certainly if it starts to 'grow' after the parent bone has stopped), it should be removed. Long-bone deformities may call for corrective osteotomy.

ACHONDROPLASIA

Achondroplasia is the most common skeletal dysplasia, with an approximate incidence of 1 : 25 000. The inheritance pattern is autosomal dominant but the majority (>80%) occur secondary to *de novo* mutation in the fibroblast growth factor receptor 3 *(FGFR3)* that is identical in 95% of patients with this condition.

Clinical features

IN INFANTS

In infancy, the most significant features are due to proximal spinal cord compression, due to narrowing of the foramen magnum and/or proximal cervical spinal canal presenting as sleep apnoea, mandating sleep studies and MRI in the first 6 months of life. Hydrocephalus may also develop, due to expression of *FGFR3* in the choroid plexus. Kyphoscoliosis is common in infancy, but resolves after independent sitting and standing.

IN OLDER CHILDREN

The most striking clinical features are disproportionate short limbs and characteristic facial features. The limb shortening is rhizomelic, with more significant shortening of the proximal segments. The average adult height is approximately 125 cm in females and 132 cm in males, intelligence is normal and lifespan is unaffected (e8.3).

Facial features are characteristic and include button nose, frontal bossing, macrocephaly, mid-face hypoplasia and small nasal bridge. Joint laxity and hypotonia are also common and lead

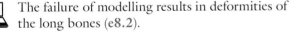

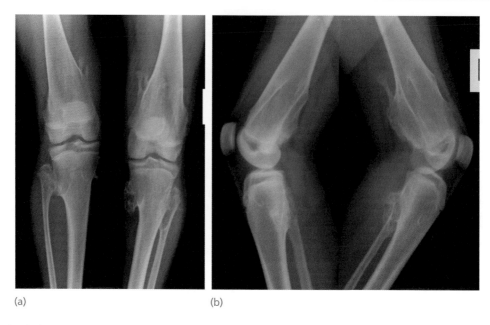

(a)   (b)

8.3 Multiple hereditary exostosis A 13-year-old girl with MHE demonstrating the characteristic appearance of multiple hereditary exostoses affecting the distal femur and the proximal tibia and fibula.

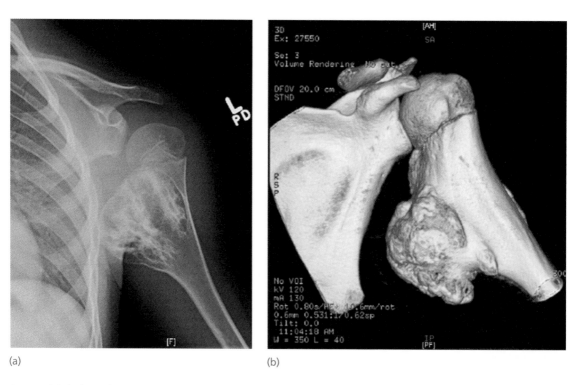

(a)   (b)

8.4 Multiple hereditary exostosis Radiograph and 3-D CT reconstruction of large exostosis of the proximal humerus.

to postural issues including flat feet, lower limb coronal malalignment, fixed hip flexion, lumbar lordosis and radial head subluxation.

IN ADULTS

Adults with achondroplasia are at significant risk of spinal stenosis, secondary to progressive distal shortening of the pedicles. This presents as spinal claudication with progressive lower limb pain, weakness, numbness and paraesthesia.

Management

- Key developments in the management of achondroplasia include the recent introduction of natriuretic peptide as a *therapeutic agent*. This has produced encouraging results in small mammal models and is entering the initial stages of human trials. The previous pharmacological approach to short stature was with growth hormone (GH), but the results of this approach have been very disappointing.
- Patients with achondroplasia and their families frequently seek advice about the *surgical management* of short stature. Advances in external fixator design and improvements in surgical technique have made this a realistic but difficult option with a high but not prohibitive risk.
- *Symptomatic lower limb malalignment*, refractory to conventional non-operative treatment modalities, may be managed with guided growth techniques in the skeletally immature patient. Skeletally mature patients may be treated with realignment osteotomies in conjunction with limb lengthening or total knee replacement.
- *Symptomatic foramen magnum or upper cervical spine stenosis* mandates urgent investigation with radiographs and an MRI. Significant stenosis should be managed with urgent decompression and stabilization.
- *Infantile kyphoscoliosis* usually resolves after the initiation of independent weight-bearing. Patients with persistent deformity may require bracing to correct the curve. Patients with symptomatic, residual kyphoses of >40 degrees may rarely require anterior strut corpectomy and posterior fusion.

- *Lumbar stenosis* in the young adult is initially managed with standard non-operative measures, including weight loss, physical therapy and activity modification. If these treatments fail, patients may be candidates for spinal decompression.

DYSPLASIAS WITH PREDOMINANTLY DIAPHYSEAL CHANGES

Most of the 'diaphyseal dysplasias' appear to be the result of defective bone modelling. Unlike the physeal and epiphyseal disorders, dwarfing is not a feature. Only the most common example, osteopetrosis, will be described here.

OSTEOPETROSIS (MARBLE BONES, ALBERS–SCHÖNBERG DISEASE)

Osteopetrosis is one of several conditions that are characterized by sclerosis and thickening of the bones which then appear unusually 'dense' on X-ray (8.5).

Osteopetrosis tarda

The common form of osteopetrosis is a fairly benign, autosomal dominant disorder that seldom causes symptoms and may only be discovered in adolescence or adulthood after a pathological fracture or when an X-ray is taken for other reasons – hence the designation *tarda*. Shape and function are unimpaired unless there are complications: pathological fracture or cranial nerve compression due to bone encroachment on foramina.

 Sufferers of osteopetrosis tarda are prone to *bone infection*, particularly of the mandible after tooth extraction.

X-rays show increased density of all the bones: cortices are widened, leaving narrow medullary canals; sclerotic vertebral end plates produce a

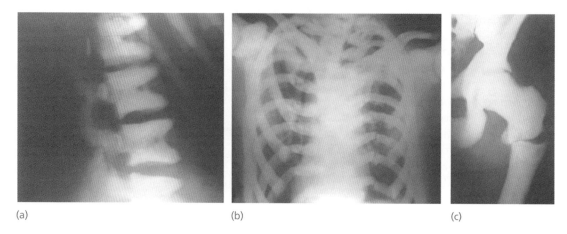

(a) (b) (c)

8.5 Osteopetrosis Despite the remarkable density, the bones fracture easily. Typical X-ray features in **(a)** the spine, **(b)** the ribs and **(c)** the femur.

striped appearance ('football-jersey spine'); the skull is thickened and the base densely sclerotic, carrying the risk of foraminal occlusion and cranial nerve entrapment.

Treatment is required only if complications occur.

Osteopetrosis congenita

This rare, autosomal recessive form of osteopetrosis is present at birth and causes severe disability. Bone encroachment on marrow results in pancytopenia, haemolysis, anaemia and hepatosplenomegaly. Foraminal occlusion may cause optic or facial nerve palsy. Osteomyelitis following, for example, tooth extraction or internal fixation of a fracture is quite common. Repeated haemorrhage or infection usually leads to death in early childhood.

Treatment has focused on methods of enhancing bone resorption and haematopoeisis (e.g. by transplanting marrow from normal donors and by long-term treatment with gamma-interferon).

CONNECTIVE-TISSUE DISORDERS

Heritable defects of collagen synthesis give rise to a number of disorders involving either the soft connective tissues or bone, or both. In many cases the specific collagen defect has now been identified.

GENERALIZED JOINT LAXITY

About 5% of people have hypermobile joints, as defined by a positive score of more than 5 (the Beighton score) in five simple tests (**8.6**).

TESTS FOR JOINT HYPERMOBILITY (BEIGHTON SCORES)

1 Passive hyperextension of the metacarpophalangeal joints to beyond 90° (*score 2*)
2 Passive stretching of the thumb to touch the radial border of the forearm (*score 2*)
3 Hyperextension of the elbows (*score 2*)
4 Hyperextension of the knees (*score 2*)
5 Ability to bend forward and place the hands flat on the floor with the knees held perfectly straight (*score 1*)

This trait runs in families and is inherited as a Mendelian dominant. The condition is not in itself disabling but it may predispose to congenital dislocation of the hip in the newborn or recurrent dislocation of the patella or shoulder in later life. Transient joint pains are common and there is an increased risk of ankle sprains.

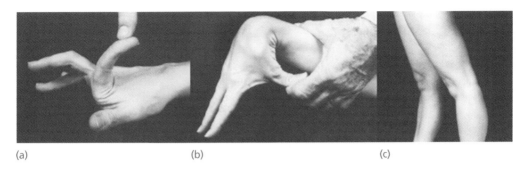

(a) (b) (c)

8.6 Generalized joint laxity Simple tests for joint hypermobility: **(a)** passive hyperextension of the metacarpophalangeal joints to beyond 90°; **(b)** passive stretching of the thumb to touch the radial border of the forearm; **(c)** hyperextension of the knees.

MARFAN'S SYNDROME

Marfan's syndrome is an autosomal dominant disorder, which is caused by a mutation in the fibrillin-1 gene *(FBN1)*. It has an approximate incidence of 1 : 10 000 and affects the musculo-skeletal, ocular and cardiovascular systems.

Affected individuals are tall and hypermobile, with long limbs and digits (**8.7**).

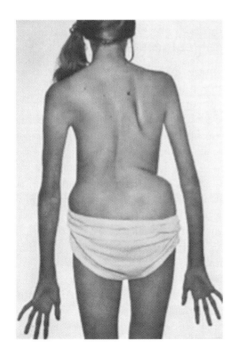

8.7 Marfan's syndrome The combination of disproportionately long arms, 'spider fingers' and scoliosis is characteristic.

Scoliosis is present in 50% of patients and is often associated with pectus excavatum. Abnormalities of acetabular development (protrusio) occur in 25% of cases. Severe ligamentous laxity produces a planovalgus foot deformity and recurrent joint dislocations. Extraskeletal manifestations include superior lens dislocation, spontaneous pneumothorax and aortic root dilatation leading to dissection. Dural ectasia is present in approximately 60% of patients.

Orthopaedic surgical treatment frequently involves scoliosis correction, and *complications* including wound infection, hardware failure and pseudarthrosis are not uncommon. Hip pain, secondary to acetabular abnormalities, may require arthroplasty but abnormalities of the feet and joint instability is generally managed without surgery. This is due to the unpredictable and generally unsatisfactory outcome that accompanies attempts at soft-tissue reconstruction.

EHLERS–DANLOS SYNDROME

Ehlers–Danlos syndrome is a group of inherited disorders caused by abnormalities of collagen formation or proteins responsible for normal collagen function. Affected individuals have fragile skin, joint hypermobility, vascular fragility and severe myalgia.

The inheritance pattern is variable and most cases have an autosomal dominant pattern. There are often abnormalities of collagen formation, commonly involving mutations of *COL5A1* or

COL5A2 with *COL1A1*, *COL1A2* and *COL3A1* also reported.

Diagnosis is often based on the constellation of clinical signs, particularly the degree of ligamentous laxity. Biochemical and genomic analysis of collagen are useful in some cases, but they cannot be guaranteed to identify an individual cause.

Affected individuals may develop cardiac anomalies including aortic root dilatation and mitral valve prolapse. Significant ligamentous laxity, elastic skin and a bruising tendency are common. Structural consequences, including congenital talipes equino-varus, progressive kyphoscoliosis and developmental dysplasia of the hips are also present. Shoulder, ankle and patella–femoral instability are common, and approximately 50% of individuals develop chronic musculoskeletal pain and are prone to early-onset OA.

> ⚠ Patients with a suspected Ehlers–Danlos syndrome diagnosis should undergo an echocardiogram to evaluate the aortic root, and all patients being considered for surgery should have a detailed cardiovascular assessment.

Specific *orthopaedic management* is directed at addressing painful or unstable joints, and physiotherapy is a central component of treatment. Persistent instability and severe and deteriorating joint pain, refractory to non-operative treatment, may require a surgical solution.

The *complications* of surgery, particularly those associated with wound healing, are increased in this condition due to fragile skin, excessive bleeding and vascular fragility. Soft-tissue procedures are ineffective and arthrodesis is occasionally necessary. Instrumented spinal fusion is required in patients with progressive scoliosis and the level is determined to prevent junctional degeneration secondary to hypermobility.

OSTEOGENESIS IMPERFECTA (BRITTLE BONES)

Osteogenesis imperfecta (OI) is a relatively common connective tissue disorder with an incidence of approximately 1 : 20 000 live births. Mutations of *COL1A1* and *COL1A2* genes cause quantitative and qualitative abnormalities of type I collagen production. All tissues that contain type I collagen are affected, including bone, ligament, teeth and sclera. This results in structurally incompetent bone, vulnerable to fracture, secondary deformity and joint laxity. Abnormalities of non-skeletal collagen produce alterations in the sclera, dentinogenesis imperfecta and deafness.

Sillence described four separate types according to scleral involvement, natural history and the perceived inheritance. Conventional wisdom was that there were clear autosomal dominant and recessive types. Contemporary understanding is that the majority of cases are caused by spontaneous mutation and that all familial mutations are inherited in an autosomal dominant fashion. Mutations previously considered to be recessive are more likely to be due to mosaicism.

Diagnosis tends to be made on clinical and radiological grounds, but DNA analysis can be used and has identified over 800 separate collagen mutations in patients with a typical phenotype.

Clinical features

The clinical manifestations are protean and are determined by the individual pattern of involvement. Recurrent fractures at multiple sites, often with trivial trauma, are a common finding and are a consequence of bone fragility. Normal bone healing is present in the majority of fractures, but progressive long bone deformity is a frequent consequence of either fracture malunion or progressive deformity due to the underlying abnormalities of collagen (8.8).

Dental abnormalities, blue sclerae (8.8d), scoliosis and kyphosis associated with flattened vertebral bodies and non-specific bone pain are common. In later life, joint degeneration can arise secondary to long-standing malalignment. A combination of protrusio, fracture and abnormal hip mechanics frequently results in painful OA, requiring total joint replacement.

Radiological features are generally non-specific and include Wormian bones, which are present in the normal population and are associated with a

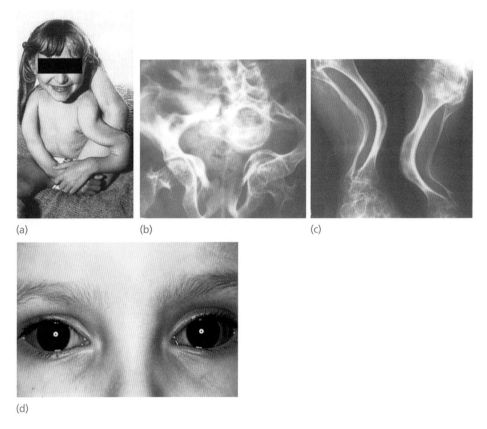

(a)   (b)   (c)

(d)

8.8 Osteogenesis imperfecta (a) This young girl had severe deformities of all her limbs, the result of multiple mini-fractures of the long bones over time. This is the classic (Type III) form of OI. **(b,c)** X-ray features in a slightly older patient with the same condition. **(d)** Blue sclerae usually occur in the milder, Type I OI.

number of skeletal abnormalities, including OI. Enlargement of frontal and mastoid sinuses are also seen in some patients with OI. The cortices of long bones are often thin and demonstrate features of general demineralization, previous fracture and previous pharmacological intervention, particularly bisphosphonates. Protrusio acetabuli and proximal femoral 'shepherd's crook' deformities of the femurs are common findings.

Treatment

Management involves physiotherapy, walking aids and orthotics to maximize mobility. Pharmaceutical agents are used to enhance bone strength, and bisphosphonates have been demonstrated to increase cortical thickness by inhibiting osteoclastic bone resorption. Cycles of intravenous bisphosphonates are used to decrease bone pain and reduce the incidence of fractures (**8.9**).

Surgical intervention to correct deformity and stabilize load-bearing bones generally utilizes intramedullary fixation systems (**8.10–8.12, e8.4**). Spinal deformity may require surgical correction.

NEUROFIBROMATOSIS

Neurofibromatosis (NF) is one of the commonest single gene disorders affecting the skeleton. Two types are recognized:

- *Type 1* (NF1) – also known as *von Recklinghausen's disease* – has an incidence of about 1 : 3500 live births. The abnormality

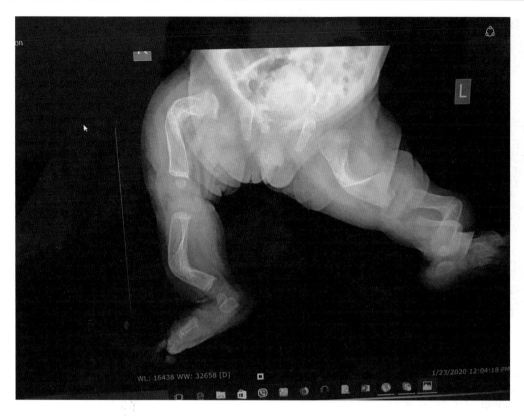

8.9 Severe osteogenesis imperfecta in an infant Multiple recent fractures are likely to be due to birth trauma. Early bisphosphonate therapy is indicated to strengthen the long bones, minimize further deformity and protect the spine from multiple wedge compression fractures.

is located in the gene which codes for neurofibromin, on chromosome 17. It is transmitted as autosomal dominant, with almost 100% penetrance, but more than 50% of cases are due to new mutation. The most characteristic lesions are neurofibromata (Schwann cell tumours) and patches of skin pigmentation (*café-au-lait spots*), but other features are remarkably protean and musculoskeletal abnormalities are seen in almost half of those affected.

- *Type 2* (NF2) is very rare and is seldom associated with skeletal defects.

Clinical features of NF1

Almost all patients have the typical widespread patches of skin pigmentation and multiple cutaneous neurofibromata, which usually appear before puberty. Less common is a single large plexiform neurofibroma, or an area of soft-tissue overgrowth in one of the limbs (**8.13**).

The orthopaedic surgeon is most likely to encounter the condition in a child or adolescent who presents with *scoliosis*; the most suggestive deformity is a very short, sharp curve. *Local tumours* in the spine can cause symptoms resembling those of disc prolapse and X-rays may show scalloping of the posterior aspects of the vertebral bodies, erosion of the pedicles or intervertebral foraminal enlargement. Correction of the deformity is often challenging due to poor bone stock and the presence of nerve impingement and dural ectasia.

Congenital pseudarthrosis is also associated with NF1 (**8.14**). The affected child presents

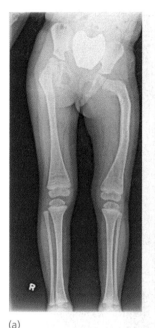
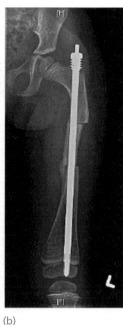

(a)   (b)

8.10 Osteogenesis imperfecta (a) AP femora: note multiple radiolucent metaphyseal lines secondary to sequential administration of bisphosphonates. There is a multilevel diaphyseal deformity, secondary to previous fractures, with an overall coxa vara. **(b)** Postoperative radiograph, following multilevel realignment osteotomies, stabilized with a Fassier–Duval intermedullary rod.

with an anterolateral tibial bow. Initial X-rays show a sclerotic region in the mid to distal third of the tibial shaft. This region typically fractures in early childhood and fails to unite without surgical intervention. This usually requires resection of the pathological bone and periosteum, intramedullary rodding and bone grafting (**8.15, 8.16**). Bone transport is sometimes required for recalcitrant cases and some patients will even require amputation such can be the challenge to achieve long-term union. (See also 'Congenital pseudarthrosis of the tibia' below.)

Malignant change occurs in 2–5% of affected individuals and is the most common complication in elderly patients.

STORAGE DISORDERS

MUCOPOLYSACCHARIDOSES

Mucopolysaccharidoses (MPS) are a group of storage disorders characterized by absence or defects of lysosomal enzymes that are responsible for the breakdown of glycosaminoglycans (GAGs). GAGs are long-chain polysaccharides, which accumulate in the liver and spleen in addition to bone, cartilage and connective tissues, leading to a spectrum of skeletal abnormalities.

Hurler (MPS type I) and *Sanfilippo (MPS type III)* are the most common, with an overall prevalence of approximately 1 : 100 000 live births. *Hunter (MPS type II)* is inherited with an X-linked recessive pattern and all the other types are inherited in an autosomal recessive pattern.

Clinical features

This condition presents in early childhood with short stature, and affected individuals tend to be less than the third percentile for height. Other generic features include characteristic 'coarse' facial features, thick inelastic skin, hepatosplenomegaly, neurological abnormalities and delayed intellectual development. Spinal abnormalities are common and include atlantoaxial instability with abnormal vertebrae producing a rigid kyphoscoliosis.

HURLER (MPS I)

MPS type I is a heterogeneous condition with significant variability of life expectancy. The rate of growth and mental development slows in the second year of life. Affected individuals walk late and develop severe joint stiffness, coxa valga, femoral head irregularities and genu valgum. Anterior vertebral wedging leads to kyphosis or thoracolumbar gibbus and, in common with most MPS, odontoid hypoplasia may develop.

Non-skeletal features include big tongues (macroglossia), hearing loss and cardiorespiratory

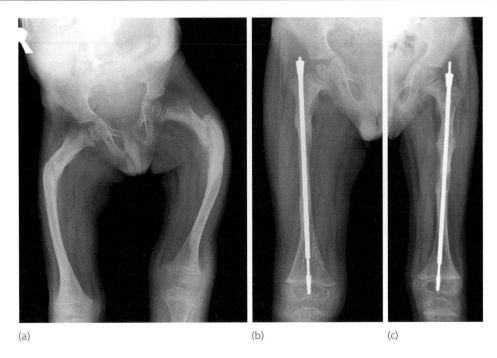

(a)　　　　　　　　(b)　　　　　　　　(c)

8.11 Osteogenesis imperfecta (a) Note the recent left proximal femoral diaphyseal shaft fracture. **(b,c)** Managed with multiple osteotomies and placement of telescopic growing rods that lengthen as the child grows, while still offering support to the pathological weak bone.

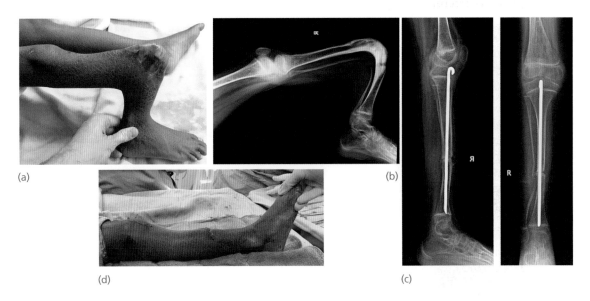

(a)　　　　　　　　　　　　　　　　　(b)

(d)　　　　　　　　　　　　(c)

8.12 Osteogenesis imperfecta (a,b) Severe tibial bow due to OI. **(c,d)** Managed with a single-level osteotomy with removal of the apex of the deformity. Use of intramedullary devices is preferable to plating as the entire length of the bone is supported and avoids a 'stress riser' at the tip of the plate.

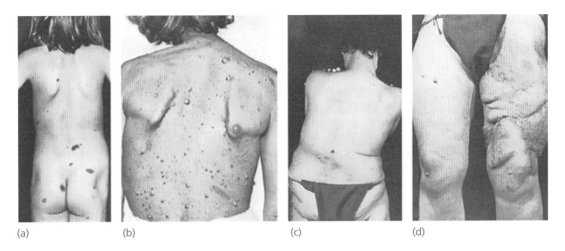

(a) (b) (c) (d)

8.13 Neurofibromatosis (a) Café-au-lait spots. **(b)** Multiple neurofibromata and slight scoliosis. **(c,d)** A patient with scoliosis and soft-tissue overgrowth ('elephantiasis').

insufficiency, which can result in death in late childhood.

HUNTER (MPS II)

MPS type II occurs only in males due to the inheritance pattern. The features are variable and are similar to those seen in type I. Macrocephaly and coarse facial features are characteristic, with marked joint contractures developing in the pre-school period leading to joint stiffness and hip arthritis in older patients. Cardiorespiratory compromise is also common, which in severe cases leads to death in the second decade.

SANFILIPPO (MPS III)

Children with MPS type III have slowing of their rate of growth after 2–3 years, at which point they also begin to develop

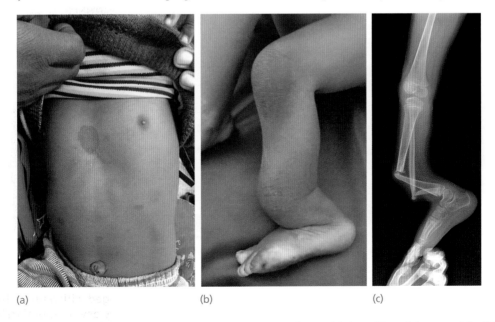

(a) (b) (c)

8.14 Neurofibromatosis A 4-year-old child with NF1. Note the multiple café-au-lait spots **(a)**, tibial deformity **(b)** and established pseudarthrosis affecting the tibia and fibula **(c)**.

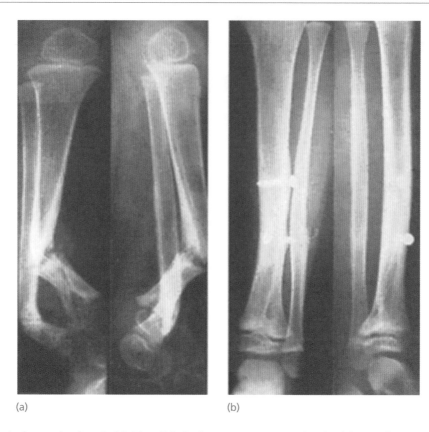

(a)   (b)

8.15 Congenital pseudarthrosis (a) The tibia is the most common site; in this case bone grafting was successful **(b).**

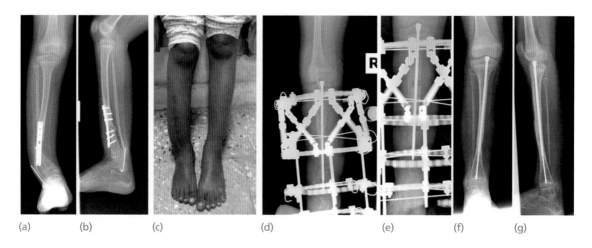

(a)   (b)   (c)   (d)   (e)   (f)   (g)

8.16 Congenital tibial pseudarthrosis (a–c) The condition was previously managed by internal fixation but failed to unite. **(d,e)** Excision of the pathological bone and periosteum performed, followed by insertion of a telescopic (growing) rod and a circular frame to 'transport' a healthy segment of tibial diaphysis to fill the defect. **(f,g)** Following frame removal, the new bone (regenerate) has formed and union is achieved.

intellectual impairment. They may become wheelchair-bound at a young age.

MORQUIO–BRAILSFORD (MPS IV)

Individuals affected with MPS IV have a normal face and intellect in contrast to most MPS subtypes and affected individuals often survive into adulthood.

The most striking features are short stature with disproportionate spinal involvement (**8.17**), barrel chest with pectus carinatum and a short neck. Limb abnormalities include coronal knee malalignment and joint stiffness.

SCHEIE SYNDROME (MPS V)

This has been reclassified as a subtype of MPS I.

MAROTEAUX–LAMY SYNDROME (MPS VI)

MPS VI presents with a similar but milder clinical picture than type I. Intellect is unaffected and the prognosis tends to be better with longer life expectancy.

Treatment

Treatment is supportive and deals with specific symptomatic areas. *Effective management* requires early, accurate biochemical diagnosis, so that the prognosis for an individual patient can be predicted. Enzyme replacement is currently available for types I and IV and has been effective in reducing non-neurological symptoms and pain. Bone marrow transplantation and umbilical cord blood transplantation have been used in selected cases with variable and unpredictable outcomes.

Surgery to remove tonsils and adenoids may improve airway obstruction. Corneal transplantation can improve vision in patients with significant corneal clouding.

Orthopaedic surgery has a role in correction of deformity in the spine, hips, knees and feet. Conditions with a slow rate of progression and a good life expectancy may benefit from corrective surgery. Surgical stabilization of the spine may be necessary to protect cardio-respiratory function and preserve sitting balance. Standing and walking function may require release of joint contractures or surgical release to produce plantigrade feet.

Gaucher's disease

Gaucher's disease is an autosomal recessive disease caused by mutation of the glucocerebrosidase gene

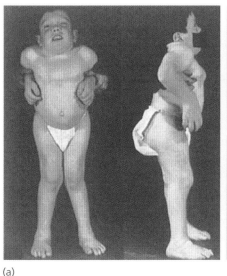
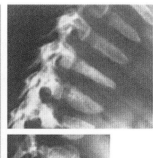
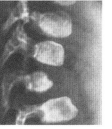
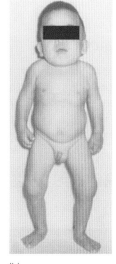

(a)   (b)

8.17 Mucopolysaccharidoses (a) A young boy showing the characteristic features of Morquio–Brailsford syndrome. **(b)** A child with Hunter's syndrome.

responsible for the breakdown of lipid-rich cell membranes in red and white blood cells. The condition is characterized by accumulation of glucocerebroside in macrophages. The estimated global prevalence is 1 : 40 000 live births and is substantially more common in the Ashkenazi population.

Clinical features

These include hepatosplenomegaly, pancytopenia and recurrent infections. Orthopaedic manifestations include stiff joints, osteopenia with vertebral compression and femoral fractures. Osteonecrosis is a frequent feature and affects femoral and humeral heads, femoral condyles and the talus (e8.5). Chronic bone pain is common and affected individuals can present acutely with a 'bone crisis' characterized by severe pain, pyrexia, leucocytosis and elevated inflammatory markers, which is difficult to discriminate from septic arthritis and osteomyelitis.

Imaging

Radiological features include areas of patchy radiolucency within cancellous bone. Flaring of the femoral condyles produces the 'Erlenmeyer flask appearance'. Plain radiographs are used to identify complications including fractures, and femoral head osteonecrosis is identified and quantified with MRI.

Treatment

- *Enzyme replacement therapy* is an effective treatment, although the skeletal abnormalities are the slowest to respond and may not recover.
- *Hip arthroplasty* is often required to manage osteonecrosis of the femoral head.

CHROMOSOME DISORDERS

Chromosome disorders are common but they usually result in fetal abortion. Of the non-lethal conditions, several produce bone or joint abnormalities. Three of the less rare conditions are described here.

DOWN'S SYNDROME (TRISOMY 21)

This condition results from having an extra copy of chromosome 21. It is much more common than any of the skeletal dysplasias, with an overall incidence of 1 : 800 live births – and 1 : 250 if the mother is over 37 years of age. Affected infants can be recognized at birth: the head is foreshortened and the eyes slant upwards, with prominent epicanthic folds; the nose is flattened, the lips are parted and the tongue protrudes (8.18). There may be abnormal palmar creases, clinodactyly and spreading of the first and second toes. The babies are unusually floppy (hypotonic) and skeletal development is delayed. Children are short and, because of their characteristic facial appearance, they tend to resemble each other. They show varying degrees of learning difficulty. Joint laxity (8.19) may lead to sprains or subluxation (e.g. of the patella).

Associated anomalies, particularly cardiac defects, are common, and there is diminished resistance to infection. The average life expectancy is about 50 years.

There is no specific treatment but surgery can offer considerable cosmetic improvement. Attentive care will allow many of these individuals to pursue a pleasant and productive life.

TURNER'S SYNDROME

Congenital female hypogonadism is a rare abnormality caused by a defective or non-functioning X chromosome. Those affected are phenotypically female, with a normal vagina and uterus, but the ovaries are markedly hypoplastic or absent. Patients are short, with webbing of the neck, barrel chest and increased carrying angle of the elbows.

Cardiovascular and renal abnormalities are common. Women have primary amenorrhoea, and hypogonadism leads to early-onset osteoporosis.

Treatment consists of oestrogen replacement from puberty onwards.

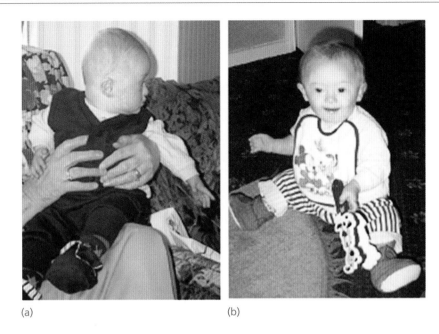

(a) (b)

8.18 Down's syndrome (a,b) An 11-month-old child with Down's syndrome. Note the shape of the head.

KLINEFELTER'S SYNDROME

Klinefelter's syndrome, a form of male hypogonadism, occurs in about 1 per 1000 males. Those affected have more than one X chromosome (as well as the usual Y chromosome). They are recognizably male, but they have eunuchoid proportions, with gynaecomastia and under-developed testicles. The condition should be borne in mind as a cause of osteoporosis in men.

Treatment with androgens may improve bone mass.

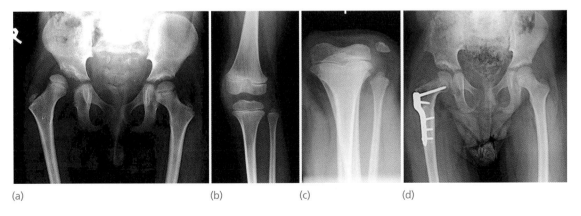

(a) (b) (c) (d)

8.19 Down's syndrome Radiographs of a 10-year-old child with Down's syndrome. The right hip was subluxing **(a)** and the left patella was dislocated laterally **(b)** due to profound associated ligamentous laxity. He underwent patella realignment **(c)** and a varus hip osteotomy with pelvic osteotomy **(d)**.

LOCALIZED MALFORMATIONS

Localized malformations of the vertebrae or limbs are common. The majority cause no disability and may be discovered incidentally during investigation of some other disorder. Some have a genetic background and similar malformations are seen in association with generalized skeletal dysplasia. Most are sporadic and probably non-genetic – i.e. caused by injury to the developing embryo, especially during the first 3 months of pregnancy. In some cases, there is a known teratogenic agent (e.g. maternal infection or drug administration). Usually, however, the exact cause is unknown.

VERTEBRAL ANOMALIES

There are three main kinds of vertebral anomaly. Associated visceral anomalies (lower intestinal and urogenital defects) are common in sacral dysgenesis and dysraphism.

TYPES OF VERTEBRAL ANOMALY	
Agenesis	Complete absence of one or more vertebrae
Dysgenesis	Errors of segmentation causing hemivertebrae, with or without vertebrae fused together
Dysraphism	Deficiencies of the neural arch (e.g. spina bifida)

CONGENITAL SHORT NECK (KLIPPEL–FEIL SYNDROME)

This condition (also known as *cervical–vertebral synostosis*) is due to failure of vertebral segmentation. Associated anomalies are common and include hemivertebrae, posterior arch defects, cervical meningomyelocele, thoracic defects, scapular elevation and visceral abnormalities involving the renal and cardiorespiratory systems.

Occasionally, a familial pattern of inheritance is noted, suggesting a genetic aetiology.

X-rays may show fusion of the lower cervical vertebrae and various combinations of the associated disorders, together with scoliosis or kyphosis. The natural history of the condition often depends on the severity of the visceral anomalies.

Orthopaedic treatment is usually unnecessary. However, cervical instability in an adjacent hypermobile segment may call for surgical fusion.

SPRENGEL'S DEFORMITY

This condition, which usually occurs sporadically, represents a failure of scapular descent from the cervical spine. The high scapula may still be attached to the spine by a tough fibrous band or a cartilaginous bar (the omovertebral bar) (**8.20**). Associated vertebral or rib anomalies are quite common.

Treatment is required only if shoulder movements are severely limited or if the deformity is particularly unsightly. Operation is best performed before the age of 6 years. The vertebroscapular muscles are released from the spine, the supraspinous part of the scapula is excised together with the omovertebral bar and the scapula is repositioned by tightening the lower muscles. Great care is needed as there is a risk of injury to the accessory nerve or the brachial plexus.

THORACOSPINAL ANOMALIES

Segmentation defects in the thoracic region usually involve the ribs as well (e.g. hemivertebrae may be associated with fusion of adjacent ribs or other types of dysplasia). Some of these disorders are of autosomal dominant inheritance.

Clinically, patients present in childhood with scoliosis or kyphoscoliosis (**8.21**), sometimes leading to paraplegia. X-rays may show various combinations of thoracic vertebral fusion or dysgenesis and rib anomalies, together with scoliosis and marked distortion of the thorax.

Operative treatment may be needed for threatened cord compression.

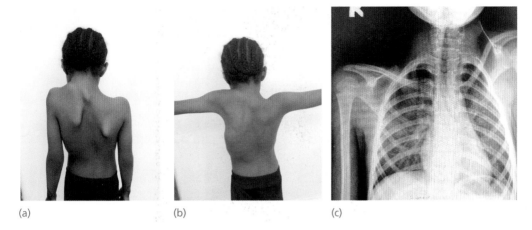

(a)   (b)   (c)

8.20 Sprengel's deformity (a,b) Note the high-riding left scapula, prominent medial border and limited shoulder abduction, due to an omovertebral bar **(c)**.

SACRAL AGENESIS

This term describes a group of conditions in which part or all of the distal spine is missing (**8.22**). Variable motor deficiencies are noted below the lowest level of normal spine but sensation is often preserved more distally. Other deformities of the lower limb may be present and, as with congenital scoliosis, there may be associated cardiac, visceral and renal abnormalities. Some cases of sacral agenesis appear to be inherited in either an autosomal or sex-linked dominant fashion.

Spina bifida is the commonest vertebral anomaly. This condition is discussed in Chapter 10.

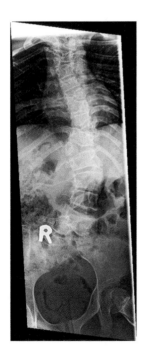

8.21 Congenital scoliosis Multiple hemivertebrae present causing the scoliosis, most clearly seen at L5 and T12.

LIMB ANOMALIES

Localized malformations of the limbs include extra bones, absent bones, hypoplastic bones and fusions. Most of the anomalies involving limb reductions are due to embryonal insults between the 4th and 6th weeks of gestation. Some are genetically determined and these usually have an autosomal dominant pattern of inheritance. Only the more important and less rare conditions will be described here.

TYPES OF LIMB ANOMALY	
Amelia	Complete absence of a limb
Phocomelia	Almost complete absence of a limb
Ectromelia	Partial absence of a limb

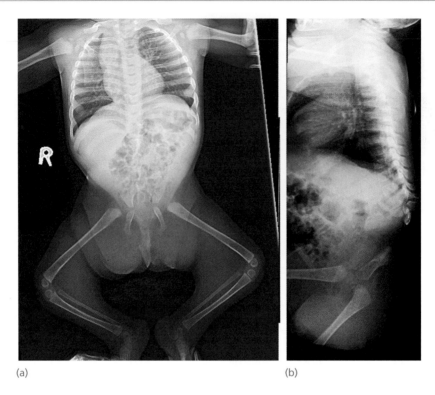

(a)   (b)

8.22 Sacral agenesis (a,b) Radiographs of an infant with complete aplasia of vertebrae below T12. The patient will often have the lower legs in a cross-legged or 'Buddha' position. The lower extremities typically have a severe neurological deficit.

A limb may be completely or partially absent; defects may be transverse or axial. In the hands and feet, *brachydactyly, syndactyly, polydactyly* and *symphalangism* are among the many possibilities.

> ⚠ Always remember that function may be satisfactory even if the appearance is not. Before any surgical treatment is considered, review what side effects there might be and how to achieve the most acceptable balance between *function*, *appearance* and *pain*. A hand that functions better but is painful may not be useful to a particular patient.

PSEUDARTHROSIS OF THE CLAVICLE

The child usually presents with a lump over the midclavicular region, almost always on the right side (**8.23**) – except in cases of dextrocardia! Sometimes there is obvious mobility at the pseudarthrosis site and, over time, this may become painful.

While occasional familial autosomal dominant cases have been described, the true aetiology is unknown; other theories such as external compression from the subclavian artery or a failure of coalescence of the two intramembranous centres of ossification have been proposed.

TRANSVERSE DEFICIENCY OF THE ARM

Transverse deficiency of the distal part of the arm will leave a simple stump below a normal elbow. This can be managed by fitting a prosthesis with a mechanical facility for grasp.

RADIAL DEFICIENCY

The forearm is short and bowed; the hand is under-developed and markedly deviated towards

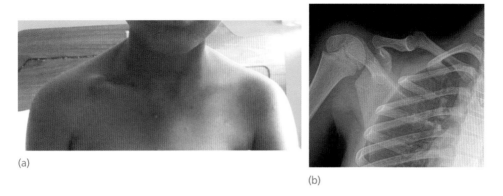

(a)

(b)

8.23 Congenital pseudarthrosis of the clavicle This child has a distinct lump over the midclavicular region **(a)** which shows clearly on X-ray **(b)**. Treatment is only advocated if there is pain or concern regarding cosmesis. Union can be reliably achieved with plate fixation and bone graft.

the radial side (*radial club hand*) and the thumb may be missing. The elbow is often also abnormal (**8.24**). In about half of cases the condition is bilateral.

The clinical deformity may look bizarre but children often acquire excellent function. If this seems unlikely, operative reconstruction

may be advisable. This could involve pollicization of a digit and other complex reconstructive procedures.

In a young child, simple stretching and splinting may help to improve hand and wrist position until further options need to be considered.

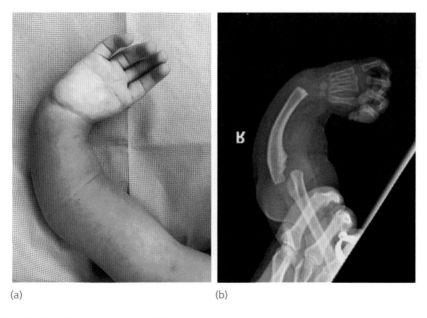

(a)

(b)

8.24 Radial dysplasia (a,b) This 2-year-old has complete absence of the radius and the thumb. The ulna has a significant bow. There is an association with cardiac and haematological pathologies, requiring preoperative evaluation. Centralizing the wrist on the ulna (with or without corrective osteotomies) and creating a thumb from the index finger (pollicization) can improve function.

ULNAR DEFICIENCY

- *Hypoplasia* of the distal end of the ulna is usually seen as part of a generalized dysplasia, but occasionally it occurs alone. The radius is bowed (as if growth is tethered on the ulnar side) and the radial head may dislocate; the wrist is deviated

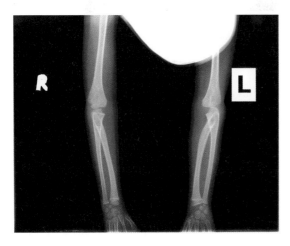

8.25 Congenital radioulnar synostosis There is an absence of the normal proximal radial head. The proximal radius is fused with the ulna resulting in a block to forearm rotation. Most patients are in a functional position and so are managed non-operatively. Rotational osteotomy through the fusion mass may be considered for a hyper-pronated hand position that interferes with normal function.

medially. Only if function is severely disturbed should wrist stabilization be advised.
- *Congenital absence* of the ulna is extremely rare; overall function is severely restricted. Operative reconstruction may provide some improvement.

RADIOULNAR SYNOSTOSIS

This is often associated with a posterolateral dislocation of the radial head (**8.25**). Clinically there is complete loss of pronation and supination. This movement cannot be regained with surgery but improvement in the resting position of the forearm (and hence of the hand) can be achieved.

DIGITAL ANOMALIES

A variety of anomalies can occur, ranging from simple soft-tissue 'extra digits' (which are easy to excise) to complex syndactylies that restrict hand function (**8.26**). They may occur alone or in conjunction with more generalized skeletal dysplasias.

FEMORAL DEFICIENCY (CONGENITAL SHORT FEMUR)

In its most benign form, femoral dysplasia consists merely of shortening of the bone with a

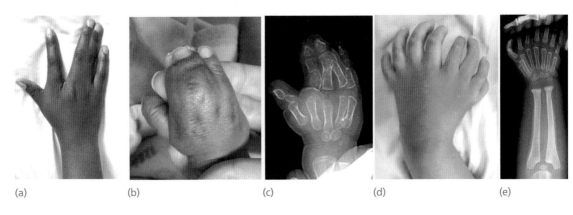

(a)　　　　　(b)　　　　　(c)　　　　　(d)　　　　　(e)

8.26 Digital anomalies (a) Simple syndactyly of the middle and ring finger with normal phalanges; **(b,c)** complex syndactyly in Apert's syndrome with fusion of the middle and ring finger phalanges and joints; **(d,e)** 'mirror hand' (ulnar dimelia) that was managed with removal of three digits and pollicization of the fourth extra digit.

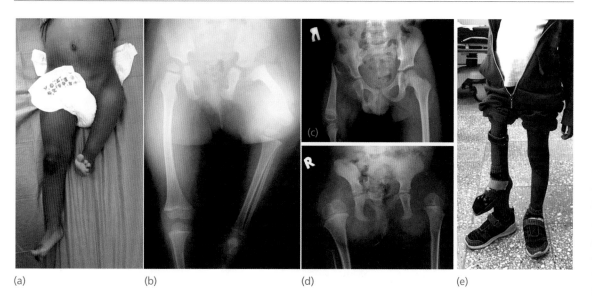

(a) (b) (d) (e)

8.27 Spectrum of pathology of congenital short femur (a,b) A 2-year-old child with a short femur and coxa vara; **(c)** congenital femoral deficiency with absence of hip joint; **(d)** bilateral absent femora; **(e)** child managed with an extension prosthesis.

normal hip and knee. This can be dealt with by limb lengthening procedures or, if shortening is very marked, by adding a distal orthosis. More severe grades of proximal femoral dysplasia are encountered, some associated with coxa vara. (The most widely used classification is that of Aitkin, as illustrated in **e8.6**.)

Coxa vara with moderate shortening of the shaft can be dealt with by corrective osteotomy and limb lengthening. Severe degrees of coxa vara, sometimes associated with pseudarthrosis of the femoral neck, may result in marked shortening of the femur.

In the worst cases, most of the femoral shaft is missing, the knee is situated at thigh level and the foot hangs where the knee is normally expected to be (**8.27**, **e8.7**). If the deformity is bilateral and symmetrical, walking is possible and some individuals acquire remarkable agility; however, they may still seek treatment to overcome the severe cosmetic problem. Unilateral deformities are not only unsightly but also very disabling. Effective limb lengthening is out of the question, and fitting a prosthesis to a short limb with flexion deformities of the 'hip' and knee and a foot jutting forwards where the knee-hinge of

the prosthesis will lie is a daunting prospect. One alternative is to fuse the knee in a functional position, amputate the foot and fit a suitable prosthesis.

TIBIAL DEFICIENCY

Tibial dysplasia (or *hemimelia*) is very rare (**8.28**): several forms exist and the condition may be associated with other limb anomalies. Prognosis, and hence treatment, depend on the quality of the knee joint and integrity of the quadriceps mechanism: if there is no ability for knee extension, a knee disarticulation must be considered. If the ankle cannot be reconstructed, a distal amputation may be required.

FIBULAR DEFICIENCY

This is the most common long-bone deficiency. Mild fibular dysplasia (or hemimelia) causes little shortening or deformity; however, complete absence of the fibula leads to considerable shortening of the leg, bowing of the tibia and valgus deformity of the unsupported ankle (**8.29**).

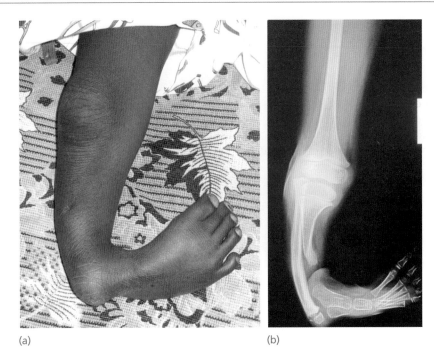

(a)   (b)

8.28 Tibia hemimelia (a,b) Short tibia, no ankle articulation but with an intact extensor mechanism. A below-knee amputation was performed and prosthesis supplied.

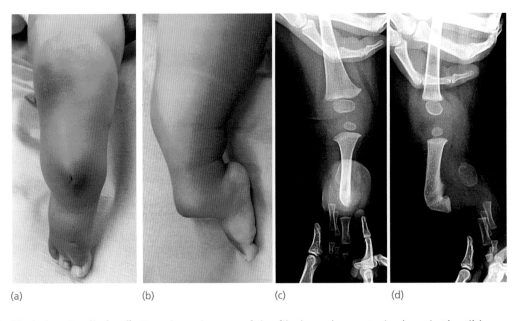

(a)   (b)   (c)   (d)

8.29 Fibula hemimelia (a–d) Complete absence of the fibula and an anterior bow in the tibia. Reconstruction is possible with correction of the tibial deformity, ankle stabilization and limb lengthening when the child is older.

There may also be absence of the fourth and fifth rays of the foot and under-development of the entire limb. Sometimes, if only the distal fibula is absent, there is a fibrous band/anlage in its place. Excision of this remnant may permit correction of the valgus deformity.

In severe cases, management is dictated by the quality of the foot and by the percentage growth inhibition. This can be calculated by a variety of methods and allows good prediction of final limb length discrepancy at skeletal maturity. Once this is known, treatment can be planned. Options range from partial amputation and the use of a prosthetic limb to epiphyseodesis of the longer limb and one or more limb lengthening procedures involving distraction osteogenesis techniques and ring external fixators. Reconstructive techniques such as these rely on a high degree of compliance from the child and their family over a long time span. In contrast, modern advances in amputation prosthetics may provide a more acceptable outcome.

CONGENITAL PSEUDARTHROSIS OF THE TIBIA

 Almost 50% of patients with congenital pseudarthrosis have some evidence of NF. The condition is discussed in more detail in 'Neurofibromatosis' above.

This rare condition is usually diagnosed in early infancy. The child may be born with a fractured tibia, or the bone may be attenuated and then fracture some months later. In either case, the fracture fails to unite, or heals very poorly, only to fracture again shortly afterwards. This is an intractable condition which will not yield to ordinary forms of fracture treatment.

Tumours

9

- Epidemiology — 161
- Classification — 161
- Staging — 162
- Clinical presentation — 163
- Investigations — 164
- Investigating the 'suspicious bone lesion' — 166
- Principles of management of primary tumours of bone — 167
- Benign lesions of bone — 169
- Primary malignant bone tumours — 179
- Metastatic bone disease — 191
- Soft-tissue tumours — 192

EPIDEMIOLOGY

Bone and soft tissue sarcomas comprise a family of tumours derived from mesenchymal tissue. Even when considered together, they are rare comprising less than 1% of all new cancer diagnoses.

Soft-tissue sarcomas occur comparatively more frequently, with an incidence of 45 cases per million of the population. The incidence of bone and soft-tissue sarcomas is marginally higher in males than females. In the case of soft-tissue sarcomas, the incidence increases with age, with the highest incidence occurring in males over 85 years. A female preponderance is seen between 50 and 60 years of age due to the higher incidence of gynaecological sarcomas in this age group.

In contrast, bone sarcomas demonstrate a bimodal distribution in both males and females, with peaks of incidence seen in both teenage/ adolescent years and the elderly.

More than 60% of tumours of bone will arise from the long bones of the lower limb, particularly around the knee. A further 18% will arise from the bones of the pelvis, sacrum or coccyx, and 13% from the upper limb or shoulder girdle.

CLASSIFICATION

Tumours of bone and soft tissue are classified on the basis of their principle cell type, and have been classified by the World Health Organization (WHO). Tissue diagnosis is essential to predict the natural history and treatment of the lesion. In the case of soft-tissue sarcomas, the histological grade of the lesion is classified according to the Federation Nationale des Centres de Lutte Contre le Cancer (FNCLCC) system, which has demonstrated correlation between grade and outcome for soft-tissue sarcomas.

In contrast to soft-tissue sarcomas, tumours of bone can vary widely in their behaviour. Their histological subtype often determines the grade of bone tumour as there is no universally accepted grading system. Ewing's sarcoma and dedifferentiated chondrosarcoma are high-grade lesions, whereas parosteal osteosarcoma, though still a malignant lesion of bone, is considered a low-grade lesion.

- *Benign lesions* are defined as those that do not invade surrounding tissue or spread elsewhere in the body. Most benign bone tumours have

SECTION 1 GENERAL ORTHOPAEDICS

a limited capacity for recurrence and when this does occur, it does so in a non-destructive manner. Surgical resection, therefore, is often curative. Benign lesions can demonstrate a wide variety of behaviours with some benign lesions being *latent* or inactive (e.g. non-ossifying fibroma (NOF)), while others are active, with a higher risk of recurrence after treatment (e.g. aneurysmal bone cyst (ABC)).

- *Intermediate (locally aggressive) lesions* can destroy bone and surrounding tissue (e.g. osteoblastoma). They often recur and are associated with an infiltrative and locally destructive growth pattern. Recurrence is frequent following limited surgical treatment and sometimes en bloc resection is required to completely remove the lesion.

- *Intermediate (rarely metastasizing) lesions* often behave in a similar way to locally aggressive lesions but occasionally demonstrate the ability to spread to distant sites. The risk of such spread is <2%, is often not fatal and is not reliably predictable from the histological appearance. The classic example is the giant-cell tumour (GCT) of bone.

- *Malignant tumours* are truly aggressive with the potential for both local extension and metastases to distant sites. The aggressiveness of a tumour is defined by the histological grade. Low-grade tumours (e.g. chordoma) have a slow rate of growth and metastases are less common, but they can arise many years after initial diagnosis. High-grade tumours have a very high risk of metastasizing, ranging from 20% to 100%, and are locally invasive (e.g. osteosarcoma and Ewing's sarcoma).

When necessary, the grade of primary malignant tumours of bone is based on the cellularity and nuclear features of the cells. In general, the higher the grade, the more cellular the tumour. Higher-grade lesions have a >25% risk of local recurrence and distant spread, whereas low-grade lesions have a <25% risk of local recurrence and metastases.

STAGING

Staging is the process of assessing the extent of a tumour both locally and distantly. As a consequence of most bone and soft-tissue sarcomas metastasizing via the bloodstream, the lungs are the most common site for metastases, although other sites may include bone, lymph nodes, liver and other soft-tissue locations.

THE BASIS OF ALL STAGING SYSTEMS

Grade of the tumour (a measure of the aggressiveness of the tumour – high, intermediate or low)
Size of the tumour
Local extent
Presence of metastases

The classic staging system for primary tumours of bone is the *Enneking system*. Developed as a reference to aid the extent of surgical resection in primary tumours of bone, the Enneking staging system classifies tumours according to whether they are high or low grade, whether there are metastases present or not, and whether the tumour has grown out of its original compartment or remains confined to a compartment. A compartment, for the purposes of this system, is defined as an enclosed tissue space, such as a bone, a joint space or a muscle group confined by its fascial envelope.

ENNEKING STAGING SYSTEM

Stage 1A	Low-grade, intracompartmental tumour
Stage 1B	Low-grade, extracompartmental tumour
Stage 2A	High-grade, intracompartmental tumour
Stage 2B	High-grade, extracompartmental tumour
Stage 3	Any of the above with metastases

More recently, the more conventional *tumour–node–metastasis (TNM) staging* has been applied to primary sarcomas of bone. This takes into consideration the histological subtype, size, continuity, grade, and local and distant spread of the tumour. This application to bone tumours has limitations (e.g. due to the rarity of lymph-node metastases), but the system has gained favour for the staging of soft-tissue sarcomas and has been adopted by the American Joint Committee on Cancer (AJCC) and the Union for International Cancer Control (UICC). In this system, size is dichotomized to small (<5 cm for soft-tissue sarcomas, <8 cm for bone sarcomas) or large (>5 cm for soft-tissue sarcomas, >8 cm for bone sarcomas).

TNM STAGING SYSTEM	
Stage 1A	Low-grade, small, no metastases
Stage 1B	Low-grade, large, no metastases
Stage 2A	Intermediate- or high-grade, small, no metastases
Stage 2B	Intermediate-grade, large, no metastases
Stage 3	High-grade, large, no metastases
Stage 4	Any with metastases

The *Kaplan–Meier survival curve* is a graphical representation of effect of stage on prognosis for bone sarcomas (**9.1**).

CLINICAL PRESENTATION

The diagnosis of bone and soft-tissue sarcomas is often delayed. Physicians, particularly

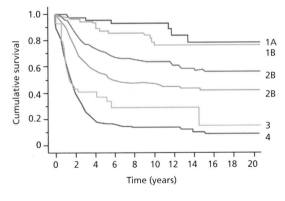

9.1 Kaplan–Meier survival curve The graph shows the effect of stage on prognosis for all bone sarcomas (Royal Orthopaedic Hospital Oncology Service data).

those dealing with children and adolescents, must maintain a high index of suspicion for malignancy. Patients may be asymptomatic until the lesion is discovered incidentally on radiographs, common for benign lesions, or for malignant lesions arising in areas where there is room for innocuous expansion, such as the pelvis, where tumours can achieve a very large size prior to presentation. In an attempt to rectify these delays in diagnosis, the National Institute for Health and Care Excellence (NICE) in the UK issued guidelines for the improvement in care for patients presenting with sarcomas.

Age is often a consistent feature for primary bone tumours; osteosarcoma and Ewing's sarcoma have preponderance in children, adolescents and young adults, while chondrosarcoma typically occurs in older patients. With increasing age, the likelihood of a bone lesion being the result of metastatic disease increases, and the investigation of any pathological lesion of bone in an elderly patient must include an attempt to identify a potential primary malignancy elsewhere.

 In patients over 70 years of age, the incidence of metastatic bone disease is greater than that of all primary bone tumours in any age group.

The most common symptom experienced by a patient with a bone tumour is *pain*. Night pain is a particularly worrying symptom that should always cause concern. Other worrisome features include family history and previous radiotherapy. Presentation with a *pathological fracture* has been reported in 5–12% of osteosarcomas and up to 21% of chondrosarcomas, and in the case of benign lesions is suggestive of a locally aggressive lesion. Prodromal symptoms of worsening functional pain are common and, in children in particular, a fracture with a disproportionate level of injury (e.g. fall from standing height) should stimulate further investigation. Certain fracture patterns should raise concern for an underlying lesion, such as supracondylar femoral fractures in children, and avulsion fractures of the lesser trochanter in adults. In elderly patients with diaphyseal long-bone fractures, the possibility of a pathological fracture should be considered.

Clinical findings in the case of primary bone tumours are often non-specific. *Swelling* and *tenderness* over the affected bone are the most common findings.

In the case of soft-tissue sarcomas, the majority present as a painless, enlarging mass. The rapidity of enlargement is often suggestive of a malignant process, though this does not accurately differentiate benign from a more sinister pathology. All superficial soft-tissue lesions measuring greater than 5 cm and all deep-seated lesions should be considered a sarcoma until proven otherwise.

INVESTIGATIONS

X-rays

All patients with the suspicion of a bone lesion should be investigated with plain X-rays. There may be an obvious abnormality in the bone (e.g. cortical thickening), a 'cyst', or ill-defined destruction (**Table 9.1**). The location within the bone and whether the lesion is solitary or multiple should be noted (**9.2**). The periphery of the lesion, whether it is well-defined or ill-defined, should also be noted.

When assessing a suspicious lesion on X-ray, there are a number of questions that should be asked.

Table 9.1 Possible diagnosis based on radiographic appearances, divided by age group

Age (years)	Well-circumscribed lesion	Ill-defined lesions	Sclerotic lesions
0–10	Eosinophilic granuloma Simple bone cyst	Eosinophilic granuloma Ewing's sarcoma Leukaemia	Osteosarcoma
10–20	Non-ossifying fibroma Osteoblastoma Fibrous dysplasia Eosinophilic granuloma Simple bone cyst Aneurysmal bone cyst Chondroblastoma Chondromyxoid fibroma	Ewing's sarcoma Eosinophilic granuloma Osteosarcoma	Osteosarcoma Fibrous dysplasia Eosinophilic granuloma Osteoid osteoma Osteoblastoma
20–40	Giant-cell tumour Enchondroma Low-grade chondrosarcoma Brown tumour Osteoblastoma	Giant-cell tumour	Enchondroma Bone island Parosteal osteosarcoma Burnt-out lesion: • Non-ossifying fibroma • Eosinophilic granuloma • Simple bone cyst • Aneurysmal bone cyst • Chondroblastoma
40+	Metastases Myeloma Geode	Metastases Myeloma High-grade chondrosarcoma	Metastases Bone island
All ages	Infection	Infection	Infection

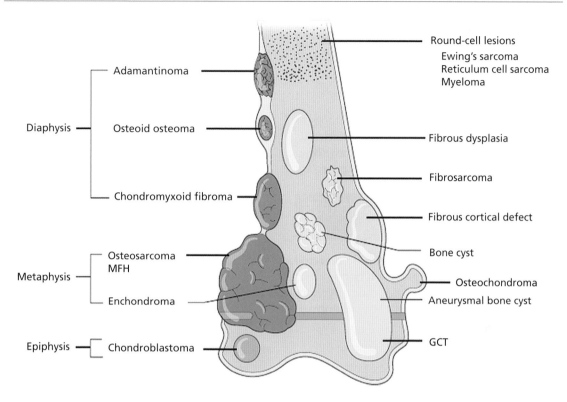

9.2 Potential diagnoses The location of the lesion within the bone is significant. MFH: malignant fibrous histiocytoma.

QUESTIONS TO ASK WHEN ASSESSING AN X-RAY

What is the age of the patient?
Which bone is affected?
Where in the bone is the lesion?
What is the lesion doing to the bone: is it osteolytic, osteoblastic or mixed?
What is the bone doing in response?
Is there a periosteal reaction?
Is there an associated soft-tissue mass?
What is the nature of the matrix: is it osteoid, chondroid or fibroid?
Is the lesion solitary or are there multiple lesions?

Radionuclide scanning

Scanning with ^{99m}Tc-methyl diphosphonate (^{99m}Tc-MDP) shows non-specific reactive changes in bone which can be helpful in revealing the site of a small tumour (e.g. an osteoid osteoma). Skeletal scintigraphy is also useful for detecting skip lesions and evidence of metastatic disease as part of the initial staging process.

Computed tomography

Computed tomography (CT) extends the range of X-ray diagnosis; it shows more accurately both intraosseous and extraosseous extension of the tumour and the relationship to surrounding structures. CT is essential to complete systemic staging and restaging in bone and soft-tissue sarcomas and metastatic disease to identify pulmonary metastases.

Magnetic resonance imaging

Magnetic resonance imaging (MRI) allows further characterization of lesions and defines the local extent of the lesion. Its greatest value is in the assessment of tumour spread:

- within the bone
- into a nearby joint
- into the soft tissues.

Blood vessels and the relationship of the tumour to the perivascular space are well defined, which aids greatly in preoperative assessment and the prediction of resection margins for limb-salvage surgery.

INVESTIGATING THE 'SUSPICIOUS BONE LESION'

In many cases, an abnormality will be detected radiologically but the diagnosis will not be clear. These patients require more specific investigation.

The differential diagnosis of a bone abnormality will depend on:

- the age of the patient
- the location of the lesion
- the radiographic or MRI characteristics of the lesion.

Investigating a suspicious bone lesion should follow well-established steps.

1. Always start with a thorough *history and examination*, looking, for instance, in an older patient at possible symptoms or signs of other malignancy. The usual primary sites that metastasize to bone are bronchus, breast, prostate, kidney and thyroid, and all of these need to be considered as possible primary sites in an older patient with a destructive bone lesion.
2. If the diagnosis is not clear on *plain X-rays*, carry out an *MRI scan* to delineate the extent of the lesion in the bone and other tissues. *CT scans* of the chest, abdomen and pelvis will be helpful to identify occult primary carcinomas.
3. *Biochemical tests* will help to exclude prostate cancer (prostate-specific antigen (PSA)) or myeloma (serum electrophoresis and urinary Bence–Jones proteins) as possible causes.
4. In older patients with the possibility of the lesion being metastatic, a *bone scan* is indicated to assess if the lesion is solitary or multiple.

5. *Other blood tests* may give useful information (e.g. raised calcium may indicate hyperparathyroidism, or raised alkaline phosphatase (ALP) may indicate Paget's disease, which is a prognostic factor in osteosarcoma). In the case of a suspected brown tumour, serum parathyroid hormone (PTH) will be elevated.

 Remember that infection can be a great mimic of tumours.

Biopsy

Biopsy remains the gold standard for obtaining a diagnosis in an abnormal lesion of bone. There are several principles in carrying out a biopsy that must be considered.

PRINCIPLES OF BIOPSY

The biopsy tract must be sited to minimize potential contamination of normal tissues and should be planned in conjunction with the surgeon who will carry out any definitive surgery.

The biopsy must be taken from representative tissue.

Image-guided biopsies should be used to reduce the risk of a sampling error.

Complete haemostasis must be achieved.

Samples should always be sent for microbiology as well as histology.

The pathologist reporting the biopsy must have an appropriate level of experience.

If there is a risk of fracture following biopsy, the bone must be appropriately splinted.

Most bone biopsies are now done with either fluoroscopic or CT guidance and in most large centres *needle biopsies* will provide adequate tissue for diagnosis (**9.3**).

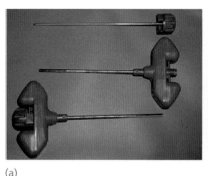
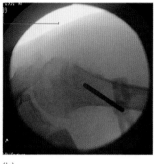
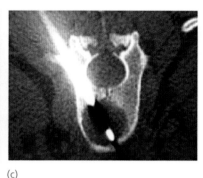

(a)   (b)   (c)

9.3 Biopsy (a) The majority of biopsies are now performed with a core needle, such as a Jamshidi needle. The procedure is often performed with radiographic guidance, either as fluoroscopy **(b)**, or under CT guidance **(c)**.

In the case of a non-diagnostic needle biopsy or if a needle biopsy could place neurovascular structures at risk, an *open biopsy* may be considered. The site is selected so that it can be included in any subsequent operation.

PRINCIPLES OF MANAGEMENT OF PRIMARY TUMOURS OF BONE

The management of patients with bone sarcomas must be carried out by a multidisciplinary team including clinicians, pathologists, radiologists and oncologists.

PRINCIPLES OF SURGICAL TREATMENT AND DEFINITION OF MARGINS

The resection of all detectable tumours, including metastases, is the cornerstone of treatment of the majority of sarcomas of bone. For primary operable tumours, the options are *tumour excision with limb salvage* or *amputation*.

Tumour resection should excise a clear margin including the pseudocapsule of the tumour and a cuff of normal tissue (e9.1).

- Many benign lesions can be managed by *intralesional excision*. This implies removal by debulking.

- A *marginal excision*, going around the edge of the lesion, will usually be sufficient to completely remove and control a benign or intermediate lesion but will usually be insufficient for a malignant tumour as there are likely to be tumour cells in the tissues left behind. This zone around a malignant tumour is known as the reactive zone and consists of tissues compressed by the expansion of the tumour, also known as the pseudocapsule. While it may appear to be a natural plane of dissection, it will often contain tumour cells. Surgical resection encroaching on the area of oedema around a tumour will also result in a high risk of local recurrence. This risk can be reduced with an effective adjuvant such as chemotherapy or radiotherapy in selected tumours, allowing a planned marginal excision of a malignant tumour (e.g. if the tumour is close to a critical structure such as a nerve or blood vessel) (9.4).
- A *wide excision* implies that the surgery has been carried out through completely normal tissue, well away from the tumour.

The key factor affecting the width of the margin is usually the closest critical structure – commonly the neurovascular bundle.

The decision between carrying out *limb salvage* or *amputation* is governed by the expected postoperative limb function, potential for complications, psychological acceptance and oncological

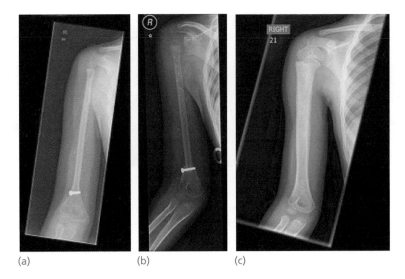

(a)   (b)   (c)

9.4 Osteosarcoma A 5-year old girl with an osteosarcoma of the proximal humerus. This was treated by neoadjuvant chemotherapy followed by resection of the tumour and reconstruction using a vascularized proximal fibular transfer, utilizing the perforating artery to the epiphysis to reconstruct the neo-humeral head **(a)**. Over time, the neo-humerus hypertrophies **(b)** and after 36 months **(c)** has achieved a comparable dimension to the contralateral humerus.

outcomes. Quality-of-life studies suggest that patients adapt equally well to amputation as limb salvage. Most importantly, no significant difference exists between the survival rates for amputation compared to limb salvage surgery.

 As survival is affected by the margins achieved at resection, limb salvage must not be favoured over amputation where the potential to compromise a complete resection exists.

> **OPTIONS FOR RECONSTRUCTION IN LIMB SALVAGE**
>
> Endoprosthetic replacement
> Allograft–prosthetic composite
> Allograft using donated bone extracorporeal sterilization and reimplantation of the patient's own bone
> Vascularized and non-vascularized autograft
> Arthrodesis

NEOADJUVANT AND ADJUVANT THERAPIES

Neoadjuvant chemotherapy

Neoadjuvant chemotherapy is used for most patients with osteosarcoma and Ewing's sarcoma.

In osteosarcoma, the principle drugs used are:

- doxorubicin
- cisplatin
- ifosfamide
- high-dose methotrexate.

The aim of this chemotherapy is to try to shrink the tumour while also treating the micrometastatic disease.

In cases of Ewing's sarcoma, most patients with apparently localized disease will have subclinical micrometastases and so any treatment must include systemic therapy in combination with local control through radiotherapy and/or surgery. As Ewing's sarcoma is often sensitive to chemotherapy, most patients will receive neoadjuvant chemotherapy, regardless of the extent of the local disease. Current regimens rely on vincristine, doxorubicin and cyclophosphamide, alternating with ifosfamide and etoposide. Multimodal neoadjuvant chemotherapy in Ewing's sarcoma will often produce a dramatic shrinkage of the tumour and reduction in symptoms.

Local control is achieved by surgical resection whenever possible.

High-energy irradiation

High-energy irradiation has long been used to destroy radiosensitive tumours or as adjuvant therapy before operation. The current indications, however, are more restricted. For highly sensitive tumours (such as Ewing's sarcoma), it offers an alternative to amputation or as an adjunct to surgery and chemotherapy.

In recent years, a number of focused conventional radiotherapy strategies, including intensity-modulated radiotherapy (IMRT), and non-conventional particle therapies (carbon ion and proton therapy) have demonstrated promising results in the treatment of primary tumours particularly in unresectable regions (especially chordomas), but also in the management of local recurrence.

LOCALLY ADVANCED DISEASE

As recurrence and hence survival is significantly affected by attaining a clear margin at local control, *amputation* must be considered for tumours which are unresectable by any other means. Such

tumours will often be extending out of the primary bone, violating a number of compartments, and will be encircling the neurovascular bundle. Amputation is required in approximately 15% of patients with primary bone tumours.

BENIGN LESIONS OF BONE

OSTEOCHONDROMA

An osteochondroma is a benign, cartilaginous neoplasm derived from an aberrant subperiosteal nest of physeal cartilage which grows and matures according to normal enchondral ossification. Osteochondromas are very frequent and more common in males. They typically present in adolescent years, during the final growth spurt, and most commonly occur in long bones, particularly the femur and humerus.

They normally present as a painless mass though can cause symptoms secondary to formation of an overlying bursa due to friction, or to activity-related discomfort. The lesion appears as a bony protuberance with well-defined limits, thin outer cortex and an inner cancellous structure. The pathognomonic feature is that the host bone flares from the cortex into the osteochondroma (**9.5, 9.6**). MRI demonstrates the classic cartilaginous cap.

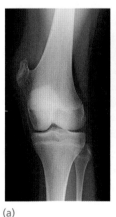
(a)

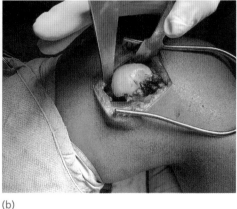
(b)

9.5 Osteochondroma (a) Radiograph demonstrating an osteochondroma of the distal femur. Note the characteristic features: pedunculated lesion growing away from the physis with cortical and medullary continuity. The lesion was removed due to discomfort. **(b)** Intraoperative image showing the cartilaginous surface on the pedunculated lesion.

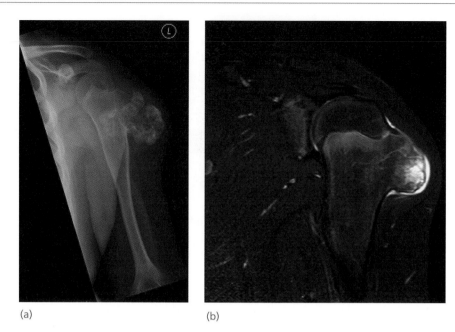

(a)   (b)

9.6 Osteochondroma A 14-year-old boy presented with a slowly enlarging mass over the left shoulder. Note the pedunculated, osseous lesion arising from the physis of the proximal humerus **(a)**. MRI demonstrates the characteristic features of a thin cartilage cap overlying a disorganized cancellous outgrowth which merges with the metaphyseal bone of the proximal humerus **(b)**.

Osteochondromas tend to grow with skeletal maturity and stop once growth stops. The risk of malignant transformation is about 1%. The risk of transformation is dependent on the size, with the cartilaginous cap being the source of neoplasia into chondrosarcoma. Malignant transformation is more common in the trunk, less common around the knee and exceptional in the extremities.

In asymptomatic lesions, *treatment* is not indicated. Excision may be warranted in large lesions where local pressure effects may occur or in adults where the risk of malignant transformation warrants removal.

For details on multiple hereditary exostosis, see Chapter 8.

Enchondroma

This is an intramedullary neoplasm made of well-differentiated hyaline cartilage. The exact incidence is unknown as the majority are asymptomatic and discovered incidentally. The commonest location is the tubular bones of the hand, followed by the femur and humerus.

Radiographically, the lesion is most commonly central with rounded, well-defined, lobulated edges and a thin rind of reactive sclerosis. MRI demonstrates the black signal voids of internal calcification and isotope bone scan is hot in most lesions.

Histologically, the lesion contains lobules of cartilage with areas of calcification. The diagnosis of an enchondroma can usually be made with X-rays (**9.7**). Treatment is usually not required although, occasionally in the hand, the lesion may be removed through curettage, particularly if there is pain or pathological fracture. Serial X-rays may be helpful if there is a suspicion of a grade 1 chondrosarcoma, as enchondromas in skeletal maturity do not grow.

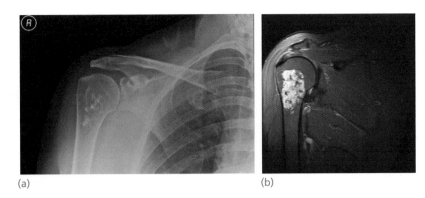

(a)   (b)

9.7 Enchondroma X-rays taken of a 65-year-old woman who presented with right shoulder pain demonstrate a 4 cm intraosseous chondroid lesion within the right proximal humerus (a). (b) Subsequent MRI demonstrates typical features of an enchondroma with a mixed cartilaginous lesion with areas of calcification but no evidence of endosteal scalloping or permeation. The shoulder pain was attributed to a full-thickness rotator cuff tear.

MULTIPLE CHONDROMAS AND ASSOCIATED CONDITIONS

Multiple chondromas are infrequent. In *Ollier's disease*, multiple chondromas may be found within the hand of one limb, or have a much wider, hemisomic distribution, or affect the entire body with a hemisomic prevalence. The disease is non-hereditary and sporadic. It most commonly affects the tubular bones of the hand or foot. Chondromas normally present as bony swellings in childhood which may cause deformities and limb length discrepancy due to epiphyseal fusion anomalies (e9.2).

In *Maffucci syndrome*, multiple chondromas are associated with multiple cutaneous or deep haemangiomas. On X-ray, the chondromas can be very large with consequent expansion of the bone, thinning of the cortex or, indeed, no cortex at all (9.8). In Maffucci syndrome, the presence of haemangioma may be seen on imaging by phleboliths.

Transformation to a secondary sarcoma is seen in both these conditions. In Ollier's disease, this may occur in 20–30% of patients; in Maffucci syndrome, in about 50%. Malignant transformation may be heralded by an increase in size of a lesion or the development of symptoms. Both conditions are associated with an increased risk of extraskeletal malignancies such as breast, liver, ovarian and central nervous system tumours.

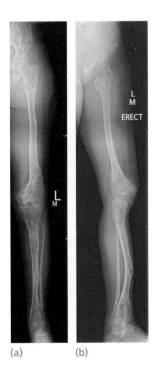

(a)   (b)

9.8 Maffucci syndrome A young woman, now in her thirties, with Maffucci syndrome with hemimelic involvement affecting virtually all the bones of her left side (a,b). Over the years she has had a number of low-grade malignancies removed with upper and lower limb ray amputations. She now presents with terrible pain from her knees and ankles due to the significant deformity resulting from her multiple chondromas.

CHONDROBLASTOMA

These are benign tumours of childhood. They occur most commonly at the epiphyses of long bones. They account for less than 1% of all bone neoplasms and are more common in males. The peak age of incidence is in teenage years, rare after the age of 35 and exceptional before the age of 10. They typically present with pain and can occasionally cause a joint effusion or stiffness. They appear as a round or oval lytic lesion ranging in size from 1 to 7 cm on X-ray. They appear within the epiphysis or apophysis and can cross the physis. The cortex may be expanded but often is not breached (e9.3).

The majority of cases can be treated with simple curettage with or without bone grafting to the defect to support the subchondral plate.

OSTEOID OSTEOMA

This is a small, benign tumour formed of osteoid and woven bone surrounded by a halo of reactive bone. These lesions are most common in young patients, but are rare below 5 years of age and equally rare over 30. They are more common in men than women. It is most commonly seen in the long bones, particularly the proximal femur. It is rare in the trunk with the exception of the spine where it is most often seen in the posterior arches. It is more often diaphyseal than metaphyseal.

Osteoid osteomas most often present with pain, which classically is worse at night and relieved by non-steroidal anti-inflammatory drugs (NSAIDs). When in close proximity to a joint, they can result in stiffness and an effusion. In the spine, they can cause muscle spasm and scoliosis.

Plain X-ray demonstrates an area of dense sclerosis with a small, rounded area of osteolysis which is often obscured by the surrounding sclerosis. Isotope bone scan is positive and the central nidus of the lesion is best seen on CT scan (9.9).

Without treatment, the lesion will slowly increase, but over time will regress and usually burns out over a variable period of a number of years. The preferred method of treatment is by CT-guided radiofrequency ablation.

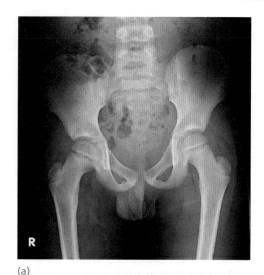

(a)

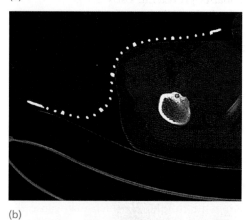

(b)

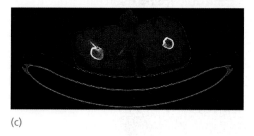

(c)

9.9 Osteoid osteoma A 9-year-old boy with a short history of worsening pain in the right groin which progressed to night pain. The pain was very responsive to non-steroidal analgesia. **(a)** X-rays demonstrate coarse trabecular thickening of the medial proximal femoral metaphysis. **(b)** CT scan demonstrates the characteristic nidus of an osteoid osteoma within the area of trabeculation. This was very effectively treated by CT-guided radiofrequency ablation **(c)**.

OSTEOBLASTOMA

This is a benign tumour of osteoblasts producing osteoid and woven bone. Similar in appearance to an osteoid osteoma, osteoblastomas are characteristically larger than osteoid osteomas. These are rare lesions most commonly seen in children and teenagers, rarely seen below the age of 8 or older than 40. Osteoblastoma have a predilection for the spine, again in the posterior arch, but can occur anywhere in the skeleton.

As with osteoid osteoma, osteoblastomas usually present with pain at the site of the tumour. In the spine, they can present with nerve root compression.

Histologically, the lesion consists of large osteoblasts producing osteoid and woven bone. Cytological activity may also be present. Of note, however, is the interface between the tumour and the surrounding normal bone which is sharp without evidence of permeation.

The majority of osteoblastomas are intraosseous at presentation although, in advanced disease, soft tissue extension is not uncommon. Reports of metastatic spread of osteoblastomas are most likely undiagnosed osteoblast-like osteosarcomas. These can be differentiated by the finding of osteoid permeating the marrow spaces and trapping the host lamellar bone.

In the majority of cases, *treatment* comprises extended intralesional curettage with radio-frequency ablation for smaller volume lesions. Rarely, en-bloc resection may be required. Consideration may be given to preoperative embolization in the case of larger lesions to reduce intraoperative haemorrhage.

NON-OSSIFYING FIBROMA

Non-ossifying fibroma (NOF), the commonest benign lesion of bone, is a developmental defect in which a nest of fibrous tissue appears within the bone and persists for some years before ossifying. It is asymptomatic and is almost always encountered in children as an incidental X-ray finding. The commonest sites are the metaphyses of long bones; occasionally there are multiple lesions. There is a more-or-less oval radiolucent area surrounded by a thin margin of dense bone (9.10). Views in different planes may show that a lesion that appears to be 'central' is actually adjacent to or within the cortex, hence the alternative name 'fibrous cortical defect'.

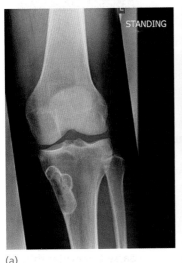 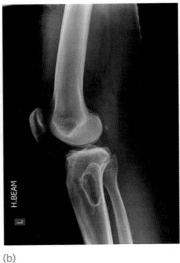 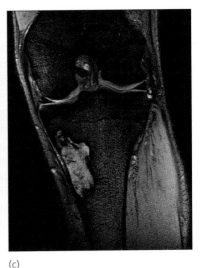

(a)   (b)   (c)

9.10 Non-ossifying fibroma Plain radiographs (a,b) demonstrate a well-circumscribed lesion of the proximal tibia of a 29-year-old man referred with knee pain. MRI (c) confirms a partially consolidated benign lesion of the proximal tibia, which, given the patient's age, is entirely in keeping with an NOF diagnosis.

Although the lesion looks cystic on X-rays, it is a solid lesion consisting of unremarkable fibrous tissue with a few scattered giant cells. As the bone grows, the defect becomes less obvious and it eventually heals spontaneously. *Treatment* is usually unnecessary.

GIANT-CELL TUMOUR OF BONE

This is a benign but locally aggressive tumour of bone composed of a proliferation of mononuclear cells with scattered macrophages. GCTs account for approximately 5% of all primary bone lesions and are most common between 20 and 45 years of age. Though they can appear in teenage years, they are rare in the immature skeleton. GCTs can occasionally be seen in conjunction with Paget's disease of bone. Malignant transformation can occur in GCTs though this is rare (<1%) and is marginally more common in females.

GCTs typically affect the metaphyses of long bones with preponderance for the distal femur, proximal tibia, distal radius and proximal humerus. When affecting the spine, they most commonly arise in the vertebral bodies of the sacrum with reduction in frequency as the spine is ascended. While flat bones are not commonly affected, GCTs affecting the pelvis are most commonly seen in the ilium. GCTs are rarely multicentric and rarely affect the tubular bones of the hands. In such cases, hyperparathyroidism (brown tumour) must be excluded.

Patients typically present with pain and, less frequently, an increasing mass, particularly around the knee. In a small number of cases (5–10%), pathological fracture is the presenting feature.

Plain X-rays classically demonstrate an eccentric, expansile, lobulated lytic lesion with a narrow zone of transition. Tumours have extended into the soft tissues at presentation and a soft-tissue mass, sometimes covered by a thin layer of sclerosis, can be seen on X-ray (9.11). GCTs usually have little or no discernible matrix calcification and little new bone formation or periosteal reaction. They are typically located within the metaphysis and are one of the few lesions to involve the physis, abutting the subchondral plate.

The lesion is driven by osteoclasts responding to RANKL, thus anti-RANKL antibodies such as denosumab can be used to stop the osteolytic process and switch the balance towards bone formation. The response of the tumour can be dramatic but the side-effect profile can result in significant morbidity, including hypocalcaemia, osteonecrosis of the jaw and atypical fracture patterns.

SIMPLE BONE CYST

This is a solitary, usually unilocular cystic bone cavity lined by a fibrous membrane and filled with serous or serosanguinous fluid. Males are more frequently affected and the majority occur within the first two decades of life. Although they can arise at any location, the vast majority of simple bone cysts (SBCs) occur in the proximal humerus, the proximal femur or the proximal tibia, most commonly affecting the metaphyseal areas close to the physis.

In the majority of cases the lesion is asymptomatic. However, fracture through the lesion is not uncommon and often this is the presenting feature. Occasionally, mild pain or swelling may be present. X-rays demonstrate a well-outlined, lytic centrally placed, metadiaphyseal lesion expanding and thinning the cortices (9.12). It often abuts but does not cross the physis. Bone septa are often present which give the impression of a multiloculated cyst. When fracture occurs, a small fragment may be seen within the cavity, the classic 'fallen leaf' sign. MRI will demonstrate the homogeneous fluid-filled cavity.

Treatment is often supportive as lesions will regress following skeletal maturity. Percutaneous injection of steroid has been reported with varying success but is best reserved for those abutting the physis in young children. Curettage and bone grafting may be required in areas at risk of fracture, and pathological fractures of the proximal femur in particular will often require fixation and stabilization. Spontaneous resolution following fracture has been reported.

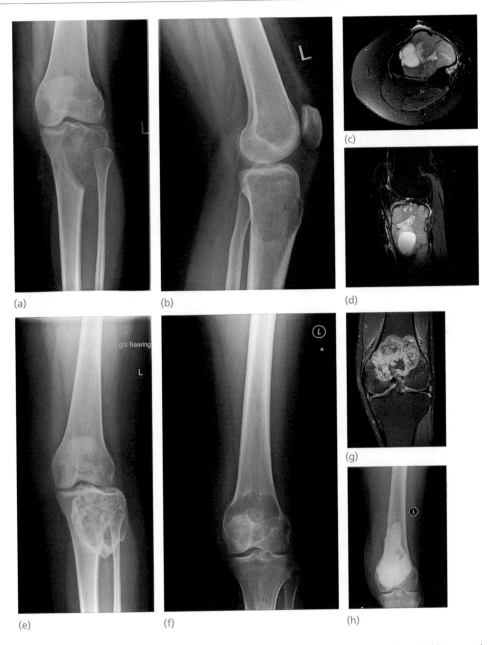

(a)

(b)

(c)

(d)

(e)

(f)

(g)

(h)

9.11 Giant-cell tumour of bone (a–e) A 29-year-old female presented with left-sided knee pain and a mass. Radiographs (a,b) demonstrate a geocentric lesion in the proximal tibia with marked destruction of the lateral proximal tibial metaphysis. MRI confirms a heterogeneous lesion in the proximal tibia which abuts the subchondral plate (c,d), with a large extraosseous, soft-tissue mass (Campanacci stage 3) and focal areas of cystic/haemorrhagic change. Biopsy confirms a giant cell-rich lesion in keeping with a GCT of bone. (e) The same patient after 4 months' treatment with the RANKL antagonist denosumab. (f–h) A similar case in the distal femur as demonstrated by X-ray (f) and MRI (g). In this case, given the lack of an extraosseous component, the patient was treated by extended intralesional curettage and cementation (h).

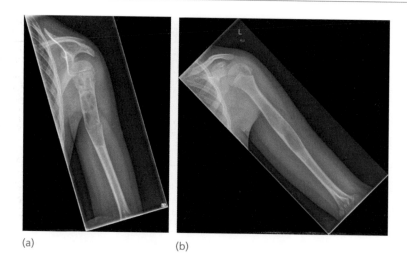

(a) (b)

9.12 Simple bone cyst A 10-year-old boy with a spontaneous fracture through the left humerus. **(a)** Plain radiographs demonstrate an expansile, lytic lesion in the humeral metadiaphysis with a pathological fracture through the base of the lesion. The imaging features are in keeping with an SBC. The fracture was managed conservatively with a humeral brace and careful observation. **(b)** Over time, the lesion consolidated and united.

ANEURYSMAL BONE CYST

ABCs are benign, expansile lesions of bone composed of blood-filled cystic spaces. They are destructive lesions and, while they are histologically benign, they can result in significant disability. They predominantly affect children and teenagers with an equal sex distribution. ABCs can affect any bone but are most commonly seen in the metaphyses of long bones, particularly the femur (**9.13**, **9.14**), tibia and humerus. They may occur in the spine where they typically affect the posterior elements.

Patients typically present with pain and swelling. When affecting the spine, presentation can be with nerve root impingement and neurological impairment.

ABCs appear as a subperiosteal, poorly defined osteolytic lesion, elevating and progressively eroding the cortex. Angiography demonstrates persistence of contrast and a blush of flow within the lesion.

The lesion may demonstrate rapid progression, but equally it may resolve spontaneously following trauma, either fracture or biopsy. Curettage of the lesion at the time of biopsy ('curopsy'),

debriding the cystic cavity wall, is often effective though recurrence can occur in up to 20% of cases. Radiation is effective at stimulating cyst calcification but must be offset by the risk of secondary sarcoma or of growth arrest due to damage to the nearby physis.

FIBROUS DYSPLASIA

This is a benign, medullary fibro-osseous lesion which may affect one bone (monostotic) or a number of bones (polyostotic). Fibrous dysplasia can affect children and adults with equal sex and race distribution. The monostotic form is considerably more frequent than the polyostotic. The craniofacial bones and the femur are the most frequently affected bones, but any bone can be affected by the monostotic form. In the polyostotic form, the pelvis, femur and tibia are commonly involved. Multiple sites of fibrous dysplasia may be seen in the same bone, particularly in the monostotic form.

The monostotic form is often discovered incidentally and is largely asymptomatic. Not infrequently, pain and fracture are the presenting

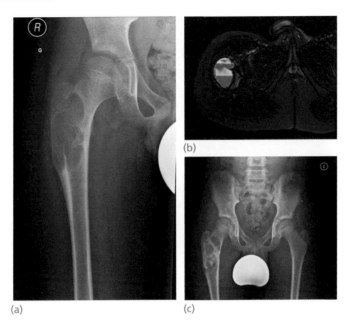

9.13 Aneurysmal bone cyst A 9-year-old boy presented with progressive right-sided hip and thigh pain on exertion. **(a)** Radiographs demonstrated an expansile, lytic, cystic lesion of the right proximal femur. **(b)** MRI demonstrated a characteristic expansile, loculated lesion of the proximal femur with thinning of the cortices but no soft-tissue component. Fluid–fluid levels are seen within the lesion, which is highly suggestive of an ABC.

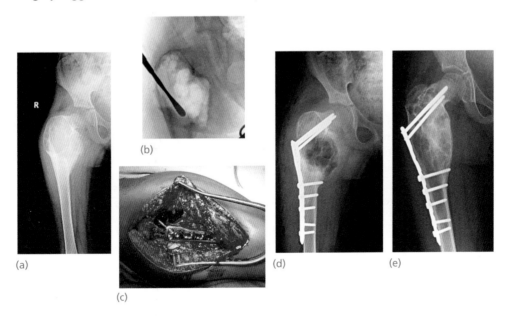

9.14 Aneurysmal bone cyst Large ABC of the right proximal femur. **(a)** Radiograph demonstrating an expansile lesion with erosion of the medial cortex. **(b,c)** Intraoperative views showing curettage of the lesion and a large cavity evident anterior to the plate (that is providing stability *in situ* while the lesion heals). No bone grafting was performed. **(d,e)** Postoperative radiographs showing gradual resolution of the lesion.

SECTION 1 GENERAL ORTHOPAEDICS

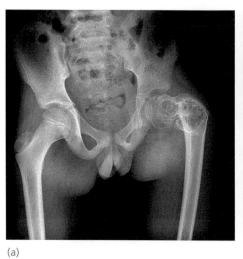

(a)

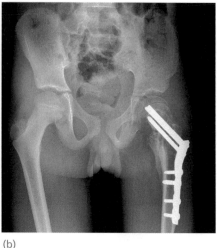

(b)

9.15 Monostotic fibrous dysplasia (a) This has caused severe varus of the right proximal femur and been managed with a valgus hip osteotomy **(b)**.

features. Bony expansion in superficial bones, deformity and growth disturbance with deformity (**9.15**) and lower-limb length discrepancy can also occur. Polyostotic fibrous dysplasia associated with café-au-lait spots (that have a characteristic 'Coast of Maine' irregular border) and endocrine abnormalities (most commonly manifesting in precocious puberty) is known as McCune–Albright syndrome (**9.16**).

X-rays often demonstrate a non-aggressive, well-circumscribed lesion with a characteristic ground-glass matrix (**9.17**). More mature lesions may show cyst formation and secondary changes. The characteristic deformity resulting from proximal femoral fibrous dysplasia is the shepherd's crook deformity. There is seldom a soft-tissue component or periosteal reaction, except in the case of fracture.

When fibrous dysplasia affects the hip, *surgical stabilization*, often with corrective osteotomies is frequently required. Intramedullary stabilization is preferred in polyostotic fibrous dysplasia where the whole femur is affected. The soft, vascular bone often makes treatment challenging. Autologous cancellous bone graft is usually rapidly replaced by the pathological woven bone (autologous cortical bone graft

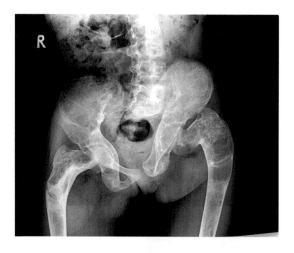

9.16 Polyostotic fibrous dysplasia In this case, both femora, the pelvis and spine are affected. The left femur has a shepherd's crook deformity. Corrective osteotomies combined with intramedullary stabilization are needed to minimize the risk of recurrence.

tends to resorb more slowly). Recurrence following treatment is not uncommon. Malignant transformation, to fibrosarcoma of bone, is rare but more frequently seen in McCune–Albright syndrome.

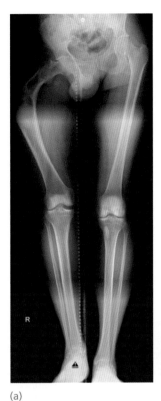
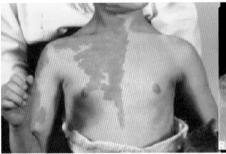
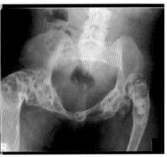

(a) (b)

9.17 Fibrous dysplasia (a) Plain radiographs of a 73-year-old male from India who presented with a long history of progressive bowing of the right thigh. He eventually sought medical advice when the pain suddenly became severe. Radiographs show a varus deformity of the proximal femur with a stress fracture on the tension side. The lesion demonstrates the typical features of mixed lytic and blastic appearances with thinning of the cortices and progressive deformity. When associated with café-au-lait spots **(b)** and polyostotic fibrous dysplasia **(c)**, as well as hyperfunctional endocrine disease, this is known as McCune–Albright syndrome.

PRIMARY MALIGNANT BONE TUMOURS

OSTEOSARCOMA

The most common primary malignant bone tumour, osteosarcoma has a bimodal age distribution peaking in adolescence (10–14 years) and again in the seventh decade. In its conventional form, osteosarcoma is a high-grade, medullary osteoid-producing tumour spreading rapidly outwards through the periosteum and into surrounding tissues. Typically metaphyseal or metadiaphyseal, the majority present at the distal femur, proximal tibia, proximal femur and humerus (i.e. where the majority of long-bone growth occurs). Patients complain of worsening pain and swelling, particularly suffering night pain, non-mechanical pain or joint restriction. Fever, elevated ALP and lactate dehydrogenase (LDH) may be useful aids to clinical assessment. The skin may be warm and erythematous with venous engorgement.

Osteosarcomas may be described as:

- *primary* (arising *de novo*)
- *secondary* (arising in abnormal bone).

SECTION 1 GENERAL ORTHOPAEDICS

Secondary osteosarcomas may be related to previous irradiation, Paget's disease, fibrous dysplasia, bone infarcts, chronic osteomyelitis or in dedifferentiated chondrosarcomas and have a less favourable prognosis. This explains the secondary elevation in the bimodal distribution of osteosarcoma.

Investigations

X-rays are generally diagnostic showing an ill-defined, permeative bone-forming lesion causing cortical destruction, periosteal reaction and expansion into the soft tissues. The tumours can be variably mineralized, and there may be a Codman's triangle where new bone forms in response to periosteal elevation and a 'sunburst' appearance when the periosteum does not have enough time to lay down a new layer and instead the Sharpey's fibres stretch perpendicular to the periosteum (**9.18**). Classically, 80% are extra-compartmental at presentation, i.e. extending through the cortex. MRI of the whole bone will delineate the medullary and extraosseous extent of the tumour. Nuclear medicine bone scintigraphy is intensively hot and may identify bone skip lesions, distant bone metastases or bone-producing chest metastases. CT chest is mandatory as lung metastases are common (up to 15%).

A biopsy should always be carried out before commencing treatment; it must be carefully planned according to the principles of performing a biopsy to allow for complete removal of the biopsy tract at definitive surgery. The neoplastic cells demonstrate severe anaplasia and pleomorphism, producing primitive woven bone and osteoid and display a permeative pattern replacing host bone.

Conventional osteosarcoma is subclassified according to the predominant extracellular matrix evident in the tissue, such as osteoblastic osteosarcoma, chondroblastic and fibroblastic variants.

Treatment

Prior to modern chemotherapy and reconstruction techniques, amputation was the standard surgical treatment for musculoskeletal sarcomas of the extremities for most of the 20th century, because of the high risks of local recurrence and associated poor survival. Advances in multi-agent chemotherapy, diagnostic imaging and surgical reconstruction enabled limb-salvage surgery, which constituted the major advancement of the last century in bone sarcoma treatment. Limb salvage has now become the preferred method of treatment for osteosarcomas, such that an amputation is considered only when attempted tumour excision would compromise safe surgical tumour margins.

The principal first-line chemotherapeutic agents used in osteosarcoma are:

- doxorubicin
- cisplatin
- ifosfamide
- methotrexate.

Multi-agent neoadjuvant chemotherapy is started immediately after diagnosis for 8–12 weeks and then, after restaging to evaluate response to induction chemotherapy and provided the tumour is resectable and there are no skip lesions, a wide resection and limb reconstruction are performed. Pulmonary metastases, especially if they are small and peripherally situated, may be completely resected with a wedge of lung tissue.

Five-year survival after wide resection and chemotherapy is about 60%.

Secondary osteosarcoma

Paget's disease affects approximately 2% of Western Europeans. Although malignant transformation is a rare complication of this disease, most osteosarcomas appearing after the age of 40 years fall into this category. The incidence of osteosarcomatous change in Paget's disease is approximately 1% and most common in the polyostotic form, usually involving the femur, pelvis, humerus and skull, and may be multifocal in up to 20%.

 Warning signs are the appearance of pain or swelling in a patient with long-standing Paget's disease.

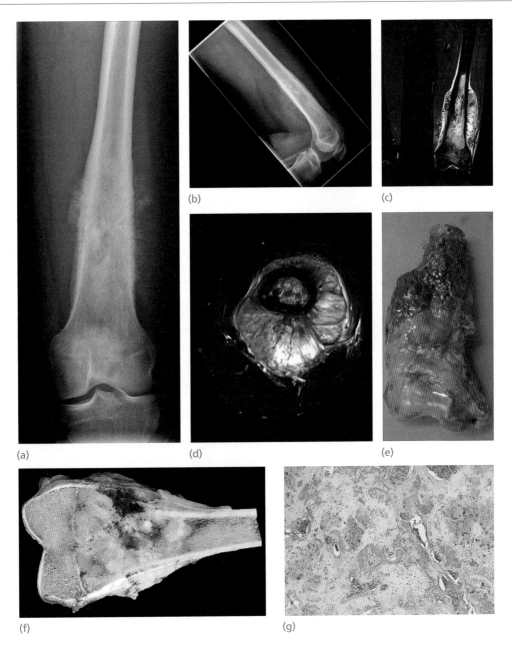

(a) (b) (c) (d) (e) (f) (g)

9.18 Osteosarcoma The characteristic features of a distal femoral osteosarcoma as seen on plain radiographs **(a,b)**. The lesion, located in the metadiaphysis, demonstrates a mixed lytic blastic appearance. There is elevation of the periosteum resulting in a Codman's triangle. The soft-tissue extension of the tumour results in bone formation within the surrounding soft tissues and the appearance of sunray spiculations. On MRI **(c,d)**, the true extent of the tumour can be seen erupting from the bone and extending into the posterior soft tissues. The patient received neoadjuvant chemotherapy with a dramatic response in the tumour volume **(i,j)** followed by resection of the tumour **(e)**. The resection specimen demonstrates a pale tumour occupying the distal femur and extending through the cortex **(f)**. The dominant histological features are those of malignant stromal tissue with areas of osteoid formation with interspersed areas of chondroid differentiation in keeping with a chondroblastic osteosarcoma **(g)** (×100).

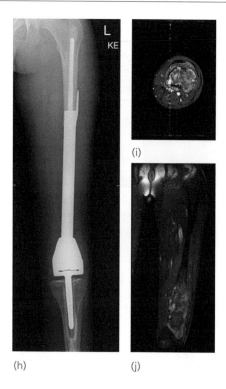

(h)   (j)

9.18 Osteosarcoma (*Continued*) The tumour was excised in its entirety and reconstruction was with a distal femoral endoprosthetic replacement (h).

Mean age at presentation is 71 years. X-rays show typical pagetic bone with a lytic destructive mass extending into the soft tissues.

The risk of post-radiation sarcoma is dose-dependent and is most common in the pelvis and scapula (reflecting radiotherapy for cervical/ ovarian and breast carcinomas respectively). The time lag between radiotherapy and subsequent development of osteosarcoma can range from 6 to 23 years. Clinically and radiologically the features are similar to conventional osteosarcoma, although post-radiation changes (trabecular coarsening and cortical lysis) may be evident.

The *treatment* principles for secondary osteosarcoma are the same as for primary, although the aggressive chemotherapeutic and surgical treatments offered to young osteosarcoma patients are less well tolerated by elderly patients. Chemotherapeutic dose reductions may be possible if there are concerns regarding cardiac and renal toxicity. Consequently, osteosarcoma in elderly patients older than 65 years has a worse prognosis than that of the younger population. Paget's osteosarcoma specifically has an abysmal prognosis; median survival is 9 months post diagnosis.

CHONDROSARCOMA

Chondrosarcomas are the second most common primary malignant bone tumours. This group of aggressive malignant cartilage tumours represents a spectrum of the same disorder that arises in enchondromas.

These tumours can present in adults from the third to the eighth decades, peaking between 40 and 70 years of age, and men are affected more often than women. They are slow-growing and are usually present for many months before being discovered. They produce deep pain and/or a gradually enlarging mass and arise in any bone derived from enchondral ossification. Most frequently located in the proximal femur, pelvis, proximal humerus, distal femur, scapula and proximal tibia, these metaphyseal lesions can extend across large segments of the involved bone. Despite the relatively frequent occurrence of benign cartilage tumours in the small tubular bones of the hands and feet, malignant lesions are rare at these sites, representing <1% of chondrosarcomas.

Chondrosarcomas take various forms, usually designated according to:

- their location in the bone (*central* or *peripheral*)
- whether they develop without benign precursor (*primary chondrosarcoma*) or by malignant change in a pre-existing benign lesion (*secondary chondrosarcoma*)
- the predominant *cell type* in the tumour.

Approximately 85% of chondrosarcomas are *primary central chondrosarcomas* occupying the medullary cavity. Radiographically these appear as large, intraosseous, osteolytic tumours with a narrow zone of transition and irregular, granular calcifications within the matrix described as 'honeycomb' or 'popcorn' (**9.19**). Endosteal scalloping of the cortex and eventual cortical destruction can occur, and there may be a faint periosteal reaction. These tumours grow along the path of least resistance, i.e. along the medullary canal, and soft-tissue extension is more common in pelvic chondrosarcomas. CT is useful for demonstrating the matrix calcifications and permeative destruction of the tumour.

Resistant to both chemotherapy and radiation, the only *treatment* for chondrosarcoma is surgical excision. In high-grade tumours, only wide excision margins are oncologically acceptable to minimize local recurrence. Prognosis is determined by the cellular grade, stage, tumour size, (axial versus appendicular) site and the resection margin. Overall survival at 5 years for low-grade tumours is 90–100%, for grade II tumours approximately 60% and for grade III approximately 30–40%.

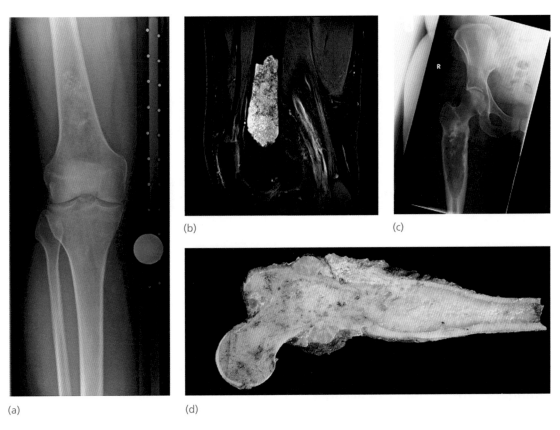

(a) (b) (c) (d)

9.19 Central chondrosarcoma The challenge of the central chondroid lesion. Plain X-rays **(a)** demonstrate an 8.5 cm chondroid lesion in the distal femur which remained unchanged on radiographs over a period of 12 months. However, on MRI **(b)**, minor endosteal scalloping of the anterior femoral cortex can be seen which, combined with the advent of pain in the thigh, warranted resection of the tumour. Histology post resection confirmed a low-grade chondrosarcoma. **(c–e)** Often, the differentiation between benign chondroid lesion and chondrosarcoma can be a little easier: radiographs **(c)** demonstrate a destructive, expansile lesion in the proximal femur with the characteristic features of a chondroid matrix. Resection histology demonstrates a pale, glistening cartilage lesion in the medullary cavity which spreads beyond the cortex **(d)**.

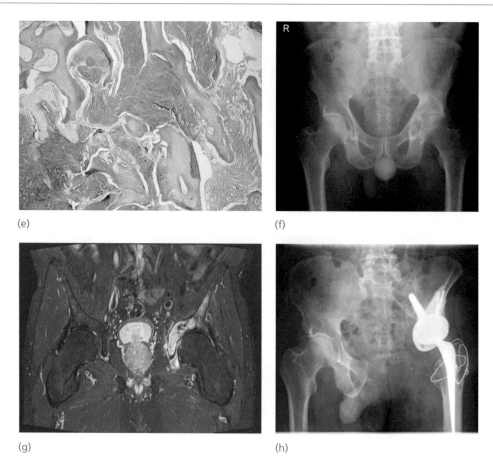

(e)

(f)

(g)

(h)

9.19 Central chondrosarcoma (*Continued*) Microscopy (×100) demonstrates lobules of highly atypical cartilage cells, including binucleate cells permeating through the surrounding bone matrix **(e)**. **(f–h)** For a 70-year-old man who presented with an 18-month history of left-sided hip pain, plain X-rays **(f)** and MRI **(g)** demonstrate a chondroid lesion in the periacetabulum which extends down the anterior column. The tumour was biopsied and found to be a chondrosarcoma. Treatment was by resection of the periacetabulum and pubis and reconstruction with an ice-cream cone prosthesis and hip replacement **(h)**.

Secondary central chondrosarcoma

These arise in previously benign enchondromas. Ollier's disease and Maffucci syndrome have a significant risk of developing secondary chondrosarcomas of approximately 20–30% and 40–50% respectively, typically in the third or fourth decade, although in Maffucci syndrome, patients are at increased risk of also developing carcinomas (e.g. breast, liver, ovary), which suggests an underlying genetic predisposition.

Secondary peripheral chondrosarcoma

These arise in the cartilage cap of an exostosis (osteochondroma) that has been present since childhood (**9.20**). Exostoses of the pelvis and scapula seem to be more susceptible than others to malignant change, because these sites permit undetected growth. Malignant transformation is associated with 1% of solitary osteochondromas and in 4% of patients with multiple osteochondromas.

SECTION 1 GENERAL ORTHOPAEDICS

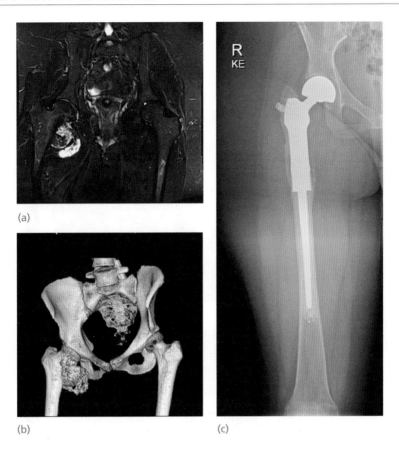

(a)

(b)

(c)

9.20 A long-standing osteochondroma arising from the proximal femur (a) MRI demonstrates a thick cartilage cap overlying the osteochondroma, which measures 3.5 cm. **(b)** 3D CT reconstruction demonstrates the calcification and speculation within the cartilage cap. The tumour was removed in its entirety and reconstructed with a proximal femoral endoprosthetic replacement **(c)**. The resection histology confirmed a low-grade chondrosarcoma.

EWING'S SARCOMA

Ewing's sarcoma is believed to arise from mesenchymal stem cells in the bone marrow. This highly malignant tumour occurs more frequently in males, typically between 10 and 20 years of age, and has a diaphyseal long-bone location but is equally as common in flat bones. The femur is the most common long-bone site, followed by the tibia, humerus and fibula, but overall, the pelvis accounts for the majority of cases.

Pain is the earliest symptom, followed by swelling and a low-grade fever. Serologically, the ESR and WCC may be elevated and haemoglobin may be reduced.

Radiographically, an aggressive, permeative, poorly defined osteolytic lesion with cortical destruction, periosteal reaction and large, radiolucent soft-tissue mass may be found. Periosteal reaction is common in young patients with the lamellar 'onion-skin' appearance causing fusiform bone enlargement (**9.21**).

Routine local and distal staging includes bone scintigraphy and chest CT. MRI demonstrates the intra- and extraosseous tumour extent, and lesions are 'hot' with bone scintigraphy. Lung, skeletal and lymph node (rare) metastases may be evident at presentation in up to 20% of cases. Bone marrow involvement is a unique feature of Ewing's sarcoma among other bone sarcomas and is associated with a worse prognosis.

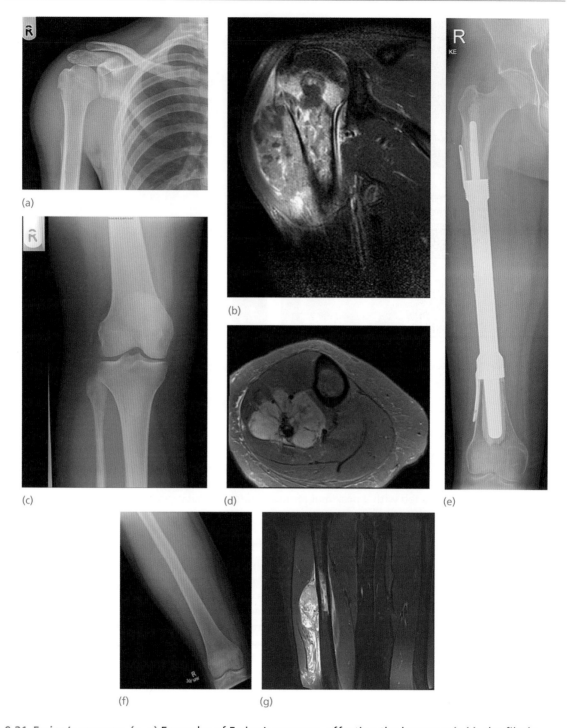

(a)

(b)

(c)

(d)

(e)

(f)

(g)

9.21 Ewing's sarcoma (a–g) Examples of Ewing's sarcoma, affecting the humerus **(a,b)**, the fibula **(c,d)**, and the femoral diaphysis **(e,f)**, treated by neoadjuvant chemo-radiotherapy and subsequent reconstruction with a diaphyseal endoprosthesis **(g)**. Note the evidence of bone destruction, which can sometimes be subtle on plain radiography, but the extensive soft-tissue component which is arising from the intramedullary compartment seen on MRI.

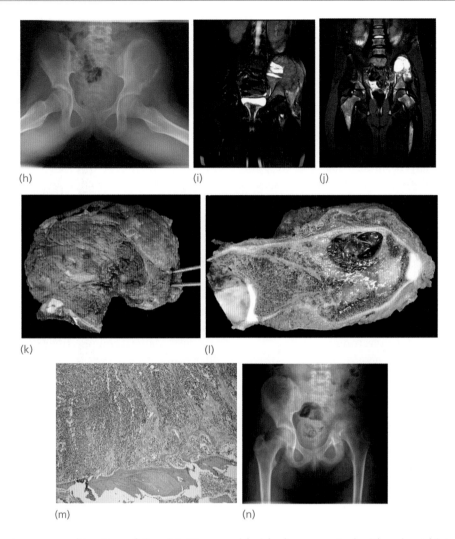

(h)   (i)   (j)

(k)   (l)

(m)   (n)

9.21 Ewing's sarcoma (*Continued*) **(h–n)** A 14-year-old girl who presented with a short history of pain and subsequently a mass in the left hemipelvis. X-rays **(h)** demonstrate a destructive lesion with a wide zone of transition in the left ileum. MRI **(i)** shows a very large soft-tissue mass with associated bone destruction arising from the left ilium extending down to the upper border of the acetabulum. The patient was treated with neoadjuvant chemotherapy and high-dose proton radiotherapy to the left ilium. Post-treatment MRI **(j)** demonstrates a dramatic response with significant reduction in the soft-tissue component. The patient underwent resection of the ilium to the level of the triradiate cartilage. The resection was assisted by computer navigation, which allowed very accurate planning of the level of the osteotomies. Note the navigation pins in the resection specimen **(k)** for mounting the navigation tracker. At sectioning, the necrotic, cystic core of the tumour can be seen **(l)**. Histology of the initial diagnostic biopsy (×100) confirms a small, round blue-cell tumour **(m)**, which is confirmed as Ewing's sarcoma by fluorescence *in situ* hybridization and the presence of the *EWS/FLI-1* translocation. Since preoperative radiotherapy was given, no implant was inserted into the pelvis due to the perceived risk of infection. Rather, a collagen matrix graft was hung from the residual acetabulum over the femoral head to form a neo-hip joint **(n)**. After a period of rehabilitation, the patient can mobilize unaided with a Trendelenburg gait. The resection histology demonstrated no evidence of viable tumour, suggesting an excellent response to neoadjuvant therapy and an excellent prognosis.

SECTION 1 GENERAL ORTHOPAEDICS

Preoperative chemotherapy frequently results in extensive tumour necrosis and shrinkage. Agents used in Ewing's sarcoma include:

- vincristine
- ifosfamide
- doxorubicin
- etoposide.

Wide excision may be combined with adjuvant radiotherapy if surgical margins are poor. Definitive radiotherapy rather than surgical excision, although associated with worse overall survival, may be advocated if non-resectable or metastasis has occurred during chemotherapy, to spare the surgical morbidity. A more favourable outcome is expected with younger age, distal appendicular sites, small tumour volume, normal ESR and greater chemotherapy necrosis response.

Five-year survival greater than 60% can be expected for appendicular tumours.

HAEMATOPOIETIC TUMOURS – MULTIPLE MYELOMA

Myeloma is a malignant proliferation of neoplastic plasma cells of B-cell lineage within the bone marrow, leading to increased production of plasma paraprotein and immunoglobulin. It arises most commonly in the marrow-containing bones of the vertebrae, pelvis and femur. The median age at diagnosis is 70 years. The commonest primary malignant lesion arising in bone, it has an estimated incidence of 3000 per annum.

Multiple myeloma arises as a result of multiple genetic mutations of plasma cells and the immunoglobulins they produce. Diagnosis of myeloma depends on the detection of para-proteins in the plasma or urine, bone marrow biopsy, and evidence of end-organ/bone damage. Serum or urinary electrophoresis measures immunoglobulins that are overproduced by the malignant plasma cells. Multiple myeloma has several effects on bone:

- focal osteolytic lesions
- generalized bone loss (osteopenia)
- elevated bone turnover.

Traditionally, a skeletal survey required X-rays of the spine, skull, pelvis, ribs/sternum, and the humerus/femurs to screen for osseous lesions, and to assess tumour burden and fracture risk. Classic 'punched-out', osteolytic lesions with cortical thinning can be seen, which in the skull may cause a 'pepper-pot' appearance (**9.22**). CT is superior for demonstrating fractures, osteolytic lesions, and soft-tissue masses and may aid in distal staging of disease. MRI scanning is useful to stage the extent of marrow infiltration, visualization of focal masses and areas most at risk of fracturing, and to highlight response to treatment. Bone scintigraphy underrepresents the extent of disease as it relies on osteoblastic activity.

Bone disease in myeloma may cause severe bone pain, spinal cord compression, diffuse osteoporosis, hypercalcaemia and pathological fractures, which occur in approximately 40% of patients. Medical complications include anaemia, hypercalcaemia, hyperviscosity, immunosuppression and renal dysfunction.

Although incurable, long-term remission can be achieved in some patients. Management comprises combined alkylating chemotherapy, a steroid such as dexamethasone or prednisolone and an immunomodulatory agent such as thalidomide. Autologous stem-cell transplantation (ASCT) involves bone marrow harvest, high-dose chemotherapy to produce myelosuppression and transfusion with stem cells, and it is the standard of care in patients up to 65 years. Bisphosphonates are used in all symptomatic patients to prevent fractures and control hypercalcaemia.

Surgery has a supportive effect on the management, long-term survival and quality of life in multiple myeloma patients. The aim is usually to decompress or stabilize vertebral fractures with instability or neurological compression, to stabilize (impending) pathological fractures and to reduce pain.

The prognosis is highly variable, but overall estimated survival has improved to 35% 5-year survival and 17% 10-year survival with the advent of new treatments.

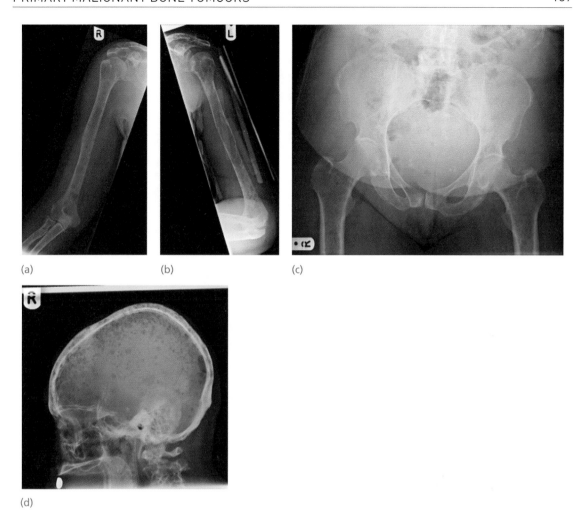

(a)   (b)   (c)

(d)

9.22 Multiple myeloma Skeletal survey **(a–c)** of a 74-year-old woman who presented with a pathological fracture through her left humerus demonstrated multiple deposits throughout the skeleton, with characteristic 'pepper-pot' appearance of the skull **(d)**. The diagnosis is multiple myeloma.

CHORDOMA

This rare, slow-growing tumour arises from primitive embryonic notochordal remnants along the spinal column, most commonly in the sacrum and less commonly at the occiput or vertebrae (**9.23**). More common in males, the mean age at presentation is 60 years. Base-of-skull chordomas present with pain and cranial nerve palsies. Sacral chordoma patients present with typically dull pain (85%), usually present for years, and worse with sitting. The classic symptoms of cauda equina (saddle anaesthesia, bladder or bowel dysfunction) occur in 70% of patients.

X-rays show ill-defined osteolysis of the sacrum, possibly with tumoural calcifications. Bone scan highlights areas of bone involvement. Bowel and bladder dysfunction relate to the anatomical level of nerve-root resection; navigated resections help to preserve nerve roots. In high sacral chordomas, with predictable surgical morbidity, proton beam and carbon-ion therapies have been used to achieve local control.

SECTION 1 GENERAL ORTHOPAEDICS

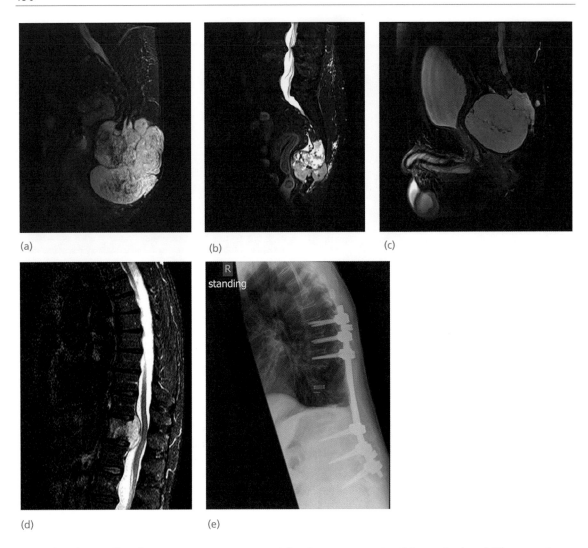

(a)   (b)   (c)

(d)   (e)

9.23 Chordoma Chordomas are rare tumours arising from remnants of the notochord. They most commonly present in the sacrum **(a,b)** where they can cause a painful mass or lower bowel and urinary symptoms which may require colostomy and bowel resection to achieve a satisfactory margin **(c)**. They can arise anywhere within the spine, in this case at the lumbar vertebrae **(d)** which was treated by en bloc resection **(e)**.

MALIGNANT VASCULAR TUMOURS OF BONE

Vascular tumours arising in bone range from benign haemangiomas, low-grade epithelioid haemangiomas, and intermediate-grade epithelioid haemangioendotheliomas to high-grade angiosarcomas.

Haemangioma

Haemangiomas are common incidental findings of spinal imaging, may be seen in the metaphysis of long bones and are more common with age. They are well demarcated and usually indolent, requiring no treatment.

Epithelioid haemangioma

These locally aggressive tumours are found in young adults in the lower limbs and spine, causing pain, and they may even metastasize. They are well-defined, lytic lesions that can erode the cortex and extend into soft tissues. Intralesional curettage is usually sufficient, and local recurrence is rare.

Epithelioid haemangioendothelioma

Rare, intermediate-grade and present in all age groups in the lower limbs, spine and pelvis, these cause pain and swelling. X-rays demonstrate expansile, lytic, invasive tumours eroding the cortex. Wide resection is advocated.

Angiosarcoma

These very rare high-grade tumours have a broad age range and wide anatomical distribution, most frequently the femur and pelvis. They can be secondary to previous irradiation of the soft tissues (e.g. breast carcinoma). Significant pain and swelling may be evident and an aggressive, osteolytic lesion with cortical destruction and soft-tissue mass is evident on radiographs and MRI. Wide surgical excision or radiation with chemotherapy is used to attempt disease control. This very aggressive tumour has a 5-year survival of 20%, although this is 0% in patients with metastases.

METASTATIC BONE DISEASE

METASTASIS DEFINED

Metastasis Transmission of pathogenic microorganisms or cancerous cells from an original site to one or more sites elsewhere in the body, usually via blood vessels or lymphatics.

Metastatic disease is the most common malignancy of bone. It is estimated that one in five cancer patients will suffer symptomatic bone metastasis, and post-mortem studies have demonstrated skeletal metastasis in 70% of patients.

The most common primary tumours to metastasize to bone are breast, lung, prostate, renal and thyroid carcinomas, which account for more than 80% of metastatic bone tumours.

PRESENTING FEATURES OF METASTATIC BONE DISEASE

Pain
Swelling
Pathological fracture
Spinal cord compression
Hypercalcaemia

- Anorexia
- Nausea
- Thirst
- Polyuria
- Abdominal pain
- General weakness
- Depression

Typically, prostatic lesions are densely osteosclerotic, in contrast to osteolytic renal and thyroid lesions (9.24). Lung and breast metastases produce mixed osteoblastic/osteolytic lesions. Routine clinical examination of all systems and screening bloods are required to exclude anaemia, renal failure, hypercalcaemia and screen PSA in males. Local and distal staging includes X-rays and MRI of the whole affected bone, bone scintigraphy and CT thorax, abdomen and pelvis. Bone scintigraphy is widely used to search for further areas of radionucleotide uptake; classically, cold lesions such as renal-cell carcinoma and myeloma do not initiate an osteoblastic response, therefore disease extent may be underestimated. Whole-body MRI has superior sensitivity to scintigraphy for identifying metastatic disease in a range of visceral tumours, particularly renal-cell carcinoma.

The prognosis for many patients with metastatic bone disease, particularly those without visceral disease, has significantly improved due to advances in medical therapy, including hormonal treatment, bisphosphonates, chemotherapy and biologically targeted agents. Radiotherapy for metastases is usually delivered in a single fraction by oncologists. Bisphosphonates are useful

SECTION 1 GENERAL ORTHOPAEDICS

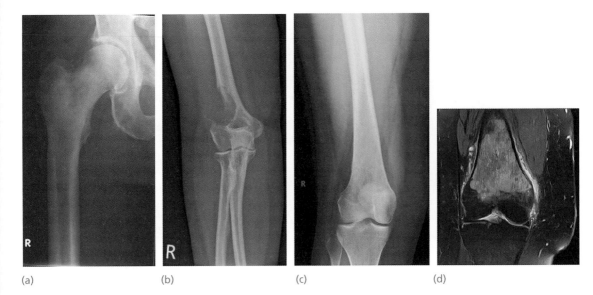

(a)   (b)   (c)   (d)

9.24 Metastatic bone disease (a) X-rays of a 75-year-old man with a past history of prostate carcinoma with a progressive, painful right hip demonstrate a sclerotic lesion in the proximal femur that
was confirmed as metastatic prostate carcinoma. **(b)** A 68-year-old woman presented with a rapid
deterioration in right elbow function with progressive pain. Radiographs demonstrate a punched-out
lesion in the distal humerus with associated soft-tissue component. Histology confirmed metastatic
renal cell carcinoma. **(c,d)** A 71-year-old woman with a past history of breast carcinoma treated 11
years previously represented with progressive pain in the left knee. X-rays demonstrate a mixed blastic and lytic lesion **(c)**, the true nature and extent of which are clearly seen on MRI **(d)**.

in metastatic breast and prostate carcinoma and
multiple myeloma. Radiofrequency ablation has
been shown to be effective, safe and well tolerated by patients.

Surgery is indicated for intractable pain, or
impending or pathological fractures (e9.4).
Surgery ranges from osteosynthesis, with or
without cement augmentation, to endoprosthetic replacement. The aims of surgery are to
provide immediate absolute stability permitting
full weight-bearing. Renal and thyroid metastases may be highly vascular lesions necessitating
preoperative embolization to avoid catastrophic
haemorrhage.

Mirels' score is commonly quoted to assess
risk of fracture in metastatic bone lesions
(**Table 9.2**). A score of 1 to 3 is given for each
of four variables. There is a high risk of fracture for total scores of 8 or above, so prophylactic fixation should be carried out prior to
radiotherapy.

Table 9.2 The Mirels' score for quantifying the
relative risk of fracture through a pathological
lesion of bone

Variable	Score		
	1	2	3
Site	Upper limb	Lower limb	Pertrochanteric
Pain	Mild	Moderate	Severe
Lesion	Blastic	Mixed	Lytic
Size*	<1/3	1/3–2/3	>2/3

* The maximum degree of cortical destruction as
  defined by the overall width of the bone, as seen on
  plain radiograph, in any view.

SOFT-TISSUE TUMOURS

Soft-tissue tumours (STTs) are a heterogeneous
group of benign and malignant diseases accounting for <4% of all tumours in adults and <8% of
all tumours in children. Soft-tissue sarcomas are

rare malignant tumours derived from mesenchymal cells at all body sites.

Patients may present with a painful or painless swelling that is growing insidiously. Almost 50% arise in the lower limbs (most commonly the adductor compartment of the thigh) and the median age for presentation is 65 years.

AGE-RELATED VARIATIONS IN STT

Embryonal rhabdomyosarcomas occur exclusively in children.
Synovial sarcomas occur in young adults.
Liposarcomas occur in older people.

Concern at the biological activity of a lesion should arise if the size is >5 cm, it is painful, deep to fascia, increasing in size, or recurrence of a previously excised lesion.

Plain X-rays of soft-tissue lesions are helpful to exclude bone lesions with soft-tissue extension and to assess bone invasion from extraosseous tumours with a risk of fracture. X-rays should be obtained as the location and presence of any periosteal reaction, erosion (e.g. glomus tumour, pigmented villonodular synovitis (PVNS)) or soft-tissue mineralization (e.g. synovial sarcoma) are useful for characterization. STTs are more difficult to diagnose specifically from imaging, but there may be characteristics which can help to determine aggressiveness or identifiable tissues such as fat, calcification or haemorrhage. Matrix calcification or ossification may be found in synovial sarcomas and in the rarer mesenchymal chondrosarcomas or soft-tissue osteosarcomas.

MRI sequencing of the affected limb is valuable to define the extent of the lesion and local invasion of critical structures and to characterize the lesion prior to biopsy. If surgery is planned, this will define the margins in relation to neurovascular structures and the involved musculature, joints or tendons.

LIPOMATOUS TUMOURS

Lipoma

Lipomas are the most common STTs encountered in clinical practice, typically presenting in middle to old age but sometimes occurring in children and adolescents (**9.25**). Benign superficial lipomas classically arise in the subcutaneous tissue of the back, shoulder, neck and proximal extremities. Intramuscular lipomas are found within or between muscles and adherent to joints, tendons, bone and nerves. In 5% of cases, lipomas can be multiple and symmetrical across the dorsum and proximal upper limbs.

Examination reveals solitary, soft, painless, mobile and slow-growing lesions. Deep lipomas may be occult and therefore larger at presentation. Excision is curative and recurrences are rare in superficial lipomas but more common with intramuscular lipomas.

Liposarcoma

Liposarcomas are the most common malignant soft-tissue sarcomas, accounting for 10% of all soft tissue sarcomas typically arising in adults after the third decade. They can arise in any location with fat, but most are found deep in the thigh, groin, calf, popliteal fossa and buttock. These insidious lesions can reach large sizes prior to presentation and a few may cause pain. Nerve compression or oedema secondary to venous occlusion can occur, particularly if involving the retroperitoneum. MRI sequences reveal heterogeneous and non-specific appearances of high and low signal regions on T2. These tumours can erode adjacent cortical bone, which responds with a modest periosteal reaction. They show diffuse uptake with scintigraphy and angiography shows dense neo-angiogenesis.

These tumours require wide excision and sometimes radical excision in the higher-grade tumours (**e9.5**). Radiotherapy is used pre- or postoperatively and chemotherapy may be used. Postoperative radiotherapy is indicated for poor

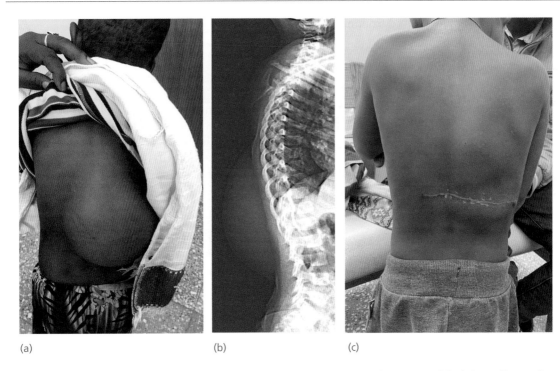

(a)   (b)   (c)

9.25 Lipomatous tumour (a) Large lipoma overlying the thoracolumbar spine. **(b)** Plain radiographs and MRI confirmed there was no spinal involvement. **(c)** The lipoma was excised.

surgical margins. Local recurrence occurs more rapidly and metastases are frequent in these high-grade liposarcomas. Mortality ranges between 30% and 50% at 5 years.

FIBROUS TUMOURS

Fibrous tumours also represent a spectrum of disease from benign to high-grade neoplasms with similar microscopic appearances.

Superficial lesions

Superficial lesions include Dupuytren's, Ledderhose, Peyronie's and Garrod's pads (Dupuytren's diathesis). They are caused by proliferation of myofibroblasts, which secrete collagen and undergo contraction by their interaction with the deposited matrix (similar to their involvement in wound healing). Palmar and plantar fibromatosis causes firm, painless nodules leading to puckering of the skin, fibrous cords and deformity. Many patients have a significant family history and treatment ranges from collagenase injections to dermofasciectomy with a significant risk of recurrence. These do not represent a premalignant condition.

Fibrosarcoma

Fibrosarcomas are deep tumours arising in the thigh, trunk, arm and forearm and are most common in adults (mean age 50 years). They present as slowly enlarging masses with and without pain. MRI demonstrates homogeneous, low-signal tumours which may erode into bone. Histologically they reveal a classic 'herringbone' pattern of dark-staining nuclei, but they may contain relatively bland areas mimicking fibromatosis. More than 80% are high-grade, necessitating systemic staging and wide excision with adjuvant radiotherapy. Fibrosarcomas metastasize to lung and bone, and chemotherapy may be indicated for systemic treatment.

Myxofibrosarcoma

These are the more common soft-tissue sarcomas in older patients with a mean age at diagnosis of 60 years, although they can arise in all age groups after skeletal maturity. Most commonly found in the lower limbs, upper limbs and girdles, they are more often subcutaneous than myofascial in origin. They present as painful enlarging masses with infiltrative margins. Low-grade myxofibrosarcomas tend not to metastasize; in intermediate-or high-grade tumours metastases are found in the lungs, bone or lymph nodes. Deeper lesions more commonly metastasize and consequently have a higher mortality rate. Wide excision and radiotherapy are the mainstays of treatment. Overall, 5-year survival is approximately 65%.

SYNOVIAL TUMOURS

Pigmented villonodular synovitis

VNS is a rare, benign and aggressive disorder arising from synovial joints and tendon sheaths capable of eroding articular structures and bone (e9.6). PVNS represents a spectrum of 'fibrohistiocytic' disorders ranging from the most common giant-cell tumour of tendon sheath (GCTTS) to localized and diffuse intra-articular PVNS lesions. Patients primarily present in the third to fifth decades with swelling and/or pain around a single joint. Articular tumours are found predominantly in the knee, hip and ankle; extra-articular tendon sheath tumours typically involve the digits.

Surgical excision is the gold standard therapy to control symptoms and prevent further joint erosion, but high recurrence rates are related to incomplete excision. Joint erosion is particularly associated with the diffuse articular form, necessitating arthroplasty in the hip and the knee. Adjunctive therapies include injection of intra-articular radiation materials and external beam radiotherapy. Alternative therapies such as tyrosine kinase inhibitors (e.g. imatinib) have demonstrated efficacy in recurrent cases although the lesions tend to recur if the therapy stops.

VASCULAR AND SMOOTH MUSCLE TUMOURS

Glomus tumour

This is a rare mesenchymal perivascular tumour usually occurring around fine peripheral neurovascular structures, particularly the nail beds of fingers or toes in young adults. These small, pea-sized blue nodules cause recurrent episodes of pain in the fingertip that are worse with cold temperatures. X-rays may show erosion of the underlying phalanx. Surgical excision from the fibrous capsule surrounding it is usually successful.

Angiosarcoma

Angiosarcoma of soft tissue is a rare, malignant tumour of cells, morphologically similar to normal endothelium, the majority of which develop as cutaneous lesions. They are often associated with previous radiotherapy and chronic lymphoedematous tissue (e.g. breast carcinoma). They may also occur adjacent to synthetic or foreign material, adjacent to arteriovenous fistulae and in Maffucci syndrome. They usually arise in the deep muscles of the thigh, calf, arm and trunk as an enlarging mass. Associated symptoms may include coagulopathy, anaemia, haematoma or bruising.

Although X-rays are usually normal, MRI demonstrates a serpentine lesion described as a 'bunch of grapes'. Fluid–fluid levels may be appreciated between fibrous septae. Histologically high-grade, complete wide excision is required as local recurrence is 20% and first-year mortality approaches 50% due to metastasis to distant bones, soft tissues and lymph nodes.

Leiomyosarcoma

This is a malignant tumour of spindle cells originating from smooth muscle, which can occur in retroperitoneal, cutaneous and vascular locations. It is the predominant sarcoma arising from larger blood vessels, most commonly the vena cava, iliac and femoral veins, causing occlusion and limb swelling. Typically arising after the fourth decade and peaking at 70 years, the retroperitoneal tumours can involve solid organs and the vertebral bodies. They present with abdominal masses, pain, weight loss, nausea and vomiting. Angiography or duplex ultrasound imaging demonstrates highly vascularized lesions, highlighting the need for vascular reconstruction after resection. These highly aggressive tumours are frequently not resectable and metastasize to lung, bone and soft tissue; consequently, survival is 25% at 5 years. Leiomyosarcoma is the commonest sarcoma giving rise to metastases of the skin.

NERVE-SHEATH TUMOURS

Neuroma

A neuroma is not a tumour but an overgrowth of fibrous tissue and randomly sprouting nerve fibrils following injury to a nerve. It is often tender, and local percussion may induce distal paraesthesia, indicating the level of the lesion (Tinel's sign).

Treatment can be frustrating. If the neuroma is excised (or as a prophylactic measure during amputation), the epineural sleeve can be freed from the nerve fascicles and sealed with a synthetic tissue adhesive or buried into muscle or bone.

Schwannoma

This is a benign tumour of the nerve sheath. It is seen in the peripheral nerves and in the spinal nerve roots. The patient complains of pain or paraesthesia; sometimes there is a small palpable swelling along the course of the nerve. MRI demonstrates a homogeneous encapsulated lesion with a 'target sign' (9.26). With careful dissection, the tumour can be shelled out from its capsule without damage to the nerve.

Neurofibroma

Neurofibromas are benign tumours of the peripheral nerve sheath. They may be solitary (90%) or multiple in neurofibromatosis type 1

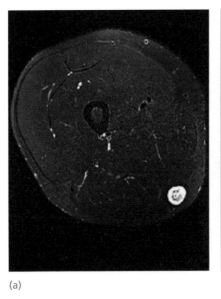
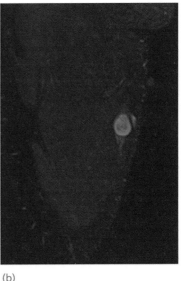

(a)   (b)

9.26 Schwannoma This patient presented with an enlarging mass in the posteromedial aspect of the right thigh. On examination, the lesion was mobile but Tinel's sign resulted in dyasthesia in a dermatomal distribution distal to the lesion. MRI scan demonstrates a well-circumscribed high-signal lesion which on axial sections (a) demonstrates a characteristic 'target' sign. The sagittal sections (b) demonstrate the nerve entering above and exiting below the lesion. Resection histology confirmed a benign peripheral nerve-sheath tumour, a schwannoma.

(NF1) and are sometimes associated with skeletal abnormalities (e.g. scoliosis, pseudarthrosis of the tibia) or overgrowth of a digit or an entire limb, in which there is no obvious neural pathology. These painless nodules can arise in all age groups, usually superficial subcutaneous growths of the lower limbs but other forms may include dumb-bell foraminal tumours or plexiform neurofibromas. In contrast to schwannomas, neurofibromas are poorly defined lesions consisting of bland spindle cells. If a nerve root is involved, symptoms can mimic those of a disc prolapse; X-rays may show erosion of a vertebral pedicle or enlargement of the intervertebral foramen. MRI may demonstrate homogeneous high signal on T1 with a 'target-sign' appearance for plexiform tumours. Malignant transformation is rare in solitary neurofibromas but occurs in up to a third of patients with neurofibromatosis. Large painful lesions are excised with marginal margins.

MUSCLE TUMOURS

Rhabdomyosarcoma

This is the most common soft-tissue sarcoma arising in children and adolescents (although it can arise in any age group) and is composed of malignant striated muscle cells. More common in the lower limbs, the most common embryonal subtype displays the rapid, infiltrative growth of an aggressive tumour. Frequently bound to bone, radiographic erosion of bone may be seen, although there may be minimal periosteal reaction.

Treatment comprises neoadjuvant chemotherapy followed by wide excision including regional lymph nodes, chemotherapy and radiation if incompletely excised. The entire muscle from origin to insertion must be excised. Five-year survival ranges from 80% if completely excised to 20% if lung metastases are present at diagnosis.

Neuromuscular disorders

10

- Nerves and muscles — 199
- Clinical assessment — 202
- Cerebral palsy — 206
- Adult acquired spastic paresis — 210
- Lesions of the spinal cord — 210
- Spina bifida — 212
- Poliomyelitis — 216
- Motor neuron disorders — 217
- Peripheral neuropathies — 219
- Muscular dystrophy — 225

Of the vast range of neurological disorders, those which most commonly give rise to orthopaedic problems are:

- cerebral palsy and stroke (upper motor neuron, spastic disorders)
- compressive lesions of the spinal cord
- neural tube defects (spina bifida)
- anterior poliomyelitis
- degenerative motor neuron disorders
- nerve root disorders
- peripheral neuropathies.

This chapter also deals with two types of 'muscle disorder':

- arthrogryposis
- muscular dystrophy.

NERVES AND MUSCLES

NEURONS

The *neuron* (**10.1**) is the defining unit of the nervous system. This is a specialized cell, capable of electrical excitation and conduction of electro-chemical impulses (action potentials) along its thread-like extensions. It consists of a *cell body* with branching processes – *dendrites* – that can receive signals from other neuronal terminals. A finer, longer branch – the *axon* – carries the action potentials to or from excitable target organs (**10.1**). Further signal transmission to the dendrites of another neuron, or neuroexcitable tissue like muscle, occurs at a *synapse* where the axon terminal releases a chemical *neurotransmitter* – typically acetylcholine.

All motor axons and the larger sensory axons serving touch, pain and proprioception are covered by a sheath – the *neurilemma* – and coated with *myelin*, a multi-layered lipoprotein substance which serves as an insulator and allows impulses to be propagated much faster than is the case in unmyelinated nerves. Depletion of the myelin sheath causes slowing – and eventually complete blocking – of axonal conduction.

NERVOUS PATHWAYS

Neurological structures can be divided into:

- the central nervous system (CNS), comprising the brain and tracts within the spinal cord
- the peripheral nervous system (PNS), which includes the cranial and spinal nerves.

SECTION 1 GENERAL ORTHOPAEDICS

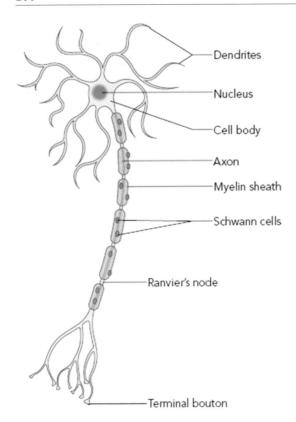

10.1 **Neuron** Diagram of a typical neuron.

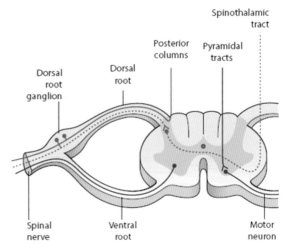

10.2 **Main nerve pathways** Simplified diagram showing the main neurological pathways to and from a typical thoracic spinal cord segment. Fibres carrying touch, sharp pain and temperature impulses (------) decussate, in some cases over several spinal segments, and ascend in the contralateral spinothalamic tracts; those carrying vibration and proprioceptive impulses (——) enter the ipsilateral posterior columns. Motor neurons (——) arise in the anterior horn of the grey matter and innervate ipsilateral muscles.

Both the CNS and the PNS have a somatic component and an autonomic component.

The *somatic nervous system* provides efferent (motor) and afferent (sensory) pathways to and from peripheral parts of the body serving, respectively, voluntary muscle contraction and sensibility (**10.2**).

- *Upper motor neurons (UMNs)* are those between the brain and the spinal cord.
- *Lower motor neurons (LMNs)* are those between the anterior horn of the spinal cord and the peripheral muscles.

Axons conveying sensory impulses from receptors in the skin and other peripheral structures enter the dorsal nerve roots, with their cell bodies in the dorsal root (or cranial nerve) ganglia, and end in synapses within the CNS. (Sensory areas (dermatomes) corresponding to the spinal nerve roots are shown in **10.4**.)

The *autonomic system* controls involuntary reflex and homeostatic activities of the various bodily organs and peripheral structures. Its two components, *sympathetic* and *parasympathetic* divisions, serve more-or-less opposing functions.

REFLEX ACTIVITY AND TONE

Sudden stretching of a muscle (e.g. by tapping sharply over the tendon) induces an involuntary muscle contraction – the stretch reflex. The sharp change in muscle fibre length is detected by the muscle spindle; the impulse is transmitted rapidly along myelinated afferent (sensory) neurons which synapse directly with the corresponding motor neurons in the spinal cord, triggering efferent signals which stimulate the muscle to contract. This is the basis of the familiar clinical tests for tendon reflexes, and is also the mechanism for maintaining normal muscle tone.

SECTION 1 GENERAL ORTHOPAEDICS

Normally this reflex activity is regulated by UMN impulses passing from the brain down the spinal cord.

> **INTERRUPTION OF MOTOR NEURON PATHWAYS**
>
> Interruption of the UMN pathways results in undamped reflex muscle contraction, clinically seen as *spastic paralysis* and hyperactive tendon reflexes. Interruption of the LMN pathways results in *flaccid paralysis*.

AUTONOMIC FUNCTIONS

The autonomic system is involved with the regulation of involuntary activities of cardiac muscle and smooth (unstriated) muscle in the lungs, gastrointestinal tract, kidneys, bladder, genital organs, sweat glands and small blood vessels. Afferent (sensory) and efferent (motor) pathways constitute a continuously active reflex arc.

The autonomic system is divided into sympathetic and parasympathetic pathways, both of which comprise efferent and afferent neurons.

Sympathetic neurons

These leave the spinal cord with the ventral nerve roots at all levels from T1 to L1, enter the paravertebral sympathetic chain of ganglia and synapse with postganglionic neurons that spread out to all parts of the body. Important functions are the reflex control of heart rate, blood flow and sweating, as well as other responses associated with conditions of 'fight and flight'.

Parasympathetic neurons

These leave the CNS (from the brainstem) with cranial nerves III, VII, IX and X and with the nerve roots of S2, 3 and 4 to reach ganglia where they synapse with postganglionic neurons close to their target organs.

PERIPHERAL NERVES

Peripheral nerves are bundles of axons conducting efferent (motor) impulses from cells in the

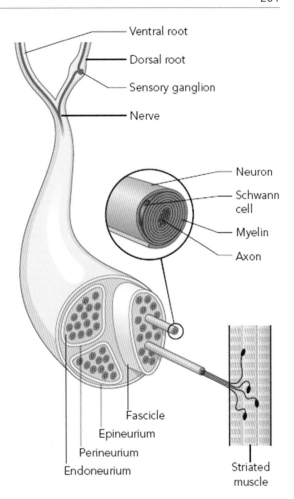

10.3 Nerve structure Diagram of the structural elements of a peripheral nerve.

anterior horn of the spinal cord to the muscles, and afferent (sensory) impulses from peripheral receptors via cells in the posterior root ganglia to the cord (**10.3**). They also convey sudomotor and vasomotor fibres from ganglion cells in the sympathetic chain. Some nerves are predominantly motor, some predominantly sensory; the larger trunks are mixed, with motor and sensory axons running in separate bundles. Peripheral nerve structure is described in Chapter 11.

SKELETAL MUSCLE

Each skeletal muscle belly consists of thousands of *muscle fibres*, separated into bundles

SECTION 1 GENERAL ORTHOPAEDICS

(or fascicles). Each fascicle is surrounded by a flimsy perimysium which envelops anything up to about 100 muscle fibres. Large muscles concerned with mass movement, like the glutei or quadriceps, have a large number of fibres in each fascicle, while muscles used for precision movements (such as those of the hand) have a much smaller number in each bundle.

Muscle fibres are of two different types:

- *Type I fibres* contract slowly and are not easily fatigued; their prime function is postural control.
- *Type II fibres* are fast-contracting but they fatigue rapidly, so they are ideally suited to intense activities of short duration.

All muscles consist of a mixture of fibre types, the balance depending mainly on genetic disposition, basic muscle function and degree of training: thus, long-distance runners have a greater proportion of type I fibres than the average.

Important terms relating to muscles are defined as follows.

- *Muscle contraction* is a complex activity. Individual myofibrils respond to electrical stimuli in much the same way as do motor neurons. When the fibres contract, internal tension in the muscle increases.
  - In *isometric contraction* there is increased tension without actual shortening of the muscle or movement of the joint controlled by that muscle.
  - In *isotonic contraction* the muscle shortens and moves the joint.
- *Muscle tone* is the state of tension in a resting muscle when it is passively stretched: tone is increased in UMN lesions (spastic paralysis) and decreased in LMN lesions (flaccid paralysis).
- *Muscle contracture* (as distinct from contraction) is the change that occurs when a normally innervated muscle is held immobile in a shortened position for a long time; for example, if a joint is habitually held flexed, it may be impossible to straighten it passively without injuring the muscle. Active exercise will eventually overcome the muscle contracture, unless the muscle has been permanently damaged.

- *Muscle wasting* follows either disuse or denervation. In the former, the fibres are intact but thinner; in the latter, they degenerate and are replaced by fibrous tissue or fat.
- *Muscle fasciculation* – or muscle twitch – is a local involuntary muscle contraction of a small bundle of muscle fibres. It is usually benign but can be due to motor neuron disease or dysfunction.

CLINICAL ASSESSMENT

HISTORY

- *Age* at presentation is important. Certain disorders are obvious at birth (e.g. spina bifida and arthrogryposis). Cerebral palsy presents during infancy; poliomyelitis usually occurs in childhood; spinal cord lesions and peripheral neuropathies are more common in adults. However, the residual effects of neurological disease, such as muscle weakness and deformity, may need attention throughout life.
- *Numbness* or *paraesthesia* is often the main complaint among adults. It is important to establish its exact distribution to help localize the level of the lesion. The rate of onset and the relationship to posture may, similarly, suggest the cause.
- *Muscle weakness* may be due to UMN or LMN lesions (spastic versus flaccid paralysis) but it may also be due to a primary muscle problem. Ask about the type and degree of weakness, the rate of onset, whether it affects part of a limb, a whole limb, upper or lower limb, one side of the body or both sides.
- *Deformity* is a common complaint in long-standing disorders. It arises as a result of muscle imbalances that may be very subtle and the deformity (such as 'claw toes') may not be recognized until it is pointed out to the patient.

EXAMINATION

Neurological examination is discussed in Chapter 1. Note that the back should always be carefully examined as it holds the key to many neurological disorders.

<table>
<tr><td>

KEY ASPECTS OF NEUROLOGICAL EXAMINATION

Patient's mental state
Natural posture
Gait
Sense of balance
Involuntary movements
Muscle wasting
Muscle tone and power
Reflexes
Skin changes
Sensibility and autonomic functions (e.g. sphincter control, peripheral blood flow and sweating)

</td></tr>
</table>

MUSCLE POWER: MRC GRADING

Grade 0	No muscle action – total paralysis
Grade 1	Barely detectable contraction
Grade 2	Not enough power to overcome gravity
Grade 3	Strong enough to act against gravity
Grade 4	Still stronger but less than normal
Grade 5	Normal power

Partial loss of power is called *paresis* and complete loss of power *paralysis*.

The type of muscle weakness is important.

- *Spastic weakness* suggests a UMN lesion.
- *Flaccid weakness* could be due to either an LMN lesion or a muscle disorder.

Gait and posture

Typical patterns can often be recognized.

- *Dystonia* refers to abnormal posturing that may affect any part of the body and is often aggravated when the patient is concentrating on a particular motor task such as walking.
- A *spastic gait* is stiff and jerky, often with the feet in equinus, the knees somewhat flexed and the hips adducted ('scissoring').
- A *drop-foot gait* is due to peripheral neuropathy or injury of the nerves supplying the dorsiflexors of the ankle. During the swing phase the foot falls into equinus ('drops') and if it were not lifted higher than usual, the toes would drag along the ground.
- A *high-stepping* gait signifies either bilateral foot drop or a problem with proprioception and balance.
- A *waddling (Trendelenburg) gait*, in which the trunk is thrown from side to side with each step, may be due to dislocation of the hips or to weakness of the abductor muscles.
- *Ataxia* produces a more obvious and irregular loss of balance, which is compensated for by a broad-based gait, or sometimes uncontrollable staggering.

Muscle weakness

Muscle power is usually graded on the Medical Research Council (MRC) scale. This is known as 'muscle charting'.

- *Monoplegia* (weakness of one limb) is usually indicative of a LMN defect, most commonly a peripheral nerve or nerve root.
- *Hemiplegia* (weakness of either the right or the left side of the body) usually denotes pathology somewhere between the cerebral cortex and the cervical segment of the spinal cord, i.e. a UMN type of weakness.
- *Diplegia* (weakness in both upper or both lower limbs) can be due to either UMN or LMN disorder.
- *Quadriplegia* (all four limbs affected) could be due to either UMN or LMN pathology (e.g. cerebral palsy, high cord damage or anterior horn cell pathology as in poliomyelitis).

Nerve root supply and muscle actions are summarized in **Table 10.1**.

Deformity

Deformity may be passively correctible or fixed. When all the muscle groups serving a particular joint are equally weak *(balanced paralysis)*, the joint simply assumes the position imposed on it by gravity. It is unstable and the limb feels floppy or flail. Deformity occurs when one group of muscles is too weak to balance the pull of antagonists *(unbalanced paralysis)*. At first the

Table 10.1 Nerve root supply and muscle action

Muscle/Muscle action	Nerve root supply
Sternomastoids	Spinal accessory C2, 3, 4
Trapezius	Spinal accessory C3, 4
Diaphragm	C3, 4, 5
Deltoid	C5, 6
Supra- and infraspinatus	C5, 6
Serratus anterior	C5, 6, 7
Pectoralis major	C5, 6, 7, 8
Elbow flexion	C5, 6
extension	C7
Supination	C5, 6
Pronation	C6
Wrist flexion	C6, (7)
extension	C6, 7, (8)
Finger flexion	C7, 8, T1
extension	C7, 8, T1
ab- and adduction	C8, T1
Hip flexion	L1, 2, 3
extension	L5, S1
adduction	L2, 3, 4
abduction	L4, 5, S1
Knee extension	L(2), 3, 4
flexion	L5, S1
Ankle dorsiflexion	L4, 5
plantarflexion	S1, 2
inversion	L4, 5
eversion	L5, S1
Toe extension	L5
flexion	S1
abduction	S1, 2

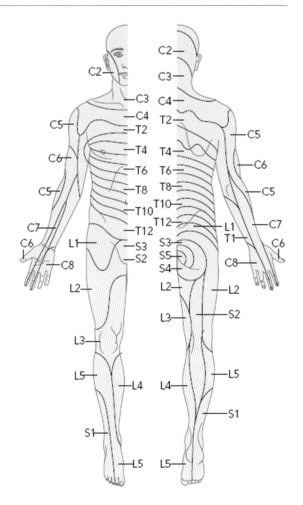

10.4 Sensory nerve root distribution Dermatomes.

Autonomic functions

The sympathetic and parasympathetic systems are concerned with functions such as involuntary muscle contraction, sphincter control, peripheral blood flow and sweating. Two classical examples of dysfunction are Horner's syndrome and the so-called cauda equina syndrome.

- *Horner's syndrome* is due to sympathetic blockade in the vicinity of C7 and T1. There is a characteristic combination of ipsilateral ptosis (drooping eyelid), miosis (contraction of the pupil), facial hyperaemia (flushing) and anhidrosis (loss of sweating).

deformity can be corrected passively but with time it becomes fixed. In children, paralysis may also affect bone growth.

Sensory changes

All sensory modalities must be tested over all dermatomes (**10.4**). Any change from the normal must be mapped to see if it fits a particular distribution pattern: dermatomal, 'glove' and 'stocking' or peripheral nerve distribution.

> Horner's syndrome is an important clue in the diagnosis of cervicothoracic tumours, cord compression, mediastinal tumours, apical tumours of the lung and preganglionic damage to the nerve roots in a brachial plexus injury.

* *Cauda equina syndrome* signals a neurological lesion of the conus medullaris or cauda equina, resulting in urinary and faecal retention and impairment of penile erection.

> The symptoms of cauda equina syndrome are important signs in patients with spinal injuries and lumbar intervertebral disc prolapse; if the neurological compression is not relieved within hours, the effects may be irreversible.

INVESTIGATION

Imaging

Plain X-rays of the skull or spine are routine for all disorders of the CNS. Specialized imaging of the brain and spinal cord may be necessary to reveal degenerative or space-occupying lesions. Narrowing of the spinal canal is best demonstrated by *computed tomography (CT)*. Destructive lesions of the spine may require both *CT* and *magnetic resonance imaging (MRI)* to show the extent of cord involvement.

Imaging of the brain is usually by *MRI*. Functional scans such as *positron emission tomography (PET)* can isolate specific areas of brain activity.

Other investigations

* *Blood and cerebrospinal fluid* (CSF) investigations may be necessary, depending on the suspected diagnosis.
* *Muscle biopsy* should be taken from a muscle that is affected but still functioning. Local anaesthetic infiltration must be avoided, the specimen must be handled gently and, depending on the tests required, it must be kept at its resting fibre length. Biopsies should be placed in special transport medium or frozen immediately.

NEUROPHYSIOLOGICAL TESTS

Neurodiagnostic techniques comprising *nerve conduction studies* and *needle electromyography* have an important role in the investigation of peripheral nerve and muscle disorders. In orthopaedic practice, most of these investigations centre on the median, ulnar, radial and sciatic nerves (motor and sensory).

Nerve conduction

MOTOR NERVE CONDUCTION

This is studied by stimulating the nerve electrically at an accessible subcutaneous site (e.g. above the medial epicondyle at the elbow for the ulnar nerve) until it propagates an action potential which travels to the innervated muscle where a surface electrode records the response (**10.5**). Measurements are displayed on an oscilloscope screen, the most informative being the time it takes in milliseconds (ms) for the impulse to reach the muscle and also the magnitude of the response in millivolts (mV). By measuring the distance from the stimulating electrode to the recording electrode one can deduce the *nerve conduction velocity* in metres per second between those two points.

In practice it is more useful to stimulate the nerve at two points – first above and then below the area thought to be abnormal – and subtract the more distal conduction velocity from the

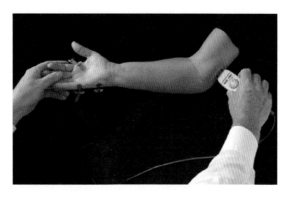

10.5 Ulnar motor nerve conduction The ulnar nerve is stimulated above the elbow, posterior to the medial epicondyle, and the impulse is recorded from the abductor digiti minimi.

proximal conduction velocity so as to obtain a truer measurement for the intervening segment of the nerve. Thus, to measure the conduction velocity of the median nerve in the carpal tunnel, one would take readings with the recording electrode first distal to the carpal tunnel and then proximal to the carpal tunnel in the forearm; this would allow one to deduce the conduction velocity in the particular segment of the nerve at the carpal tunnel. A reduced velocity is typical of the common carpal tunnel compression syndrome. By contrast, conduction slowing throughout the length of the nerve suggests a demyelinating neuropathy.

SENSORY NERVE CONDUCTION

Sensory nerve conduction can be studied in a similar manner, by stimulating the nerve at a distal site and recording the findings at a suitably placed proximal electrode.

Electromyography

Electromyography (EMG) is used to record the electrical discharge of motor units in a muscle: a needle electrode is inserted into the muscle and connected to an oscilloscopic screen and a loudspeaker. At rest, a normal muscle is silent. As the patient slowly contracts the muscle there is recruitment of more and more motor units; this is reflected first as a progressive increase in the number and then also as increased amplitude of motor unit action potentials, with recognizable patterns. In a denervated muscle (e.g. the result of spinal nerve root entrapment) the number of motor units recruited will be reduced proportional to disrupted axons. Instead of the white noise of full recruitment, one sees a reduced pattern of muscle potentials.

Diagnostic evaluation

Nerve conduction and EMG studies are concentrated in the appropriate anatomical territory and, whenever possible, the findings are compared to those in other nerve root territories in the same as well as the contralateral (usually asymptomatic) limb.

The electrophysiological findings should always be interpreted in conjunction with the clinical evaluation. Nerve conduction and EMG tests alone, without a provisional diagnosis, are less helpful.

Spinal monitoring

Spinal cord monitoring with neurophysiological tests is now considered an essential part of any spinal surgery that includes deformity correction to ensure that no neurological damage occurs. The techniques used are based on the principles defined above but often in combination with techniques employed in electroencephalography (EEG), such as *averaging*. A peripheral nerve in the upper or the lower limb (usually the median or posterior tibial) is stimulated but, instead of recording from the nerve or the muscle twitch, one records from the scalp overlying the patient's sensory parietal cortex.

The somatosensory-evoked responses (SSEPs) from the recorded cortex are miniscule and one must therefore *average* the obtained responses from at least 100–200 stimuli in order to differentiate the time-linked evoked response from the background brain EEG activity. Averaging 200 or more responses at a stimulus rate of 3 per second to demonstrate a reproducible response may take 1–2 minutes, assuming all other factors are even and perfect. The surgeon should be aware of this drawback.

One can also measure potentials developed in the cervical spinal cord at C7 level and the L1 level as well as distally in the brachial plexus at Erb's point, resulting from peripheral nerve stimulation.

CEREBRAL PALSY

The term 'cerebral palsy' includes a group of disorders which result from non-progressive brain damage during early development. The incidence is about 2 : 1000 live births.

The main consequence is the development of neuromuscular incoordination, dystonia (abnormal posturing and movement), weakness and muscle spasticity; in addition, there may be

KNOWN CAUSAL FACTORS OF CEREBRAL PALSY
Prematurity Perinatal anoxia Kernicterus Postnatal brain infections or injury

convulsions, perceptual problems, speech disorder and mental retardation.

Early diagnosis

A history of perinatal difficulties may suggest the diagnosis, but at birth the disease is rarely recognized. Early symptoms include difficulty in sucking and swallowing, with dribbling at the mouth; the mother may notice that the baby feels stiff or wriggles awkwardly. It gradually becomes apparent that the developmental milestones are delayed: the normal child usually holds its head up by 6 months, sits up by 9 months and begins walking by 18 months. Neonatal reflexes also may be delayed.

Late diagnosis

The clinical picture emerges slowly and varies considerably from case to case. Some patients have severe athetosis; others are ataxic; but the large majority have a spastic paresis. As the name implies, there is both spasticity and weakness, although the presence of the former may make it difficult to assess the latter. Tendon reflexes are brisk and plantar responses extensor. Sensation is normal. The children are often emotionally unstable and sometimes suffer from fits. Intelligence may be impaired.

TYPES OF MOTOR DYSFUNCTION

Cerebral palsy is usually classified according to the type of motor disorder. Those most readily recognized are spastic paresis, athetosis and ataxia.

* *Spastic paresis* is the commonest variety, accounting for over 60% of all cases. It may appear as:
  - *hemiplegia* (affecting one side of the body)
  - *diplegia* (affecting mainly the lower limbs)
  - *total body* involvement, in which all four limbs and the head and neck are affected (often associated with a low IQ)
  - *isolated asymmetrical paresis.*
* *Athetosis* manifests as continuous, involuntary writhing movements. Tongue and speech muscles may also be involved.
* *Ataxia* appears as muscular incoordination during voluntary movements. Balance is poor and the child walks with a characteristic wide-based gait.

CHARACTERISTIC DEFORMITIES

The combination of muscle imbalance and spasticity gives rise to characteristic deformities and postures, which are exaggerated when the child attempts to stand or walk (**10.6**):

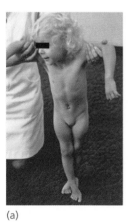 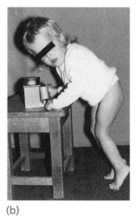 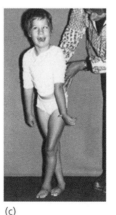 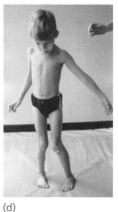

(a)   (b)   (c)   (d)

10.6 Cerebral palsy (a) Adductor spasm (scissors stance); **(b)** flexion deformity of hips and knees with equinus of the feet; **(c)** general posture and characteristic facial expression; **(d)** ataxic type of palsy.

- flexion of the elbows and wrists, with fingers clasped
- tight adduction of the hips (scissors posture)
- knees slightly flexed and unable to be straightened
- ankles and feet in equinus.

POSTURE AND GAIT

 Attempts to correct one deformity may often aggravate another and it is important to establish which deformity is the primary one and which are compensatory.

The child should be carefully observed sitting, standing, walking and lying.

- *Sitting* unsupported can be difficult and sometimes impossible. Children with a hypotonic trunk may slump into a kyphotic posture and others may 'fall' to one side. There may also be an obvious scoliosis or pelvic obliquity.
- *Standing* can be equally problematic. In the typical case of a spastic diplegia, the child stands with hips flexed, adducted and internally rotated, the knees are also flexed and the feet are in equinus. With tight hamstrings, the normal lumbar lordosis may be obliterated and the child may have difficulty staying upright.
- Many patients show pelvic obliquity and a scoliosis. Balance reactions are often poor and a gentle push that would force a normal child to take a step in the appropriate direction to maintain their balance may simply knock over a child with cerebral palsy.
- *Gait* should be observed with and without shoes or orthotic supports. Dystonic, athetoid and ataxic movements may become more noticeable during walking. In the spastic diplegic patient, lack of free rotation at the hip means that the entire trunk has to move from side to side as each leg swings through, and with the adduction it leads to a 'scissoring' action (one leg crossing in front of the other). Walking aids may help. Computerized gait analysis requires specialized skills and facilities.

Management

Treatment is best carried out in a special centre where the child can enjoy the benefits of combined surgical skills, physiotherapy, occupational therapy, speech therapy and educational support. Parents and children must be helped to understand the problems that they will encounter and realistic goals should be set.

MANAGEMENT PRIORITIES

Ability to communicate with others
Ability to cope with the activities of daily living
Independent mobility – which may mean a
    walking aid or even a motorized wheelchair

- *For the child who from an early age is recognized to be 'non-walking'* (e.g. someone with total body involvement), the goals should be:
  - a straight spine with a level pelvis
  - located, mobile and painless hips that flex to 90 degrees (for comfortable sitting) and extend sufficiently to allow comfortable sleeping and participation in standing/swivel transfers
  - knees that are mobile enough for sitting, sleeping and transferring
  - plantigrade feet that fit into shoes and rest on the footplates of the wheelchair comfortably.
- *For the child who is able to walk*, careful assessment is needed to decide whether medical management, physiotherapy, orthotics and surgery could improve their function. The multidisciplinary team will work to develop a personalized treatment plan for the patient. In recent years, specialist centres have used a 3D gait laboratory as part of the assessment to inform the treatment decision (**10.7**).

MEDICAL TREATMENT

Medications   The most generally effective medications are anticonvulsants for seizures, short-term benzodiazepine for postoperative pain and trihexyphenidyl for dystonia. Analgesics are used, when necessary, to reduce pain.

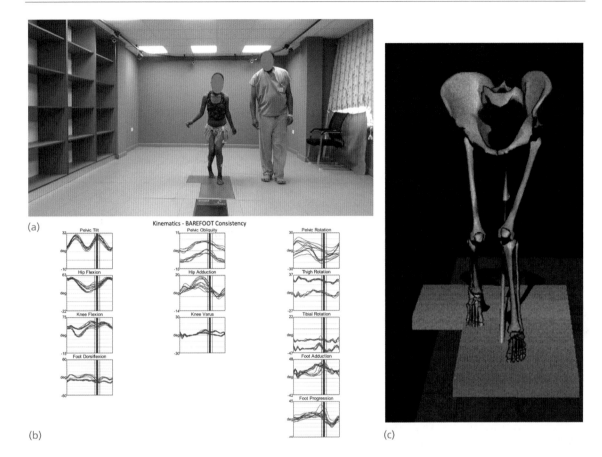

10.7 3D gait laboratory (a) Reflective markers are placed on bony prominences. Motion is captured by overhead cameras, and force and pressure plates record kinetic information. The data is processed and the graphic output **(b,c)** helps the multidisciplinary team analyse the patient's gait accurately, helping guide treatment decisions.

Botulinum A toxin Botulinum is used to reduce muscle tone in children who have marked spasticity that is interfering with their gait. It acts by blocking acetylcholine release at the neuromuscular junction. The preparation is injected into the 'spastic' muscle at (or as near as possible to) the motor end point. The usual targets are the hip adductors, hamstrings, gastrocnemius and tibialis posterior. Muscle weakness takes a few days to become obvious; the effect is temporary and after 10–14 weeks there is a return of muscle tone. In the meantime, physiotherapy and orthotics (splints) are continued. Even a temporary reduction in spasticity can help defer surgery until the child is older as well as informing the surgical plan.

Selective dorsal rhizotomy Division of selected dorsal nerve roots from L1 to S2 has recently gained wider acceptance. This aims to reduce spasticity and rebalance muscle tone by selectively reducing the input from the muscle spindles, thus leading to less excitation of the anterior horn cells. Good results have been obtained in children aged 3–8 years who can walk, have good intellectual function and good voluntary control but have significant spasticity.

 Fixed contractures are a contraindication to selective dorsal rhizotomy.

SECTION 1 GENERAL ORTHOPAEDICS

Physical therapy   This has an important role in all treatment programmes, particularly for children up to the age of 7–8 years and following surgery.

Positioning and splinting   These also play an important part. Care must be taken at all times to ensure that the child sits and sleeps, works and eats in a good position and with good posture. Splints can prevent muscle contractures, maintain joint position and improve movement and hence function.

Operative treatment   Surgery plays a crucial role.

INDICATIONS FOR SURGERY

A spastic deformity which cannot be controlled by conservative measures
Fixed deformity that interferes with function
Secondary problems including rotational deformities of the femur and tibia, dislocation of the hip and joint instability

---

Weak muscles can be augmented by tendon transfers but, because of the muscle imbalance, expertise is needed to avoid both undercorrection and overcorrection. Correction of bony deformity at the hip, knee and ankle is an important part of the management in older children.

The timing of surgical intervention is often crucial. Development of the CNS and the gait pattern matures around the age of 7–8 years. Many orthopaedic surgeons therefore advocate non-operative management until this age and offer surgical intervention when the child is older and is showing signs of a deteriorating gait. In the past, 'birthday surgery' was performed where the child would have annual surgery to improve function at the ankle, knee and hip. Surgery is usually now undertaken on the same admission with 'single-event multilevel surgery'.

Patients with *hemiplegia* respond well to both conservative and operative treatment, and all of them should eventually be able to walk unaided. Those with *diplegia* are more difficult to manage but most of them will eventually be able to walk. Patients with *total body involvement* have a poor prognosis for walking, yet even in this group

surgery may be needed to improve spinal alignment, hip instability, perineal care or to alleviate pain.

For a regional survey of corrective operations, the reader is referred to *Apley & Solomon's System of Orthopaedics and Trauma*, 10th edition, CRC Press (2017).

ADULT ACQUIRED SPASTIC PARESIS

Cerebral damage following a stroke may cause persistent spastic paresis in the adult; disturbance of proprioception and stereognosis may coexist.

In the early recuperative stage, physiotherapy and splintage are important in preventing fixed contractures; all affected joints should be put through a full range of movement every day, and deformities should be corrected and splinted until controlled muscle power returns.

Proprioception and coordination can be improved by occupational therapy. Once maximal motor recovery has been achieved – usually by 9 months – residual deformity or joint instability may need surgical correction or permanent splinting. In general, treatment is similar to that of spastic deformity in the child, and is summarized in **Table 10.2**.

LESIONS OF THE SPINAL CORD

With lesions of the spinal cord, patients complain of muscle weakness, numbness or loss of balance; bladder and bowel control may be impaired and men may complain of impotence. Examination reveals a spastic UMN paresis, with exaggerated reflexes and a Babinski response. There may be a fairly precise boundary of sensory change, suggesting the level of cord involvement. Extradural compression may also involve nerve roots and cause LMN signs.

Patterns of cord dysfunction

The pattern of motor and sensory impairment suggests the level of cord involvement (**Table 10.3**).

Table 10.2 Treatment of principal deformities of the limbs

	Deformity	Splintage	Surgery
Foot	Equinus	Spring-loaded dorsiflexion	Lengthen tendo Achillis
	Equinovarus	Bracing in eversion and dorsiflexion	Lengthen tendo Achillis and transfer lateral half of tibialis anterior to cuboid
Knee	Flexion	Long caliper	Hamstring release
Hip	Adduction	–	Obturator neurectomy Adductor muscle release
Shoulder	Adduction	–	Subscapularis release
Elbow	Flexion	–	Release elbow flexors
Wrist	Flexion	Wrist splint	Lengthen or release wrist flexors; may need fusion or carpectomy
Fingers	Flexion	–	Lengthen or release flexors

Table 10.3 Cord involvement and motor/sensory impairment

Cord involvement	Motor/sensory impairment
Cervical cord	LMN weakness and sensory loss in arms UMN signs in the lower limbs
Thoracic cord	UMN paresis in lower limbs Variable sensory impairment
Lumbar cord	Combination of UMN and LMN signs in lower limbs
Cauda equina	LMN signs and sensory loss in lower limbs, plus urinary retention with overflow
Spinal shock	Acute cord lesions may present with a flaccid paralysis which resolves over time, usually to reveal the typical UMN signs associated with cord injury

Diagnosis and management

The more common causes of spinal cord dysfunction are listed in the box. Traumatic and compressive lesions are the ones most likely to be seen by orthopaedic surgeons. Plain X-rays will show structural abnormalities of the spine; cord compression can be visualized by myelography, alone or combined with CT. Intrinsic lesions of the cord require further investigation by blood tests, CSF examination and MRI.

COMMON CAUSES OF SPINAL CORD DYSFUNCTION

Acute injury
- Vertebral fracture
- Fracture-dislocation

Infection
- Epidural abscess
- Poliomyelitis

Intervertebral disc prolapse
- Sequestrated disc
- Disc prolapse in spinal stenosis

Vertebral canal stenosis
- Congenital stenosis
- Acquired stenosis

Spinal cord tumours
- Neurofibroma
- Meningioma

Intrinsic cord lesions
- Tabes dorsalis
- Syringomyelia
- Other degenerative disorders

Miscellaneous
- Spina bifida
- Vascular lesions
- Multiple lesions
- Multiple sclerosis
- Haemorrhagic disorders

Urgent diagnosis and treatment are needed for the following traumatic and compressive lesions:

- acute compressive lesions
- epidural abscess
- acute disc prolapse.

Compressive lesions

- *Acute compressive lesions* require urgent diagnosis and treatment if permanent damage is to be prevented.

 Bladder dysfunction is ominous: whereas motor and sensory signs may improve after decompression, loss of bladder control, if present for more than 24 hours, is usually irreversible.

- With *chronic lesions*, one can afford to temporize. Once the diagnosis is certain, appropriate treatment can be applied.

Epidural abscess   This is a surgical emergency. The patient rapidly develops acute pain and muscle spasm, with fever, leucocytosis and elevation of the erythrocyte sedimentation rate (ESR). X-rays may show disc space narrowing and bone erosion. Treatment is by immediate decompression and antibiotics.

Acute disc prolapse   This usually causes unilateral symptoms and signs. However, complete lumbar disc prolapse may present as a cauda equina syndrome. Spinal canal obstruction is demonstrated by MRI. Operative discectomy is urgent.

Chronic discogenic disease   Often associated with narrowing of the intervertebral foramina and compression of nerve roots, diagnosis is usually obvious on X-ray and MRI. Operative decompression may be needed.

Spinal stenosis   This produces a typical clinical syndrome, due partly to direct pressure on the cord or nerve roots and partly to vascular obstruction and ischaemic neuropathy during hyperextension of the lumbar spine. The patient complains of pain and paraesthesia in one or both lower limbs after standing or walking for a few minutes, symptoms that are relieved by bending forward, sitting or crouching so as to flex the lumbar spine. Congenital narrowing of the spinal canal is rare, except in developmental disorders such as achondroplasia. Treatment calls for bony decompression of the nerve structures.

Vertebral disease   Conditions such as tuberculosis or metastatic disease, may cause cord compression and paraparesis. The diagnosis is usually obvious on X-ray, but a needle biopsy may be necessary for confirmation. Management is usually by anterior decompression and, if necessary, internal stabilization.

Spinal cord tumours   Tumours are a comparatively rare cause of progressive paraparesis. X-rays may show bony erosion, widening of the spinal canal or flattening of the vertebral pedicles. Widening of the intervertebral foramina is typical of neurofibromatosis. Treatment usually involves operative removal of the tumour.

Intrinsic lesions of the cord   These lesions produce slowly progressive neurological signs. Two conditions in particular – *tabes dorsalis* and *syringomyelia* – may present with orthopaedic problems because of neuropathic joint destruction. In tabes dorsalis, the posterior column is affected resulting in loss of proprioception and balance. In syringomyelia a long cavity (the syrinx) filled with CSF develops within the spinal cord, most commonly in the cervical region. Symptoms and signs are most noticeable in the upper limbs. The expanding cyst presses on the anterior horn cells, producing weakness and wasting of the hand muscles. Destruction of the spinothalamic fibres in the centre of the cord produces a characteristic dissociated sensory loss in the upper limbs: impaired response to pain and temperature but preservation of touch. CT may reveal an expanded cord and the syrinx can be defined on MRI. Deterioration may be slowed by decompression of the foramen magnum.

SPINA BIFIDA

Spina bifida is a congenital disorder in which the two halves of the posterior vertebral arch (or

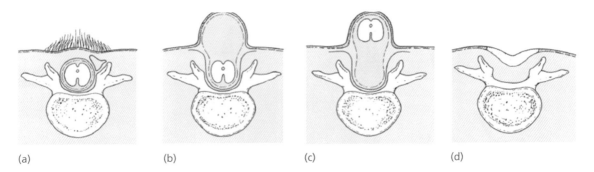

(a)   (b)   (c)   (d)

10.8 Dysraphism **(a)** Spina bifida occulta; **(b)** meningocele; **(c)** myelomeningocele; **(d)** open myelomeningocele.

several arches) have failed to fuse. This is often associated with maldevelopment of the neural tube and the overlying skin; the combination of faults is called dysraphism (**10.8**). It usually occurs in the lumbar or lumbosacral region. If neural elements are involved there may be paralysis and loss of sensation and sphincter control.

SPINA BIFIDA OCCULTA

In the mildest forms of dysraphism there is a midline defect between the laminae and nothing more; hence the term *occulta* (meaning secret). However, there may be tell-tale defects in the overlying skin: a dimple, a pit or a tuft of hair.

SPINA BIFIDA CYSTICA

In severe forms of dysraphism the vertebral laminae are missing and the contents of the vertebral canal prolapse through the defect – either as a CSF-filled meningeal sac or *meningocele* or as a sac containing part of the spinal cord and nerve roots, a *myelomeningocele* (the commonest lesion). The cord may be in its primitive state, the unfolded neural plate forming part of the roof of the sac; this is an *'open' myelomeningocele* or rachischisis. In a *'closed' myelomeningocele* the neural tube is fully formed and covered by membrane and skin.

HYDROCEPHALUS

Distal tethering of the cord may cause herniation of the cerebellum and brainstem through the foramen magnum, resulting in obstruction to CSF circulation and hydrocephalus. The ventricles dilate and the skull enlarges by separation of the cranial sutures. Persistently raised intracranial pressure may cause cerebral atrophy and mental retardation.

NEUROLOGICAL DYSFUNCTION

Myelomeningocele is always associated with neurological deficit below the level of the lesion. This may also occur – though less frequently and much less severely – in spina bifida occulta.

Incidence and screening

Isolated laminar defects are seen in over 5% of lumbar spine X-rays. By comparison, cystic spina bifida is rare at 2–3 per 1000 live births, but if one child is affected the risk for the next child is 10 times greater.

Neural-type defects are associated with high levels of alpha-fetoprotein in the amniotic fluid and serum. This offers an effective method of antenatal screening during the 15th to 18th week of pregnancy.

Clinical features

Antenatal tests and scans may already have revealed the defect.

- *Spina bifida occulta*, marked by isolated laminar defects, is often seen in normal people and can usually be ignored. However, a posterior midline dimple, a tuft of hair or a pigmented naevus is more serious; patients may present at any age with neurological symptoms and signs.

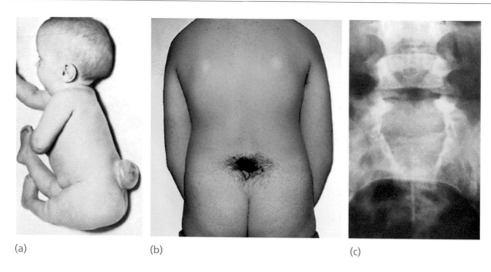

(a)   (b)   (c)

10.9 Spina bifida (a) Baby with spina bifida cystica (a myelomeningocele). **(b)** Tuft of hair over the lumbosacral junction; X-ray in this case showed a sacral defect **(c)**.

- *Spina bifida cystica* is obvious at birth in the shape of a sacular lesion over the lumbar spine (**10.9**). It may be covered only with membrane, or with membrane and skin. In *open myelomeningoceles* the neural elements form the roof of the cyst. *Hydrocephalus* is common.

The baby's posture may suggest the type of paralysis and sometimes indicates its neurological level. There is generally a flaccid weakness of muscle groups in the lower limbs; sensibility is impaired and there may be urinary and bowel incontinence. The precise neurological deficit varies according to the level of the lesion (the 'neurosegmental level'). Deformities such as hip dislocation, genu recurvatum and talipes may also be present at birth, or they may develop later due to muscle imbalance.

In about one-third of infants with myelomeningocele there is complete LMN paralysis and loss of sensation and sphincter control below the affected level; in one-third there is a complete lesion at some level but a distal segment of cord is preserved, giving a mixed neurological picture with intact segmental reflexes and spastic muscle groups; in the remaining one-third the cord lesion is incomplete and some movement and sensation are preserved.

X-rays and CT will show the extent of the bony lesion as well as other vertebral anomalies. *MRI* may be helpful to define the neurological defects.

Management

FOLIC ACID AND NEURAL TUBE DEFECTS

Folic acid, taken daily before conception and continuing through the first 12 weeks of pregnancy, reduces the risk of neural tube defects in the fetus. All mothers who have an infant born with spina bifida should be counselled to take supplementation prior to a subsequent pregnancy.

Selection of patients for operative closure is tailored to the clinical needs of each individual child.

A few weeks later, when the back has healed, the degree of hydrocephalus is assessed. Most children also have the Arnold–Chiari malformation with displacement of the posterior fossa structures through the foramen magnum and will require management of their real or potential hydrocephalus in the form of a ventriculoperitoneal shunt (VP shunt) to reduce the risk of further damage to their CNS. A chronically raised intracranial pressure may be associated with learning difficulties and other problems. Later, if the child's neurological status changes unexpectedly, shunt problems such as infection or blockage should be considered. VP drainage can be maintained for 5–6 years, by which time the tendency to hydrocephalus usually ceases.

Subsequent management requires intermittent bladder catheterization to minimize the risk of hydronephrosis and ascending infection due to the hypertonic bladder. There can also be a need for urological surgery (for bladder incontinence or urinary retention and hydronephrosis) and orthopaedic surgery (for muscle imbalance and joint deformity).

 Surgical treatment must always be supported by prolonged and skilled physiotherapy, occupational therapy and splintage, ideally in a specialized centre.

Except in the mildest cases, the late functional outcome cannot be predicted with any confidence until the child's neuromuscular condition is assessed at the age of 3–4 years. Patients with a low lumbar (L5) or sacral-level spina bifida will be functionally independent but those with spina bifida in the low thoracic, high and mid-lumbar area will need ongoing support.

 More important than walking is the development of upper limb function and intellectual skills and the ability to cope with the basic activities of daily living. These objectives can be achieved from a wheelchair just as well as from unsteady legs.

JOINT DEFORMITIES

Joint deformities should be corrected – initially by gentle physiotherapy (beware of causing iatrogenic fractures!) and later by splintage with lightweight orthoses. Surgical correction may be needed if these measures fail. Prolonged immobilization carries the risk of pathological fracture and should therefore be avoided.

SPINAL DEFORMITY

Spinal deformity (scoliosis and/or kyphosis) is common in children with myelomeningocele, due to a combination of muscle weakness, associated congenital vertebral anomalies and the tethered cord syndrome. Indications for operative

release of the tethered cord are increasing pain and neurological dysfunction or progressive spinal deformity.

Kyphosis may be severe enough to need localized vertebral resection and arthrodesis. Paralytic scoliosis is usually progressive and makes sitting particularly difficult. It is unlikely to respond to the use of a brace. Moulded seat inserts for the wheelchair are essential to aid sitting balance and independence and may help reduce the rate of curve deterioration. Surgery via an anterior, a posterior or a combined approach is often necessary and fusion to the pelvis may be required. The operation is always difficult and carries a high risk of complications, particularly postoperative infection and implant failure.

HIP PROBLEMS

Hip problems may also call for operative treatment. However, if the neurological level of the lesion is above L1, all muscle groups are flaccid and splintage is the only option; in the long term, the child will use a wheelchair. For lower lesions, hip instability or dislocation can be a challenge. Retaining hip movement may be more useful than striving for hip reduction by multiple operations, with their attendant complications and uncertain prognosis. There is little evidence to suggest that function is improved significantly by operative hip relocation.

KNEE PROBLEMS

Unlike the hip, the knee usually presents few problems. Children with lesions below L4 will have quadriceps control and active knee extension; they should therefore be encouraged to walk. In others the objective is simple: a straight knee suitable for wearing calipers and using gait-training devices. Children with high lumbar lesions may start off walking with the aid of lower limb braces but they will eventually opt for a wheelchair.

FIXED FLEXION

In older children prolonged sitting may result in fixed flexion. If stretching fails to correct this deformity, one or more of the hamstrings may be lengthened, divided or reinserted into the femur or patella.

FOOT DEFORMITIES

Foot deformities are among the most common problems. The aim of treatment is a mobile foot, with healthy skin and soft tissues that will not break down easily, that can be held or braced in a plantigrade position. Flail feet are relatively easy to treat and only require the use of accurately made orthoses. Equinovarus deformity is likely to be more severe (and more resistant to treatment) than the 'ordinary' club foot. This subject is dealt with in the section on talipes equinovarus in Chapter 21.

POLIOMYELITIS

Poliomyelitis is an acute infectious viral disease that has been the target of a global WHO-lead programme to eradicate the condition. It is fortunately now rarely seen in high-income countries. Acute infections are still encountered in parts of Africa and Asia and survivors present with challenging sequelae. In a small percentage of cases the CNS is involved, the effects falling on the anterior horn cells in the spinal cord and brainstem, leading to flaccid (LMN) paralysis of isolated groups of muscles.

Clinical features

Following a trivial and often unrecognized minor illness (a sore throat or diarrhoea), the patient develops symptoms resembling those of meningitis. They lie curled up with the joints flexed; the muscles are painful and tender and passive stretching provokes painful spasms.

Soon muscle weakness appears; it reaches a peak in the course of 2–3 days and may give rise to difficulty with breathing and swallowing. If the patient does not succumb from respiratory paralysis, pain and pyrexia subside after 7–10 days and the patient enters the convalescent stage but may continue to be infective for at least 4 weeks from the onset of illness.

Some anterior horn cells will have been destroyed by the virus; others, merely damaged by oedema, survive, and the muscles they supply can regain their lost power. Such recovery may continue for about 2 years but after that any residual weakness is permanent.

If recovery is not complete, the patient is left with some degree of asymmetrical flaccid paralysis or unbalanced muscle weakness that can lead to joint deformity and growth defects (**10.10**). If the trunk muscles were involved, they may have respiratory difficulty and/or scoliosis. An affected limb often looks bluish, wasted and deformed; there are frequently extensive chilblains and the skin feels cold. However, sensation is unaffected.

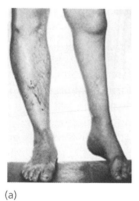
(a)

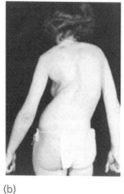
(b)

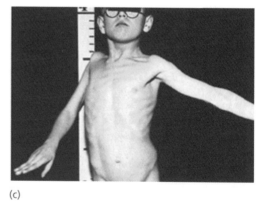
(c)

10.10 Poliomyelitis (a) Shortening and wasting of the left leg, with equinus of the ankle. **(b)** This long curve is typical of a paralytic scoliosis. **(c)** Paralysis of the right deltoid and supraspinatus makes it impossible for this boy to abduct his right arm.

Paralysis may be obvious, but lesser degrees of weakness are discovered only by systematic examination.

Principles of treatment

In some countries immunization has been so successful that poliomyelitis has become a rare disease. However, the victims of earlier epidemics continue to pose challenging problems.

ACUTE PHASE

During the acute phase, the patient is isolated and kept at complete rest, with symptomatic treatment for pain and muscle spasm. Active movement is avoided but gentle passive stretching helps to prevent contractures. Respiratory paralysis calls for artificial respiration.

RECOVERY PERIOD

During the period of recovery, physiotherapy is stepped up and every effort is made to regain maximum power; because of the associated trophic changes, hydrotherapy also is useful. Between exercise periods splintage may be needed to prevent fixed deformities. Muscle charting (see 'Examination' above) is carried out at regular intervals until no further recovery is detected.

LATE STAGE

In the late stage, orthopaedic treatment comes into its own. Six types of problem in particular may need attention.

- *Isolated muscle weakness without deformity* may affect important movements and joint stability. Quadriceps paralysis may make weight-bearing and walking impossible; it can be managed by using a splint or calliper which holds the knee straight. Elsewhere isolated weakness (e.g. of thumb opposition) may be treated by tendon transfer. Muscle charting is essential: a muscle usually loses one grade of power when it is transferred, so to be really useful it should have grade 4 or 5 power; however, even a grade 3 muscle may act as a kind of tenodesis and reduce the deformity caused by gravity.
- *Passively correctible deformity* (due to unbalanced paralysis) can at first be counteracted by

splintage. An appropriate tendon transfer may solve the problem permanently.
- *Fixed deformities* cannot be corrected by either splintage or tendon transfer alone; alignment must be restored operatively to stabilize the joint (if necessary, by arthrodesis). This is especially applicable to fixed deformities of the ankle and foot, but the same principle applies in treating paralytic scoliosis (**10.11**).

 Occasionally, fixed deformity is an advantage. For example, a stable equinus foot may help to compensate mechanically for quadriceps weakness and, if so, it should not be corrected.

- *A flail joint*, because it causes no deformity, may need no treatment. However, if the joint is unstable, it must be stabilized, either by permanent splintage or by arthrodesis.
- *Leg length inequality* of up to 3 cm can be compensated for by building up the shoe. Anything more is unsightly and operative lengthening of the femur or tibia (or shortening of the opposite limb) might be preferable.
- *Vascular dysfunction* may need treatment. Sensation is intact but the paralysed limb is often cold and blue. Large chilblains sometimes develop and sympathectomy may be needed.

For a detailed regional survey, consult *Apley & Solomon's System of Orthopaedics and Trauma*, 10th edition, CRC Press (2017).

MOTOR NEURON DISORDERS

Rare degenerative disorders of the CNS motor neurons and/or anterior horn cells of the cord cause progressive and sometimes fatal paralysis.

Spinal muscular atrophy

This term applies to a rare group of heritable disorders in which there is *widespread anterior horn cell degeneration* leading to progressive LMN weakness. In the worst cases, the infant is weak and floppy at birth and death usually occurs

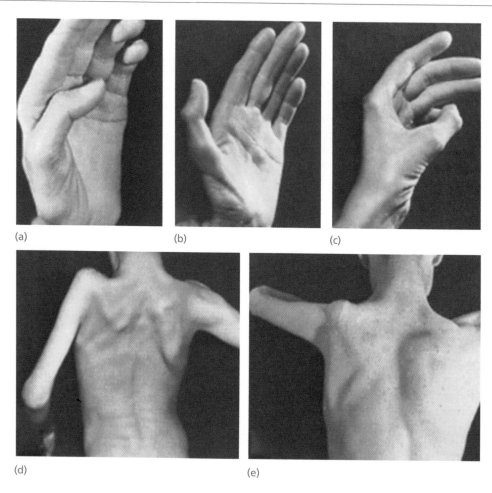

(a)   (b)   (c)

(d)   (e)

10.11 Poliomyelitis – treatment (a–c) Superficialis tendon transfer for opponens paralysis. In **(b)** the tendon can be seen in action at the start of thumb opposition **(c)**. **(d,e)** Arthrodesis of the left shoulder to restore abduction after paralysis of the deltoid.

within 1 year. In less severe forms, adolescents or young adults present with limb weakness, proximal muscle wasting and 'paralytic' scoliosis. Patients may live to 30–40 years of age but are usually confined to a wheelchair. Spinal braces are used to improve sitting ability; if this cannot prevent the spine from collapsing, operative instrumentation and fusion is advisable.

Motor neuron disease (amyotrophic lateral sclerosis)

Motor neuron disease *affects both UMNs and anterior horn cells*, causing widespread symptoms and signs. Patients may present in middle age with muscle weakness (e.g. clumsy hands or unexplained foot drop) and wasting in the presence of exaggerated reflexes. Sensation and bladder control are normal. The disease is progressive and incurable. Patients usually end up in a wheelchair and have increasing difficulty with speech and eating. Most of them die within 5 years from a combination of respiratory weakness and aspiration pneumonia.

Supportive treatment includes nursing, occupational therapy and the use of various mechanical and electronic aids to assist in essential activities.

PERIPHERAL NEUROPATHIES

Disorders of the peripheral nerves may affect motor, sensory or autonomic functions, may be localized to a short segment or may involve the full length of the nerve fibres. In some cases, spinal cord tracts are involved as well.

There are over 100 types of neuropathy; here we consider those conditions that are of most interest to orthopaedic surgeons.

Classification

Classification by anatomical level and distribution is the simplest. In over 40% of cases, no specific cause has been found!

- *Radiculopathy* shows involvement of nerve roots, most commonly by vertebral trauma, intervertebral disc herniation and nerve root infections such as herpes zoster.
- *Plexopathy* includes brachial plexus injury or viral infection (neuralgic amyotrophy).
- *Distal neuropathy* shows involvement of neurons in distinct peripheral nerves:
  - mononeuropathy – involvement of a single nerve (e.g. nerve injury, or nerve compression)
  - multiple mononeuropathy – involvement of several nerves (e.g. leprosy)
  - polyneuropathy – widespread symmetrical dysfunction (e.g. diabetic neuropathy, alcoholic neuropathy and various hereditary neuropathies).

Pathology

Abnormalities may be predominantly sensory (e.g. diabetic polyneuropathy), predominantly motor (e.g. peroneal muscular atrophy) or mixed. Chronic motor loss with no sensory component is usually due to anterior horn cell disease rather than more esoteric pathology.

There are three basic types of peripheral neuronal pathology:

- acute interruption of axonal continuity
- chronic axonal degeneration
- demyelination.

In all three, conduction is disturbed or completely blocked, with consequent loss of motor and/or sensory and/or autonomic functions.

ACUTE AXONAL INTERRUPTION

Acute axonal interruption occurs most typically after nerve division (described in Chapter 11). Loss of motor and sensory functions is immediate and complete. The distal segments of axons that are crushed or severed will degenerate – as will the muscle fibres which are supplied by motor neurons – if nerve conduction is not restored within 2 years. Axonal regeneration, when it occurs, is slow (the new axon grows by about 1 mm per day) and is often incomplete.

CHRONIC (NON-TRAUMATIC) AXONAL DEGENERATION

Chronic (non-traumatic) axonal degeneration is slow and typically progressive. Most large-fibre disorders affect both sensory and motor neurons causing 'stocking' and 'glove' numbness, altered postural reflexes and ataxia as well as muscle weakness and wasting, beginning distally and progressing proximally. Symptoms tend to appear in the feet and legs before the hands and arms. Some disorders are predominantly either motor or sensory.

DEMYELINATING NEUROPATHIES

These neuropathies occur most commonly in nerve entrapment syndromes and blunt soft-tissue trauma. The main effects are slowing of conduction and sometimes complete nerve block, causing sensory and/or motor dysfunction distal to the lesion. These changes are potentially reversible; recovery usually takes less than 6 weeks, and in some cases only a few days. Demyelinating polyneuropathies are rare, with the exception of Guillain–Barré syndrome. Other conditions include the hereditary motor and sensory neuropathies (HMSNs).

Clinical features

Patients usually complain of 'pins and needles' (paraesthesiae), numbness or 'restless legs'. They may also notice weakness or loss of balance in walking. Occasionally (in the predominantly motor neuropathies) the main complaint is of progressive deformity (e.g. claw hand or cavus foot).

The onset may be rapid (over a few days) or very gradual (over weeks or months). Sometimes there is a history of injury, infection, a known disease such as diabetes or malignancy, alcohol abuse or nutritional deficiency.

Examination may reveal weakness in a particular muscle group and/or loss of peripheral sensation. In the polyneuropathies, the limbs are involved symmetrically, usually legs before arms and distal before proximal parts. In mononeuropathy, sensory loss follows the 'map' of the affected nerve. In polyneuropathy, there is a symmetrical 'glove' or 'stocking' distribution.

Trophic skin changes may be present. Deep sensation is also affected and some patients develop ataxia. If pain sensibility and proprioception are depressed, there may be joint instability or breakdown of the articular surfaces (neuropathic joint disease or 'Charcot joints').

Clinical examination alone may establish the diagnosis. Further help is provided by EMG (which may suggest the type of abnormality) and nerve conduction studies (which may show exactly where the lesion is).

The mononeuropathies (mainly nerve injuries and entrapment syndromes) are discussed in Chapter 11. Some of the more common polyneuropathies are described below.

DIABETIC NEUROPATHY

Diabetes is one of the commonest causes of peripheral neuropathy. The metabolic disturbance associated with hyperglycaemia interferes with axonal and Schwann cell function, leading to mixed patterns of demyelination and axonal degeneration. Autonomic dysfunction and vascular disturbance also play a part.

The onset is insidious and the condition often goes undiagnosed until the patient starts complaining of numbness and paraesthesiae in the feet and lower legs. Even at that early stage there may be areflexia and diminished vibration sense. Another suspicious pattern is an increased susceptibility to nerve entrapment syndromes. Later, muscle weakness becomes more noticeable in proximal parts of the limbs. In advanced cases, trophic complications can arise:

* neuropathic ulcers of the feet
* regional osteoporosis
* insufficiency fractures of the foot bones
* Charcot joints in the ankles and feet.

Treatment

Treatment starts with proper control of the underlying disorder. Local measures consist of skin care, management of fractures and splintage or arthrodesis of grossly unstable or deformed joints. Management of the diabetic foot is discussed in Chapter 21.

NEURALGIC AMYOTROPHY (ACUTE BRACHIAL NEURITIS)

This unusual cause of severe shoulder girdle pain and weakness is believed to be due to a parainfectious disorder of one or more of the cervical nerve roots and the brachial plexus, sometimes producing a pseudomononeuropathic pattern (e.g. scapular winging or wrist drop). There is often a history of an antecedent viral infection or antiviral inoculation; sometimes a small epidemic occurs among several residents of an institution.

The history alone often suggests the diagnosis. Pain in the shoulder and arm is typically sudden in onset, intense and unabating; the patient can often recall the exact hour when symptoms began. Pain may extend into the neck and down as far as the hand; usually it lasts for 2–3 weeks. Other symptoms are paraesthesiae in the arm or hand and weakness of the muscles of the shoulder, forearm and hand.

Winging of the scapula (due to serratus anterior weakness) (**10.12**), wasting of the shoulder girdle muscles, and occasionally involvement of more distal arm muscles may be profound, becoming evident as the pain improves. Shoulder movement is initially limited by pain but this is superseded by weakness due to muscle atrophy. Sensory loss and paraesthesiae in one or more

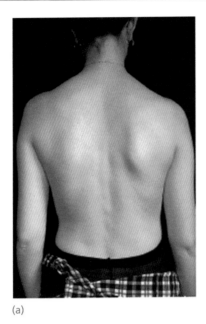
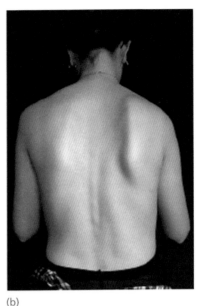

(a)   (b)

10.12 Neuralgic amyotrophy A common feature of neuralgic amyotrophy is winging of the scapula due to serratus anterior weakness. Even at rest **(a)** the right scapula is prominent in this young woman. When she thrusts her arms forwards against the wall **(b)**, the abnormality is more pronounced.

of the cervical dermatomes are not uncommon. Involvement of overlapping root territories of the brachial plexus is a feature that helps to distinguish neuralgic amyotrophy from an acute cervical disc herniation which is monoradicular.

Treatment

There is no specific treatment; pain is controlled with analgesics. The prognosis is usually good but full neurological recovery may take months or years.

GUILLAIN–BARRÉ SYNDROME

Guillain–Barré syndrome describes an acute demyelinating motor and sensory polyneuropathy. It can occur at any age and usually appears 2–3 weeks after an upper respiratory or gastrointestinal infection – probably as an autoimmune reaction.

The typical history is of aching and weakness in the legs, often accompanied by numbness and paraesthesiae, which steadily progresses upwards over a period of hours, a few days or a few weeks.

Symptoms may stop when the thigh and pelvic muscles are reached, and then gradually retreat, or may go on ascending to involve the upper limbs, facial muscles and diaphragm, resulting in quadriplegia and respiratory failure. In the established case, there will be areflexia and loss of position sense. In severe cases, patients may develop features of autonomic dysfunction.

CSF analysis may show a characteristic pattern: elevated protein concentration in the presence of a normal cell count (unlike an infection, in which the cell count would also be elevated). Neurophysiological studies may show conduction slowing or block; in severe cases there may be EMG signs of axonal damage.

Treatment

Treatment consists essentially of bed rest, pain-relieving medication and supportive management to monitor, prevent and deal with complications such as respiratory failure and difficulty with swallowing. In severe cases, specific treatment with intravenous immunoglobulins or plasmapheresis should be started as soon as possible. Once the acute disorder is under control,

SECTION 1 GENERAL ORTHOPAEDICS

physiotherapy and splintage will help to prevent deformities and improve muscle power.

Most patients recover completely, though this may take 6 months or longer; about 10% are left with long-term disability and about 3% are likely to die.

LEPROSY

Although uncommon in Europe and North America, this is still a frequent cause of peripheral neuropathy in Africa and Asia.

Mycobacterium leprae, an acid-fast organism, causes a diffuse inflammatory disorder of the skin, mucous membranes and peripheral nerves. Depending on the host response, several forms of disease may evolve.

The most severe neurological lesions are seen in *tuberculoid leprosy*. Anaesthetic skin patches develop over the extensor surfaces of the limbs; loss of motor function leads to weakness and deformities of the hands and feet (**10.13**).

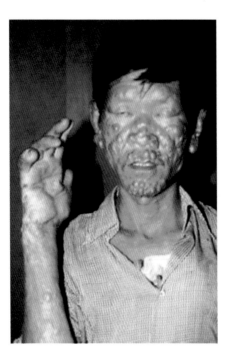

10.13 Leprosy ulnar nerve paralysis Ulnar nerve paralysis is relatively common in long-standing leprosy. This patient has the typical ulnar claw-hand deformity.

Thickened nerves may be felt as cords under the skin or where they cross the bones (e.g. the ulnar nerve behind the medial epicondyle of the elbow). Trophic ulcers are common and may predispose to osteomyelitis. *Lepromatous leprosy* is associated with a symmetrical polyneuropathy, which occurs late in the disease.

Treatment

Treatment by combined chemotherapy (mainly rifampicin and dapsone) is continued for 6 months to 2 years, depending on the response. Muscle weakness, particularly intrinsic muscle paralysis due to ulnar nerve involvement, may require multiple tendon transfers.

HEREDITARY NEUROPATHIES

These rare disorders present in childhood and adolescence, usually with muscle weakness and deformity.

Hereditary sensory neuropathy

Congenital insensitivity to pain and temperature is inherited as either a dominant or a recessive trait. Patients are prone to painless injury and may develop ulceration of the feet or neuropathic joint disease.

Hereditary motor and sensory neuropathy

HMSNs comprise a group of conditions which includes peroneal muscular atrophy and Charcot–Marie–Tooth disease, the commonest of the inherited neuropathies, which are usually passed on as autosomal dominant disorders.

- *HMSN Type I* is seen in children who have difficulty walking and develop claw toes and pes cavus or cavovarus. There may be severe wasting of the legs and (later) the upper limbs, but often the signs are quite subtle. Spinal deformity may occur in severe cases. This is a demyelinating disorder; nerve conduction velocity is markedly slowed and the diagnosis can be confirmed by finding demyelination on sural nerve biopsy.

- *HMSN Type II* occurs in adolescents and young adults and is less disabling than Type I. It affects only the lower limbs, causing mild pes cavus and wasting of the peronei (**10.14**). Nerve conduction velocity is only slightly reduced, indicating primary axonal degeneration.

TREATMENT

Treatment during the early stages of HMSN may call for foot and ankle orthoses. If the deformities are progressive or disabling, operative correction may be indicated. Claw toes (due to intrinsic muscle weakness) can be corrected by transferring the toe flexors to the extensors, with or without fusion of the interphalangeal joints. Clawing of the big toe is best corrected by transfer of the extensor hallucis longus to the metatarsal neck and fusion of the interphalangeal joint (the Robert Jones procedure). The cavus deformity needs treatment only if it causes pain; it can be improved by calcaneal or dorsal midtarsal osteotomy or (in severe cases) triple arthrodesis.

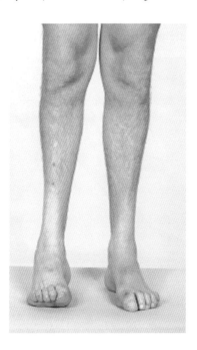

10.14 Hereditary neuropathies This patient with peroneal muscular atrophy has the typical wasting of the legs, cavus feet and claw toes.

Friedreich's ataxia

This autosomal recessive condition is the classic archetype of a large group of genetic disorders – the spinocerebellar ataxias – characterized by spinocerebellar dysfunction, but there may also be degeneration of the posterior root ganglia and peripheral nerves. Many of these disorders have now been genotypically defined. Patients generally present at around the age of 6 years with gait ataxia, lower limb weakness and deformities similar to those of severe Charcot–Marie–Tooth disease. The muscle weakness, which may also involve the upper limbs and the trunk, is progressive; by the age of 20 years the patient has usually taken to a wheelchair and is likely to die of cardiomyopathy before the age of 45. Despite the potentially poor prognosis, surgical correction of deformities is worthwhile.

ARTHROGRYPOSIS MULTIPLEX CONGENITA

This unwieldy term is applied to a group of rare congenital disorders characterized by multiple (often symmetrical) non-progressive soft-tissue contractures and restriction of joint movement. Deformities and contractures develop *in utero* and remain largely unchanged throughout life. Myopathic and neuropathic features may coexist in the same muscle.

The incidence is said to be about 1 : 3000 live births; in some cases, a genetic linkage has been demonstrated. A more proximate cause may be an intrauterine lack of sufficient room for movement during fetal development.

Three major categories are recognized:

- children with total body involvement (the condition traditionally known as arthrogryposis multiplex congenita and now termed *amyoplasia*)
- those with predominantly hand or foot involvement – *distal arthrogryposis*
- patients with *pterygia syndromes*: conditions characterized by arthrogrypotic joint contractures with soft-tissue webs, usually across the flexor aspects of the knees and ankles.

SECTION 1 GENERAL ORTHOPAEDICS

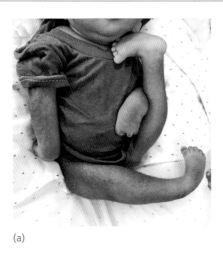

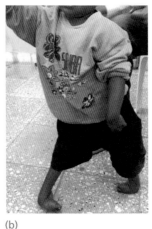

(a)   (b)

10.15 Arthrogryposis multiplex congenita (a) An infant with the amyoplasia form of arthrogryposis multiplex congenital. **(b)** A 3-year-old child with untreated amyoplasia who is able to walk despite bilateral club feet and stiff, extended knees. The upper limbs have the characteristic stiff, extended elbows and flexed wrists and digits.

Clinical features

Involved joints are tubular and featureless and although the normal skin creases are absent there are often deep dimples over the joints. Muscle mass is markedly reduced. In some cases there is true muscle weakness.

In the classic form of *amyoplasia*, the shoulders are adducted and internally rotated, the elbows usually extended and the wrists/hands flexed and deviated ulnarwards. In the lower limbs, the hips are flexed and abducted, the limbs externally rotated, the knees usually extended and the feet showing equinovarus or vertical talus deformities (**10.15, e10.1**). While affected children and adults have (sometimes considerable) physical restrictions, intelligence is often unaffected.

Distal arthrogryposis often manifests an autosomal dominant pattern of inheritance. Common deformities are ulnar deviation of the metacarpophalangeal joints, fixed flexion of the proximal interphalangeal joints and tightly adducted thumbs. Foot deformities are likely to be resistant forms of equinovarus or vertical talus.

Treatment

Treatment begins soon after birth and initially consists of gentle manipulation and muscle stretching exercises, later combined with splintage to prevent

(or slow down) recurrence of joint contractures. If progress is slow, tendon release, tendon transfers and osteotomies may become necessary. In the pterygia syndromes, physiotherapy can be tried but early release of the popliteal contractures should be considered (**10.16**). Great care is needed to avoid injury to tight neurovascular structures.

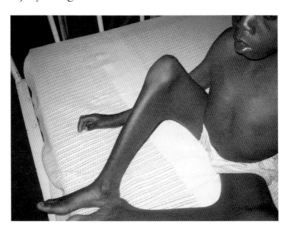

10.16 Arthrogryposis multiplex congenita Popliteal pterygium in an 8-year-old child. Bilateral webs behind each knee limit extension beyond 90°. The sciatic nerve is located within the web, creating a challenge to safely achieve knee extension. When popliteal pterygium is associated with elbow and neck webbing, it is known as Escobar syndrome.

Arthrogrypotic club foot usually demands operative correction. Dislocation of the hip, likewise, often defies conservative treatment and open reduction is needed. Whatever the form of treatment, parents should be warned that recurrent deformity is common.

 Remember that the aims of treatment are to provide these children with the ability to walk and upper limb function adequate to the needs of their most important daily activities, rather than the restoration of full movement.

MUSCULAR DYSTROPHY

The muscular dystrophies are a group of about 30 extremely rare inherited disorders characterized by progressive muscle weakness and wasting. Pathological changes include malformation of muscle fibres, death of muscle cells and replacement of muscle by fibrous tissue and fat. Only one of them will be considered here: *pseudohypertrophic muscular dystrophy (Duchenne dystrophy)*.

This is a progressive disease of sex-linked inheritance with recessive transmission. It is therefore seen only in boys, affecting 1 : 3500 male births. A defect at locus p21 on the X chromosome results in failure to code for the dystrophin gene, which is essential for maintaining the integrity of cardiac and skeletal muscle cells. Absence of functional dystrophin leads to cell membrane leakage, muscle fibre damage and replacement by fat and fibrous tissue.

Clinical features

The condition is usually unsuspected until the child starts to walk. He has difficulty standing, he cannot run properly and he falls frequently. A characteristic feature is the boy's method of rising from the floor by climbing up his own legs (Gowers' sign, e10.2); this is due to weakness of the gluteus maximus and thigh muscles.

Shoulder girdle weakness follows about 5 years after the clinical onset of the disease. By the age of 10 the child has usually lost the ability to walk and has to use a wheelchair; from then on there is rapid deterioration in spinal posture with the development of scoliosis and, subsequently, further deterioration in lung function. Cardiopulmonary failure is the usual cause of death, generally before the age of 30 years.

The diagnosis is usually based on the clinical features and family history and by testing for serum creatinine phosphokinase levels which are 200–300 times the normal in the early stages of the disease. Muscle biopsy and genetic testing confirms the diagnosis.

Family counselling is important. Up to 20% of families already have a younger affected sibling by the time the proband is diagnosed.

Treatment

While the child can still walk, physiotherapy and splintage or tendon operations may help to prevent or correct joint deformities and so prolong the period of mobility. Corticosteroids (deflazacort and prednisolone) have been shown to preserve muscle strength and delay the loss of independent mobility, respiratory function and onset of scoliosis, but there are significant side effects such as osteoporosis, increased risk of fractures and cataract formation.

If scoliosis is marked (more than 30 degrees), instrumentation and spinal fusion helps to maintain pulmonary function and improves quality of life. Preoperative cardiac and pulmonary function should be reviewed.

Peripheral nerve injuries

11

- Pathology of nerve injuries 228
- Clinical features 230
- Principles of treatment 231
- Nerve injuries affecting the upper limb 232
- Nerve injuries affecting the lower limb 238
- Nerve entrapment syndromes 242

Peripheral nerves are bundles of *axons* conducting efferent (motor) impulses from cells in the anterior horn of the spinal cord to the muscles, and afferent (sensory) impulses from peripheral receptors, via cells in the posterior root ganglia, to the cord. They also convey sudomotor and vasomotor fibres from ganglion cells in the sympathetic chain. Some nerves are predominantly motor, some predominantly sensory; the larger trunks are mixed, with motor and sensory axons running in separate bundles.

A single motor neuron supplies ten to several thousand muscle fibres, the ratio depending on the degree of dexterity demanded of the particular muscle (the smaller the ratio, the finer the movement). Similarly, the peripheral branches of each sensory neuron may serve anything from a single muscle spindle to a comparatively large patch of skin; here again, the fewer the end receptors served by a single axon, the greater the degree of discrimination.

The signal, or action potential, carried by motor neurons is transmitted to the muscle fibres by the release of a chemical transmitter, acetylcholine, at the terminal bouton of the nerve. Sensory signals are similarly conveyed to the dorsal root ganglia and from there up the ipsilateral column of the spinal cord, through the brainstem and thalamus, to the opposite (sensory) cortex. Proprioceptive impulses from the muscle spindles and joints bypass this route and are carried to the anterior horn cells as part of a local reflex arc. The economy of this system ensures that 'survival' mechanisms such as balance and sense of position in space are activated with great speed.

In the peripheral nerves, all motor axons and the large sensory axons serving touch, pain and proprioception are coated with *myelin*, a multi-layered lipoprotein membrane derived from the accompanying *Schwann cells*. Every few millimetres the myelin sheath is interrupted, leaving short segments of bare axon called the *nodes of Ranvier*. Nerve impulses leap from node to node with the speed of electricity, much faster than would be the case if these axons were not insulated by the myelin sheaths. Depletion of the myelin sheath causes slowing – and eventually complete blocking – of axonal conduction.

Most axons – in particular the small-diameter fibres carrying crude sensation and the efferent sympathetic fibres – are unmyelinated but wrapped in Schwann cell cytoplasm. Damage to these axons causes unpleasant or bizarre sensations and various sudomotor and vasomotor effects.

Outside the Schwann cell membrane the axon is covered by a connective tissue stocking, the

SECTION 1 GENERAL ORTHOPAEDICS

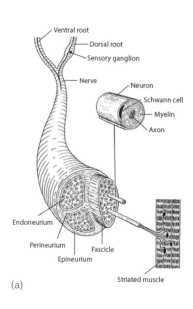

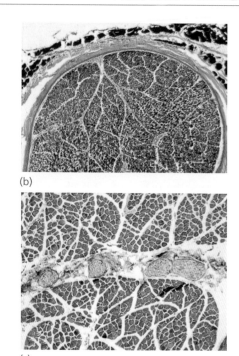

11.1 Nerve structure (a) Diagram of the structural elements of a peripheral nerve. **(b)** Histological section through a large nerve. The epineurium and perineurial septa are well defined; axons appear as tiny black dots. **(c)** High-power view, showing blood vessels in the perineurium.

endoneurium. The axons that make up a nerve are separated into bundles (fascicles) by fairly dense membranous tissue, the *perineurium.* In a transected nerve, these fascicles are seen pouting from the cut surface, their perineurial sheaths well defined and strong enough to be grasped by fine instruments. The groups of fascicles that make up a nerve trunk are enclosed in an even thicker connective tissue coat, the *epineurium* (**11.1**).

The nerve is richly supplied by *blood vessels* that run longitudinally in the epineurium before penetrating the various layers to become the *endoneurial capillaries.* These fine vessels may be damaged by stretching or rough handling.

PATHOLOGY OF NERVE INJURIES

Nerves can be injured by ischaemia, compression, traction, laceration, burning or chemicals. Damage varies in severity from transient and quickly recoverable loss of function to complete interruption and degeneration. A nerve injury can be classified by Seddon (1943) and Sunderland (1978) according to the amount of nerve dysfunction and the eventual degree of recovery (**Table 11.1**).

Transient ischaemia

Acute nerve compression causes numbness and tingling within 15 minutes, loss of pain sensibility after 30 minutes and muscle weakness after 45 minutes. Relief of compression is followed by intense paraesthesiae lasting up to 5 minutes (the familiar 'pins and needles' after a limb 'goes to sleep'); feeling is restored within 30 seconds and full muscle power after about 10 minutes. These changes are due to transient endoneurial anoxia and they leave no trace of nerve damage.

Neurapraxia

This is a reversible block to nerve conduction in which there is loss of sensation and muscle power, followed by spontaneous recovery after a few

Table 11.1 Classification of nerve injuries

Seddon	Structural damage	Sunderland	Recovery
Neurapraxia	None	I	Full
Axonotmesis	Axons	II	Full
	+ endoneurium	III	Some
	+ perineurium	IV	None
Neurotmesis	Discontinuity	V	None

days or weeks. The nerve is intact but mechanical pressure has caused demyelination of axons in a limited segment. This reversible lesion is also called a 'first-degree' injury.

Axonotmesis

This is a more severe form of injury in which there is interruption of the axons in a segment of nerve. It is seen typically after closed fractures and dislocations. Although there is loss of conduction due to axon loss, the nerve is in continuity because the outer neural tubes are intact. Distal to the lesion, and for a few millimetres proximal to it, axons disintegrate and are resorbed by phagocytes. This *Wallerian degeneration* (named after the physiologist Augustus Waller) takes only a few days and is accompanied by proliferation of Schwann cells and fibroblasts lining the endoneurial tubes. The denervated motor endplates and sensory receptors gradually atrophy and, if they are not reinnervated within 2 years, they will never recover (**11.2**).

Axonal regeneration starts within hours of nerve damage. The proximal stumps sprout numerous unmyelinated tendrils, many of which find their way into the cell-clogged endoneurial tubes. These new axonal processes grow at a speed of 1–2 mm per day, the larger fibres slowly acquiring a new myelin coat. Eventually they join to the denervated end-organs, which enlarge and start functioning again.

Depending on the degree of damage within the axonotmesis, there may be full recovery (second-degree injury), partial recovery (third-degree) or no recovery (fourth-degree).

Neurotmesis

This means division of the nerve trunk, such as may occur in an open wound. Severe injury can

be inflicted without actually dividing the nerve; in such cases there may be degrees of damage between that of axonotmesis, which is potentially recoverable, and complete neurotmesis, which will never recover without surgical intervention. Neurotmesis is therefore a fifth-degree injury. As in axonotmesis, there is rapid Wallerian degeneration, but here the endoneurial tubes are destroyed over a variable segment and scarring

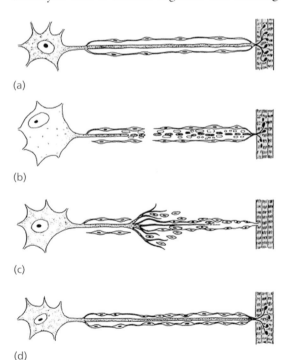

(a)

(b)

(c)

(d)

11.2 Nerve injury and regeneration (a) Normal axon and target organ (striated muscle). **(b)** Following nerve injury, the distal part of the axon disintegrates and the myelin sheath breaks up. **(c)** New axonal tendrils grow into the mass of proliferating Schwann cells. One of the tendrils will find its way into the old endoneurial tube and **(d)** the axon will slowly regenerate.

thwarts any hope of regenerating axons entering the distal segment and regaining their target organs. Instead, regenerating fibres mingle with proliferating Schwann cells and fibroblasts in a jumbled knot, or 'neuroma', at the site of injury. Even after surgical repair many new axons fail to reach the distal segment; those that do may not find suitable Schwann tubes, or may not reach the correct end-organs in time, or may remain incompletely myelinated. Function may be adequate but is never normal.

CLINICAL FEATURES

Acute nerve injuries are easily missed, especially if associated with fractures or dislocations, the symptoms of which may overshadow those of the nerve lesion.

> ⚠ Always test for nerve injuries following any significant trauma. And test again after manipulation or operation, in case the nerve has been damaged during treatment!

Ask the patient if there is numbness, tingling or muscle weakness in the target area. Then examine the injured limb systematically for signs of abnormal posture (e.g. a wrist-drop in radial nerve palsy), weakness in specific muscle groups and changes in sensibility. The pattern of change is usually sufficiently characteristic to provide an anatomical diagnosis (see **Table 11.1**).

> ⚠ If a nerve injury is present, it is crucial also to look for an accompanying vascular injury.

Diagnosis

> **DIAGNOSIS: QUESTIONS TO ASK**
>
> Are there neurological symptoms?
> Are there neurological signs?
> What is the level of the lesion?
> What type of lesion is it?
> Are there signs of nerve recovery?

Having established the presence of a *nerve injury* and, in most cases, the likely anatomical *level* of the injury, it is still necessary to diagnose the *type* of injury and the *degree* of damage. Nerve loss in low-energy injuries is likely to be due to neurapraxia, and in high-energy injuries and open wounds to axonotmesis or neurotmesis. In doubtful cases, one may have to wait a few weeks to see if signs of recovery appear, which would exclude complete nerve division. The grading may therefore not be known until the nerve reaches its final recovery. Muscles supplied by the nerve should be tested repeatedly: assuming that nerve regeneration occurs at the rate of 1 mm per day, one can estimate the expected time of recovery in muscles closest to the site of injury. With open wounds, however, early exploration is the best policy.

TESING FOR MUSCLE POWER

Muscles innervated by the injured nerve (**e11.1**) should be carefully examined for wasting and power. Muscle power should be recorded using the Medical Research Council (MRC) scale.

> **MUSCLE POWER: MRC GRADING**
>
> *Grade 0* No contraction
> *Grade 1* A flicker of muscle activity
> *Grade 2* Muscle contraction but inability to overcome gravity
> *Grade 3* Contraction able to overcome gravity
> *Grade 4* Contraction and movement against resistance
> *Grade 5* Normal power

SENSATION

This should be mapped out according to the territory of the damaged nerve. If the injury is more central, then the specific dermatome is examined (**e11.2**). Sensation includes light touch or pinprick.

SWEATING

Absence of sweating indicates loss of nerve function in that territory – a useful sign in the young or unconscious.

TINEL'S SIGN

A classic sign of progressive nerve recovery is peripheral tingling provoked by percussing the nerve at the site of injury (where regenerating axons are most sensitive). After a delay of a few weeks, the sensitive spot should begin to advance down the limb at a rate of about 1 mm per day. Failure of Tinel's sign to advance suggests a severe degree of nerve injury and the need for operative exploration.

TWO-POINT DISCRIMINATION

The density of sensory axonal recovery can be determined by measuring the ability to sense the distance between two pinpoints (**e11.3**) or the pressure applied through fine filaments (**e11.4**).

STEREOGNOSIS

The ability to recognize objects by touch alone can also be gauged asking the patient to handle a number of small commonly used items.

ELECTRODIAGNOSTIC TESTS

Nerve conduction tests and insertion electromyography may help to establish the level and severity of the injury, as well as the progress of nerve recovery. Remember, though, that these tests are not very accurate during the first few weeks after nerve injury.

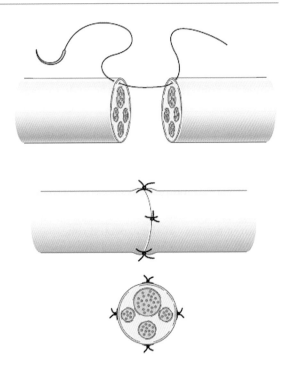

11.3 Nerve repair The stumps are correctly oriented and attached by fine sutures through the epineurium.

PRINCIPLES OF TREATMENT

Open injuries

The earlier a nerve is repaired, the better the recovery. This is skilled surgery, which must be performed under magnification using very delicate instruments. Nerve injuries associated with an open wound (even a small stab wound) should be explored and, if necessary, repaired as part of the patient's primary treatment. If the nerve is cleanly divided, end-to-end suture may be possible (**11.3**). A ragged cut will need paring of the stumps with a sharp blade. If this leaves too large a gap, or if the nerve stumps have retracted so that they cannot be brought together without tension, some slack can be gained by mobilizing the nerve, but if it is still difficult to bring the ends together without tension, nerve grafts (usually from the sural nerve) are inserted with special glue (**e11.5**) or very fine sutures; an alternative is to use artificial nerve conduits to span the interval.

Postoperatively, physiotherapy is applied to retain joint movement. However, if there is the least doubt about tension on the nerve, the limb should be splinted in a position which keeps the nerve relaxed for about 2 weeks before starting physiotherapy.

Closed injuries

With closed nerve lesions it is more difficult to decide what to do, especially during the first few weeks after injury. In most cases, if the history suggests that the force of injury was low, the nerve sheath is likely to be intact (neurapraxia or axonotmesis), so one can afford to wait at least until the muscle whose nerve supply arises just below the injury should have recovered. If at

SECTION 1 GENERAL ORTHOPAEDICS

that time there is still no sign of recovery, the nerve should be explored. If the history suggests a higher degree of force, or if the nerve could be trapped (e.g. in a fracture), then early exploration should be considered because the earlier a nerve is repaired, the better its recovery.

Delayed repair

Late repair – i.e. weeks or months after the injury – may be indicated because:

- a closed injury was left alone but showed no sign of recovery at the expected time
- the diagnosis was missed and the patient presented late
- primary repair has failed.

The options must be weighed carefully: if the patient has adapted to the functional loss, if it is a high lesion and reinnervation is unlikely within the critical 2-year period, or if there is a pure motor loss which can be treated by tendon transfer, it may be best to leave well alone. Excessive scarring and intractable joint stiffness may, likewise, make nerve repair questionable; yet in the hand it is still worthwhile simply to regain protective sensation.

The lesion is exposed under high magnification, working from normal tissue above and below towards the scarred area. If the nerve is in continuity, only slightly thickened and soft, or if there is conduction across the lesion, resection is not advised; if the nerve is scarred and there is no conduction on electrical stimulation, the scar should be resected, paring back the stumps until healthy fascicles are exposed. Nerve suture or grafting is then performed as described above.

Care of paralysed parts

 While recovery is awaited, the anaesthetic skin must be protected from friction damage and burns. The joints should be moved through their full range several times daily to prevent stiffness and minimize the work required of muscles when they recover.

Tendon transfers

Motor recovery may not occur if the regenerating axons fail to reach the muscle within 18–24 months of injury. In such circumstances, tendon transfers should be considered, observing specific principles.

PRINCIPLES FOR TENDON TRANSFER

The donor muscle should be expendable and have adequate power.
The recipient site must be mobile and stable.
The transferred tendon should be routed subcutaneously in a straight line of pull.
The patient should be well motivated.
Dedicated physiotherapy is important.

NERVE INJURIES AFFECTING THE UPPER LIMB

BRACHIAL PLEXUS INJURIES

The brachial plexus is formed by the confluence of nerve roots from C5 to T1 (**11.4**). The network is most vulnerable to injury where the nerves run from the cervical spine, between the muscles of the neck and beneath the clavicle en route to the arm – either a stab wound or severe traction caused by a fall on the side of the neck or the shoulder.

- *Supraclavicular lesions* typically occur in motorcycle accidents.
- *Infraclavicular lesions* are usually associated with fractures or dislocations of the shoulder.

Fractures of the clavicle rarely damage the plexus, and then only if caused by a direct blow.

The injury may affect any level of the plexus.

- *Preganglionic lesions* (i.e. disruption of nerve roots proximal to the dorsal root ganglion) cannot recover and are surgically irreparable.
- *Postganglionic lesions* can be repaired and are capable of recovery. Lesions in continuity have a better prognosis than complete ruptures.

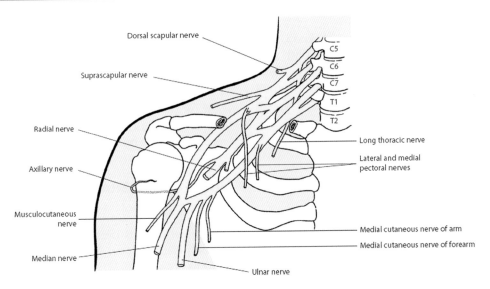

11.4 Brachial plexus Diagram of the brachial plexus and its relationship to the clavicle.

Clinical features

Clinical examination should establish:

- the level of the lesion
- whether it is preganglionic or postganglionic
- the type of damage.

LEVEL OF THE LESION

- Upper plexus injuries (C5 and C6) cause paralysis of the shoulder abductors and external rotators and the forearm supinators; typically, the arm hangs close to the body and internally rotated. Sensation is lost along the outer aspect of the arm and forearm.
- *Pure lower plexus injuries* are rare; the intrinsic hand muscles are paralysed, resulting in clawing, and sensation is lost along the inner (ulnar) aspect of the arm.
- *Total plexus lesions* result in paralysis and numbness of the entire limb (e11.6).

PREGANGLIONIC OR POSTGANGLIONIC

It is important to establish whether the lesion is proximal or distal to the dorsal root ganglion.

- *Proximal (preganglionic) damage* is irreparable.
- *Distal (postganglionic) damage* can be repaired and may recover.

> **FEATURES SUGGESTING PREGANGLIONIC ROOT AVULSION**
>
> Burning pain in an anaesthetic hand
> Paralysis of scapular muscles or diaphragm
> Horner's syndrome
> Severe vascular injury
> Associated fractures of the cervical spine
> Spinal cord dysfunction

The *histamine test* is helpful. Intradermal injection of histamine normally causes a reflex triple response in the surrounding skin (central capillary dilatation, a wheal and a surrounding flare).

- If the flare reaction persists in an anaesthetic area of skin, the lesion must be proximal to the posterior root ganglion – i.e. it is probably a root avulsion.
- With a postganglionic lesion, the test will be negative because nerve continuity between the skin and the dorsal root ganglion is interrupted.

CT myelography or *MRI* may show pseudomeningoceles produced by root avulsion (e11.7).

TYPE OF DAMAGE

In postganglionic lesions it helps to know how severely the nerve has been damaged. With low-velocity injuries, a period of observation is justified; neurapraxia and axonotmesis should show signs of recovery by 6–8 weeks. If neurotmesis seems likely, early operative exploration is called for.

Management

Emergency surgery is best performed by a team specializing in this kind of work.

INDICATIONS FOR EMERGENCY PLEXUS SURGERY

Penetrating wounds
Vascular injury
Severe (high-energy) soft-tissue damage, whether open or closed

---

Clean-cut nerves should be repaired or grafted.

All other brachial plexus injuries are left until detailed examination and special investigations have been completed. Patients with root avulsion or severe mutilating injuries of the limb will be unsuitable for nerve surgery, at least until the prognosis for limb function becomes clear.

Progress of the neurological features is carefully monitored. As long as recovery proceeds at the expected rate, watchful observation is in order. If recovery falters, or if special investigations suggest neurotmesis, the patient should be referred to a special centre for surgical exploration of the brachial plexus and nerve repair, grafting or a nerve transfer procedure. The sooner this decision is made, the better: during the early days, operative exposure is easier and the response to repair more reliable. Repairs performed after 6 months are unlikely to succeed.

Prognosis

Pure upper plexus lesions have the best prognosis. Hand function is spared and muscles innervated from the upper roots often recover quite well after plexus repair, nerve grafting or nerve transfer. With avulsion of C7, C8 and T1, even if shoulder and elbow movements are restored, the loss of hand function causes severe disability.

Late reconstruction

If the patient is not seen until very late after injury, or if plexus reconstruction has failed, tendon transfers may restore a moderate level of function.

OBSTETRICAL BRACHIAL PLEXUS INJURIES

Obstetrical palsy is caused by excessive traction on the brachial plexus during childbirth. Three patterns are seen:

- upper root injury *(Erb's palsy)*, typically in overweight babies with shoulder dystocia at delivery
- lower root injury *(Klumpke's palsy)*, usually after breech delivery of smaller babies
- *total plexus injury.*

 In cases of prolonged labour and/or shoulder dystocia, examine for brachial plexus injury.

Clinical features

The diagnosis is usually obvious at birth: after a difficult delivery the baby has a floppy or flail arm. Further examination a day or two later will define the type of brachial plexus injury.

- *Erb's palsy* is caused by injury of C5, C6 and (sometimes) C7. The abductors and external rotators of the shoulder as well as the forearm supinators are paralysed. The arm is held to the side, internally rotated and pronated.
- *Klumpke's palsy* is due to injury of C8 and T1. The baby lies with the arm supinated and the elbow flexed; there is loss of intrinsic muscle power in the hand. Reflexes are absent and there may be a unilateral Horner's syndrome (**11.5**).
- With a *total plexus injury*, the baby's arm is flail and pale; all finger muscles are paralysed and there may also be vasomotor impairment and a unilateral Horner's syndrome.

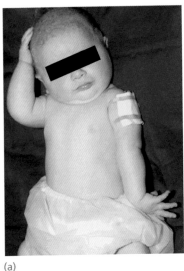
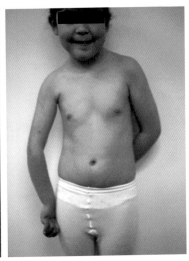

(a) (b)

11.5 Obstetrical brachial plexus palsy (a) Paralysis of the abductors and external rotators of the shoulder, as well as the forearm supinators, results in the typical posture demonstrated in this baby with Erb's palsy of the left arm. **(b)** Young boy with Klumpke's palsy of the right arm.

X-rays should be obtained to exclude fractures of the shoulder or clavicle, which can be mistaken for obstetrical palsy.

Treatment

Over the next few weeks, one of the following may happen:

- *Paralysis may recover completely.* Upper root lesions often recover spontaneously. A reliable indicator is return of biceps activity by the third month.
- *Paralysis may improve and then remain static.* A total lesion may partially resolve, leaving the infant with either an upper or a complete root syndrome which is unlikely to change.
- *Paralysis may remain unaltered.* This is more likely with complete lesions, especially in the presence of Horner's syndrome.

While waiting for recovery, physiotherapy is applied to keep the joints mobile.

If there is no biceps recovery by 3 months, operative intervention should be considered. Unless the roots are avulsed, it may be possible to excise the scar and bridge the gap with free sural nerve grafts; if the roots are avulsed, nerve transfer may give a worthwhile result. This is very demanding surgery which should be undertaken only in specialized centres.

The shoulder is prone to fixed internal rotation and adduction deformity. If diligent physiotherapy does not prevent this, a subscapularis release will be needed, sometimes supplemented by a tendon transfer. In older children, the deformity can be treated by rotation osteotomy of the humerus.

LONG THORACIC NERVE

The nerve to serratus anterior may be damaged in shoulder or neck injuries, or by carrying heavy loads on the shoulder (**11.6**).

The classic sign of serratus anterior palsy is winging of the scapula. This is displayed by asking the patient to push forward forcefully against a wall.

Except after direct injury or division, the nerve usually recovers spontaneously, though this may take a year or longer.

SPINAL ACCESSORY NERVE

The spinal accessory nerve supplies the sterno-mastoid muscle and then runs obliquely across

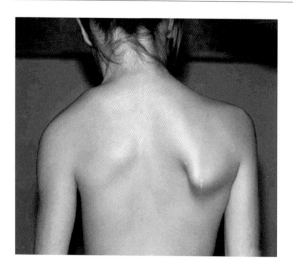

11.6 Long thoracic nerve palsy Winging of the scapula is demonstrated by the patient pushing forwards against the wall. If the serratus anterior is paralysed, the scapula cannot be held firmly against the ribcage.

the posterior triangle of the neck to innervate the upper half of the trapezius. Because of its superficial course, it is easily injured in stab wounds and operations in the posterior triangle of the neck (**11.7a**).

Following an open wound or operation, the patient complains of pain in the shoulder and weakness on abduction of the arm. There is mild winging of the scapula on active abduction against resistance. In late cases there may be wasting of the trapezius and drooping of the shoulder.

Stab injuries and operative injuries should be explored immediately and the nerve repaired. If the exact cause of injury is uncertain, it is prudent to wait for 6 weeks for signs of recovery. If this does not occur, the nerve should be repaired or grafted (**e11.8**).

AXILLARY NERVE

The axillary nerve is sometimes injured during shoulder dislocation, fractures of the humeral neck or inept surgery (**11.7b**). The patient can initiate shoulder abduction with supraspinatus muscle but cannot maintain it owing to deltoid weakness (**e11.9, e11.10**). The deltoid muscle is wasted. There may be a small patch of numbness over the 'Sergeant's stripes'.

The nerve usually recovers spontaneously, but if there is no sign of recovery by 8 weeks and electrodiagnostic tests suggest denervation, the nerve should be explored and grafted. A good result can be expected if surgery is performed within 12 weeks of injury.

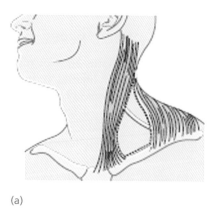

(a)

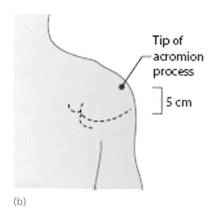

(b)

11.7 Dangerous landmarks (a) The accessory nerve runs across the middle of the posterior triangle of the neck and is easily damaged during lymph node biopsy in this area. (b) The axillary nerve runs from behind the shoulder around the outer aspect of the arm about 5 cm below the tip of the acromion process. Incisions across the top of the shoulder must stop short of this level if injury to the axillary nerve is to be avoided.

SECTION 1 GENERAL ORTHOPAEDICS

RADIAL NERVE

The radial nerve may be injured at the elbow, in the upper arm or in the axilla.

- *Low lesions* are usually due to fractures or dislocations at the elbow, or an open wound or surgical accident. The patient cannot extend the metacarpophalangeal joints.
- *High lesions* occur with fractures of the humerus or after prolonged tourniquet pressure. They are also seen in patients who fall asleep with the arm dangling over the back of a chair ('Saturday night palsy'). There is an obvious wrist-drop due to weakness of the wrist extensors and a small patch of sensory loss on the back of the hand at the base of the thumb.
- *Very high lesions* are usually due to pressure in the axilla ('crutch palsy'). The triceps muscle is wasted and paralysed.

For injuries caused by pressure (a crutch, tourniquet, Saturday night palsy, fractured humerus), the lesion is usually an axonotmesis and spontaneous recovery is the rule. One can therefore afford to wait. However, if there is no sign of recovery by 8–12 weeks, the nerve should be explored and repaired or grafted.

Open wounds should be explored and the nerve repaired or grafted as soon as possible (11.8, 11.9).

With a fractured humerus, if it is certain that there was no nerve injury on admission and the signs appear only after manipulation or operative treatment, the chances of an iatrogenic injury are high so the nerve should be explored and repaired.

 If a nerve is not working following manipulation or surgery, exploration is needed.

In all cases, while recovery is awaited, the wrist should be splinted in extension and the metacarpophalangeal and finger joints kept moving.

In radial nerve lesions that do not recover, the disability can be largely overcome by suitable tendon transfers (**e11.11**).

ULNAR NERVE

Injuries of the ulnar nerve are usually either near the wrist or near the elbow, although open wounds may damage it at any level.

- *Low lesions* may be caused by pressure (e.g. from a deep ganglion) or a laceration at the wrist. There is hypothenar wasting and the hand is clawed due to paralysis of the intrinsic muscles. Finger abduction is weak, and the loss of thumb adduction makes pinch difficult.

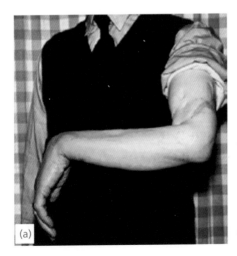
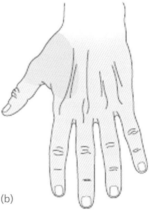

11.8 Radial nerve injury (a) This man developed a complete drop-wrist palsy following a severe open fracture of the humerus and division of the radial nerve. **(b)** The typical area of sensory loss.

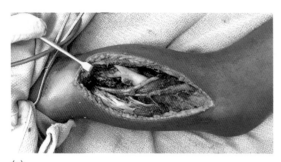

(a)

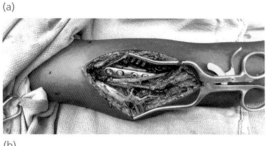

(b)

11.9 Radial nerve palsy A 10-year-old child with an open humeral fracture and dense radial nerve palsy. Radial nerve exploration (via posterior approach) **(a)** confirmed the nerve was intact. The humeral shaft was plated **(b)** and a full recovery was noted 6 weeks postoperatively.

Sensation is lost over the ulnar one and a half fingers.

• *High lesions* occur with elbow fractures; they are also seen (much later) if malunion produces marked cubitus valgus with tension on the nerve where it skirts the medial epicondyle. Remember that ulnar nerve symptoms can also be caused by nerve entrapment in the cubital tunnel, especially in patients lying for long periods with the elbows flexed and pressing on the bed. Curiously, the visible deformity is not marked, because the ulnar half of flexor digitorum profundus is paralysed and the fingers are therefore less 'clawed'. This is known as 'ulnar paradox'. Otherwise motor and sensory loss are the same as in low lesions.

Exploration and suture of a divided ulnar nerve are more easily achieved than with most other nerves; large gaps can be bridged because one can gain length by transposing the nerve to the front of the elbow. If recovery does not occur, hand function is significantly impaired because of the loss of power in metacarpophalangeal flexion, finger abduction, pinch and grip. Tendon transfers are possible, but usually restore only a modest level of function.

MEDIAN NERVE

The median nerve is commonly injured near the wrist or high up in the forearm.

• *Low lesions* may be caused by cuts in front of the wrist or by carpal dislocations. The thenar eminence is wasted and thumb abduction and opposition are weak. Sensation is lost over the radial three and a half digits, and trophic changes may be seen (**11.11**, **11.12**).
• *High lesions* are generally due to forearm fractures or elbow dislocation, but stabs and gunshot wounds may damage the nerve at any level (**e11.12**). The signs are the same as those of low lesions but, in addition, the long flexors to the thumb, index and middle fingers are paralysed.

NERVE INJURIES AFFECTING THE LOWER LIMB

FEMORAL NERVE

The femoral nerve may be injured by a gunshot wound, by traction during an operation or by bleeding into the thigh. There is weakness of knee extension (quadriceps) and numbness of the anterior thigh and medial aspect of the leg. The knee jerk is depressed.

> ⚠ A femoral nerve injury is a disabling lesion and early treatment is essential.

A thigh haematoma may need to be evacuated. A clean cut of the nerve may be treated by careful suturing or grafting but results can be disappointing.

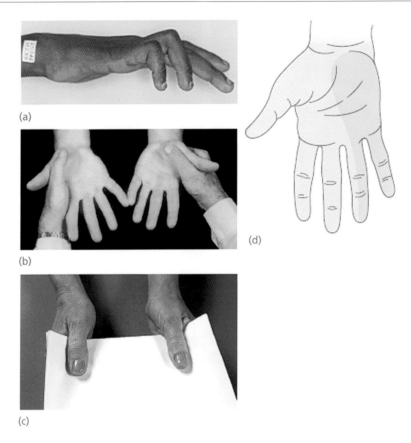

(a)

(b)

(c)

(d)

11.10 Ulnar nerve palsy (a) Clawing of the ring and little fingers and wasting of the intrinsic muscles. **(b)** A good test for interosseous muscle weakness. Ask the patient to spread their fingers (abduct) as strongly as possible and then force the hands together with the little fingers apposed; the weaker side will collapse (the left hand in this case). **(c)** Froment's sign: the patient is asked to grip a card firmly between thumbs and index fingers; normally this is done using the thumb adductors while the interphalangeal joint is held extended. In the right hand, because the adductor pollicis is weak, the patient grips the card only by acutely flexing the interphalangeal joint of the thumb (flexor pollicis longus is supplied by the median nerve). **(d)** Typical area of sensory loss.

SCIATIC NERVE

Division of the main sciatic nerve is rare except in gunshot wounds or operative (iatrogenic) accidents usually during hip replacement. Traction and compression are more common and they occur with local trauma.

The patient complains of foot drop, numbness and paraesthesia in the leg and foot; if there has been direct injury to the nerve, the limb may also be painful. Muscles below the knee are paralysed and sensation is absent in most of the leg. If only the deep (peroneal) component of the nerve is affected, paralysis is incomplete and the signs are easily mistaken for those of a common peroneal nerve injury. Late features are wasting of the calf and trophic ulcers.

Open wounds should be explored and the nerve repaired. While recovery is awaited, a drop-foot splint should be fitted.

The chances of recovery are generally poor and, at best, it will be long-delayed and incomplete. Partial lesions can sometimes be managed by tendon transfers. However, if there is no recovery whatever, amputation may be preferable to a flail, deformed, insensate limb (**11.13**).

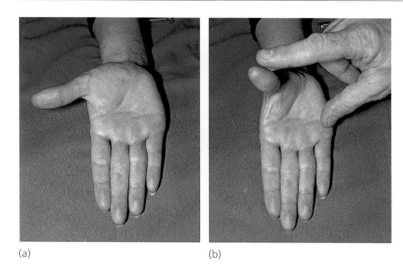

(a)   (b)

11.11 Median nerve – testing for abductor power (a) The hand must remain flat, palm upwards. **(b)** The patient is told to point the thumb towards the ceiling against the examiner's resistance.

IATROGENIC LESIONS

Sciatic nerve palsy is one of the recognized complications of hip replacement. Usually, it is a partial lesion, which is sometimes misdiagnosed as a common peroneal compression injury. There is little to guide one as to whether the sciatic injury is due to direct trauma or to traction on the nerve. If direct injury is suspected, the nerve should be explored. Otherwise it is best to wait for spontaneous recovery, which may take several weeks. In all cases the foot should be splinted to prevent a permanent equinus (foot-drop) deformity.

> ⚠ Following hip surgery, symptoms and signs of 'peroneal nerve injury' are usually due to partial sciatic nerve injury.

PERONEAL NERVES

The *common peroneal nerve* may be damaged in lateral ligament injuries when the knee is forced into varus, or by pressure from a splint or a plaster cast, or from lying with the leg externally rotated (**e11.13**). The patient develops a drop foot in

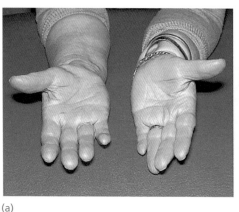

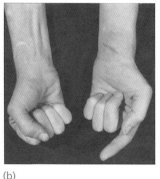

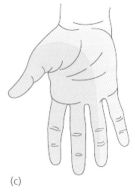

(b)

(c)

(a)

11.12 Median nerve lesions (a) Wasting of the thenar eminence on the right side. **(b)** In high median nerve lesions, the long flexors to the thumb and index fingers are also paralysed and the patient shows the 'pointing index sign'. **(c)** Typical area of sensory loss.

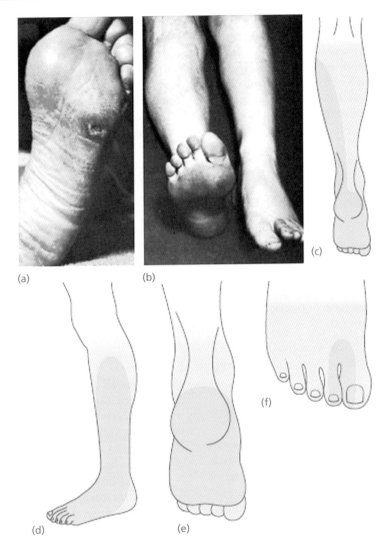

11.13 Sciatic and peroneal nerve lesions (a) One of the late complications is trophic ulceration due to loss of sensibility in the foot. **(b)** Loss of dorsiflexion causes foot drop. Characteristic areas of sensory loss are shown: **(c)** complete sciatic nerve injury; **(d)** common peroneal nerve injury; **(e)** posterior tibial nerve injury and **(f)** anterior tibial (deep peroneal) nerve injury.

which both dorsiflexion and eversion are weak, causing a tendency to trip and fall while walking. Sensation is lost over the front and outer half of the leg and the dorsum of the foot.

If only the *superficial branch* is involved, the peroneal muscles are paralysed and eversion is lost, but dorsiflexion is intact. There is loss of sensation over the outer side of the leg and foot.

The *deep branch* may be threatened in an anterior compartment syndrome. The patient complains of pain, abnormal sensation and weakness of dorsiflexion; on testing, there may be an area of sensory loss around the first web space on the dorsum of the foot.

Treatment

Treatment depends on the local circumstances. A threatened compartment syndrome must be treated as an emergency and may need immediate decompression. If there is an open wound, the nerve should be explored and sutured.

SECTION 1 GENERAL ORTHOPAEDICS

While recovery is awaited, a splint is worn to control the foot drop; the skin must be protected against ulceration. If recovery does not occur, disability can be improved by transferring the tibialis posterior tendon to the dorsum of the foot (so that it acts as a dorsiflexor); alternative solutions are operative stabilization of the hindfoot or permanent splintage.

NERVE ENTRAPMENT SYNDROMES

Wherever peripheral nerves traverse fibro-osseous tunnels, they are at risk of entrapment or compression, especially if the soft tissues increase in bulk, as they may in pregnancy, myxoedema or rheumatoid arthritis, or if there is a local obstruction (e.g. a ganglion or osteophytic spur). The most common sites are:

- the *carpal tunnel* at the wrist (median nerve)
- the *cubital tunnel* at the elbow (ulnar nerve).

Less common sites are:

- the *Guyon's canal* where the ulnar nerve enters the wrist
- the *radial tunnel* in the forearm as the posterior interosseous nerve enters supinator muscle
- the *tarsal tunnel* below the ankle (posterior tibial nerve)
- the lateral part of the *inguinal ligament* (lateral cutaneous nerve of the thigh).

A special case is the *thoracic outlet*, where the subclavian vessels and trunks of the brachial plexus cross the first rib between the scalenus anterior and medius muscles. In these cases, there may be vascular as well as neurological signs in the upper limb.

Patients with long-standing, mild, possibly unrecognized polyneuropathies (e.g. due to diabetes or alcohol abuse) are particularly prone to symptoms of localized nerve compression. A general neurological assessment is therefore advisable in all patients with features of local nerve compression.

Clinical features

The patient complains of unpleasant tingling or pain or numbness in the territory of the compressed nerve. Symptoms are usually intermittent and related to specific postures which compromise the nerve. Areas of altered sensation, motor weakness and muscle wasting are so characteristic that the diagnosis and the site of compressive trauma are immediately suggested. The clinical features of altered peripheral nerve function are described in the preceding pages.

The likely site of compression should be carefully examined for any local cause, for example in ulnar nerve entrapment a long-standing valgus deformity of the elbow, or in carpal tunnel following a Colles' fracture.

The diagnosis may be confirmed by measuring nerve conduction velocity, which is likely to be impaired in the affected segment of the nerve. It is well to remember, though, that this test is not infallible and it should not be used as a substitute for careful clinical assessment.

Treatment

In early cases, simple measures such as advising the patient to avoid compromising postures of the affected limb, or preventing flexion of the wrist or elbow with a light-weight splint, may help. If an inflammatory disorder is suspected, corticosteroid injection into the entrapment area can reduce local tissue swelling. The condition is often self-limiting, so there is no hurry about operative treatment. If symptoms persist, or if there is muscle weakness and wasting, operative decompression is indicated. Once axonal degeneration occurs, tunnel decompression may fail to give complete relief.

CARPAL TUNNEL SYNDROME

This is the most common compressive neuropathy, caused by compression of the median nerve beneath the transverse carpal ligament. It is described in detail in Chapter 15.

ULNAR NERVE COMPRESSION

At the elbow

Compression of the ulnar nerve usually occurs behind the medial epicondyle at the elbow. It usually occurs spontaneously, more commonly in middle-aged men (as opposed to carpal tunnel syndrome which is more common in women). It is sometimes associated with a post-traumatic valgus deformity of the elbow or swelling from arthritis. Most patients complain only of a tingling sensation in the fifth and the ulnar side of the fourth finger; this is most likely to occur when the elbow is held flexed for long periods or when leaning on the inner side of the flexed elbow.

On examination there is usually a positive Tinel's sign when percussing the nerve behind the elbow.

> ⚠ Beware! Anyone may experience sharp 'tingling' when they suffer a bump on the 'funny bone' at the medial edge of the elbow – so always examine the normal side for comparison.

Objective numbness and weakness in the ulnar nerve distribution denotes axonal damage; in that case the nerve should be decompressed, and sooner rather than later.

Treatment may simply be a matter of avoiding the provocative posture such as flexing the elbow when sleeping, leaning on the flexed elbow in more refractory cases, and always if there is established numbness or muscle wasting, the nerve should be released through an incision behind the epicondyle. If the nerve is unstable, it can be gently transposed in front of the epicondyle (**e11.14**).

At the wrist

The ulnar nerve is occasionally compressed as it runs in front of the wrist just radial to the pisiform. The cause is usually a ganglion from the underlying joint, but neurological symptoms may also be produced by external pressure (e.g. in cyclists who lean too heavily on their handlebars). MRI may define a local compressive lesion; the nerve can then be carefully explored and any causal pathology removed (**e11.15**).

RADIAL (POSTERIOR INTEROSSEOUS) NERVE COMPRESSION

The radial nerve itself is rarely the source of 'entrapment' symptoms. Just above the elbow, it divides into a superficial branch (sensory to the skin over the anatomical snuffbox) and the posterior interosseous nerve, which dives between the two heads of the supinator muscle before supplying motor branches to extensor carpi ulnaris and the metacarpophalangeal extensors (branches to extensor carpi radialis longus and brevis arise above the elbow).

Posterior interosseous nerve compression may occur at five sites, represented by the mnemonic FREAS.

FREAS: SITES OF POSTERIOR INTEROSSEOUS NERVE COMPRESSION

Fibrous bands around radiocapitellar joint
Recurrent arterial branches
Extensor carpi radialis brevis
Arcade of Frohse (a thickening at the proximal edge of supinator)
Distal edge of **S**upinator

It may also be caused by a space-occupying lesion pushing on the nerve – a ganglion, a lipoma or severe radiocapitellar synovitis.

Two clinical patterns are encountered:

- posterior interosseous syndrome
- radial tunnel syndrome.

POSTERIOR INTEROSSEOUS SYNDROME

This is a pure motor disorder and there are no sensory symptoms. Gradually emerging weakness of metacarpophalangeal extension affects first one or two and then all the digits. Wrist extension is preserved (the nerves to extensor carpi radialis longus arise proximal to the supinator) but the wrist veers into radial deviation because of the weak extensor carpi ulnaris (**11.14**).

Surgical exploration is warranted if the condition does not resolve spontaneously within

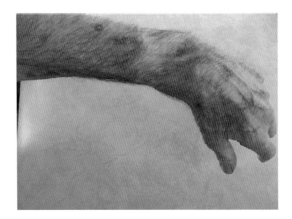

11.14 Posterior interosseous nerve compression Wrist in radial deviation; fingers dropped.

3 months or earlier if MRI shows a swelling. Recovery after surgery is slow; if there is no improvement by the end of a year, and if muscle weakness is disabling, tendon transfer is needed.

Radial tunnel syndrome

This syndrome is controversial. Although a motor nerve is involved, the patient presents with pain, often work-related or at night, just distal to the lateral aspect of the elbow. Resisted wrist extension may precipitate the pain. Unlike posterior interosseous syndrome, there is no weakness and there is not an association with a mass lesion. Electrodiagnostic tests are not helpful.

If the symptoms do not resolve with prolonged non-operative measures (modification of activities and splintage), surgery is considered to free the nerve, but the patient should be warned that surgery often fails to relieve the symptoms.

Thoracic outlet syndrome

Neurological and vascular symptoms and signs in the upper limbs may be produced by compression of the lower trunk of the brachial plexus (C8 and T1) and subclavian vessels between the clavicle and the first rib. These neurovascular structures are made taut when the shoulders are braced back and the arms held tightly to the sides; an extra rib (or its fibrous equivalent extending from a large costal process) exaggerates this effect by forcing

the vessel and nerve upwards. Such anomalies are present at birth, yet symptoms are rare before the age of 30. This is probably because, with increasing age, the shoulders sag, thus putting more traction on the neurovascular bundle.

Clinical features

The patient, typically a woman in her thirties, complains of pain and paraesthesiae extending from the shoulder, down the ulnar aspect of the arm and into the medial two fingers. Symptoms tend to be worse at night and are also aggravated by bracing the shoulders (wearing a backpack) or working with the arms above shoulder height. Examination may show weakness and slight wasting of the intrinsic muscles in the hand. Vascular signs are uncommon, but there may be cyanosis, coldness of the fingers and increased sweating (e11.16, e11.17).

Symptoms and signs can sometimes be reproduced by certain provocative manoeuvres, such as Adson's test and Wright's test, although these tests are neither specific nor sensitive enough to clinch the diagnosis.

TESTS FOR THORACIC OUTLET SYNDROME

Adson's test   The patient's neck is extended and turned towards the affected side while they breathe in deeply. This compresses the interscalene space and may cause paraesthesia and obliteration of the radial pulse.

Wright's test   The arms are abducted and externally rotated. Again, the symptoms recur and the pulse disappears on the abnormal side.

Investigations

- *X-rays* of the neck occasionally demonstrate a cervical rib or an abnormally long C7 transverse process. However, similar features are sometimes encountered as purely incidental findings in asymptomatic people, and the demonstration of a cervical rib should not be

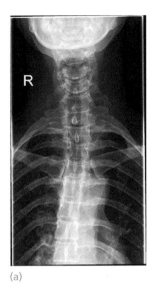
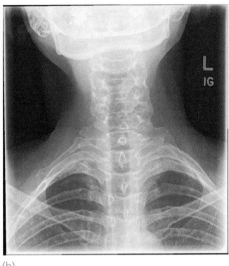

(a)   (b)

11.15 Cervical ribs (a) Elongated transverse process of C7 associated with cervical band and **(b)** bilateral cervical ribs.

taken as 'proof positive' of a thoracic outlet problem. Equally important are X-rays of the lungs (is there an apical tumour?) and the shoulders (to exclude any local lesion) (**11.15**).

- *Electrodiagnostic tests* are helpful mainly to exclude peripheral nerve lesions such as ulnar or median nerve compression which may confuse the diagnosis.
- *Angiography* and *venography* are reserved for the few patients with vascular symptoms (e11.18).

Differential diagnosis

The diagnosis of thoracic outlet syndrome is not easy. Indeed, some clinicians doubt its very existence as a pathological entity!

Tumours of the lower cervical cord or cervical vertebrae and compressive lesions affecting the lower cervical nerve roots These must always be excluded. The presence of Horner's syndrome is a valuable clue.

Cervical spondylosis Although sometimes discovered on X-ray, this seldom involves the T1 nerve root.

Pancoast's syndrome This is due to apical carcinoma of the bronchus with infiltration of the structures at the root of the neck, and it includes pain, numbness and weakness of the hand. A hard mass may be palpable in the neck, and X-ray of the chest shows a characteristic opacity.

Ulnar nerve compression This can be excluded by electromyography and nerve conduction studies.

Treatment

CONSERVATIVE TREATMENT

This suffices for most patients: exercises to strengthen the shoulder-girdle muscles; postural training; instruction in work practices; and other ways of preventing shoulder droop and muscle fatigue. Analgesics may be needed for pain.

OPERATIVE TREATMENT

Surgery is indicated if pain is severe, if muscle wasting is obvious or if there are vascular disturbances. The thoracic outlet is decompressed by removing the first rib (or the cervical rib). This can be accomplished by either a supraclavicular approach or a transaxillary approach (e11.19).

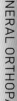

Orthopaedic operations

12

- Preparation — 247
- Intraoperative radiography — 248
- The 'bloodless field' — 249
- Measures to reduce risk of infection — 250
- Thromboprophylaxis — 251
- **Operations on bones** — 254
- Osteotomy — 254
- Bone fixation — 254
- Bone grafts and substitutes — 257
- Distraction osteogenesis and limb reconstruction – Ilizarov method — 259
- **Operations on joints** — 262
- Arthrotomy — 262

- Arthrodesis — 262
- Arthroplasty — 263
- **Limb replantation** — 264
- **Amputations** — 264
- Amputations at sites of election — 264
- Prostheses — 266
- **Implant materials** — 267
- Metals — 267
- Ultra-high molecular weight polyethylene — 269
- Carbon — 269
- Acrylic cement — 269
- Hydroxyapatite — 270

This chapter discusses the principles applying to orthopaedic operations and describes the fundamental techniques of soft-tissue and bone repair. For detailed descriptions of the various operative procedures, the reader is referred to standard textbooks on operative orthopaedic surgery and monographs dealing with specific regional subjects.

PREPARATION

PLANNING

Operations upon the musculoskeletal system must be carefully planned in advance, when accurate measurements can be made, bones can be compared for symmetry with those on the other side of the axis or with those of the opposite limb. This stage allows the surgeon to plan for appropriate equipment, expertise and support to be available. Imaging with digital templating software may be needed to help size and select the most appropriate implant.

MINIMUM EQUIPMENT REQUIREMENTS FOR ORTHOPAEDIC OPERATIONS

Drills – for boring holes
Osteotomes – for cutting cancellous bone
Saws – for cutting cortical bone
Chisels – for shaping bone
Gouges – for removing bone
Plates, screws and screwdrivers – for fixing bone

EQUIPMENT

Many operations such as joint replacement, spinal fusion and the various types of internal fixation require more specialized implants and instruments.

INTRAOPERATIVE RADIOGRAPHY

Intraoperative radiography is often helpful and sometimes essential. Fracture reduction, osteotomy alignments and the positioning of implants and fixation devices can be checked before completing the procedure (**12.1**). Fluoroscopy, where available, is quick and easy to use. Angiography may be needed to diagnose a vascular injury or demonstrate the success of a vascular repair.

IMAGING GUIDANCE SYSTEMS

By using a navigation system based on techniques such as optical tracking, implanted markers and intraoperative radiography with suitable computer software, surgeons may be able to improve their accuracy and consistency in placing implants correctly. Examples are insertion of screws into vertebral pedicles and positioning of joint replacement components.

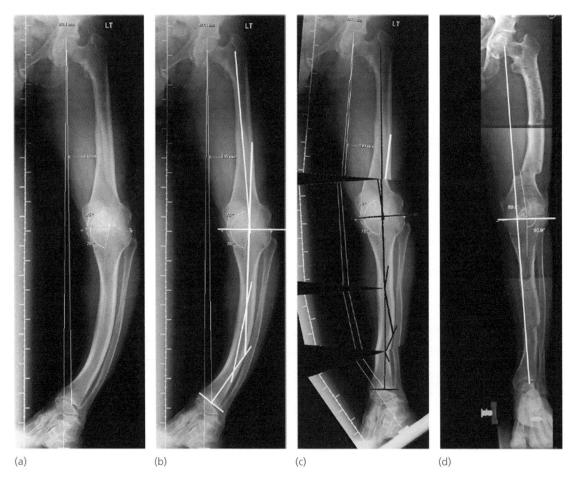

(a)   (b)   (c)   (d)

12.1 Preoperative planning on digitized X-ray images The computer software allows the deformity to be analysed **(a,b)** and the correction simulated **(c)**. The end result then mimics the simulation **(d)**.

ROBOTICALLY ASSISTED SURGERY

In an attempt to improve the accuracy and reproducibility of certain surgical procedures (e.g. joint replacement), robotically assisted surgery can be considered. There are a variety of different ways in which surgeons can interact with robots including haptic feedback, force constraint and telemanipulation.

RADIATION EXPOSURE

Intraoperative radiography involves the risks to both patient and members of the theatre team of radiation exposure. The recommended dose limit for the general public is 1 mSv per year, which is the equivalent of 1000 chest X-rays. Fluoroscopic images acquired during operations are usually pulsed exposures rather than continuous screening, thus reducing total exposure and amounting to a negligible additional risk of developing cancer.

Total exposure varies with the type of procedure performed (operations on limb extremities produce the least, hip operations, midline and spine operations the most), the number of procedures needing X-ray assistance and the protective measures used. The latter influence the cumulative exposure significantly and lead aprons are therefore compulsory; further attenuation of radiation exposure is gained through the use of thyroid shields and, if practical, eye goggles.

MAGNIFICATION

Magnification is an integral part of peripheral nerve and hand surgery. The improved view minimizes the risk of inadvertent injury to structures and allows more accurate apposition of tissues during reconstruction.

Operating loupes range in power from 2× to 6× magnification. As the magnification increases, the field of view decreases and the interruption by unwanted head movements becomes more apparent.

The operating microscope allows much greater magnification with a stable field of view.

THE 'BLOODLESS FIELD'

Many operations on limbs can be done more rapidly and accurately if bleeding is prevented and a 'bloodless field' is created. This is usually achieved by the application of a tourniquet.

WIDE AWAKE LOCAL ANAESTHETIC NO TOURNIQUET

A bloodless field can be achieved by slowly infiltrating large volumes of very dilute lidocaine and adrenaline (epinephrine). The advantage of the procedure called wide awake local anaesthetic no tourniquet (WALANT) is that there is no paralysis from the tourniquet. This allows the surgeon to assess the effect of a tenolysis, the tension of a tendon transfer, the rotation of a fixed finger fracture throughout range of movement, and the alignment and offset of a small joint replacement.

TOURNIQUET CUFF

Only a pneumatic cuff should be used and it should be at least as wide as the diameter of the limb. Wide cuffs reduce the pressure needed for vascular occlusion. A protective layer should be applied to the skin prior to placement of the tourniquet.

 During skin preparation, it is essential that the sterilizing fluid does not leak beneath the cuff as this can cause a chemical burn. Isolating the tourniquet with a plastic drape can help prevent this complication.

EXSANGUINATION

Elevation of the lower limb at 60 degrees for 30 seconds will reduce the blood volume by 45%; increasing the elevation time does not alter the percentage significantly. This simple manoeuvre will therefore suffice to 'drain' the tissues if a truly bloodless field is not essential, or when surgery is being undertaken for tumour or infection and forceful exsanguination might squeeze pathological tissue into the proximal part of the limb. If a clearer field is required, exsanguination can be achieved by pressure using a rubber tubular exsanguinator prior to skin preparation, or if tourniquet time is to be kept to a minimum, a sterile Esmarch or gauze bandage wrapped from distal to proximal.

TOURNIQUET PRESSURE

A tourniquet pressure of 150 mmHg above systolic is recommended for the lower limb and 80–100 mmHg above systolic for the upper limb. This may need to be increased in hypertensive, obese or very muscular patients.

> Higher pressures are unnecessary and will increase the risk of damage to underlying muscles and nerves.

Tourniquet time

Tourniquet time is ischaemia time and thus an absolute maximum tourniquet time of 2.5 hours is allowed. Transient nerve-related symptoms may occur with 3-hour tourniquet times, but full recovery is usual by the fifth day. Time can be saved by ensuring that the limb is shaved, prepared, draped and marked before inflating the cuff. The time of application of the tourniquet should be recorded and the surgeon should be informed of the elapsed time at regular intervals.

Deflating and reinflating the tourniquet

This has serious local and systemic effects.

- *Locally*, deflation is followed by a hyperaemic response that reduces by half in 5, 12 and 25 minutes respectively after ischaemic times of 1, 2 and 3 hours. This information is useful to the surgeon trying to obtain haemostasis after tourniquet release. There is also a variable amount of swelling, unrelated to the length of the ischaemic period; it is therefore wise not to use a tourniquet when it is not

required to perform the procedure safely and for those limbs where significant swelling is already evident.

- *At the systemic level*, tourniquet deflation induces a free radical-mediated reperfusion syndrome, which adds to any muscle damage already produced by the ischaemic period.

MEASURES TO REDUCE RISK OF INFECTION

SKIN PREPARATION AND DRAPING

Hair removal

Shaving the limb is more likely to be harmful than helpful. Shaving before surgery causes superficial skin damage and leads to local bacterial proliferation.

Skin cleaning

A 'social wash' with a soap solution removes particulate matter and grease. This is particularly useful in:

- visibly contaminated cases
- managing open fractures
- cases where the limb has been wrapped in a cast or splint for some time.

Skin preparation prior to surgery should be carried out with an alcohol-based preparation where safe.

> Alcohol skin-cleaning preparations should not be applied over open wounds, exposed joints or nerve tissue.

Iodine or chlorhexidine preparations are available, but there is evidence that chlorhexidine is more effective after a single application, having longer residual activity and maintaining efficacy in the presence of blood and serum.

Drapes

Drapes function to isolate the surgical field from the rest of the patient and reduce contamination from outside. Disposable drapes have been shown to be superior at preventing passage of bacteria and strike through of fluids.

ESSENTIAL QUALITIES OF OPERATIVE DRAPES AND GOWNS

Barrier effectiveness throughout the
  length of the procedure
Configurability to cover the appropriate
  areas of body or limb
Tear-resistance
Non-allergenicity
Reasonable cost

SURGICAL ATTIRE

Gowns

Gowns need to share the requisite qualities of drapes but should also be comfortable to wear. An anterior panel with increased resistance to fluid penetration is an advantage.

Gloves

Gloves are available in latex and non-latex varieties. The latter are needed if either the surgeon or the patient has a latex hypersensitivity. Double gloving, with a coloured inner glove (so-called 'indicator glove') reduces the number of inner-glove perforations and allows outer-glove perforations to be picked up more quickly. Reassuringly, studies have shown that very small penetrations to inner gloves do not lead to significant passage of bacteria.

Face mask

This hallmark of the surgeon in theatre has been questioned in its ability to reduce surgical site infections. Certainly, the mouth is a potent source of bacterial contamination of theatre air. As studies provide conflicting views as to whether masks reduce infection rates rather than just decrease bacterial counts in the theatre air, for the time being at least, face masks should continue to be used if only for protection of the surgical staff. Modern face masks incorporate visors (eye shields), which substantially reduce the risk of contact with blood.

Glasses and eye protection

For procedures in which blood and bone may be splattered, or if the patient carries a blood-borne virus, protective eye wear should be worn.

THROMBOPROPHYLAXIS

Venous thromboembolism (VTE) is one of the commonest complications of lower limb surgery. It comprises three associated disorders:

- *deep vein thrombosis* (*DVT*)
- *pulmonary embolism* (*PE*)
- the later complication of *chronic venous insufficiency* in some cases.

Approximately one in 30–40 patients operated on for hip fractures or hip and knee replacements will develop a symptomatic thromboembolic complication despite the use of prophylaxis during their hospital stay.

MOST IMPORTANT RISK FACTORS FOR VTE

Increasing age
Obesity
Prolonged immobility
Malignancy
In particular, a personal or family history
  of previous thrombosis

PATHOPHYSIOLOGY

According to Virchow, thrombosis results from an interaction between vessel wall damage, alterations in blood components and venous stasis. DVT occurs most frequently in the veins of the calf and less often in the proximal veins of the thigh and pelvis. It is from the larger and more proximal thrombi that fragments sometimes get carried to the lungs, where they may give rise to symptomatic PE and, in a small percentage of cases, fatal pulmonary embolism (FPE).

CLINICAL FEATURES AND DIAGNOSIS

Deep vein thrombosis

DVT is usually asymptomatic, although some patients present with pain in the calf or thigh. An increase in temperature and pulse rate may develop. There are usually no signs but there may be calf swelling and tenderness.

Pulmonary embolism

Patients may develop pleuritic pain in the chest and shortness of breath, but other conditions, such as myocardial infarction or fulminant pneumonia, can be mistaken for PE. In most cases, PE is asymptomatic and FPE usually presents as a sudden collapse without any prior symptoms.

Imaging studies help to confirm the diagnosis in patients who have a moderate or high clinical probability of thromboembolism. Ultrasound or venography is important for demonstrating DVT and computerized tomographic pulmonary angiography or ventilation–perfusion (V/Q) scans are helpful in the diagnosis of PE.

INCIDENCE OF THROMBOEMBOLIC EVENTS

The incidence of symptomatic post-surgical thromboembolism and FPE is decreasing with time, due to more efficient surgery as well as earlier mobilization and the widespread use of prophylaxis and regional anaesthesia. In particular, the risk of death from PE following common procedures such as hip and knee replacement is now very low (**Table 12.1**).

PREVENTION

The overall risk of DVT and PE can be reduced by prophylaxis. Patients admitted for surgery, whether electively or in emergency, need an individualized risk assessment.

General measures

Neuraxial anaesthesia Spinal or epidural anaesthesia reduces mortality, enhances perioperative analgesia and reduces the risk of VTE by about 50%. It is wise to avoid giving neuraxial anaesthesia and chemical prophylaxis too close together to avoid a spinal haematoma.

Surgical technique Rough surgical technique will potentiate thromboplastin release. Prolonged torsion of a major vein, when maintaining a dislocated hip for purposes of replacement or during aggressive dorsal retraction of the tibia during knee replacement, inhibits venous return and damages the endothelium.

Tourniquet A tourniquet probably does not change the risk; clotting factors that accumulate while the tourniquet is inflated are flushed out by the hyperaemia on tourniquet deflation.

Table 12.1 Risk of VTE

Procedure or condition	FPE	Symptomatic VTE	Asymptomatic DVT
Hip fracture	1%	4%	60%
Hip replacement	0.2–0.4%	3–4%	55%
Knee replacement	0.2%	3–4%	60%
Isolated lower limb trauma	Unknown	0.4–2%	10–35%
Spinal surgery	Unknown	0.4–2%	10–35%
Knee arthroscopy	Unknown	0.2%	7%
Major trauma	Unknown	Unknown	58%
Spinal cord injury	Unknown	13%	35%
Upper limb surgery	Unknown	Very rare	Very rare
Minor lower limb surgery	Very rare	Very rare	Very rare

Derived from the International Consensus Statement 2013 and ACCP Guidelines 2015.

Early mobilization This is a simple physiological means of improving venous flow.

Physical methods

Graduated compression stockings These can halve the incidence of DVT when they are correctly sized and fitted compared to no prophylaxis.

Intermittent plantar venous compression This takes advantage of the fact that blood from the sole of the foot is normally expressed during weight-bearing by intermittent pressure on the venous plexus around the lateral plantar arteries, which, in turn, increases venous blood flow in the leg. A mechanical foot pump can reproduce the physiological mechanism in patients who are confined to bed.

 Plantar venous compression should not be used in combination with compression stockings as these impair refill of the venous plexus after emptying by the foot pump.

Intermittent pneumatic compression of the leg This has also been shown to reduce the risk of 'radiological DVT' after hip replacements and in trauma. It is, however, impractical for patients undergoing operations at or below the knee.

Inferior vena cava filters Resembling an umbrella, these are passed percutaneously through the femoral vein and lodged in the inferior vena cava. They merely catch an embolus to prevent it from reaching the lungs. They have a specific role in the occasional case where the risk of embolism is high yet anticoagulation is contraindicated (e.g. in a patient with a pelvic fracture who has already developed a DVT but needs major surgical reconstruction).

 The complication rate, which includes death from proximal coagulation, should restrict use of these filters.

Electrical stimulation A small device over the peroneal nerve at the knee may enhance blood flow.

Chemical methods

These are generally safe, effective, easy to administer (tablet or injection) and can be used for extended periods. However, all chemical methods incur a risk of bleeding. Methods include the following.

Aspirin Use of aspirin is contentious. Some recent guidelines (American Academy of Orthopaedic Surgeons, Australian Orthopaedic Association, American College of Chest Physicians) recommend aspirin in conjunction with mechanical methods for joint surgery with average risk of VTE. Other guidelines (e.g. NICE in the United Kingdom and the International Consensus Statement) advise against its use.

Unfractionated heparin

 Heparin carries a risk of increased bleeding after operation and is contraindicated in elderly people.

Low molecular weight heparin (LMWH) This class of drug has haematological and pharmacokinetic advantages over unfractionated heparin including ready bio-availability and a wide window of safety; therefore monitoring is not required.

Pentasaccharide This synthetic injectable antithrombotic drug (fondaparinux) precisely inhibits activated Factor X. It is at least as effective as LMWH and is best given 6–8 hours *after surgery*.

 Pentasaccharide must not be given too close to surgery or bleeding may become a significant problem. The drug is excreted by the kidneys rather than metabolized by the liver and so must be used carefully or avoided in those with poor renal function.

Direct anti-Xa inhibitors (e.g. rivaroxaban) and direct thrombin inhibitors (e.g. dabigatran) These drugs are given orally and have a broad therapeutic and safety window (so that no monitoring is required). They are given after surgery and should be continued for as long as the patient is at risk of VTE.

Warfarin Warfarin has been used fairly widely, particularly in North America. It reduces the prevalence of DVT after hip and knee replacement and FPE is extremely rare.

 It is difficult to establish appropriate dosage levels and constant monitoring is needed. If it is used at all, warfarin must be maintained at an international normalized ratio (INR) level of 2–3.

Timing and duration of prophylaxis

Risk factors for thromboembolism are most pronounced during surgery, but in some patients (particularly those with hip or major long-bone fractures of the lower limb), immobility and a hypercoagulable state may begin before the operation. In general, prophylaxis is given on admission to hospital in this group, particularly if surgery will be delayed beyond 24 hours.

 Chemical prophylaxis should not be given too close to surgery because there is a risk of provoking a bleeding complication.

The ideal duration of thromboprophylaxis is not known. Current recommendations are that prophylaxis is continued for 14–35 days following knee replacement and 35 days following hip replacement.

OPERATIONS ON BONES

OSTEOTOMY

Osteotomy may be used to correct deformity, to change the shape of the bone, or to redirect load trajectories in a limb so as to influence joint function. Preoperative planning is essential.

Knowledge of the limb axes and their relation to the joints is the foundation for analysing skeletal deformity. Deformity is 3D and should be addressed as such.

The use of 3D printing from computed tomography (CT) data now allows very accurate

planning, especially if scans of the normal limb are reversed to match the deformed limb as a template. 3D printing of customized fixation plates will enhance accuracy even further.

Complications of osteotomy include:

- under- and overcorrection
- neuropraxia (from stretching of nerves)
- non-union
- compartment syndrome.

BONE FIXATION

Stabilizing two or more segments or fragments of bone is usually by internal or external fixation methods. In internal fixation, this may involve screws, wires, plates or intramedullary rods. External fixators come in a variety of types.

INTERNAL FIXATION BY SCREWS

Simple screw

Screws are devices that convert rotational movement into longitudinal movement. Turning of the head causes the screw to advance. They can be used to hold two fragments of bone in close proximity to allow healing or to fix an implant such as a plate to bone.

Lag screw

Screws are also used to compress two fragments together through what is called the 'lag principle' (**12.2**). By overdrilling the near fragment, the threads of the screw only engage the far fragment; when the screw is tightened, the head of the screw pushes the near fragment towards the far fragment and causes compression between the two.

The lag screw works best if passed at right angles to the plane between the bone fragments. If there is a long fracture line, several screws can be inserted at different levels with each screw at right angles to the fracture plane at their respective sites. A similar lag effect is achieved if the screw is threaded only near its tip – a partially threaded screw. The pull-out strength of a screw fixed in bone depends on factors involving both the screw and the bone. It increases:

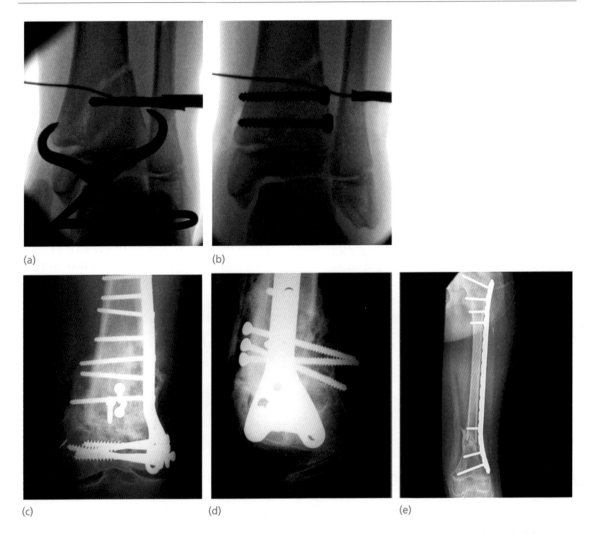

(a) (b)

(c) (d) (e)

12.2 Lag screw fixation This is accomplished through design of the screw (being unthreaded for part of the shank) or through overdrilling the near fragment **(a,b)**. Lag screws are thus used individually or in conjunction with a plate **(c,d)**. Plates can be applied to control twisting forces (here they are used in conjunction with lag screws) or simply as long internal splints, as in indirect submuscular plating of fractures **(e)**.

- with the diameter of screw thread and the length of screw embedded
- with the thickness and density of the bone in which it is embedded
- if both cortices are engaged by the screw.

Most screws are inserted after drilling a pilot-hole and tapping, although self-drilling and self-tapping screws are available.

Cannulated variable pitch screws

A pragmatic alternative to lag screw fixation involves screws with a variable pitch along the length. As the screw is advanced the ends are compressed together. The devices were first used in the scaphoid (Herbert screw) but are invaluable for other carpal fractures, capitellum fractures and metacarpal head fractures.

INTERNAL FIXATION BY PLATES AND SCREWS

Plates have various designs and purposes.

> ### TYPES OF FIXATION PLATE
>
> Simple *straight compression plates* allow compression along the axis of the plate.
> *Contoured plates* fit specific bones.
> *Low-profile plates* reduce the 'footprint' on the bone so as to preserve local vascularity.
> *Locked plates* enable the screw to engage the plate by a secure mechanism so as to create a rigid 3D construct which prevents toggling of the screw in the hole.
> *Bridge plates* span a comminuted defect without disturbing the fracture haematoma or periosteum and do not apply compression.
> *Neutralization plates* do not apply compression but add some extra stability to a fracture that has been primarily compressed and stabilized by a lag screw.

The plate may be applied sub-periosteally by a formal exposure of the fracture or osteotomy, or extra-periosteally in the submuscular plane so as to span the site. These are internal splints that should not be used as load-bearing devices. The ability to control loads across the bone will depend on the degree of contact between the bone ends; it is important that this should be accomplished, usually by compression across the bone ends by a lag screw or through compression with the plate itself.

INTERNAL FIXATION BY INTRAMEDULLARY DEVICES

Two major design types are used: those with and those without interlocking capabilities.

Interlocked intramedullary nails

Interlocking nails have become a standard fixation method for most diaphyseal fractures of the tibia and femur in adults. Stability from these nails is due to a combination of an interference (frictional) fit within the medullary canal and the capture of bone to nail by means of the interlocking screws, which act as

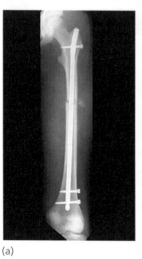
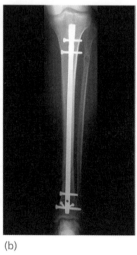
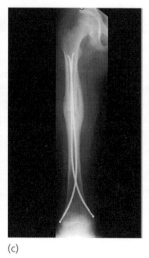
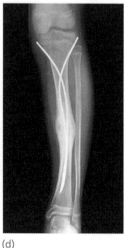

(a)　　　　　　　　　(b)　　　　　　　　　(c)　　　　　　　　　(d)

12.3 Intramedullary nails These are excellent for stabilizing shaft fractures of the major long bones: **(a)** femur; **(b)** tibia. Locked nails have the added benefit of controlling length and torsion. Flexible and elastic nails work by three-point fixation and are suitable for paediatric fractures where damage to the physis can be avoided **(c,d)**.

bolts. Interlocked intramedullary nails offer better control of length and torsion than the unlocked varieties of this device.

The medullary canals of the femur and tibia are not simple cylinders and there are variations between individuals. None of the present-day nail designs is anatomically contoured; therefore, intramedullary reaming to a diameter greater than the nail to be used allows unimpeded insertion of the device. Insufficient reaming potentially risks the bone splitting during nail insertion as a result of hoop stresses (expansile forces) generated.

Unlocked intermedullary nails

Unlocked intramedullary nails are increasingly used in the treatment of long-bone shaft fractures in children. These flexible rods are inserted so as not to damage the physes at either end of the long bone and they function as internal splints by achieving three-point fixation until callus formation takes over (**12.3**). *Intramedullary wires* have a role in metacarpal fractures.

EXTERNAL FIXATION

Static external fixators are useful for temporary stabilization of fractures with severe soft-tissue injuries, for open fractures and for reconstruction of limbs using methods such as the Ilizarov method. They may also be used during emergency stabilization of multiple long-bone fractures in the polytraumatized patient (**12.4**).

The fixator functions as an exoskeleton through which the patient's own skeleton can be supported and adjusted. The basic components are wires or pins inserted into bone to which rods or rings are attached and interconnected.

BONE GRAFTS AND SUBSTITUTES

Bone grafts are both *osteoinductive* and *osteoconductive*.

- They are able to stimulate osteogenesis through the differentiation of mesenchymal cells into osteoprogenitor cells.

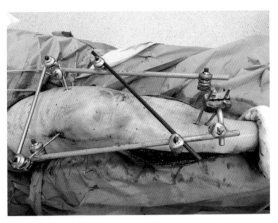

(a)

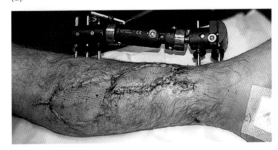

(b)

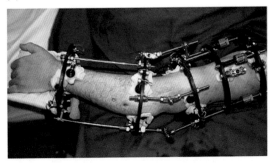

(c)

12.4 External fixators (**a**) These are useful for provisional fracture control, as in severe open fractures. Fixators are also used for definitive fracture treatment (**b**) and for Ilizarov limb reconstruction surgery (**c**).

- They provide linkage across defects and a scaffold upon which new bone can form.

Osteogenesis is brought about partly by the activity of cells surviving on the surface of the graft but mainly by the action of osteoprogenitor cells in the host bed.

BASIC REQUIREMENTS FOR OSTEOGENESIS

The presence of osteoprogenitor cells
A bone matrix
Growth factors

AUTOGRAFTS (AUTOGENOUS GRAFTS)

Bone is transferred from one site to another in the same individual (12.5). These are the most commonly used grafts and are satisfactory provided that sufficient bone of the sort required is available and that, at the recipient site, there is a clean vascular bed.

Cancellous autografts

DONOR SITES FOR CANCELLOUS BONE

Ilium
Greater trochanter
Proximal metaphysis of the tibia
Calcaneum
Lower radius
Olecranon

Cortical autografts can be harvested from any convenient long bone or from the iliac crest; they usually need to be fixed with screws, sometimes reinforced by a plate and can be placed on the host bone, or inlaid, or slid along the long axis of the bone. Cancellous grafts are more rapidly incorporated into host bone than cortical grafts, but sometimes the greater strength of cortical bone is needed to provide structural integrity.

The autografts undergo necrosis, though a few surface cells remain viable. The graft stimulates an inflammatory response with the formation of a fibrovascular stroma; through this, blood vessels and osteoprogenitor cells can pass from the recipient bone into the graft. Apart from providing a stimulus for bone growth (osteoinduction), the graft also provides a passive scaffold for new bone growth (osteoconduction).

Vascularized grafts

This is theoretically the ideal graft; bone is transferred complete with its blood supply, which is anastomosed to vessels at the recipient site. The technique is difficult and time-consuming and requires microsurgical skills.

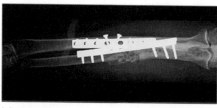

(a)

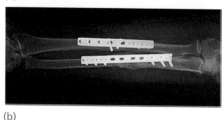

(b)

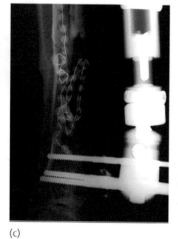

(c)

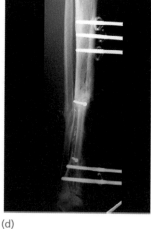

(d)

12.5 Autogenous cancellous bone grafts (a) Autogenous grafts are used here to fill a defect of the ulna and they unite with the host bone in 4 months **(b).** Free vascularized bone transfer (in this case a portion of fibula) is also helpful when larger defects need to be filled **(c,d).**

DONOR SITES FOR VASCULARIZED GRAFTS
Iliac crest (complete with one of the circumflex arteries) Fibula (with the peroneal artery) Radial shaft

ALLOGRAFTS

Allografts consist of bone transferred from one individual (alive or dead) to another of the same species. They can be stored in a bone bank and, as supplies can be plentiful, are particularly useful when large defects have to be filled.

 Sterility must be ensured.

The graft must be harvested under sterile conditions and the donor should be screened for malignancy and blood-borne viruses. Sterilization of the donor material can be done by exposure to ethylene oxide or by ionizing radiation, but the physical properties and potential for osteoinduction are considerably altered by these processes.

Fresh allografts, though dead, are not immunologically acceptable. They induce an inflammatory response in the host and this may lead to rejection. However, antigenicity can be reduced by freezing (at –70 °C), freeze-drying or by ionizing radiation. Demineralization is another way of reducing antigenicity and it may also enhance the osteoinductive properties of the graft. Acid extraction of allograft bone yields *demineralized bone matrix*, which contains collagen and growth factors.

Allografts are most often used in reconstructive surgery where pieces are inserted for structural support; an example is revision hip arthroplasty where bone loss from prosthesis loosening is replaced.

BONE MORPHOGENETIC PROTEINS

Bone morphogenetic proteins (BMPs) are naturally occurring osteoinductive proteins from the Transforming Growth Factor Beta family. BMP-2 and BMP-7 are manufactured using recombinant techniques and are available commercially. There is evidence to support their use in the treatment of non-union and open tibial fractures where the success rate is equivalent to that of autogenous bone grafts.

CALCIUM-BASED SYNTHETIC SUBSTITUTES

Calcium phosphate, hydroxyapatite (HA) and calcium sulphate are primarily osteoconductive and provide a scaffold along which new bone can be formed. Various forms of the material are available, including granules, chips and paste (**12.6**). These synthetic substitutes do not usually possess sufficient compressive strength to withstand high loads and they should be used as void fillers and not as a means of contribution to stability. Compression strength can be increased by altering the ratio of calcium phosphate to HA, by increasing the scintering temperature and by decreasing porosity. Calcium phosphate materials are usually absorbed completely by 6–9 months, but HA substitutes are still visible on X-ray after several years.

DISTRACTION OSTEOGENESIS AND LIMB RECONSTRUCTION – ILIZAROV METHOD

Distraction osteogenesis is a form of tissue engineering founded on the principle of *tension-stress*, which is the generation of new bone in response to gradual increases in tension. Discovered in the 1950s by Gavril Ilizarov in Russia, the *'Ilizarov method'* embraces the various applications of this principle, emphasizing minimally invasive surgery (many of the techniques are performed percutaneously) and an early return of function.

DISTRACTION OSTEOGENESIS

Callus distraction, or *callotasis*, is the single most important application of the tension-stress principle. It is used for limb lengthening or filling of large segmental defects in bone, either through bone transport or other strategies. The basis of the technique is to produce a careful fracture of bone, followed by a short wait before the young callus is gradually distracted via a circular or unilateral external fixator (**12.7**).

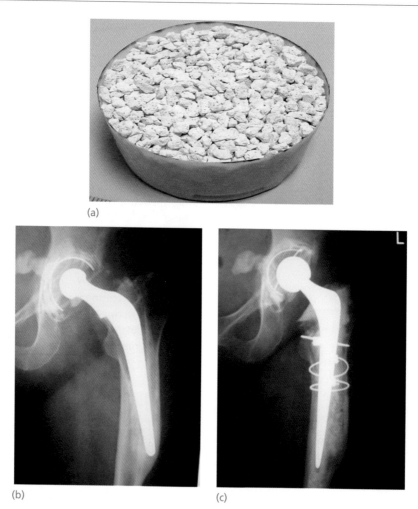

(a)

(b)   (c)

12.6 Synthetic bone substitutes These are used primarily as osteoconductive agents or as a delivery medium for antibiotics, but can be used in weight bearing situations such as revision hip and knee replacement. Several forms are available, including putties, injectable pastes and granules (a). Loose total hip replacement with large potential femoral defect caused by cantilevering of stem (b). Femoral component revised and defect grafted with HA/TCP biphasic bone graft substitute (c).

The external fixator is applied, then a surgical fracture performed. After an initial wait of 5–10 days, distraction is begun and proceeds at 1 mm a day, with small (usually 0.25 mm) increments spaced evenly throughout the day. When the desired length is reached, a second wait follows, which allows the new bone to consolidate and harden. Weight-bearing is permitted throughout this period and it assists the consolidation process. When cortices of even thickness are seen on X-ray and weight-bearing is not painful, the fixator is removed.

CORRECTING BONE DEFORMITIES AND JOINT CONTRACTURES

Angular deformities are corrected by carefully planned osteotomies. However, the amount of correction needed may induce, if undertaken acutely, an unwanted sudden tension on soft tissues, particularly nerves. The correction is performed gradually with the aid of an external fixator; length, rotation and translation deformities can be dealt with simultaneously (**12.8**).

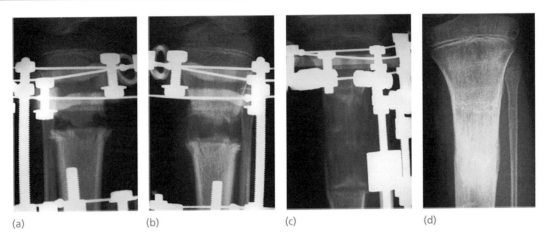

(a)   (b)   (c)   (d)

12.7 Distraction osteogenesis Early on, there is little activity in the distracted gap **(a)**. A little later, columns of bone are seen reaching for the centre of the distracted zone, leaving a clear space in between – the fibrous interzone **(b)**. When the columns bridge the gap, the regenerate bone matures and, finally, a medullary cavity is re-established **(c,d)**.

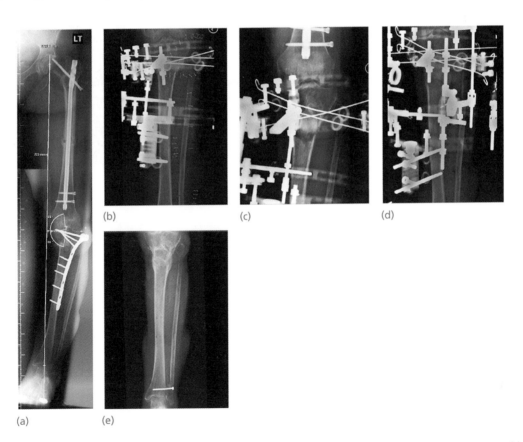

(a)   (e)

12.8 Correction of deformity **(a)** Varus malunion in a fracture of the proximal tibia was corrected by osteotomy and gradual realignment in a circular external fixator **(b–d)**. A cuneiform-shaped mass of bone formed after the axes were aligned **(e)**.

OPERATIONS ON JOINTS

ARTHROTOMY

Arthrotomy, the opening of a joint, may be indicated for a number of reasons.

INDICATIONS FOR ARTHROTOMY

To inspect the interior or perform a synovial biopsy
To drain a haematoma or an abscess
To remove a loose body or damaged structure (e.g. a torn meniscus)
To excise inflamed synovium

ARTHRODESIS

Arthrodesis is a reliable operation for a painful or unstable joint; where stiffness does not seriously affect function, this is may be the treatment of choice.

Arthrodesis involves four basic stages.

STAGES IN ARTHRODESIS

1 *Exposure* – both joint surfaces need to be well visualized and often this means an extensile incision, but some smaller joints are now accessible by arthroscopic means.
2 *Preparation* – both articular surfaces are denuded of cartilage and sometimes the subchondral bone is 'feathered' to increase the contact area.
3 *Coaptation* – the prepared surfaces are apposed in the optimum position, ensuring good contact.
4 *Fixation* – the surfaces are held rigidly by internal or external fixation. Sometimes bone grafts are added in the larger joints to promote osseous bridging (**12.9**).

The main *complication* after arthrodesis is nonunion with the formation of a pseudoarthrosis.

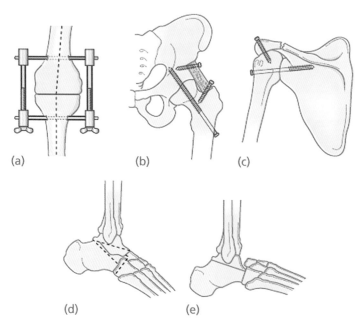

(a)   (b)   (c)

(d)   (e)

12.9 Arthrodesis (a) Compression arthrodesis; **(b)** screw plus bone graft; **(c)** similar technique using the acromion. **(d,e)** Subtalar mid-tarsal fusion.

ARTHROPLASTY

Arthroplasty, the surgical refashioning of a joint, aims to relieve pain and to retain or restore movement. The main varieties are:

- *excision arthroscopy*
- *partial replacement*
- *total joint replacement* (**12.10**).

EXCISION ARTHROPLASTY

Sufficient bone is excised from the articulating parts of the joint to create a gap at which movement can occur (e.g. Girdlestone's excision arthroplasty, trapeziectomy, proximal row carpectomy). This movement is limited and occurs through intervening fibrous tissue, which forms in the gap.

Partial replacement

One articulating part only is replaced (e.g. a femoral prosthesis or hemiarthroplasty for an intracapsular hip fracture, without an acetabular component); or one compartment of a joint is replaced (e.g. the medial or lateral half of the tibiofemoral joint in a unicompartmental knee replacement). The prosthesis is kept in position either by acrylic cement or by initial press-fit stability between implant and bone and later osseointegration, i.e. bonding at a molecular level between the implant and the bone.

Total joint replacement

Both the articulating parts of the joint are replaced by prosthetic implants. Bearings may be hard-on-soft (e.g. metal-on-polyethylene) or hard-on-hard (e.g. ceramic-on-ceramic). All joint replacements have articulations (parts that move against each other) and all articulations produce wear. Usually the harder material causes wear of the softer material. Wear can be accelerated by roughening of the surfaces, such as by scratching, or by interposition of third bodies, such as cement fragments becoming trapped in the joint. Metal-on-metal bearings became popular in hip replacement with over one million such devices implanted worldwide, but they have been associated with higher incidences of failure, due to production of cobalt and chrome debris, and their use has been almost entirely abandoned. Irrespective of type, these components are fixed to the host bone, either with acrylic cement or by a cementless press-fit technique.

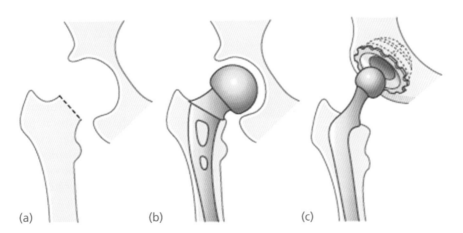

12.10 Arthroplasty The main varieties as applied to the hip joint: **(a)** excision arthroplasty (Girdlestone's); **(b)** partial replacement – an Austin Moore prosthesis has been inserted after removing the femoral head; **(c)** total replacement – both articular surfaces are replaced.

Using hip replacement as an example, the rationale, indications and complications of total joint replacement are discussed in detail in Chapter 19.

LIMB REPLANTATION

Microsurgical techniques are used in repairing nerves and vessels, transplanting bone or soft tissue with a vascular pedicle, transferring a less essential digit (e.g. a toe) to replace a lost essential one (e.g. a thumb) and, occasionally, for reattaching a severed limb or digit.

 Replantation is time-consuming, expensive and often unsuccessful.

Two teams dissect, identify and mark each artery, nerve and vein of the stump and the limb. Following careful debridement, the bones are shortened to reduce tension and are stabilized internally. Next the vessels are sutured – veins first and (if possible) two veins for each artery. Nerves and tendons are sutured next. Only healthy ends of approximately equal diameter should be joined; tension, kinking and torsion must be prevented. Decompression of skin and fascia, as well as thrombectomy, may be needed in the postoperative period (**12.11**).

AMPUTATIONS

Alan Apley, in characteristic style, encapsulated the indications for amputation in the never-to-be forgotten 'three Ds'.

> ## INDICATIONS FOR AMPUTATION: APLEY'S 'THREE DS'
>
> Dead
> Dangerous
> Damned nuisance!

Dead (or dying)   Limb death can result from:

- peripheral vascular disease (accounts for almost 90% of all amputations)
- severe trauma
- burns
- frostbite.

Dangerous   'Dangerous' disorders are:

- malignant tumours
- potentially lethal sepsis
- crush injury.

Damned nuisance   In some cases, retaining the limb may be worse than having no limb at all. This may be because of:

- pain
- gross malformation
- recurrent sepsis
- severe loss of function.

 In crush injury, releasing the compression may result in renal failure (*crush syndrome*).

The combination of deformity and loss of sensation is particularly trying, and in the lower limb it is likely to result in pressure ulceration.

AMPUTATIONS AT SITES OF ELECTION

Most lower-limb amputations are for ischaemic disease and are performed through the site of election below the most distal palpable pulse. The selection of amputation level can be aided by Doppler indices; if the ankle/brachial index is greater than 0.5, or if the occlusion pressures at the calf and thigh are greater than 65 mmHg and 50 mmHg respectively, there is a greater likelihood the below-knee amputation will succeed. The knee joint should be preserved if clinical examination and investigations suggest this is at all feasible – energy expenditure for a transtibial amputee is 10–30% greater as compared to a 40–67% increase in transfemoral cases.

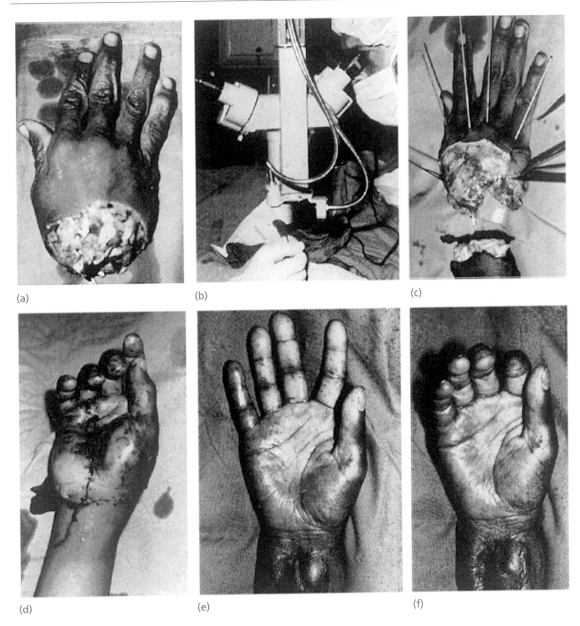

(a)   (b)   (c)

(d)   (e)   (f)

12.11 Microsurgery and limb replantation (a) The problem: a severed hand. **(b)** The solution: replantation with microsurgical techniques. **(c)** The bones of the severed hand have been fixed with K-wires as a preliminary to suturing vessels and nerves. **(d)** The appearance at the end of the operation. **(e,f)** The limb 1 year later; the fingers extend fully and bend about halfway. But the hand survived, has moderate sensation and the patient was able to return to work – as a guillotine operator in a paper works!

The sites of election are determined also by the demands of prosthetic design and local function.

- *Too short a stump* may tend to slip out of the prosthesis.

- *Too long a stump* may have inadequate circulation and can become painful, or ulcerate; moreover, it complicates the incorporation of a joint in the prosthesis (**12.12**).

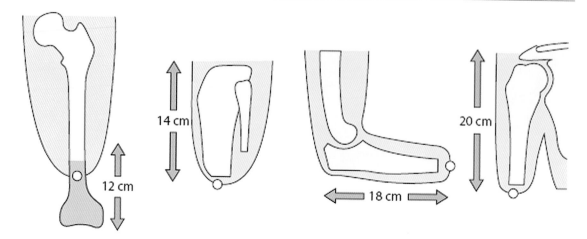

12.12 Amputations The traditional sites of election; the scar is made terminal because these are not end-bearing stumps.

PRINCIPLES OF TECHNIQUE

A tourniquet is used unless there is arterial insufficiency. Skin flaps are cut so that their combined length equals 1.5 times the width of the limb at the site of amputation. As a rule, anterior and posterior flaps of equal length are used for the upper limb and for transfemoral (above-knee) amputations; below the knee, a long posterior flap is usual.

Muscles are divided distal to the proposed site of bone section; subsequently, opposing groups are sutured over the bone end to each other and to the periosteum, thus providing better muscle control as well as better circulation. Nerves are divided under tension proximal to the bone with a sharp blade cut to ensure a cut nerve end will not bear weight.

The bone is sawn across at the proposed level. In transtibial amputations the front of the tibia is usually bevelled and filed to create a smoothly rounded contour; the fibula is cut 3 cm shorter.

The main vessels are tied, the tourniquet is removed and every bleeding point meticulously ligated. The skin is sutured carefully without tension and the stump covered without constricting passes of bandage.

PROSTHESES

All prostheses must fit comfortably, should function well and should look presentable.

 The patient accepts and uses a prosthesis much better if it is fitted soon after operation.

Upper limb

In the *upper limb*, the distal portion of the prosthesis is detachable and can be replaced by a 'dress hand' or by a variety of useful terminal devices. Electrically powered limbs are activated by detection of impulses in the stump muscles. The absence of sensory feedback limits their use, as the right amount of pressure for each object cannot be properly judged. In the hand, remarkably lifelike cosmetic prostheses can transform a patient's confidence although, again, the absence of sensory feedback limits their functional benefit.

Lower limb

In the *lower limb*, weight can be transmitted through the ischial tuberosity, patellar tendon, upper tibia or soft tissues. Combinations are permissible; recent developments in silicon and gel materials provide improved comfort in total-contact self-suspending sockets.

IMPLANT MATERIALS

METALS

Metals used

Metals used in implants should be tough, strong, non-corrosive, biologically inert and easy to sterilize. Those commonly used are:

- *stainless steel*
- *cobalt-chromium alloys*
- *titanium alloys.*

No one material is ideal for all purposes.

STAINLESS STEEL

Because of its relative plasticity, stainless steel can be cold-worked. This is a process in which the metal is reshaped or resized, usually at room temperature, which increases its hardness and strength. The form of stainless steel used in orthopaedic surgery is 316L; in addition to iron, it contains chromium (which forms an oxide layer providing resistance to corrosion), carbon (which adds strength but needs to be in low concentrations – hence the L suffix – or else it offsets corrosion resistance), nickel and molybdenum as the main elements used in the alloy. The tensile plasticity (ductility) of stainless steel makes it possible to bend plates to required shapes during an operation without seriously disturbing their strength.

COBALT–CHROMIUM-BASED ALLOYS

These alloys are widely used in joint prosthesis manufacture. Chromium is added to cobalt for *passivation*; an adherent oxide layer formed by the chromium provides corrosion resistance, as it does in stainless steel. Other elements are sometimes added, such as tungsten and molybdenum, to improve strength and machining ability.

TITANIUM ALLOYS

These are used in fracture fixation devices and joint prostheses. They usually contain aluminium and vanadium in low concentrations for strength; passivation (and thus corrosion resistance) is obtained by creating a titanium oxide layer. The elastic modulus of the metal is close to that of bone and this reduces the stress concentrations that can occur when stainless steel or cobalt chromium alloys are used. Additionally, the corrosion resistance (which is superior to that of the other two alloys) augments this metal's biocompatibility.

A *disadvantage* of titanium alloy is notch sensitivity; this is when a scratch or sharp angle created in the metal, either at manufacture or during insertion of the implant, can significantly reduce its fatigue life.

Implant failure

Metal implants may fail for a variety of reasons.

REASONS FOR METAL IMPLANT FAILURE

Defects during manufacture
Incorrect implant selection for the intended purpose
Exposure to repeated high stresses from incorrect seating of the implant or from exceeding the fatigue life (**12.13**), e.g. when there is delay in a fracture union

---

Corrosion

Corrosion is inevitable unless the implanted metal is treated, for example by passivation, which creates a protective passive layer; this is usually an oxide layer formed from chemical treatment. In stainless steel and cobalt–chromium, it is the chromium component that helps in creating an oxide layer; in titanium, the element itself forms it. With passivated metal alloys used in orthopaedic surgery, corrosion is rarely a problem except when damage to the passive layer occurs; it may be initiated by abrasive damage or minute surface cracks due to fatigue failure. The products of corrosion, metal ions and debris,

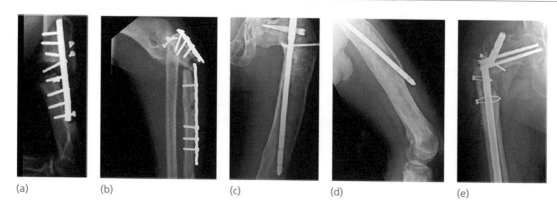

(a)   (b)   (c)   (d)   (e)

12.13 Fatigue failure of implants Fatigue failure can be due to **(a,b)** incorrect implant selection (too small or too weak) or **(c,d)** incorrect positioning. Other factors are also involved: infection may delay union and lead to eventual implant fracture **(e)**.

cause a local inflammatory response that accelerates loosening.

Dissimilar metals

Dissimilar metals immersed in solution in contact with one another may set up galvanic corrosion with accelerated destruction of the more reactive (or 'base') metal.

Friction and wear

These mechanical concepts are relevant to understanding joint function and prosthesis design. *Friction* between two sliding surfaces will not be affected by the area of contact or the speed of movement but will depend on the applied load. Therefore, any two surfaces can have a coefficient of friction derived to represent this interaction – it is the ratio of the force needed to start a sliding movement to the normal compression force between the surfaces.

Normal human joints possess coefficients of friction that are about ten times lower than those of various combinations of prosthesis-bearing materials. Metal on ultra-high molecular weight polyethylene (UHMWPE – see below) produces a better (lower) coefficient of friction, and this is improved further if the metal is replaced by a ceramic, such as alumina or zirconium.

An important modulator of friction characteristics in joints is *lubrication*. Synovial fluid reduces the coefficient of friction by forming either a layer of fluid that is greater in thickness than the surface irregularities on normal articular cartilage (fluid film lubrication) or, in the absence of this interposed fluid layer, a molecular-width coating that resists abrasion (boundary lubrication).

Friction and joint lubrication are related to *wear*, which is the loss of surface material due to sliding motion under load. Wear is proportional to the load and distance of movement between the two surfaces, and it may be caused in several ways.

CAUSES OF WEAR BETWEEN SURFACES

Abrasion, where a harder surface erodes the surface of the softer material
Adhesion, where the two surfaces bond more tightly than particles within one of the surfaces
Debris that becomes trapped between articulating surfaces and causes abrasion (third-body wear)

Metal wear particles may cause local inflammation and scarring and, occasionally, a toxic or allergic reaction; most importantly, however, they may cause implant loosening following their uptake by macrophages and subsequent activation of osteoclastic bone resorption. Metal wear particles may provoke a lymphocyte-dominated vasculitis-associated reaction locally and their presence has also been demonstrated in lymph nodes and other organs far distant from the implant; the significance of this finding is uncertain.

ULTRA-HIGH MOLECULAR WEIGHT POLYETHYLENE

UHMWPE is an inert thermoplastic polymer. Its density is close to that of the low-density polyethylenes but the very high molecular weight provides increased strength and wear resistance. The material is most commonly used in orthopaedics for hip (acetabular cup) and knee (tibial tray) prostheses and is sterilized by gamma irradiation.

DISADVANTAGES OF UHMWPE

The cross-linked form may have improved wear properties but poorer yield strength, which may influence crack development and propagation.
Being a viscoelastic material, it is susceptible to deformity (stretching) and creep.
It is easily abraded, a reflection of poor hardness, and chips of bone or acrylic cement trapped on its surface cause accelerated wear.

When in contact with a polished metal as part of a bearing, UHMWPE has a low coefficient of friction and it therefore seemed ideal for joint replacement. This has proved to be true in hip reconstruction with a simple ball-and-socket articulation. However, UHMWPE has several *disadvantages* (see Box).

CARBON

Carbon fibre

This is extensively used for the manufacture of external fixation devices, such as connecting rods and even circular rings, as the combination of lightweight, rigidity and radiolucency is attractive. Carbon fibre is also sometimes used to replace ligaments; it induces the formation of longitudinally aligned fibrous tissue, which substitutes for the natural ligament. However, a *disadvantage* is that the carbon fibres tend to break up and, if particles find their way into the synovial cavity, they induce a synovitis.

Pyrocarbon

For small joint components in the hand and foot, a graphite core is moulded and then coated with a carbon deposit in a very high temperature chamber. These implants are very smooth with negligible wear against another implant and probably induce less wear if articulating directly with joint cartilage. A *disadvantage* is that it does not formally osseo-integrate and over time the implants do tend to erode and loosen.

ACRYLIC CEMENT

In joint replacement, prostheses are often fixed to the bone with acrylic cement (polymethylmethacrylate – PMMA). It is usually presented as a liquid (the PMMA monomer) and powder (the PMMA polymer plus copolymers or other additives), which is mixed to set off an exothermic polymerization reaction. Before the mixture cures, it is applied to the bone in which the prosthesis is embedded. The application of pressure causes interdigitation into the bony interstices and, when fully polymerized, the now hard compound prevents movement between prosthesis and bone. It can withstand large compressive loads but is easily broken by tensile stress.

Cement mixing and cement introduction techniques have been shown to influence the tensile strength. An almost 50% increase in tensile strength can be obtained by vacuum mixing. Additionally, cleaning of the bone and pressurization of the cement within the bone cavity, prior to introduction of the implant, improves interdigitation of the cement into interstices of the bone surface. When the partially polymerized cement is forced into the bone, there is often a drop in blood pressure; this is attributed to the uptake of residual monomer, which can cause peripheral vasodilatation, and fat embolization from the bone marrow. This is seldom a problem in fit patients with osteoarthritis, but can be very serious in less fit or elderly patients.

 In elderly patients undergoing treatment for hip fracture, monomer and marrow fat may enter the circulation very rapidly when the cement is compressed, and the fall in blood pressure can be fatal, particularly in a dehydrated under-resuscitated patient.

HYDROXYAPATITE

The mineral phase of bone exists largely in the form of crystalline HA. It is not surprising, therefore, that this material has been used to reproduce the osteoinductive and osteoconductive properties of bone grafts. HA can also be plasma sprayed onto implants; the HA coating promotes rapid osseointegration. HA coating is used in uncemented joint replacement prostheses and with external fixator pins.

Section 2

Regional Orthopaedics

13	The shoulder and pectoral girdle	273
14	The elbow	297
15	The wrist	309
16	The hand	325
17	The neck	345
18	The back	359
19	The hip	393
20	The knee	421
21	The ankle and foot	453

■ Clinical assessment	273	■ Atraumatic instability	289
■ Disorders of the rotator cuff	277	■ Posterior instability of the shoulder	289
■ Lesions of the biceps tendon	284	■ Disorders of the glenohumeral joint	290
■ 'Slap' lesions	285	■ Disorders of the scapula and clavicle	293
■ Adhesive capsulitis (frozen shoulder)	285	■ Operations	295
■ Anterior instability of the shoulder	286		

CLINICAL ASSESSMENT

HISTORY

- *Pain* is the commonest symptom. However, 'pain in the shoulder' is not necessarily 'shoulder pain'! Pain from the shoulder or its surrounding tendons is felt anterolaterally and at the insertion of the deltoid; sometimes it radiates down the arm. Pain on top of the shoulder suggests acromioclavicular dysfunction or a cervical spine disorder.

 Beware the trap of *referred pain* – the shoulder is a common site of referred pain from the neck, heart, mediastinum and diaphragm.

- *Stiffness* may be progressive and severe – so much so as to merit the term 'frozen shoulder'.
- *Deformity* may consist of muscle wasting, prominence of the acromioclavicular joint or winging of the scapula.
- *Instability* is a feeling that the shoulder might come out of its socket.
- *Loss of function* is expressed as inability to reach behind the back and difficulty with combing the hair or dressing.

THE PAINFUL SHOULDER

Referred pain syndromes

- Cervical spondylosis
- Mediastinal pathology
- Cardiac ischaemia

Joint disorders

- Glenohumeral arthritis
- Acromioclavicular arthritis

Bone lesions

- Infection
- Tumours

Rotator cuff disorders

- Tendinitis
- Rupture
- Frozen shoulder

Instability

- Dislocation
- Subluxation

Nerve injury

- Suprascapular nerve entrapment

SECTION 2 REGIONAL ORTHOPAEDICS

EXAMINATION

The patient should always be examined from in front and from behind. Both upper limbs, the neck and the chest must be visible. Because shoulder and neck symptoms are often felt in the same areas, examination of the shoulder must include a full examination of the neck, and vice versa.

Look

Skin Scars or sinuses are noted; don't forget the axilla!

Shape Asymmetry of the shoulders, winging of the scapula, wasting of the deltoid or short rotators and acromioclavicular dislocation are best seen from behind; joint swelling or wasting of the pectoral muscles is more obvious from in front. The typical 'Popeye' bulge of a ruptured biceps is more easily seen if the elbow is flexed.

Position If the arm is held persistently internally rotated, think of posterior dislocation of the shoulder.

Feel

Because the joint is well covered, inflammation rarely influences skin temperature. The soft tissues and bony points are carefully palpated, following a mental picture of the anatomy. Start with the sternoclavicular joint, then follow the clavicle laterally to the acromioclavicular joint, onto the anterior edge of the acromion and around the acromion to the back of the joint. The supraspinatus tendon lies just below the anterior edge of the acromion. Tenderness and crepitus can usually be accurately localized to a particular structure.

Move

ACTIVE MOVEMENTS

A range of active movements should be tested (13.1, 13.2, e13.1).

Abduction Ask the patient to raise both arms sideways until the fingers point to the ceiling. Abduction may be:

- difficult to initiate
- diminished in range
- altered in rhythm, the scapula moving too early and creating a shrugging effect.

If movement is painful, the arc of pain must be noted:

- Pain in the mid range of abduction suggests a rotator cuff tear or supraspinatus tendinitis.
- Pain at the end of abduction is often due to acromioclavicular arthritis.

Flexion and extension These are examined by asking the patient to raise the arms forwards and then backwards.

Adduction To test adduction, ask the patient to move the arm across the front of the body.

Rotation This is tested as follows:

1 With the arms close to the body and the elbows flexed to 90 degrees, the hands are separated as widely as possible (external rotation) and brought together again across the body (internal rotation).
2 The patient is asked to clasp their fingers behind their neck (external rotation in abduction).
3 The patient is asked to reach up the back with their fingers (internal rotation in adduction).

PASSIVE MOVEMENTS

These can be deceptive because even with a stiff shoulder the arm can be raised to 90 degrees by scapulothoracic movement. To test true glenohumeral abduction, the scapula must first be anchored; this is done by pressing firmly down on the top of the shoulder with one hand while the other hand moves the patient's arm.

POWER

The deltoid is examined while the patient abducts against resistance. To test serratus anterior (long thoracic nerve), ask the patient to push forcefully against a wall with both hands; if the muscle is weak, the scapula is not stabilized on the thorax and stands out prominently (*winged scapula*). Pectoralis major is tested by having the patient thrust both hands firmly into the waist. Any difference in muscle bulk between the two sides is noted at the same time.

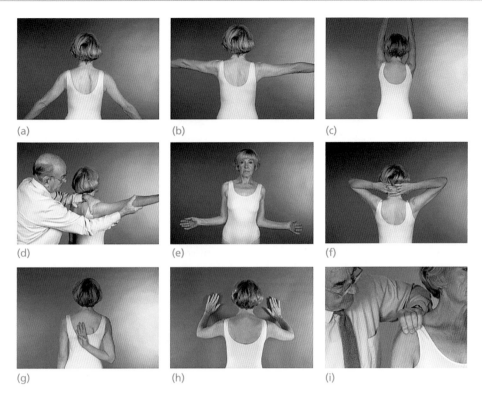

13.1 Examination Active movements are best examined from behind the patient, paying careful attention to symmetry and the coordination between scapulothoracic and glenohumeral movements. **(a)** Abduction; **(b)** limit of glenohumeral abduction; **(c)** full abduction and elevation, a combination of scapulothoracic and glenohumeral movement. **(d)** The range of true glenohumeral movement can be assessed by blocking scapular movement with a hand placed firmly on the top edge of the scapula. **(e)** External rotation. **(f,g)** Complex movements involving abduction, rotation and flexion or extension of the shoulder. **(h)** Testing for serratus anterior weakness. **(i)** Feeling for supraspinatus tenderness.

OTHER SYSTEMS

The cervical spine should be examined as it is a common source of referred pain. If the shoulder feels unstable, look for generalized joint laxity. If weakness is the main complaint, a neurological examination is needed.

INVESTIGATION

Imaging

X-RAYS

At least two X-ray views should be obtained:

- an anteroposterior in the plane of the glenoid
- an axillary projection with the arm in abduction to show the relationship of the humeral head to the glenoid (**13.3a–c**).

Look for evidence of:

- subluxation or dislocation
- joint space narrowing
- bone erosion
- calcification in the soft tissues.

Special views can show the acromioclavicular joint and the subacromial space.

MAGNETIC RESONANCE IMAGING

Magnetic resonance imaging (MRI) is useful to identify osteonecrosis of the humeral head, or a bone tumour. It can also identify labral tears and rotator cuff tears (**13.3d**) although the accuracy for these latter two is enhanced by combining the scan with arthrography.

SECTION 2 REGIONAL ORTHOPAEDICS

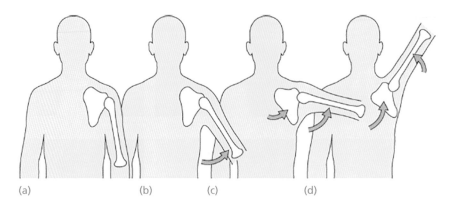

(a)   (b)   (c)   (d)

13.2 Abduction and elevation (a–c) During the early phase of abduction, most of the movement takes place at the glenohumeral joint. As the arm rises, the scapula begins to rotate on the thorax **(c)**. In the last phase of abduction, the movement is almost entirely scapulothoracic **(d)**.

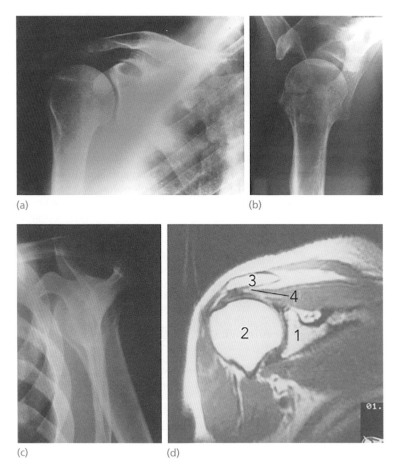

(a)   (b)

(c)   (d)

13.3 Imaging (a) Normal anteroposterior X-ray. **(b)** Axillary view showing the humeral head opposite the shallow glenoid fossa. **(c)** True lateral view; the head of the humerus should lie where the coracoid process, the spine of the scapula and the blade of the scapula meet. **(d)** MRI. (1, Glenoid; 2, head of the humerus; 3, acromion process; 4, supraspinatus.) The high signal in the supraspinatus suggests degenerative change.

COMPUTED TOMOGRAPHY SCAN

Computed tomography (CT) is helpful for planning fracture surgery and shoulder joint replacement.

ULTRASOUND

This is a simple and accurate test for identifying rotator cuff tears and calcific tendinitis. It can also be useful in guiding injections or barbotage (aspirating calcific deposits in the rotator cuff).

Arthroscopy

Arthroscopy is useful for diagnosing and treating subacromial impingement, intra-articular lesions, detachment of the glenoid labrum and rotator cuff tears.

DISORDERS OF THE ROTATOR CUFF

The commonest causes of pain around the shoulder are disorders of the rotator cuff, chiefly the rotator cuff syndrome, calcific tendinitis and adhesive capsulitis.

Anatomy

The rotator cuff is a sheet of conjoined tendons closely applied over the shoulder capsule and inserting mainly into the greater tuberosity of the humerus (subscapularis is inserted into the lesser tuberosity) (**13.4**). The cuff is made up of subscapularis in front, supraspinatus above and infraspinatus and teres minor behind (the 'rotator' muscles), which have an important function in stabilizing the head of the humerus by pulling it firmly into the glenoid whenever the deltoid lifts the arm forwards or sideways.

Arching over the cuff is a fibro-osseous canopy – the coracoacromial arch – formed by the acromion process posterosuperiorly, the coracoid process anteriorly and the coracoacromial ligament joining them. Separating the tendons from the arch, and allowing them to glide, is the subacromial bursa. Normally, when the shoulder is abducted, the conjoint tendon passes under the arch. There should be enough room for it to do so, but if there is not, due to either pathology

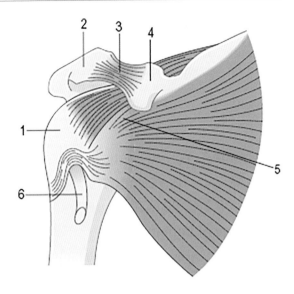

13.4 Anatomy The tough coracoacromial ligament stretches from the coracoid to the underside of the anterior third of the acromion process; the humeral head moves beneath this arch during abduction and the rotator cuff may be irritated or damaged as it glides in this confined space. (1, Rotator cuff; 2, acromion process; 3, coracoacrominal ligament; 4, coracoid process; 5, suscapularis; 6, LHB.)

within the tendon (e.g. swelling from inflammation) or to narrowing of the space (e.g. by osteoarthritis (OA) of the acromioclavicular joint), pain or awkward shoulder movement may result.

Rotator cuff syndrome

The commonest cause of pain and weakness around the shoulder is a disorder of the rotator cuff – the so-called *rotator cuff syndrome* – which comprises four conditions with distinct clinical features and natural history.

CONDITIONS COMPRISING ROTATOR CUFF SYNDROME
Supraspinatus impingement and tendinitis – subacute and chronic Tears of the rotator cuff Acute calcific tendinitis Biceps tendinitis and/or rupture

In all these conditions the patient complains of pain. The pain will be over the front and lateral aspect of the shoulder with weakness on abduction for supraspinatus involvement, tears of the cuff and tendinitis and over the front for biceps pathology. If the cuff or biceps has ruptured, there will also be weakness.

SUPRASPINATUS IMPINGEMENT, SUPRASPINATUS TENDINITIS AND TEARS OF THE ROTATOR CUFF

Pathology of impingement

Rotator cuff impingement is a painful disorder which is thought to arise from repetitive compression or rubbing of the tendons (mainly supraspinatus) under the coracoacromial arch (13.5). Normally, when the arm is abducted, the conjoint tendon slides under the coracoacromial arch. As abduction approaches 90 degrees, there is a natural tendency to externally rotate the arm, thus allowing the rotator cuff to occupy the widest part of the subacromial space. If the arm is held persistently in abduction and then moved to and fro in internal and external rotation (as in cleaning a window, painting a wall or polishing a flat surface), the rotator cuff may be compressed and irritated as it comes in contact with the anterior edge of the acromion process and the taut coracoacromial ligament. This attitude (abduction, slight flexion and internal rotation) has been called the 'impingement position'.

The development of impingement is thought to be due to *intrinsic* and *extrinsic* factors.

- *Intrinsic factors* include degeneration of the tendon, changes in the presence of highly sulphated glycosaminoglycans and changes in the collagen composition with loading. Tendon degeneration may be age-related and a cell-mediated response. Changes in vascularity may also contribute.

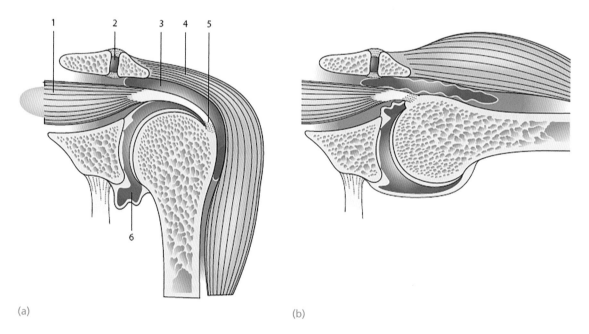

(a)   (b)

13.5 Rotator cuff impingement Coronal sections through the shoulder to illustrate show how the subdeltoid bursa and supraspinatus tendon can be irritated by repeated impingement under the coracoacromial arch or a rough acromioclavicular joint during abduction. **(a)** Joint at rest. **(b)** In abduction. (1, Supraspinatus muscle; 2, acromioclavicular joint; 3, subdeltoid bursa; 4, deltoid muscle; 5, supraspinatus tendon; 6, synovial joint.)

- *Extrinsic factors* that may cause impingement include spurs growing down the coracoacromial ligament and osteoarthritic thickening of the acromioclavicular joint.

SUPRASPINATUS TENDINITIS – SUBACUTE AND CHRONIC

The mildest injury is a type of friction, which may give rise to localized oedema and swelling ('tendinitis'). This is usually self-limiting, but with prolonged or repetitive impingement and especially in older people, minute tears can develop and these may be followed by scarring and fibrocartilaginous metaplasia. Healing is accompanied by a vascular reaction and local congestion (in itself painful) which may contribute to further impingement in the constricted space under the coracoacromial arch whenever the arm is elevated.

ACUTE CALCIFIC TENDINITIS

Sometimes the inflamed tendon becomes calcified.

TEARS OF THE ROTATOR CUFF

Sometimes – perhaps where healing is slow or following a sudden strain – the microscopic disruption extends, becoming a partial or full-thickness tear of the cuff; shoulder function is then more seriously compromised and active abduction may be impossible.

BICEPS TENDINOPATHY

The tendon of the long head of biceps (LHB), lying adjacent to the supraspinatus, may also be involved and is often torn.

SECONDARY ARTHROPATHY

Large tears of the cuff may eventually lead to serious disturbance of shoulder mechanics. The humeral head migrates upwards, abutting against the acromion process, and passive abduction is severely restricted. Abnormal movement predisposes to OA of the glenohumeral joint.

Clinical features

In all these conditions the patient is likely to complain of pain and/or weakness during certain movements of the shoulder. Pain may have started recently, sometimes quite suddenly, after a particular type of exertion; the patient may know precisely which movements now reignite the pain and which to avoid, providing a valuable clue to its origin. 'Rotator cuff' pain typically appears over the front and lateral aspect of the shoulder during activities with the arm abducted and medially rotated, but it may be present even with the arm at rest. Tenderness is felt at the anterior edge of the acromion.

Pain and tenderness directly in front along the deltopectoral boundary could be associated with the biceps tendon. Localized pain over the top of the shoulder is more likely to be due to acromioclavicular pathology, and pain at the back along the scapular border may come from the cervical spine. All these sites should be inspected for muscle wasting, carefully palpated for local tenderness and constantly compared with the opposite shoulder.

The rotator cuff syndrome may develop through three phases.

PHASES OF DEVELOPMENT OF ROTATOR CUFF SYNDROME

1 *Subacute tendinitis* – the 'painful arc syndrome', due to vascular congestion, microscopic haemorrhage and oedema
2 *Chronic tendinitis* – recurrent shoulder pain due to tendinitis and fibrosis
3 *Cuff disruption* – recurrent pain, weakness and loss of movement due to tears in the rotator cuff

---

The fourth component of rotator cuff syndrome – *biceps tendinopathy* – may occur at any stage.

SUBACUTE TENDINITIS (PAINFUL ARC SYNDROME)

The patient develops anterior shoulder pain after vigorous or unaccustomed activity, such as competitive swimming or a weekend of house decorating. The shoulder looks normal but may be tender along the anterior edge of the acromion. Point tenderness is most easily elicited by palpating this spot with the arm held in extension, thus placing the

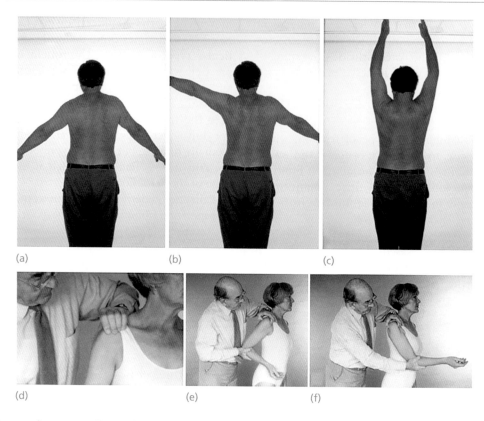

(a)   (b)   (c)

(d)   (e)   (f)

13.6 Supraspinatus tendinitis (a–c) The painful arc. During active abduction, the scapulohumeral rhythm is disturbed on the right and the patient starts to experience pain at about 60° **(a)**. As the arm passes beyond 120° **(b)** the pain eases and the patient is able to abduct and elevate up to the full 180° **(c)**. **(d–f)** The tender spot is at the anterior edge of the acromion process. With the shoulder extended **(e)** tenderness is more acute. When the shoulder is flexed **(f)**, the painful tendon disappears under the acromion process and tenderness disappears.

supraspinatus tendon in an exposed position anterior to the acromion process; with the arm held in flexion the tenderness disappears **(13.6)**.

Subacute tendinitis is often reversible, settling down gradually once the initiating activity is avoided.

CHRONIC TENDINITIS

The patient, usually aged between 40 and 50, gives a history of recurrent attacks of subacute tendinitis, the pain settling down with rest or anti-inflammatory treatment, only to recur when more demanding activities are resumed.

Characteristically pain is worse at night; the patient cannot lie on the affected side and often finds it more comfortable to sit up out of bed. Pain and slight stiffness of the shoulder may restrict even simple activities such as hair grooming or dressing. The physical signs described above should be elicited. In addition, there may be signs of bicipital tendinitis: tenderness along the bicipital groove and crepitus on moving the biceps tendon.

> A disturbing feature is *coarse crepitation or palpable snapping* over the rotator cuff when the shoulder is passively rotated; this may signify a partial tear or marked fibrosis of the cuff.

TEARS OF THE ROTATOR CUFF

The most advanced stage of the disorder is progressive fibrosis and disruption of the cuff, resulting in either a partial or full-thickness tear. The patient is usually aged over 45 and gives a history of refractory shoulder pain with increasing stiffness and weakness.

- *Partial tears* may occur within the substance or on the deep surface of the cuff. The remaining cuff fibres permit active abduction with a painful arc, making it difficult to tell whether chronic tendinitis is complicated by a partial tear.
- A *full-thickness tear* may follow a long period of chronic tendinitis, but occasionally it occurs spontaneously after a sprain or jerking injury of the shoulder. There is sudden pain and the patient is unable to abduct the arm. If the diagnosis is in doubt, pain can be eliminated by injecting a local anaesthetic into the subacromial space. If active abduction is now possible, the tear must be only partial. If active abduction remains impossible, then a complete tear is likely. With time there may be some recovery of active abduction, though power in both abduction and external rotation is weaker than normal. There is usually wasting of the supraspinatus and infraspinatus, and on testing the biceps there may be an old tear of the LHB tendon. There is often tenderness of the acromioclavicular joint.

In long-standing cases of partial or complete rupture, secondary OA of the shoulder may supervene and movements are then severely restricted.

Clinical tests for supraspinatus tendinitis

The painful arc On active abduction, scapulohumeral rhythm is disturbed and pain is aggravated as the arm traverses an arc between 60 and 120 degrees. Repeating the movement with the arm in full external rotation may be much easier for the patient and relatively painless (see **13.6**).

Neer's impingement sign The scapula is stabilized with one hand while with the other hand the examiner raises the affected arm to the full extent in passive flexion, abduction and internal rotation, thus bringing the greater tuberosity directly under the coracoacromial arch. The test is positive when pain, located to the subacromial space or anterior edge of acromion, is elicited by this manoeuvre. If the previous manoeuvre is positive, it may be repeated after injecting 10 mL of 1% lidocaine into the subacromial space; if the pain is abolished (or significantly reduced), this will help to confirm the diagnosis (**13.7, e13.2**).

Hawkins–Kennedy test The patient's arm is placed in 90 degrees of elevation in the scapular plane with the elbow also flexed to 90 degrees. The examiner then stabilizes the upper arm with one hand while using the other hand to internally rotate the arm fully. Pain around the anterolateral aspect of the shoulder is noted as a positive test. As with the Neer's sign, this test is highly sensitive but weakly specific.

Jobe's test The arm is elevated in the scapular plane. The elbow is extended and the thumb points to the floor in full internal rotation. The patient is then asked to hold this position with downward pressure by the examiner. Pain indicates irritation of the supraspinatus tendon.

Clinical test for weakness from a rotator cuff tear

With a complete tear of the supraspinatus, initiation of active abduction is impossible even when pain subsides or has been abolished by injection; but once the arm is passively abducted, the patient can hold it up with their deltoid muscle.

Imaging

X-RAYS

X-rays are usually normal in the early stages of the cuff dysfunction, but with chronic tendinitis there may be erosion, sclerosis or cyst formation at the site of cuff insertion on the greater tuberosity, or overgrowth of the anterior edge of the acromion, thinning of the acromion process and upward displacement of the humeral head (see **13.7**). OA of the acromioclavicular joint is common in older patients and, in late cases, the glenohumeral joint also may show features of OA. Sometimes there is calcification of the supraspinatus, but this is coincidental and not the cause of the pain.

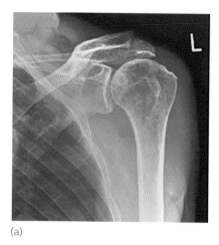 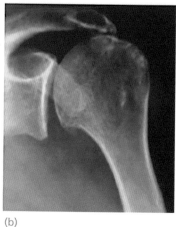

(a)   (b)

13.7 Supraspinatus tendinitis – X-rays (a) X-ray of the shoulder showing a typical thin band of sclerosis at the insertion of supraspinatus and narrowing of the subacromial space. The rest of the joint looks normal. **(b)** X-ray at a later stage showing upward displacement of the humeral head due to a large cuff rupture. There is almost complete loss of the subacromial space.

MRI

MRI can effectively show cuff pathology but it should be remembered that up to one-third of asymptomatic individuals also have abnormalities of the rotator cuff on MRI (**13.8**). Changes on MRI always need to be correlated with the clinical examination.

ULTRASONOGRAPHY

This has comparable accuracy to MRI for identifying and measuring the size of full thickness and partial thickness rotator cuff tears, but it is not as accurate in predicting the reparability of the tendons.

Treatment of rotator cuff syndrome

CONSERVATIVE TREATMENT

Uncomplicated impingement syndrome (or tendinitis) is often self-limiting and symptoms settle down once the aggravating activity is eliminated.

- Patients should be taught ways of avoiding the 'impingement position'.
- Physiotherapy may tide the patient over the painful healing phase. A short course of non-steroidal anti-inflammatory drugs (NSAIDs) sometimes brings relief.
- If all these methods fail, and before disability becomes marked, the patient should be given

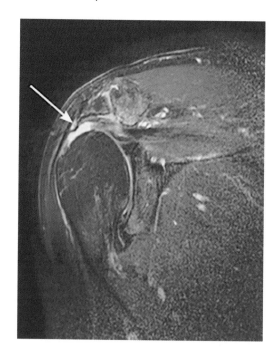

13.8 Rotator cuff tear – MRI High signal on MRI, indicating a full-thickness tear of the rotator cuff.

one or two injections of depot corticosteroids into the subacromial space. In most cases, this will relieve the pain and it is then important to persevere with protective modifications of shoulder activity for at least 6 months.

Healing is slow, and a hasty return to full activity will often precipitate further attacks of tendinitis.

SURGICAL TREATMENT FOR IMPINGEMENT

If the patient has a useful range of movement, adequate strength and well-controlled pain, non-operative measures are adequate. If symptoms do not subside after 3 months of conservative treatment, or if they recur persistently after each period of treatment, an operation is considered preferable to prolonged and repeated treatment with NSAIDs and local corticosteroids. The indication is more pressing if there are signs of a partial rotator cuff tear and in particular if there is good clinical evidence of a full-thickness tear in a younger patient. The object is to decompress the rotator cuff by removing the structures pressing upon it, i.e. the coracoacromial ligament, the anterior part of the acromion process and osteophytes at the acromioclavicular joint (13.9). This can be achieved by open surgery or

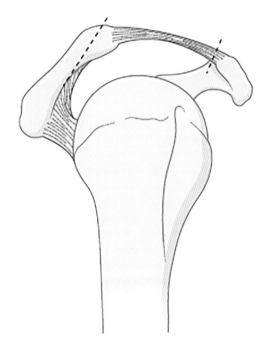

13.9 Impingement syndrome – surgical treatment The coracoacromial ligament and underside of the anterior third of the acromion are removed to enlarge the space for the rotator cuff. This can be performed by open surgery or arthroscopically.

arthroscopically. If tears are encountered, they can be repaired.

Arthroscopy allows good visualization inside the glenohumeral joint and therefore detection of other abnormalities which may cause shoulder pain. This procedure also allows earlier rehabilitation than open surgery because there is no need to detach the deltoid muscle.

REPAIR OF ROTATOR CUFF TEARS

INDICATIONS FOR OPERATIVE REPAIR OF ROTATOR CUFF TEARS
Chronic pain Weakness of the shoulder Significant loss of function

The younger and more active the patient, the greater is the justification for surgery. The operation always includes acromioplasty, as described above. The repair can be performed either by open techniques or by arthroscopy. Advantages of arthroscopy include less soft-tissue damage, faster rehabilitation and a better cosmetic appearance.

Massive tears which cannot be approximated might be treated by decompression and debridement alone, or with tendon transfer or tendon grafts.

CALCIFIC TENDINITIS

Acute calcific tendinitis

Calcium hydroxyapatite crystals are deposited in the supraspinatus tendon, probably due to fibro-cartilaginous metaplasia from local ischaemia. Calcification alone is probably not painful; symptoms, when they occur, are due to the florid vascular reaction which produces swelling and tension in the tendon. Resorption of the calcific material is rapid and it may soften or disappear entirely within a few weeks.

CLINICAL FEATURES

The condition affects 30–50 year olds. Aching, sometimes following overuse, develops and increases in severity within hours, rising to an

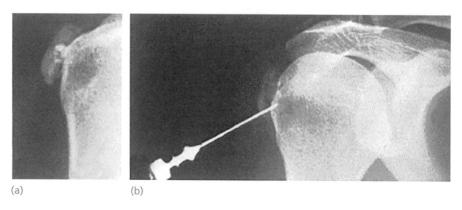

(a)   (b)

13.10 Acute calcification (a) Calcific deposit in the subdeltoid bursa. **(b)** Treatment by needle aspiration; best done under ultrasound control.

agonizing climax. After a few days, pain subsides and the shoulder gradually returns to normal. In some patients, the process is less dramatic and recovery slower. During the acute stage the arm is held immobile; the joint is usually too tender to permit palpation or movement.

X-RAYS

Calcification just above the greater tuberosity is always present. As pain subsides, the dense blotch lightens and may then disappear (**13.10**).

TREATMENT

* If symptoms are not very severe, the arm is rested in a sling and the patient is given a short course of NSAIDs. If pain is more intense, then corticosteroid is injected into the subacromial space.
* Extracorporeal shockwave therapy, to disintegrate the calcium crystals, is also an effective option.
* An alternative approach is to drain the pasty calcium deposit under ultrasound guidance (a process known as 'barbotage').
* For patients with disabling or recurrent symptoms unresponsive to conservative measures, relief can be obtained by an operation to remove the calcific material. While this can be performed by open surgery, arthroscopy is preferable with a simultaneous decompression.

Chronic calcification

Asymptomatic calcification of the rotator cuff is common and often appears as an incidental finding in shoulder X-rays. When it is seen in association with the impingement syndrome, it is tempting to attribute the symptoms to the only obvious abnormality – supraspinatus calcification. However, the connection is spurious and treatment should be directed at the impingement lesion rather than the calcification.

LESIONS OF THE BICEPS TENDON

Tendinitis

Though not part of the rotator cuff, the tendon of LHB lies adjacent to the rotator cuff and may be involved in the impingement syndrome. Rarely, it presents as an isolated problem in young people after unaccustomed shoulder strain. Pain and tenderness are localized to the bicipital groove. Stressing the biceps tendon (resisted elbow flexion and supination) will provoke the pain.

Rest, local heat and deep transverse frictions usually bring relief; if recovery is delayed, a corticosteroid injection will help. For refractory cases, surgery is considered.

Ruptured long head of biceps

Degeneration and disruption of the tendon of LHB is fairly common and is often associated with rotator cuff problems. The patient is usually middle-aged or elderly. While lifting a heavy object, he or she feels something snap; the shoulder, which previously felt normal, aches for a time

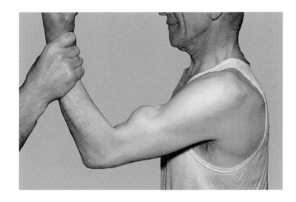

13.11 Ruptured long head of biceps The lump in the front of the arm becomes even more prominent when the patient contracts the biceps against resistance.

and bruising appears over the front of the arm. Soon the ache subsides and good function returns, but when the elbow is flexed actively the belly of the muscle contracts into a prominent lump. Sometimes the initial episode passes unremarked and the patient presents for the first time with a 'lump' in the arm, which is easily mistaken for tumour. Ask the patient to flex the elbow against resistance; this will show that the 'lump' is actually the bunched-up belly of biceps (**13.11**).

Function is usually so little disturbed that treatment is unnecessary, unless the associated rotator cuff symptoms need attention.

'SLAP' LESIONS

A fall on the outstretched arm can sometimes damage the superior part of the glenoid labrum anteriorly and posteriorly (SLAP) (**e13.3**). There is usually a history of a fall followed by pain in the shoulder. As the initial acute symptoms settle, the patient continues to experience a painful 'click' on lifting the arm above shoulder height, together with loss of power when using the arm in that position. They may also complain of an inability to throw with that arm.

MRI arthrography is the modality of choice, though the diagnosis is best confirmed by arthroscopic examination; at the same time the lesion is treated by reattachment or debridement (**e13.4**).

ADHESIVE CAPSULITIS (FROZEN SHOULDER)

The term *frozen shoulder* should be reserved for a well-defined disorder characterized by progressive pain and stiffness which usually resolves spontaneously after about 18 months. The cause and pathogenesis are still topics of heated debate. The histological features are reminiscent of Dupuytren's disease, with active fibroblastic and myofibroblastic proliferation in the rotator interval, anterior capsule and coracohumeral ligament.

CONDITIONS PARTICULARLY ASSOCIATED WITH FROZEN SHOULDER
Diabetes
Dupuytren's disease
Hyperlipidaemia
Hyperthyroidism
Cardiac disease
Hemiplegia

Clinical features

The patient, aged 40–60 years, may give a history of trauma, often trivial, followed by pain. Gradually it increases in severity and often prevents sleeping on the affected side. After several months it begins to subside, but as it does so stiffness becomes more and more of a problem. Untreated, stiffness persists for another 6–12 months. Gradually movement is regained, but may not return to normal (**13.12**).

Usually there is nothing to see except slight muscle wasting; there may also be some tenderness, but movements are always limited and in a severe case the shoulder is extremely stiff.

X-rays are normal. The main role of an X-ray is to exclude other causes of pain and stiffness.

Differential diagnosis

Post-traumatic stiffness After any severe shoulder injury, stiffness (without much pain) may persist for some months. It is maximal at the start and gradually lessens, unlike the pattern of a frozen shoulder.

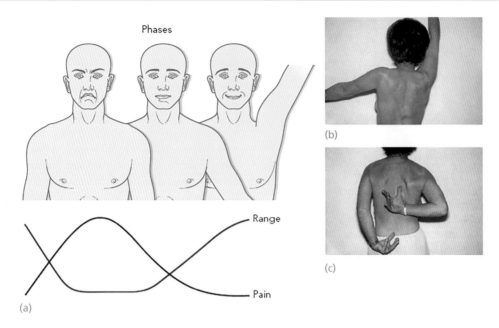

13.12 Frozen shoulder (a) Natural history of frozen shoulder. The face tells the story. **(b,c)** This patient has hardly any abduction but manages to lift her arm by moving the scapula. She cannot reach her back with her left hand.

Disuse stiffness   If the arm is nursed overcautiously (e.g. following a wrist fracture) the shoulder may stiffen. Again, the characteristic pain pattern of a frozen shoulder is absent.

Complex regional pain syndrome   This condition, formerly known as *reflex sympathetic dystrophy*, may follow acute trauma; it is also seen in patients with myocardial infarction or a stroke. The features can be similar to those of a frozen shoulder.

Arthritis   Both rheumatoid arthritis (RA) and OA can affect the shoulder, and either of these can develop bilaterally. The diagnosis is usually obvious on X-ray. In the case of RA, there may also be characteristic generalized symptoms and signs.

Treatment

CONSERVATIVE TREATMENT
Treatment with analgesics, NSAIDs, local heat and exercise aims at relieving pain and preventing further stiffening while recovery is awaited. The role of physiotherapy and steroid injections is unproven. Once the acute pain has subsided, manipulation under anaesthesia often hastens recovery. This can be accompanied by distending the joint with saline until the capsule ruptures. Active exercises should recommence immediately afterwards.

OPERATIVE TREATMENT
Operative treatment is occasionally called for. Arthroscopic division of the interval between supraspinatus and infraspinatus may dramatically improve the range of movement.

ANTERIOR INSTABILITY OF THE SHOULDER

The shoulder achieves its uniquely wide range of movement at the cost of stability. The glenoid socket is very shallow and the joint is held secure by the fibrocartilaginous glenoid labrum and the surrounding ligaments and muscles. If these structures give way, the shoulder becomes unstable and prone to recurrent dislocation or subluxation.

DISLOCATION OR SUBLUXATION?	
Dislocation	Complete separation of the glenohumeral surfaces
Subluxation	Symptomatic separation of the surfaces without dislocation

One must distinguish between the laxity and the instability of a joint.

JOINT LAXITY OR JOINT INSTABILITY?	
Joint laxity	A degree of translation in the glenohumeral joint which falls within a physiological range and which is asymptomatic
Joint instability	Abnormal symptomatic motion for that shoulder which results in pain, subluxation or dislocation of the joint

There are two broad reasons why shoulders become unstable:

- There may be *structural changes* due to major trauma such as acute dislocation or recurrent microtrauma.
- *Unbalanced muscle recruitment* (as opposed to muscle weakness) can result in the humeral head being displaced upon the glenoid.

From a clinical and therapeutic point of view, three polar types of disorder can be identified.

TYPES OF INSTABILITY	
Type I	Traumatic structural instability
Type II	Atraumatic (or minimally traumatic) structural instability
Type III	Atraumatic non-structural instability (altered muscle patterning)

TRAUMATIC STRUCTURAL INSTABILITY

Anterior instability is far and away the commonest type of instability, accounting for over 95% of cases. It usually occurs as sequel to acute anterior dislocation of the shoulder, with detachment or stretching of the glenoid labrum and capsule. It usually follows an acute injury in which the arm is forced into abduction, external rotation and extension. In *recurrent dislocation* the labrum and capsule are often detached from the anterior rim of the glenoid (the classic Bankart lesion). In those over 50 years of age, dislocation is often associated with a rotator cuff tear.

Clinical features

The typical patient is a young man who describes an initial episode of the shoulder coming out of joint following an injury. The first episode of *acute dislocation* is a landmark. An initial, acute episode of dislocation goes on to *recurrent dislocation* in over one-third of patients under the age of 30 years and in about one-fifth of those over 50 years. The patient complains of the shoulder repeatedly 'coming out of joint' during over-arm movements (lifting the arm in abduction, extension and external rotation), and each time having to have it manipulated back into position.

Recurrent *subluxation* is less obvious. The patient may describe a 'catching' sensation (rather than complete displacement), followed by 'numbness' or 'weakness' – the so-called dead arm syndrome – when attempting to throw a ball or serve at tennis.

Between episodes, the diagnosis rests on demonstrating the *apprehension sign* (13.13).

THE APPREHENSION TEST
With the patient seated, the examiner cautiously lifts the arm into abduction, external rotation and then extension. At the crucial moment, the patient senses that the humeral head is about to slip out anteriorly and their body tautens in apprehension.

Imaging

- The classic *X-ray* feature is a depression in the posterosuperior part of the humeral head (the Hill–Sachs lesion), where the bone has been

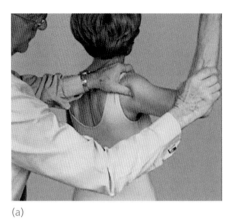
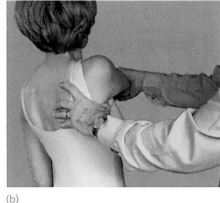

(a)   (b)

13.13 Shoulder instability – the apprehension test (a) This is the apprehension test for anterior subluxation or dislocation. Abduct, externally rotate and extend the patient's shoulder while pushing on the head of the humerus. If the patient feels that the joint is about to dislocate, she will forcibly resist the manoeuvre. **(b)** Posterior dislocation can be tested for in the same way by drawing the arm forward and across the patient's body (adduction and internal rotation).

damaged by repeated impact with the anterior rim of the glenoid. Subluxation is more difficult to demonstrate; an axillary view may show the humeral head riding on the anterior lip of the glenoid.

- *MRI arthrography* and *arthroscopy* may reveal a detached glenoid labrum (the Bankart lesion) and/or the Hill–Sachs lesion (**13.14**).
- *Examination under anaesthesia* can help to determine the direction of instability. This forms an essential part of assessing instability. Both shoulders need to be examined.

Treatment

If dislocation recurs only at long intervals, the patient may choose to put up with the inconvenience.

> **INDICATIONS FOR OPERATIVE REPAIR OF TRAUMATIC STRUCTURAL INSTABILITY**
>
> Frequent dislocations, especially if these are painful
>
> Fear of recurrent subluxation or dislocation sufficient to prevent participation in everyday activities, including sport

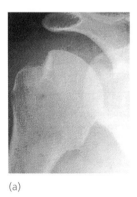
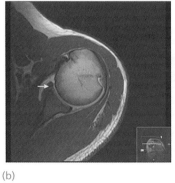
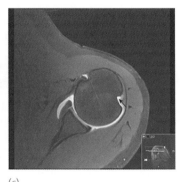

(a)   (b)   (c)

13.14 Anterior instability – imaging (a) The plain X-ray shows a large depression in the posteriosuperior part of the humeral head (the Hill–Sachs lesion). **(b,c)** MRI shows both a Bankart lesion, with a flake of bone detached from the anterior edge of the glenoid, and the Hill–Sachs lesion (arrows).

Surgery aims to restore the anatomy. The glenoid labrum is reattached, together with tightening of the anterior capsule. This is usually achieved by open operation, although with advanced equipment and specialized sutures, arthroscopic repair is an option.

ATRAUMATIC INSTABILITY

ATRAUMATIC (OR MINIMALLY TRAUMATIC) STRUCTURAL INSTABILITY

In this condition, the patient complains of the shoulder going 'out of joint' with remarkable ease. This can occur in athletes such as swimmers and throwers who overload and fatigue the stabilizing muscles around the shoulder, leading to pain and subluxation in various directions. This is usually treated by physiotherapy to strengthen the muscles and to restore proprioception. Just occasionally surgery is needed to tighten the capsule.

ATRAUMATIC NON-STRUCTURAL INSTABILITY (ALTERED MUSCLE PATTERNING)

The stability of the shoulder joint throughout its large range of motion comes partly from precise synchronized muscle contractions and relaxations during movement. If this pattern is altered, instability can occur. This is associated with individuals who are able to voluntarily subluxate or dislocate their shoulders (often demonstrated as a 'party trick') (e13.5). This can then become involuntary (e13.6).

Treatment requires physiotherapy and sometimes even psychological counselling.

> ⚠ Surgery for atraumatic non-structural instability should be avoided.

POSTERIOR INSTABILITY OF THE SHOULDER

This condition is usually due to a violent jerk in an unusual position or following an epileptic fit or a severe electric shock. Posterior instability sometimes persists after an acute posterior dislocation (13.15). It usually takes the form of recurrent subluxation rather than full-blown dislocation. The shoulder subluxates when the arm is held in flexion and internal rotation.

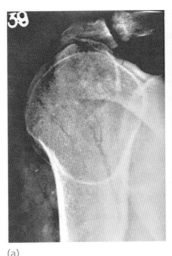
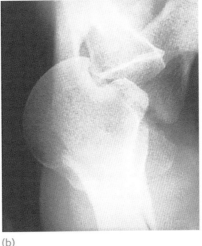

(a)   (b)

13.15 Posterior dislocation (a) In the anteroposterior view, the humeral head looks globular – the so-called 'light bulb' appearance. **(b)** In the lateral view, one can see the humeral head is lying behind the glenoid fossa, with an impaction fracture on the anterior surface of the head.

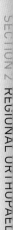

Clinical features

On examination, the posterior drawer test (scapular spine and coracoid process in one hand, humeral head pushed backwards with the other) and posterior apprehension test (forward flexion and internal rotation of the shoulder with a posterior force on the elbow) confirm the diagnosis.

Treatment

- Treatment is usually *conservative*, i.e. muscle-strengthening exercises and voluntary control of the joint.
- *Operative reconstruction* is indicated only if disability is marked, there is no gross joint laxity and a structural abnormality is found on investigation with CT or MRI.

DISORDERS OF THE GLENOHUMERAL JOINT

TUBERCULOUS ARTHRITIS

Tuberculosis of the shoulder is uncommon. It usually starts as an osteitis but is rarely diagnosed until arthritis has supervened. This may proceed to abscess and sinus formation; in some cases, fibrous ankylosis develops.

Clinical features

Patients are usually adults. They complain of a constant ache and stiffness lasting many months. The striking feature is wasting of the muscles around the shoulder. In neglected cases, a sinus may be present. There is diffuse warmth and tenderness, and all movements are limited and painful. Axillary lymph nodes may be enlarged.

X-rays

Early signs are generalized rarefaction of bone on both sides of the joint and erosion of the joint surfaces. In late cases, there may be 'cystic' destruction of the humeral head and/or glenoid fossa (**13.16**).

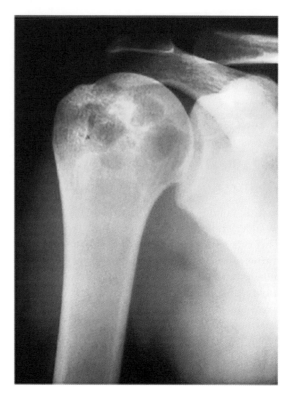

13.16 Tuberculosis X-ray of the shoulder showing tuberculous abscesses in the head of the humerus.

Treatment

In addition to systemic treatment with antituberculous drugs, the shoulder should be rested until acute symptoms have settled. Thereafter, movement is encouraged and, provided the articular cartilage is not destroyed, the prognosis for painless function is good. If there are repeated flares, or if the articular surfaces are extensively destroyed, the joint should be arthrodesed.

RHEUMATOID ARTHRITIS

The acromioclavicular joint, the glenohumeral joint and the various synovial pouches around the shoulder are frequently involved in rheumatoid disease. Chronic synovitis leads to rupture of the rotator cuff and progressive joint erosion (**13.17**).

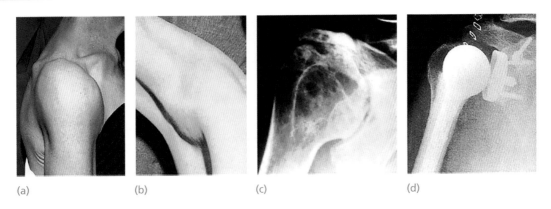

(a)   (b)   (c)   (d)

13.17 Rheumatoid arthritis (a) Large synovial effusions cause easily visible swelling; small ones are likely to be missed, especially if they are present in the axilla **(b)**. **(c)** X-rays show progressive erosion of the joint. **(d)** X-ray appearance after total joint replacement.

Clinical features

The patient, who usually has generalized arthritis, complains of pain in the shoulder and difficulty with tasks such as combing their hair or washing their back.

Active movements are limited, and passive movements are painful and accompanied by marked crepitus. If the supraspinatus is involved, the features are similar to those of post-traumatic cuff lesions.

X-rays

There are three patterns of RA on X-ray.

PATTERNS OF RA ON X-RAY	
Wet	Periarticular erosions, rapid progress, early cuff rupture
Dry	Subchondral sclerosis, osteophytes, slow progress, cuff intact
Resorptive	Marked bone loss, few erosions

Often the acromioclavicular joint is involved. Although it may start on one side, the condition usually becomes bilateral.

Treatment

If general measures do not control the synovitis, corticosteroid may. If synovitis persists, operative synovectomy is carried out and at the same time cuff tears may be repaired. Excision of the lateral end of the clavicle may relieve acromioclavicular pain.

In advanced cases, pain and stiffness can be very disabling and may call for either arthroplasty or arthrodesis. Shoulder replacement gives good pain relief and improved function, even though the range of movement remains well below normal. If there is inadequate bone stock for a shoulder replacement, then the shoulder may have to be arthrodesed.

OSTEOARTHRITIS

Primary glenohumeral OA is not uncommon, affecting 30% of those over 60. Primary OA is when there are no predisposing factors but secondary OA may be secondary to local trauma, recurrent subluxation or long-standing rotator cuff lesions.

Clinical features

Patients, usually 50–60 years old, complain of pain; they may give a history of previous shoulder problems. The most typical sign is progressive restriction of shoulder movements (**13.18**).

X-rays show the characteristic features of loss of the articular space, distortion of the joint, subchondral sclerosis and marginal osteophyte formation.

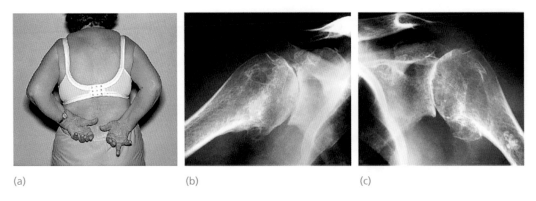

(a)   (b)   (c)

13.18 Osteoarthritis of the shoulder **(a)** This woman has advanced OA of both shoulders. Movements are so restricted that she has difficulty dressing herself and combing her hair. **(b,c)** X-rays show the severe degree of articular destruction.

Treatment

Medication   Most patients manage to live with the restrictions imposed by stiffness, provided pain is not severe. Analgesics and anti-inflammatory drugs relieve pain, and exercises may improve mobility.

Steroid injection   There is little evidence to support the routine use of steroid injection. These may give short-term relief and can be useful as a diagnostic aid.

Surgery   If pain and stiffness become intolerable, joint replacement is justified. It may not improve mobility much, but it does relieve pain.

13.19 Milwaukee shoulder The X-ray features are remarkable. There is gross destruction of the joint and calcification in the soft tissues around the shoulder.

RAPIDLY DESTRUCTIVE ARTHROPATHY (MILWAUKEE SHOULDER)

Occasionally, in the presence of long-standing or massive cuff tears, patients develop a rapidly progressive and destructive form of OA in which there is severe erosion of the glenohumeral joint, the acromion process and the acromioclavicular joint – a *cuff tear arthropathy*. The changes are attributed to hydroxyapatite crystal shedding from the torn rotator cuff and a synovial reaction involving the release of lysosomal enzymes (including collagenases) which lead to cartilage breakdown. A similar condition is seen in other joints such as the hip and knee. The shoulder disorder, however, has come to be known as *Milwaukee shoulder* (**13.19**).

There is no satisfactory treatment. Arthroplasty may relieve pain but will not improve function because the joint is unstable.

OSTEONECROSIS

The shoulder is the second most common site of steroid-induced osteonecrosis (**e13.7**). The condition may also be seen in association with marrow storage disorders, sickle-cell disease and caisson disease, or following irradiation of the axilla.

DISORDERS OF THE SCAPULA AND CLAVICLE

CONGENITAL ELEVATION OF THE SHOULDER

The scapulae normally complete their descent from the neck by the third month of foetal life; occasionally one or both scapulae remain incompletely descended. Associated abnormalities of the cervical spine are common and sometimes there is a family history of scapular deformity. Two similar, and possibly related, conditions are encountered:

* *Sprengel's shoulder/deformity* (13.20a)
* *Klippel–Feil syndrome* (13.20b).

Sprengel's shoulder

The shoulder on the affected side is elevated; the scapula looks and feels abnormally high, smaller than usual with a prominent superomedial pole that can be palpated in the neck. Movements are painless, but abduction may be limited due to an abnormal connection between the medial scapula and cervical spine (an omovertebral bar). Associated deformities (e.g. fusion of cervical vertebrae, kyphosis or scoliosis) may be present.

Mild cases are best left untreated. Marked limitation of abduction or severe deformity may necessitate an operation to lower the scapula.

Klippel–Feil syndrome

This is usually a more widespread disorder. There is bilateral failure of scapular descent associated with marked anomalies of the cervical spine and failure of fusion of the occipital bones. The neck is unusually short and may be webbed; cervical mobility is restricted.

The condition is usually left untreated.

WINGING OF THE SCAPULA

In this condition, also known as winged scapula, the scapula juts out under the skin, like a small wing (13.20c). It is due to weakness of the serratus anterior, the muscle which stabilizes the scapula on the thoracic cage. It may cause asymmetry of the shoulders, but it is often not apparent until the patient tries to contract the serratus anterior against resistance (e.g. pushing hard against a wall).

There are several causes of weakness or paralysis of the serratus anterior muscle.

> **CAUSES OF SERRATUS ANTERIOR MUSCLE WEAKNESS**
>
> Neuralgic amyotrophy
> Injury to the brachial plexus (e.g. a blow to the top of the shoulder, severe traction on the arm or carrying heavy loads on the shoulder)
> Direct damage to the long thoracic nerve (e.g. during radical mastectomy or first rib resections)
> Fascioscapulohumeral muscular dystrophy

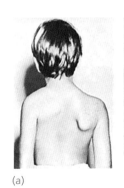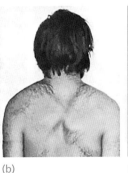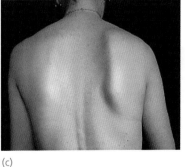

(a) (b) (c)

13.20 Scapular disorders (a) Sprengel's shoulder; (b) Klippel–Feil syndrome; (c) winged scapula.

A less obvious form of scapular instability may be caused by weakness of the trapezius following injury to the spinal accessory nerve.

Treatment

Some of the disorders causing winging of the scapula are self-limiting and the condition gradually improves. Even if it doesn't, disability is usually slight and is best accepted. However, if function is markedly impaired, the scapula can be stabilized by tendon transfer.

CONGENITAL PSEUDARTHROSIS OF THE CLAVICLE

This rare condition occurs due to failure of fusion of the medial and lateral ossification centres of the clavicle. Patients have a painless mass over the region and normal glenohumeral motion (13.21). The condition is typically noted on the right side and is thought to be due to external compression from the subclavian artery. Left-sided lesions are associated with situs inversus.

Treatment

When asymptomatic, no treatment is indicated. If there is associated pain or an unacceptable cosmetic deformity, excision of the pseudarthrosis with plate fixation and bone graft is indicated.

GRATING SCAPULA

This is found in about one-third of normal people; a cause is usually not found but occasionally a tangential X-ray (or better still a CT scan) will show a bone lesion such as an osteochondroma.

ACROMIOCLAVICULAR INSTABILITY

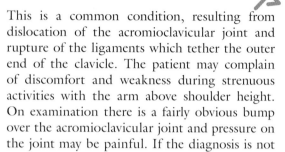

This is a common condition, resulting from dislocation of the acromioclavicular joint and rupture of the ligaments which tether the outer end of the clavicle. The patient may complain of discomfort and weakness during strenuous activities with the arm above shoulder height. On examination there is a fairly obvious bump over the acromioclavicular joint and pressure on the joint may be painful. If the diagnosis is not obvious on plain X-ray, re-examination with the patient standing up and holding a heavy weight (to drag the shoulder downwards) will show the displacement.

Treatment

The condition causes little disability during non-strenuous activities and treatment is therefore unnecessary. However, certain types of work activity may be seriously curtailed and in such cases reconstructive surgery should be considered.

OSTEOARTHRITIS OF THE ACROMIOCLAVICULAR JOINT

Clinical features

OA of the acromioclavicular joint generally affects two groups of people.

- *People in their thirties* who are involved in sports or carry out heavy manual activities may be affected. Early presentation in this group may be damage to the cartilaginous disc due to previous injury or repetitive stress

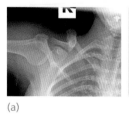
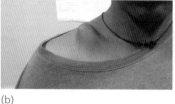
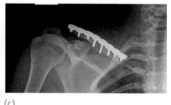

(a)   (b)   (c)

13.21 Pseudarthrosis of the clavicle (a,b) 17-year-old patient with a prominent pseudarthrosis, managed with excision, iliac crest bone grafting and plate fixation (c).

(e.g. habitually carrying weights on the shoulder or working with pneumatic hammers or drills).

- *In older people*, the condition is due to degenerative changes and usually develops spontaneously.

The patient complains of pain over the top of the shoulder, particularly while using the arm above shoulder height. Tenderness and swelling are localized to the acromioclavicular joint (13.22). Shoulder movements are usually not restricted.

X-rays

These show the characteristic features of OA.

Treatment

If analgesics and corticosteroid injections are ineffectual, pain may be relieved by excision of the lateral end of the clavicle. Trimming of the bony roughness, or excision of the outer end of the clavicle, may also be needed during subacromial decompression for rotator cuff impingement.

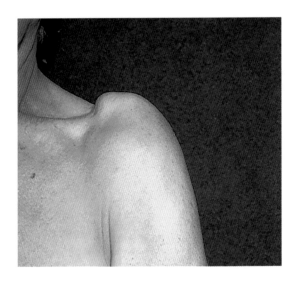

13.22 Osteoarthritis of the acromioclavicular joint Osteophytic thickening of the acromioclavicular joint produces a small (but very tender) bump on top of the left shoulder. Occasionally the joint capsule herniates, producing a large 'cyst' over the acromioclavicular joint.

OPERATIONS

ARTHROSCOPY

Arthroscopy is useful for the *diagnosis* of periarticular and intra-articular disorders, such as rotator cuff disruption and instability. At the same time a *biopsy* can be taken which may assist in the diagnosis of synovial disorders such as RA or pigmented villonodular synovitis.

Arthroscopic surgery is now well established. Because it is safer and recovery is quicker, it is the first-line surgical option for subacromial decompression, acromioclavicular joint excisions, debridement of rotator cuff tears and release of frozen shoulder. Arthroscopic repair of anterior shoulder instability produces results comparable to those obtained by open surgery.

ARTHROPLASTY OF THE SHOULDER

Shoulder replacement was initially introduced for the treatment of complex proximal humeral fractures but technical advances have allowed it to be used for end-stage glenohumeral OA and RA if non-operative treatment fails. The options are replacement of either just the humeral head or of both the head and the glenoid socket (13.23).

Complications

COMMONEST COMPLICATIONS OF SHOULDER ARTHROPLASTY
Loosening of the components
Glenohumeral instability
Rotator cuff failure
Periprosthetic fracture
Infection
Implant failure

Glenoid fixation remains a challenge; radiographic lucent lines around the glenoid component (usually regarded as a sign of implant loosening) are very common, although not always symptomatic.

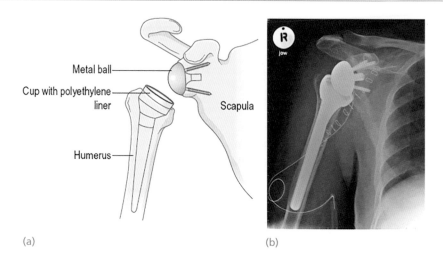

Metal ball
Cup with polyethylene liner
Humerus
Scapula

(a)   (b)

13.23 Shoulder replacement (a) Illustration showing principles of total shoulder replacement. (b) Postoperative X-ray of this type of implant. Other ball-and-socket configurations are also available.

Outcome

The outcome depends largely on the indications for surgery. Generally, pain relief is excellent but range of movement is often disappointing.

Arthrodesis

Arthrodesis of the glenohumeral joint is now seldom performed, but it is still a useful operation for severe shoulder dysfunction associated with:

- paralysis of the scapulohumeral muscles
- infective disorders of the glenohumeral joint (including tuberculous arthritis)

- advanced erosive arthritis with massive disruption of the rotator cuff
- failed total shoulder arthroplasty
- uncontrolled instability.

A prerequisite is stable and powerful scapulothoracic movement, because with a fused shoulder 'movement' is achieved entirely by rotation of the scapula on the thorax.

The optimal position is 30 degrees of flexion, 30 degrees of abduction and 30 degrees of internal rotation. The arthrodesis is held by internal fixation with a plate and screws.

The elbow

14

■ Clinical assessment	297	
■ Congenital conditions	300	
■ Acquired elbow deformities	300	
■ Tuberculosis	301	
■ Rheumatoid arthritis	302	
■ Osteoarthritis	302	

■ Loose bodies	304	
■ Osteochondritis dissecans	305	
■ Olecranon bursitis	305	
■ Recurrent elbow instability	306	
■ Tendinopathies around the elbow	307	

CLINICAL ASSESSMENT

HISTORY

- *Pain* may be felt diffusely on the medial side of the joint (ulnohumeral), the posterolateral side (radiohumeral) or acutely localized to one of the humeral epicondyles ('tennis elbow' on the lateral side and 'golfer's elbow' on the medial side). Pain over the back of the elbow is often due to an olecranon bursitis. Pain over the front is likely to be due to a biceps tendinopathy.
- *Stiffness*, if severe, can be very disabling; the patient may be unable to reach to the mouth (loss of flexion) or the perineum (loss of extension); limited supination makes it difficult to hold something in the palm or to carry large objects.
- *Swelling* may be due to injury or inflammation; a soft lump on the back of the elbow suggests an olecranon bursitis.
- *Deformity* is usually the result of previous trauma: *cubitus varus* due to a malunited supracondylar fracture, or *cubitus valgus* due to an old displaced and malunited fracture of the lateral condyle.
- *Instability* is not uncommon in the late stage of rheumatoid arthritis (RA).
- *Ulnar nerve symptoms* (tingling and numbness in the little and ring fingers, weakness of the hand) may occur in elbow disorders because the nerve is so near to the joint.
- *Loss of function* is notable because the role of the elbow is to position the hand in space to manipulate the environment and bring objects towards the individual.

EXAMINATION

Both upper limbs must be completely exposed and it is essential to look at the back as well as the front. The neck, shoulders and hands should also be examined (**14.1**).

Look

Look at the patient from the front, with his or her arms outstretched alongside the body and the palms facing forwards. In this position,

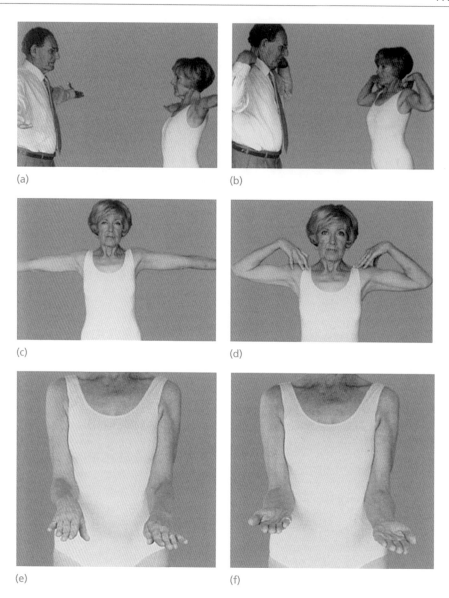

(a) (b) (c) (d) (e) (f)

14.1 Initial examination (a,b) The best way to examine active movement is to stand in front of the patient and show them what to do. **(c,d)** The normal range of flexion is from 0° (full extension) to 140° (full flexion). **(e,f)** To test pronation and supination, ask the patient to tuck their elbows tightly in to the body with the elbows flexed to 90° and then turn their hands from palm up to palm down. The normal range is 90° in both directions, although this is a composite of forearm and carpal rotation.

the forearms are normally angled slightly outward relative to the line of the arm – a valgus or *carrying angle* of 5–15 degrees. 'Varus' or 'valgus' *deformity* is determined by angular deviation towards the body or away beyond those limits or, in unilateral abnormalities, by comparison with the normal side. The most common swelling is in the olecranon bursa at the back of the elbow.

Feel

Important bony landmarks are the medial and lateral condyles and the tip of the olecranon (**14.2**).

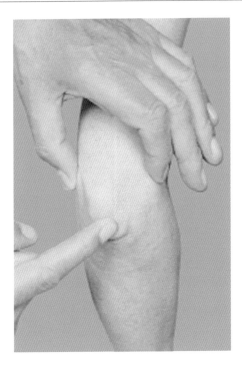

14.2 Examination Feeling begins with the skin. Is there undue warmth? Next, feel the bony landmarks. With the elbow flexed, the tips of the medial and lateral epicondyles and the olecranon process form an isosceles triangle. With the elbow extended, they lie transversely in line with each other. These relationships may be disturbed by trauma.

These are palpated to determine whether the joint is correctly positioned. Tenderness is caused by tendinitis.

Superficial structures are examined for warmth and subcutaneous nodules. The joint

line (including the radioulnar joint depression) is located and palpated for synovial thickening.

The ulnar nerve is fairly superficial behind the medial condyle and here it can be rolled under the fingers to feel if it is thickened or tapped to find if it is hypersensitive.

Move

Flexion and extension are compared on the two sides. Then, with the elbows tucked into the sides and flexed to a right angle, the radioulnar joints are tested for pronation (palms downwards 0–90 degrees) and supination (palms upwards 0–90 degrees) (14.3).

General examination

If the symptoms and signs do not point clearly to a local disorder, other parts are examined: the neck (for cervical disc lesions), the shoulder (for cuff lesions) and the hand (for nerve lesions).

INVESTIGATION

Imaging

X-RAYS

The position of each bone is noted, then the joint line and space. Next, the individual bones are inspected for evidence of old injury or bone destruction. Finally, loose bodies are sought.

In children, while the epiphyses are still incompletely ossified the anatomy has to be

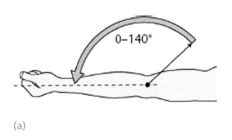

(a)

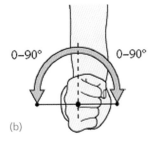

(b)

14.3 Normal range of movement (a) The extended position is recorded as 0° and any hyperextension as a minus quantity; flexion is full when the arm and forearm make contact. (b) From the neutral position, the palm rotates 90° into pronation and 90° into supination. This is a composite of radioulnar motion (80°) and carpal rotation (10°). The functional range of motion where most activities of daily living can be performed is 30° to 130° flexion and 50° of pronation–supination.

SECTION 2 REGIONAL ORTHOPAEDICS

deduced from the shape and position of the emerging secondary ossific centres; the average ages at which they appear can be remembered by the mnemonic CRITOE.

CRITOE: AVERAGE AGE AT WHICH SECONDARY OSSIFIC CENTRES APPEAR	
Capitellum	2 years
Radial head	4 years
Internal epicondyle	6 years
Trochlea	8 years
Olecranon	10 years
External epicondyle	12 years

COMPUTED TOMOGRAPHY SCAN

Computed tomography (CT) is used mainly for planning trauma reconstruction but it can be used, with or without arthrography, to look for loose bodies or detail changes in osteoarthritis (OA).

MAGNETIC RESONANCE IMAGING

Magnetic resonance imaging (MRI) is used mainly for the investigation of soft-tissue lesions around the elbow such as ligament tears and tendinopathies. The addition of arthrography improves sensitivity for detecting loose bodies and chronic ligament lesions.

CONGENITAL CONDITIONS

CONGENITAL RADIOULNAR SYNOSTOSIS

This painless condition is a result of failure of separation of the radius and ulna anlage *in utero*. The radius and ulna are connected (synostosis) in the proximal forearm. There is an absence of forearm rotation (flexion is preserved) with the forearm typically in fixed pronation. This condition may not be identified until later in childhood when the lack of forearm rotation causes some difficulty in playing a musical instrument or some sports. Surgical intervention is usually reserved for those with a bilateral radioulnar

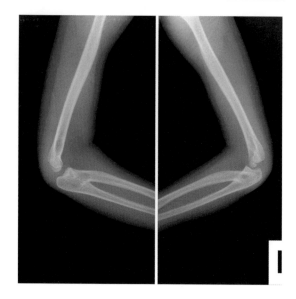

14.4 Bilateral radioulnar synostosis

synostosis (**14.4**) when bilateral fixed pronation is limiting activities.

ACQUIRED ELBOW DEFORMITIES

CUBITUS VARUS

Varus (or 'gunstock') deformity is most obvious when the elbows are extended and the arms are elevated (**14.5**). The most common cause is malunion of a supracondylar fracture. The deformity can be corrected by a wedge osteotomy of the lower humerus.

CUBITUS VALGUS

The most common cause is non-union of a fractured lateral condyle; this may give gross deformity and a bony knob on the inner side of the joint (**14.6**). The importance of valgus deformity is the liability for delayed ulnar palsy to develop; years after the causal injury, the patient notices weakness of the hand with numbness and tingling of the ulnar fingers. The deformity itself needs no treatment, but for delayed ulnar palsy the nerve should be transposed to the front of the elbow.

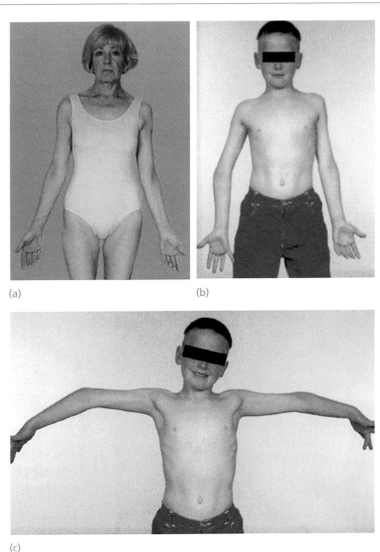

(a)

(b)

(c)

14.5 Cubitus varus (a) Note that the elbows are normally held in approximately 10° of valgus (the carrying angle). **(b)** This young boy ended up with varus angulation after a supracondylar fracture of the distal humerus. The deformity is much more obvious **(c)** when he raises his arms (gunstock deformity) and increases his risk of developing posterolateral rotatory instability and a snapping triceps.

STIFF ELBOW

A stiff elbow can be a severe impediment. Patients may be unable to reach out to, or bring back from, their environment; others, again, cannot turn the hand palm downwards to pick up something, or palm upwards to lift something. Causes include congenital disorders, trauma (**14.7**) and arthritis (**e14.1**). If physiotherapy does not help, surgery may.

TUBERCULOSIS

Clinical features

Although the disease begins as synovitis or osteomyelitis, tuberculosis of the elbow is rarely seen until arthritis supervenes. The onset is insidious, with a long history of aching and stiffness. The most striking physical sign is the marked

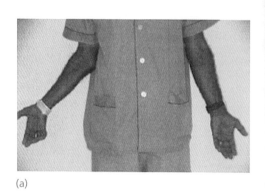
(a)

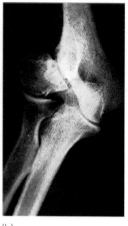
(b)

14.6 Cubitus valgus (a) This man has excessive valgus of the right elbow but his main complaint was of weakness and deformity in the hand, which was caused by a tardy ulnar nerve palsy secondary to the elbow deformity. **(b)** Valgus deformity from an un-united fracture of the lateral condyle.

wasting. While the disease is active, the joint is held flexed, looks swollen, feels warm and is diffusely tender; movement is considerably limited and accompanied by pain and spasm.

X-rays

These typically show generalized rarefaction and an apparent increase of joint space because of bone erosion (e14.2).

Treatment

In addition to antituberculous drugs, the elbow is rested, at first in a splint, but later simply by applying a collar and cuff. Surgical debridement is rarely needed.

RHEUMATOID ARTHRITIS

Clinical features

The elbow is involved in more than 50% of patients with RA. Rheumatoid nodules can often be detected over the olecranon (14.8). There is pain and tenderness, especially around the head of the radius. Eventually the whole elbow may become swollen and unstable. Often both elbows are affected.

X-rays

Bone erosion, with gradual destruction of the radial head and widening of the trochlear notch of the ulna, is typical of chronic inflammatory arthritis.

Treatment

In addition to general treatment, the elbow should be splinted during periods of active synovitis and steroid injections should be considered. For chronic, painful arthritis of the radiohumeral joint, resection of the radial head and partial synovectomy give reasonably good results. If the entire joint is severely damaged, joint replacement should be considered (e14.3). The result is often excellent, at least compared to the preoperative situation. With modern techniques complications such as infection, instability and implant loosening are much less common than in the past. The results are more reliable in RA than OA, because the lower functional demands of the former, often restricted by multiple joint problems in the same limb, put less stress on the device.

OSTEOARTHRITIS

The elbow is an uncommon site for OA. When it does occur, it may be secondary to trauma.

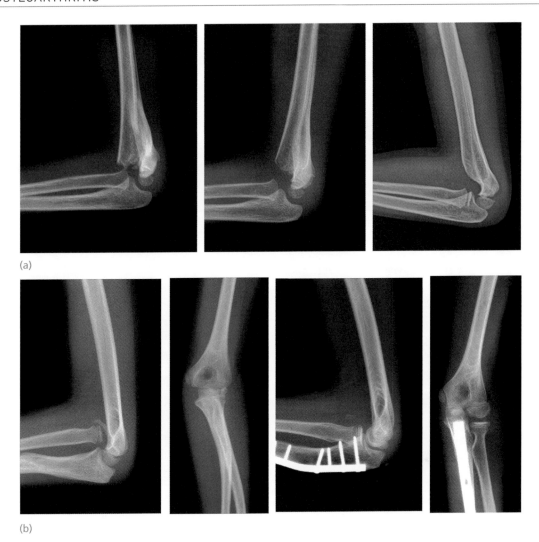

14.7 Two post-traumatic conditions in childhood that resulted in a flexion block (a) Supracondylar elbow fracture malunion: severe untreated posterior translation of the distal humerus resulted in anterior impingement. Over 18 months, remodelling occurred with resultant restoration of elbow flexion without the need for surgical intervention. **(b)** Untreated Monteggia fracture–dislocation: proximal ulna shaft fracture with dislocation of the radial head. Radiocapitellar joint reduced following a corrective ulna osteotomy, open reduction of the radial head and annular ligament reconstruction.

'Primary' OA of the elbow should suggest an underlying disorder such as pyrophosphate arthropathy or congenital dysplasia, but usually occurs spontaneously.

Clinical features

The usual symptoms are pain and stiffness, but in late cases the joint may become unstable. Occasionally, ulnar palsy is the presenting feature. The elbow may look and feel enlarged and movements are limited.

X-rays

These show diminution of the joint space with subchondral sclerosis and marginal osteophytes; one or more loose bodies may be seen (e14.4).

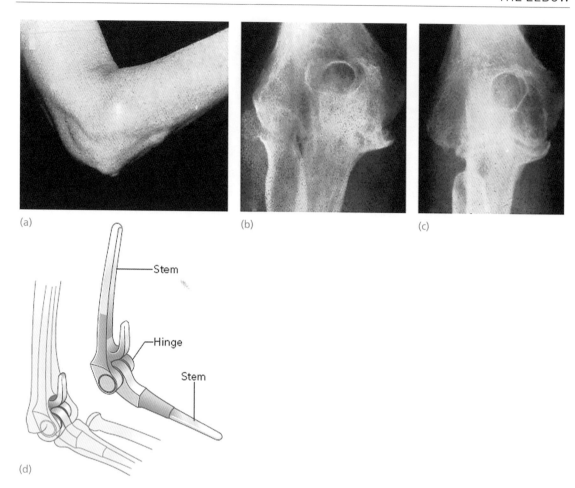

(a)   (b)   (c)

Stem

Hinge

Stem

(d)

14.8 Rheumatoid arthritis (a) This patient has a painful elbow as well as the typical rheumatoid nodules over the olecranon. **(b)** His X-rays show deformity of the radial head and marked erosion of the rest of the elbow joint. **(c)** Excision of the radial head combined with synovectomy relieved the pain. **(d)** Total elbow arthroplasty: hinged implants.

Treatment

OA of the elbow rarely requires more than symptomatic treatment; loose bodies, however, should be removed arthroscopically if they cause locking (**14.9**). If stiffness is sufficiently disabling, removal of osteophytes (by either open or arthroscopic surgery) can improve the range of movement. If there are signs of ulnar neuritis, the nerve may have to be transposed to the front of the elbow. Joint replacement can be considered but the complication rate is rather high and the durability is uncertain.

LOOSE BODIES

COMMONEST CAUSES OF LOOSE BODIES

Acute trauma
Osteochondritis dissecans
Synovial chondromatosis
Osteoarthritis

The cardinal clinical feature is sudden locking of the elbow.

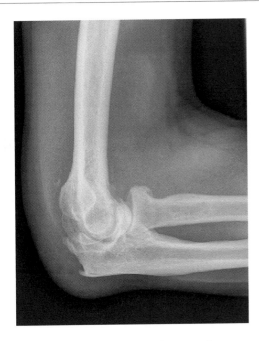

14.9 **Osteoarthritis** X-ray with osteophytes, joint narrowing, sclerosis and loose bodies typically seen after trauma or in manual workers.

Imaging

A plain *X-ray* may or may not show the loose body. A *CT or MR arthrogram* (**14.10**) is more sensitive.

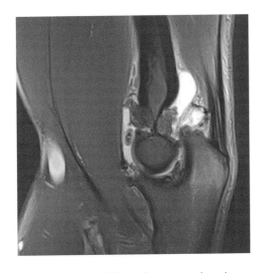

14.10 **Loose body** MRI arthrogram showing a loose body in the elbow joint.

Treatment

If the loose body is troublesome, it can be removed arthroscopically. This is the most common indication for arthroscopy.

 The risk of this operation is devastating injury to the ulnar nerve, median nerve and posterior interosseous nerve, each of which lies less than 1 cm from the joint and very close to the portals used for access.

OSTEOCHONDRITIS DISSECANS

The capitellum is a common site of osteochondritis dissecans. This may be due to repeated stress but can occur spontaneously. The diagnosis should be excluded in any active adolescent complaining of lateral elbow pain. They may complain of loss of range of movement, usually equal loss of flexion and extension, due to an effusion of the elbow. A history of locking may be elicited due to a loose body in the elbow from fragmentation of the articular surface.

Imaging

X-rays may show fragmentation or, at a later stage, flattening of the capitellum (**14.11**). *CT and MRI* are more useful for defining the lesion.

Treatment

Treatment is symptomatic. The lesion can heal and symptoms resolve with a repeat MRI at 3 months to assess resolution. A small loose body floating in the joint should be removed with an arthroscope or, if too large, through a small incision. A larger fragment which is still partly attached to the capitellum can sometimes be repaired back with a small screw.

OLECRANON BURSITIS

The olecranon bursa sometimes becomes enlarged as a result of pressure or friction (**14.12**). When it is also painful, the cause is more likely to be infection, gout or RA.

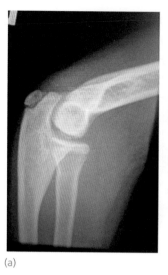
(a)

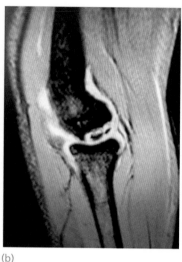
(b)

14.11 Osteochondritis dissecans (a) The capitellum is fragmented and slightly flattened. **(b)** Sometimes the fragment separates and lies in the joint.

- *Gout* is suspected if there is a history of previous attacks, if the condition is bilateral, if there are tophi, or if X-ray shows calcification in the bursa. Even then it is not easy to distinguish from acute infection, unless pus is aspirated.
- *RA* causes both swelling and nodularity over the olecranon. In almost all cases this will be associated with a typical symmetrical polyarthritis. In the late stages, erosion of the elbow joint may cause marked instability.

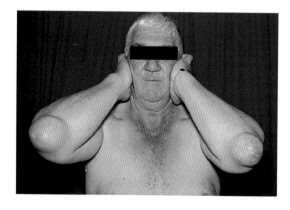

14.12 Olecranon bursitis The enormous red lumps over the points of the elbows are due to swollen olecranon bursae; the patient's ruddy complexion completes the typical picture of gout.

Treatment

The underlying disorder must be treated. Septic bursitis may need local drainage. Occasionally, a chronically enlarged bursa has to be excised.

RECURRENT ELBOW INSTABILITY

Recurrent elbow instability occurs as a result of injury to the lateral collateral ligament complex of the elbow, causing the radial head to rotate posterolaterally off the humerus. It presents with lateral elbow pain and with locking or 'clunking' of the elbow. Various tests have been described including the varus stress test, push-up test and table-top test.

Flail elbow may also be caused by gunshot wounds and neuropathic arthritis (e14.5).

Treatment

The lateral collateral ligament can be repaired, if identified acutely, or reconstructed with tendon autograft, allograft or synthetic graft with satisfactory results.

TENDINOPATHIES AROUND THE ELBOW

'TENNIS ELBOW' AND 'GOLFER'S ELBOW'

These conditions are common, affecting about 15% of 40- to 55-year-olds at some time. The cause of these common disorders is unknown, but they are seldom due to either tennis or golf. Most cases occur spontaneously as part of a natural degenerative process in the tendon aponeuroses attached to either the lateral or medial humeral epicondyle. Pain is probably due to a repair process similar to that of rotator cuff tendinitis around the shoulder. There is often a history of occupational stress or unaccustomed activity, such as house painting, carpentry or other activities that involve strenuous wrist movements and forearm muscle contraction.

Clinical features

'TENNIS ELBOW'

Pain is felt over the outer side of the elbow, but in severe cases it may radiate widely. It is initiated or aggravated by movements such as pouring tea, turning a stiff door-handle, shaking hands or lifting with the forearm pronated. The elbow looks normal and flexion and extension are full and painless. Tenderness is localized to a spot just in front of the lateral epicondyle, and pain is reproduced by getting the patient to extend the wrist against resistance, or simply by passively flexing the wrist so as to stretch the common extensors (14.13).

'GOLFER'S ELBOW'

Similar symptoms occur around the medial epicondyle and, owing to involvement of the common tendon of origin of the wrist flexors, pain is reproduced by passive extension of the wrist in supination.

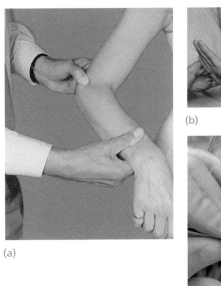
(a)

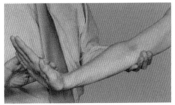
(b)

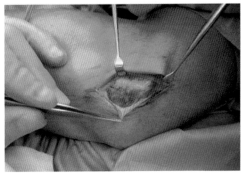
(c)

14.13 Tennis elbow (a) Tenderness over the lateral epicondyle. **(b)** Pain is provoked by resisted wrist extension. **(c)** Extensor carpi radialis brevis origin may have to be released.

Treatment

Rest, or avoiding the precipitating activity, may allow the lesion to heal. Most will fade away over a few to several months. A splint and physiotherapy may help. Steroid injection will provide short-term pain relief but recurrence rates are high and the elbow is more likely to be painful in the long term. Alternatives are platelet-rich plasma and shockwave therapy.

Persistent pain which fails to respond to conservative measures may call for operative treatment. The affected common tendon on the lateral or medial side of the elbow is detached from its origin at the humeral epicondyle; about 80% are improved.

DISTAL BICEPS TENDINOPATHY

This is an increasing problem due to the growing number of individuals going to the gym to lift weights into their forties and fifties. It is one of the few causes of anterior elbow pain, with pain reproduced on resisted forearm supination.

Treatment is as for tennis elbow, except that, if surgery is required, the tendon is reattached after debridement (a substantial undertaking).

BASEBALL PITCHER'S ELBOW

Repetitive, vigorous throwing activities can cause damage to the bones of soft-tissue attachments around the elbow. In adolescents, traction apophysitis of the medial epicondyle, or 'little leaguer's elbow', became so prevalent that limits are now placed on the number of pitches that juniors are permitted to make. *Treatment* is rest and avoidance of pitching activities.

In adults, persistent valgus strain causes attenuation of the medial collateral ligament and posteromedial impingement – valgus extension overload. This often requires arthroscopic debridement and medial ligament reconstruction.

The wrist

15

■ Clinical assessment	309
■ Wrist deformities	311
■ Tuberculosis	313
■ Rheumatoid arthritis	314
■ Osteoarthritis of the radiocarpal joint	314
■ Osteoarthritis of the first carpometacarpal joint	315
■ Scaphotrapeziotrapezoid arthritis	315
■ Distal radioulnar joint arthritis	316

■ Kienböck's disease	316
■ Tears of the triangular fibrocartilage	318
■ Ulnocarpal impaction and TFCC degeneration	318
■ Chronic carpal instability	318
■ Tenosynovitis and tenovaginitis	319
■ Occupational disorders	321
■ Ganglia	321
■ Carpal tunnel syndrome	322

CLINICAL ASSESSMENT

HISTORY

- *Pain* may be localized to the radial side (e.g. tenovaginitis of the thumb tendons or thumb base arthritis, in distal radioulnar joint arthritis and pisotriquetral arthritis) or to the dorsum (e.g. radiocarpal arthritis, Kienböck's disease and occult dorsal wrist ganglion).
- *Stiffness* is often not noticed until it is severe. Loss of rotation (pronation means palm down and supination means palm up) is more readily noticed and may be very disabling.
- *Swelling* may signify involvement of either the joint or the tendon sheaths.
- *Deformity* is a late symptom except after trauma.
- *Loss of function* affects both the wrist and the hand. Firm grip is possible only with a strong, stable, painless wrist that has a reasonable range of movement.

EXAMINATION

Examination of the wrist is not complete without also examining the elbow, forearm and hand. Both upper limbs should be completely exposed.

Look

Inspect the skin for scars. Compare both wrists and forearms to see if there is any deformity. If there is swelling, note whether it is diffuse or localized to one of the tendon sheaths.

Feel

Note any undue warmth. Tender areas must be accurately localized and the bony landmarks compared with those of the normal wrist (15.1, e15.1).

SECTION 2 REGIONAL ORTHOPAEDICS

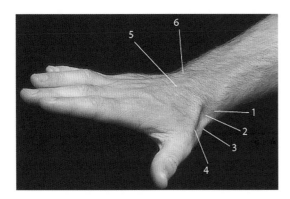

15.1 Tender points at the wrist (1) Tip of the radial styloid process; (2) anatomical snuff-box, bounded on the radial side by (3) the extensor pollicis brevis and on the ulnar side by (4) the extensor pollicis longus; (5) the extensor tendons of the fingers; and (6) the head of the ulna.

Move

PASSIVE MOVEMENTS

Passive flexion and extension of the wrist Measure these on each side in turn. To view both sides simultaneously and compare them, ask the patient first to place their palms together in a position of prayer, elevating the elbows, then to repeat the manoeuvre with the wrists back-to-back. The normal range for both flexion and extension is 100–130 degrees (e15.2).

Radial deviation and ulnar deviation Measure these in the palms-up position:

- ulnar deviation is normally about 50 degrees
- radial deviation is only about 15 degrees.

Pronation and supination These are included in wrist movements, although they depend also on the condition of the elbow and movement between the forearm bones (**15.2**). The normal range is 0–90 degrees in both directions.

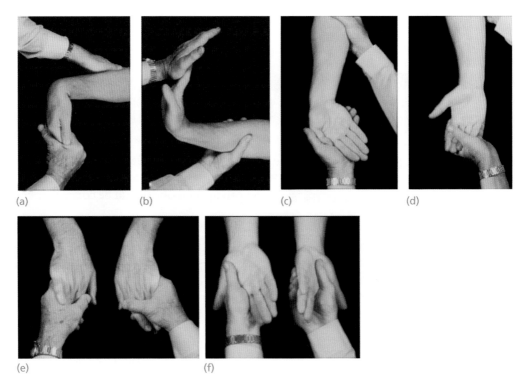

(a)   (b)   (c)   (d)

(e)   (f)

15.2 Wrist movements (a) Flexion; (b) extension; (c) ulnar deviation; (d) radial deviation; (e) pronation; (f) supination.

SECTION 2 REGIONAL ORTHOPAEDICS

ACTIVE MOVEMENTS

Active movements should be tested against resistance; *loss of power* may be due to pain, tendon rupture or muscle weakness. *Grip strength* can be gauged by having the patient squeeze the examiner's hand; mechanical instruments allow more accurate assessment.

INVESTIGATION

Imaging

- *X-rays* are routinely obtained (15.3). Special oblique views are necessary to show up difficult scaphoid fractures. Note the position of the carpal bones and look for evidence of joint-space narrowing, especially at the carpometacarpal (CMC) joint of the thumb.
- *Computed tomography (CT) scans* are helpful in defining hook of hamate fractures and planning scaphoid reconstruction.
- *Magnetic resonance imaging (MRI)* is useful for demonstrating soft-tissue lesions or the early signs of avascular necrosis in one of the carpal bones.

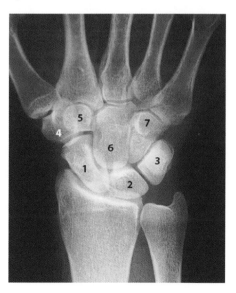

15.3 X-ray Note the shape and position of the bones which make up the normal carpus: (1) scaphoid, (2) lunate, (3) triquetrum overlain by pisiform, (4) trapezium, (5) trapezoid, (6) capitate, (7) hamate.

- *Fluoroscopy* may demonstrate some patterns of carpal instability.

Arthroscopy

This is the most reliable way of diagnosing tears of the triangular fibrocartilage complex (TFCC), synovitis, ligament tears and early changes of osteoarthritis (OA). Many of these conditions can be treated through the arthroscope.

WRIST DEFORMITIES

CONGENITAL VARIATIONS

Embryonic abnormalities of the upper limb are likely to affect more than one segment (or indeed the whole) of the limb; therefore, congenital anomalies often appear together in the forearm, wrist and hand. Furthermore, other organs developing during the same period may be affected and thus there may be associated congenital abnormalities.

These are rare conditions; the overall incidence of upper limb anomalies is estimated to be about 1 : 600 live births, but in only a fraction of those affected are the defects severe enough to require corrective surgery. A few of the least unusual deformities affecting the wrist are described here.

Transverse deficiency

This can exist anywhere between the shoulder and the phalanges. The most common levels of absence are at the proximal forearm and mid-carpus, then at the metacarpals and humerus. Associated anomalies are unusual.

Radial longitudinal deficiency

The infant is born with the wrist in marked radial deviation, hence the common name *radial club hand*; one-half of the patients are affected bilaterally. There is absence of the whole or part of the radius, and usually also the thumb.

Treatment in the neonate consists of gentle stretching and splintage. Serious cases can be treated by distraction prior to a tension-free soft-tissue correction. Prolonged splintage is still required to avoid recurrence of the deformity.

 Always examine the elbow. Surgical correction of a radially deviated wrist in cases where the elbow is stiff can be disastrous.

Always examine the elbow: if the joint is stiff, a radially deviated wrist can actually be advantageous, as the child can then get the hand to their mouth (for eating) and the perineum (for toilet care). Surgical correction of the wrist in these cases can be disastrous. This condition is associated with cardiac septal anomalies and blood dyscrasias, hence the need for careful preoperative workup.

Madelung's deformity

In Madelung's deformity (15.4) the lower radius curves forwards (ventrally), carrying with it the carpus and hand but leaving the distal end of the ulna projecting on the back of the wrist. Although the abnormality is present at birth, the deformity is rarely seen before the age of 10 years, after which

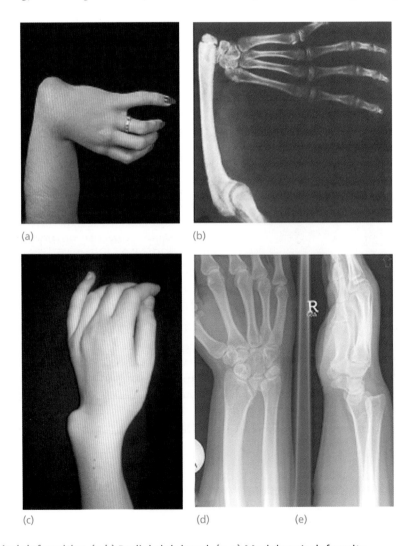

(a)   (b)

(c)   (d)   (e)

15.4 Congenital deformities (a,b) Radial club hand. **(c–e)** Madelung's deformity.

it increases until growth is complete. Despite the deformity, function is usually undisturbed.

Treatment may be unnecessary, but if the deformity is severe, the lower end of the ulna can be shortened; this is sometimes combined with osteotomy of the radius.

ACQUIRED DEFORMITY

Physeal injuries can result in malunited fractures or subluxation of the distal radioulnar joint. Osteotomy of the radius or stabilization of the ulna may be needed (e15.3, e15.4).

Non-traumatic deformities are seen typically in rheumatoid arthritis (RA) and cerebral palsy. These disorders are discussed in Chapters 3 and 10, respectively.

A drooping wrist is typical of a radial nerve palsy.

TUBERCULOSIS

Clinical features

Tuberculous arthritis sometimes occurs at the wrist. Pain and stiffness come on gradually and the hand feels weak. The forearm looks wasted; the wrist is swollen and feels warm. Involvement of the flexor tendon compartment may give rise to a large fluctuant swelling that crosses the wrist into the palm (what used to be called a 'compound palmar ganglion'). Movements are restricted and painful. In a neglected case, there may be a sinus.

X-ray examination shows localized osteoporosis and irregularity of the radiocarpal and intercarpal joints, and sometimes bone erosion (15.5).

Diagnosis

The condition must be differentiated from RA. Bilateral arthritis of the wrist is nearly always rheumatoid in origin; when only one wrist is affected, the signs resemble those of tuberculosis. X-rays and serological tests may help, but sometimes a biopsy is necessary (e15.5).

Treatment

Antituberculous drugs are given and the wrist is splinted. If an abscess forms, it must be drained. If the wrist is destroyed, systemic treatment should be continued until the disease is quiescent and the wrist is then arthrodesed.

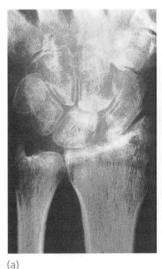 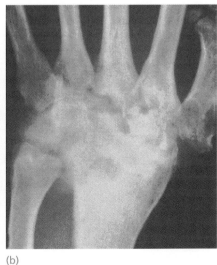

(a)   (b)

15.5 Tuberculosis (a) Subacute tuberculous arthritis; note the marked osteoporosis in the distal radius and the carpus. **(b)** A much more advanced case of tuberculous arthritis giving rise to extensive bone destruction.

RHEUMATOID ARTHRITIS

Clinical features

After the metacarpophalangeal joints, the wrist is the most common site of RA (**15.6**). Pain, swelling and tenderness may at first be localized to the radioulnar joint, or to one of the tendon sheaths. Sooner or later the whole wrist becomes involved and tenderness is much more ill defined. In late cases, the wrist is deformed and unstable. Extensor tendons may rupture where they cross the dorsum of the wrist, causing one or more of the fingers to drop into flexion (e15.6).

X-rays show the characteristic features of osteoporosis and bony erosions. Tell-tale signs are usually more obvious in the metacarpophalangeal joints (e15.7).

Treatment

EARLY

Management in the early stage consists of splintage and local injection of corticosteroids, combined with systemic treatment. Persistent synovitis (usually affecting the extensor tendon sheaths) may call for synovectomy and soft-tissue stabilization of the wrist. If the radioulnar joint is involved, synovectomy can be combined with excision of the distal end of the ulnar head. Flexor synovitis may cause median nerve compression (carpal tunnel syndrome), which should be treated by operative release of the flexor retinaculum.

LATE

In the late stage, tendon ruptures at the wrist, joint destruction, instability and deformity may require reconstructive surgery, including either arthroplasty or arthrodesis (e15.8).

OSTEOARTHRITIS OF THE RADIOCARPAL JOINT

OA of the radiocarpal joint may occur spontaneously or may follow an old, sometimes forgotten injury or a condition such as Kienböck's or infection. The patient complains of pain, progressive stiffness and weakness of grip.

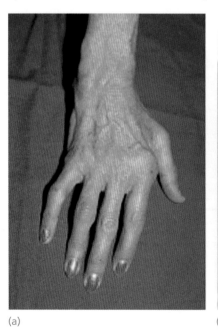
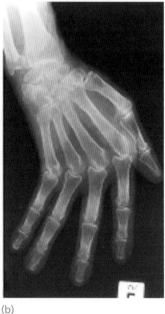

(a)   (b)

15.6 Rheumatoid arthritis (a) The wrist is deviated radialwards and the fingers ulnarwards; this is the typical zigzag deformity of established RA in the wrist and hand. **(b)** X-ray of the same patient.

The appearance is usually normal, but the wrist is tender and movements are restricted and painful.

X-rays

Radiological features are:

- narrowing of the radiocarpal joint
- bone sclerosis
- irregularity of one or more of the proximal carpal bones.

There may also be signs of the old injury or Kienböck's disease.

Treatment

Rest in a splint and an occasional steroid injection may suffice. Surgery depends on the joint

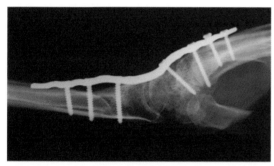

(a)

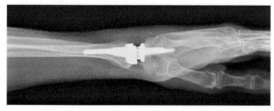

(b)

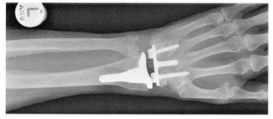

(c)

15.7 Osteoarthritis of the radiocarpal joint
(a) Total wrist fusion; **(b,c)** wrist replacement.

affected; partial or total wrist fusion, or wrist replacement, may be indicated (**15.7**, **e15.9**, **e15.10**).

OSTEOARTHRITIS OF THE FIRST CARPOMETACARPAL JOINT

OA of the thumb CMC joint is common in postmenopausal women. The patient complains of pain and swelling around the proximal end of the thumb metacarpal. Careful examination will show that tenderness is sharply localized to the CMC joint, about 1 cm distal to the radial styloid process. The condition is often bilateral, and Heberden's nodes of the finger joints are common. In late cases, fixed adduction of the first metacarpal produces a characteristic deformity.

X-ray examination shows the usual features of joint-space narrowing, sclerosis and osteophyte formation.

Treatment

Local injection of corticosteroid usually relieves pain, and movements may improve. If this fails, operation may be advisable. The most reliable way of abolishing pain and preserving function is to excise the trapezium. A more sophisticated, but rather experimental, option is joint replacement. Joint arthrodesis is difficult and causes stiffness (**15.8**).

SCAPHOTRAPEZIOTRAPEZOID ARTHRITIS

The joint between the distal end of the scaphoid and the underside of the trapezium and trapezoid ('the triscaphe joint') can develop arthritis either in isolation or in association with arthritis of the CMC joint.

Late middle-aged females are most commonly affected. The patient points to the front of the scaphoid tubercle as the source of the pain (whereas in CMC arthritis the patient points to the back of the thumb base).

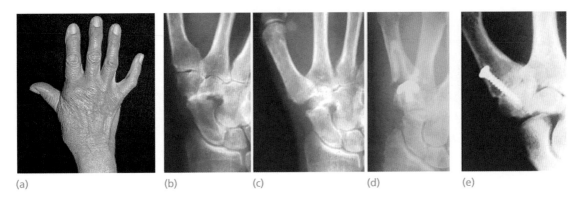

(a)   (b)   (c)   (d)   (e)

15.8 Osteoarthritis of the first carpometacarpal joint (a) Typical deformity: note the swelling over the first CMC joint. **(b)** X-ray changes. Choice of treatment is between **(c)** trapeziectomy, **(d)** replacement arthroplasty and **(e)** arthrodesis.

Treatment

Treatment is initially along standard lines, i.e. adaptive measures, anti-inflammatory medication, cortisone injection and splintage. Injections are best performed under ultrasound or fluoroscopic control.

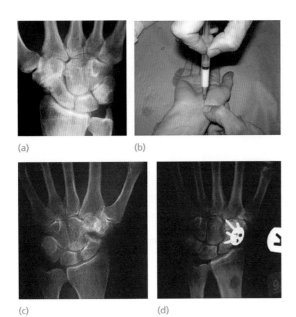

(a)   (b)

(c)   (d)

15.9 Scaphotrapeziotrapezoid arthritis (a) Changes on X-ray; **(b)** steroid injection; **(c)** distal pole of scaphoid excision (do not remove too much!); **(d)** soft-tissue tumour fusion.

Patients with severe symptoms may benefit from surgery (**15.9**). However, there is as yet no completely satisfactory operation.

DISTAL RADIOULNAR JOINT ARTHRITIS

Degenerative changes are seen either with no obvious cause or after long-standing instability of the joint.

If pain and loss of function cannot be controlled by conservative measures, the patient may benefit from ulnar head replacement (although, like all implants in the hand and wrist, there is a risk of significant early complications and the durability is uncertain). Operations that involve excision of the ulnar head should be undertaken with extreme caution and avoided if possible because of the high risk of causing severe and intractable instability (**15.10**).

KIENBÖCK'S DISEASE

The lunate bone sometimes develops a patchy avascular necrosis. A predisposing factor may be relative shortening of the ulna (negative ulnar variance), which could result in excessive stress being applied to the lunate where it is squeezed between the distal surface of the (overlong) radius and the second row of carpal bones.

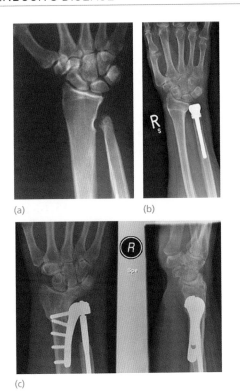

(a)   (b)

(c)

15.10 Distal radioulnar joint arthritis – operative treatment (a) Excising too much of the distal ulna may cause painful radioulnar impingement. **(b)** One alternative is an ulnar head replacement. **(c)** Total distal radioulnar joint replacement for arthritis and instability.

The patient, usually a young adult, complains of aching and stiffness. Tenderness is localized to the centre of the wrist on the dorsum; wrist extension may be limited.

Imaging

The earliest signs of osteonecrosis can be detected only by MRI (e15.11). Typical X-ray signs are increased density in the lunate and, later, flattening and irregularity of the bone. Ultimately there may be features of OA of the wrist.

Treatment

EARLY

During the early stage, while the shape of the lunate is more or less normal, osteotomy of the distal end of the radius may reduce pressure on the bone and thereby protect it from collapsing. Microsurgical revascularization of the bone is also worth considering if the necessary expertise is available.

LATE

In late cases, partial wrist arthrodesis or proximal row excision or even joint replacement are considered (**15.11**).

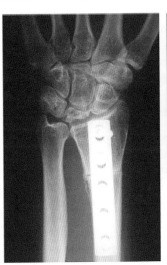

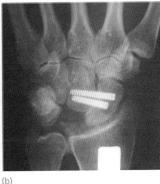

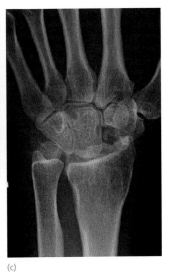

(a)   (b)   (c)

15.11 Kienböck's disease – treatment (a) Radial shortening; **(b)** scaphocapitate fusion; **(c)** proximal row carpectomy.

TEARS OF THE TRIANGULAR FIBROCARTILAGE

The TFCC fans out from the base of the ulnar styloid process to the medial edge of the distal radius, acting somewhat like a meniscus in the wrist joint (15.12). A central perforation can occur after trauma but usually occurs as a degenerative process (see 'Ulnocarpal impaction and TFCC degeneration' below). An avulsion from the ulnar styloid causes instability of the distal radioulnar joint (e15.12). The diagnosis is confirmed by MRI and arthroscopy.

Treatment

Operative treatment may be needed if the symptoms are marked. Peripheral tears can be reattached by either open or arthroscopic techniques; central tears, in the absence of ulnocarpal impaction (see below) are best managed by arthroscopic debridement to remove the ragged fragments.

ULNOCARPAL IMPACTION AND TFCC DEGENERATION

Chronic degeneration of the TFCC may be associated with a relatively long ulna, impaction of the ulnar head against the ulnar side of the lunate and ulnocarpal arthritis (*the ulnocarpal impaction syndrome*). This may result when an impacted Colles' fracture leaves the radius relatively shorter than usual. X-ray examination shows a relatively long ulna ('positive ulnar variance') and in late cases there may be arthritic changes in the ulnolunate articulation.

Treatment

Treatment starts with simple analgesics, splintage and steroid injections.

- *If the positive ulnar variance is slight* (<3 mm), arthroscopic excision of the distal dome of the ulnar head may be successful (15.13c).
- *If the variance is great* (>3 mm), the long ulna can be shortened using a special jig and compression plate (15.13d,e).

CHRONIC CARPAL INSTABILITY

The wrist functions as a system of intercalated segments (i.e. adjacent congruous bones) stabilized by ligaments and by the scaphoid, which bridges the two rows of carpal bones (e15.13). Following trauma to the carpus, there may be partial collapse of this structure, a condition which is not always recognized at the time. Some years later, the patient complains of progressive pain and weakness in the wrist.

Diagnosis

The most easily spotted example is a rupture of the scapholunate ligament, which appears on X-ray as an unusual gap between the scaphoid and lunate and foreshortening of the scaphoid image (15.14).

Treatment

The best form of treatment is prevention. Acute 'wrist sprains' should be carefully assessed for signs of carpal displacement and instability (see Chapter 27). Carpal displacement must be reduced, the ligament repaired and the bones held in position with Kirschner wires (K-wires).

Patients with chronic instability can often be treated by splintage, analgesics and specific physiotherapy. Occasionally, operative treatment is indicated, involving soft-tissue augmentation or partial fusion of the wrist.

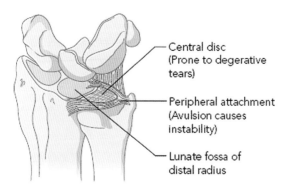

Central disc (Prone to degerative tears)

Peripheral attachment (Avulsion causes instability)

Lunate fossa of distal radius

15.12 Triangular fibrocartilage complex

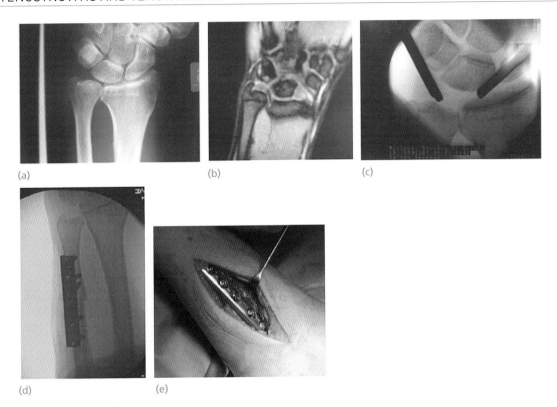

15.13 Ulnocarpal impaction **(a)** X-ray; **(b)** MRI shows the long ulna and signal change in the lunotri-quetral region; **(c)** intraoperative X-ray during arthroscopic removal of the distal dome of the ulna; **(d)** intraoperative image of ulnar shortening; **(e)** plate used to hold the shortened ulna.

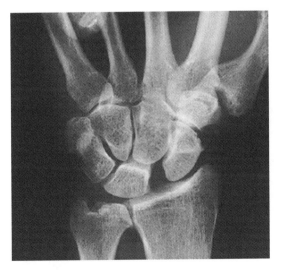

15.14 Carpal instability The scapholunate ligament has ruptured. The X-ray shows a large gap between the two bones and the scaphoid is foreshortened.

TENOSYNOVITIS AND TENOVAGINITIS

The extensor retinaculum contains six compartments which transmit tendons lined with synovium. Although tenosynovitis is most associated with RA, it can be caused by unaccustomed movement; sometimes it occurs spontaneously. The resulting synovial inflammation causes secondary thickening of the sheath and stenosis of the compartment, which further compromises the tendon. Early treatment, including rest, anti-inflammatory medication and injection of corticosteroids, may break this vicious circle.

The first dorsal compartment (enclosing abductor pollicis longus and extensor pollicis brevis) and the second dorsal compartment (extensor carpi radialis longus and brevis) are the ones most commonly affected.

SECTION 2 REGIONAL ORTHOPAEDICS

De Quervain's disease

Tenovaginitis of the first dorsal compartment is usually seen in women between the ages of 30 and 50 years. There may be a history of unaccustomed activity, such as pruning roses, cutting with scissors or wringing out clothes. It is quite common shortly after childbirth.

Clinical features

Pain, and sometimes swelling, is localized to the radial side of the wrist. The tendon sheath feels thick and hard. Tenderness is most acute at the very tip of the radial styloid (15.15).

The pathognomonic sign is elicited by *Finkelstein's test*.

> **FINKELSTEIN'S TEST FOR DE QUERVAIN'S DISEASE**
>
> Hold the patient's hand firmly, keeping the thumb tucked in close to the palm, then turn the wrist sharply towards the ulnar side. A stab of pain over the radial styloid is a positive sign. Repeating the movement with the thumb left free is relatively painless.

Treatment

In early cases, symptoms can be relieved by ultrasound therapy or a corticosteroid injection into the tendon sheath, sometimes combined with splintage of the wrist. Resistant cases need an operation, which consists of slitting the thickened tendon sheath. Care should be taken to prevent injury to the dorsal sensory branches of the radial nerve, which may cause intractable dysaesthesia.

Other sites of tenosynovitis

- Tenosynovitis of *extensor carpi radialis brevis* (the most powerful extensor of the wrist) or *extensor carpi ulnaris* may cause pain and point tenderness just medial to the anatomical snuffbox or immediately distal to the head of the ulna, respectively.
- The *flexor carpi radialis* can become inflamed, often in association with arthritis of the adjacent triscaphe joint.
- *Flexor carpi ulnaris* can become inflamed (e15.14).

Treatment with splintage and corticosteroid injections is usually effective.

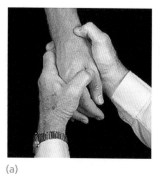
(a)
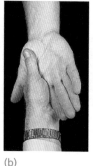
(b)
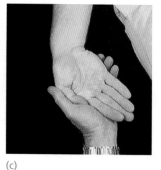
(c)
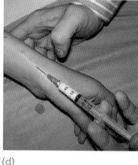
(d)

15.15 De Quervain's disease (a) There is point tenderness at the tip of the radial styloid process. **(b,c)** Finkelstein's test: ulnar deviation with the thumb left free is relatively painless **(b)**, but if the movement is repeated with the thumb held close to the palm **(c)**, the pull on the thumb tendons causes intense pain. **(d)** Injecting the tendon sheath.

OCCUPATIONAL DISORDERS

Inappropriate terms such as *repetitive stress injury* and *cumulative trauma disorder* have been used in the past for a controversial syndrome comprising ill-defined and unusually disabling pain around the wrist and forearm (and sometimes the entire limb) which is usually ascribed to a particular work practice. There is no good evidence to suggest that using the hands causes harm – after all, training makes muscles and tendons less vulnerable to damage. Other defined and treatable conditions such as carpal tunnel syndrome, thumb base arthritis, tenosynovitis from sudden unaccustomed use and De Quervain's should be excluded and treated accordingly. Epidemiological studies suggest that these conditions are no more common among keyboard operators than in the general population. There are often social and psychological aspects which confound the picture. The term 'work-relevant upper limb disorder' is preferred as it acknowledges that the symptoms are noticed at work, but it does not imply causation.

GANGLIA

The ubiquitous ganglion is seen most commonly on the back of the wrist. It is less common, but usually more painful, on the front (15.16). It arises from cystic degeneration in the joint capsule or tendon sheath. The distended cyst contains a glairy fluid.

The patient, often a young adult, presents with a painless lump, usually on the back of the wrist, but sometimes on the front. Occasionally there is a slight ache. The lump is well defined, cystic and not tender. It may be attached to one of the tendons. Sometimes the ganglion is so small that it can only be appreciated properly on an MRI (e15.15).

The ganglion often disappears after some months, so there should be no haste about treatment. If the lesion continues to be troublesome, it can be aspirated; if it recurs, excision is justified, but the patient should be told that there is a 30% risk of recurrence, even after careful surgery.

Sometimes mistaken for a ganglion is a hard bony bump over the back of the second CMC joint – the so-called 'carpometacarpal boss' (15.17). This can be left alone but if symptomatic the bony bump is excised.

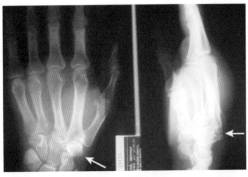
(a)

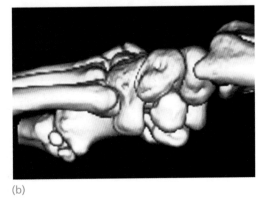
(b)

15.17 Carpometacarpal boss (a) X-ray; **(b)** 3D CT.

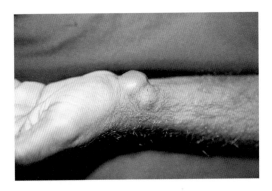

15.16 Volar wrist ganglion

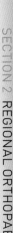

CARPAL TUNNEL SYNDROME

This is the commonest and best known of all the nerve entrapment syndromes. In the normal carpal tunnel there is barely room for all the tendons and the median nerve; consequently, any swelling is likely to result in compression and ischaemia of the nerve. Usually the cause eludes detection; the syndrome is, however, common in women at the menopause, in RA, in pregnancy and in myxoedema. The usual age group is 40–50 years.

Clinical features

The history is most helpful in making the diagnosis. Pain and paraesthesia occur in the distribution of the median nerve in the hand (15.18). Night after night the patient is woken with burning pain, tingling and numbness. Patients tend to seek relief by hanging the arm over the side of the bed or shaking the arm; however, merely changing the position of the wrist will usually help.

Early on, there is little to see, but there are two helpful tests that can reproduce sensory symptoms: *Tinel's sign* and *Phalen's test*.

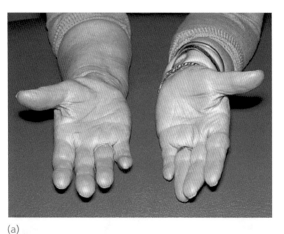

(a)

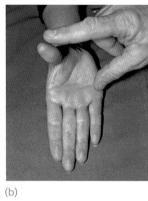

(b)

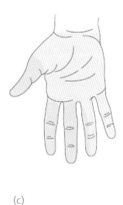

(c)

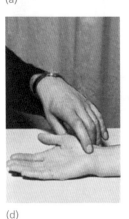

(d)

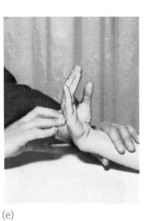

(e)

15.18 Median nerve compression (a) In the right hand there is wasting of the thenar eminence. **(b)** Testing for abductor power shows that it is weaker than that in the normal hand. **(c)** Area of diminished sensibility. **(d)** Tapping on the nerve may cause tingling in the hand (Tinel's sign), and holding the wrist flexed for 1 minute may also produce tingling in the median nerve distribution (Phalen's test) **(e)**.

TESTS FOR CARPAL TUNNEL SYNDROME	
Tinel's sign	Percuss over the median nerve.
Phalen's test	Hold the wrist fully flexed for 1 minute.

In late cases, there is wasting of the thenar muscles, weakness of thumb abduction and sensory dulling in the median nerve territory.

Electrodiagnostic tests, which show slowing of nerve conduction across the wrist, are reserved for those with atypical symptoms.

Radicular symptoms of cervical spondylosis may confuse the diagnosis and may coincide with carpal tunnel syndrome.

Treatment

Night splints   Preventing wrist flexion can help those with night pain or with pregnancy-related symptoms.

Steroid injection   Injection into the carpal canal, likewise, provides temporary relief.

Open surgical division   Division of the transverse carpal ligament usually provides a quick and simple cure; this can usually be done under local anaesthesia. The incision should be kept to the ulnar side of the thenar crease so as to avoid accidental injury to the palmar cutaneous (sensory) and thenar motor branches of the median nerve.

Endoscopic carpal tunnel release   This offers an alternative with slightly quicker postoperative rehabilitation.

SECTION 2 REGIONAL ORTHOPAEDICS

The hand

16

■ Clinical assessment   325
■ Congenital variations   329
■ Acquired deformities   329
■ Acute infections of the hand   336

■ Rheumatoid arthritis   340
■ Osteoarthritis   342
■ Vascular disorders of the hand   342
■ Other general disorders   344

CLINICAL ASSESSMENT

The hand is (in more senses than one) the medium of introduction to the outside world. Deformity and loss of function are quickly noticed – and often bitterly resented.

HISTORY

- *Pain* is usually felt in the palm or in the finger joints. A poorly defined ache may be referred from the neck, shoulder or mediastinum.
- *Swelling* may be localized, or may occur in many joints simultaneously. Characteristically, rheumatoid arthritis (RA) causes swelling of the proximal joints and osteoarthritis (OA) the distal joints.
- *Deformity* can appear suddenly (due to tendon rupture) or slowly (suggesting bone or joint pathology).
- *Loss of function* is particularly troublesome in the hand. The patient may have difficulty handling eating utensils, holding a cup or glass, grasping a doorknob (or a crutch), dressing or (most trying of all) attending to personal hygiene.

- *Sensory symptoms and motor weakness* provide clues to neurological disorders affecting the lower cervical nerve roots and their peripheral extensions.

EXAMINATION

Both upper limbs should be bared for comparison. Examination of the hand needs patience and meticulous attention to detail.

Look

Skin   The skin may be scarred, altered in colour, dry or moist, and hairy or smooth. Wasting and deformity, and the presence of any lumps, should be noted; a crimped appearance of the skin in the palm is characteristic of Dupuytren's contracture.

Position   The resting posture of the hand and fingers is an important clue to nerve or tendon damage.

Swelling   Swelling may be in the subcutaneous tissue, in a tendon sheath or in a joint – typically

SECTION 2 REGIONAL ORTHOPAEDICS

the metacarpophalangeal (MCP) joints in RA or the interphalangeal (IP) joints in OA.

Feel

Note the temperature and texture of the skin. Swelling or thickening may be in the subcutaneous tissue, a tendon sheath, a joint or one of the bones. If a nodule is felt, the underlying tendon should be moved by flexing the finger to discover if the nodule is attached to that tendon. Tenderness should be accurately localized to one of these structures.

Move

PASSIVE MOVEMENTS

Passive movements should be tested first, to see whether the joints are 'movable' before you ask the patient to move them actively. The range of movement for each digit is recorded, starting with the MCP joints and then going on to the proximal interphalangeal (PIP) and distal interphalangeal (DIP) joints.

ACTIVE MOVEMENTS

Active movements reflect, simultaneously, the state of the joints, the integrity of the tendons and motor nerve function in each digit.

Ask the patient to place both hands with palms facing upwards and the fingers extended, then to curl the fingers into full flexion; a 'lagging finger' is immediately obvious (16.1).

MCP flexion and IP extension are activated by the intrinsic muscles (lumbricals and interossei). This is tested by asking the patient to extend the fingers with the MCP joints flexed (the 'duckbill' position).

The interossei also motivate finger abduction and adduction (fingers together and then spread widely apart). Active power can be roughly gauged by having the patient abduct the fingers while the examiner presses against the spread-out index and little fingers, trying to force them back to the neutral position. A better way is to ask the patient to spread the fingers of both hands to the maximum; the examiner then grasps the patient's hands, pushes them towards each other and forces the two little fingers against each other; the weaker (non-dominant) side will normally give way first, but if the difference in one or other hand is marked it signifies true abductor weakness, a sign of ulnar nerve or T1 root dysfunction.

Thumb movements (and their nomenclature) are unusual, comprising the combined mobility of both the first carpometacarpal (CMC) and the first MCP joint. With the hand lying flat, palm upwards, five types of movement are recognized (16.2).

TYPES OF THUMB MOVEMENT	
Extension	Sideways movement in the plane of the palm
Abduction	Upward movement at right angles to the palm
Adduction	Pressing against the palm
Flexion	Sideways movement across the palm
Opposition	Touching the tips of the fingers

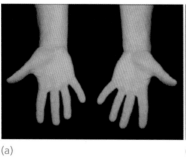 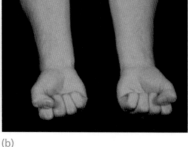 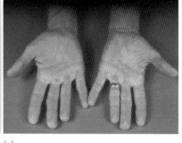

(a)   (b)   (c)

16.1 Examination – active movement **(a)** Extension. **(b)** Full flexion. **(c)** Testing finger abduction. The abducted little fingers are forced against each other; the weaker one will collapse 'lagging finger'.

Weakness of abduction (tested simply by pressing against the abducted thumb of each hand) is a cardinal feature of median nerve dysfunction. In advanced cases there will also be obvious wasting of the thenar eminence.

Pain, deformity and loss of motion at the base of the thumb (the first CMC joint) are common symptoms of OA.

Testing for musculotendinous function

FLEXOR DIGITORUM PROFUNDUS

Flexor digitorum profundus (*FDP*) is tested by simply immobilizing the PIP joint and then asking the patient to bend the tip of the finger (16.3).

FLEXOR DIGITORUM SUPERFICIALIS

Flexor digitorum superficialis (*FDS*) is more complicated. The FDP must first be inactivated, otherwise it is not possible to tell which of the two tendons is flexing the PIP joint. This is done by grasping all the fingers, except the one being examined, and holding them firmly in full extension; because the profundus tendons share a common muscle belly, this manoeuvre automatically prevents *all* the profundus tendons from

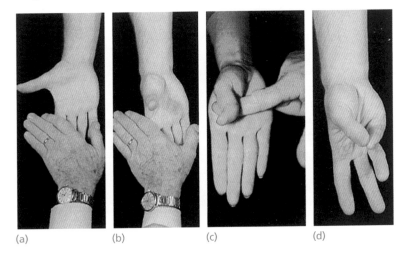

(a) (b) (c) (d)

16.2 Thumb movements Hold the patient's hand flat on the table and ask them to 'stretch to the side' (extension); **(b)** 'point to the ceiling' (abduction); **(c)** 'pinch my finger' (adduction); and **(d)** 'touch your little finger' (opposition).

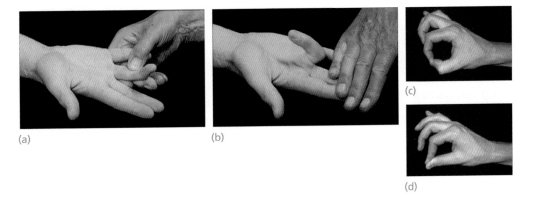

(a) (b) (c) (d)

16.3 Testing musculotendinous function (a) FDP lesser finger; **(b)** FDS lesser fingers; **(c)** FDP index; **(d)** FDS index.

participating in finger flexion. Then ask the patient to flex the isolated finger which is being examined; this movement must be activated by FDS.

There are two exceptions to this rule:

- The little finger sometimes has no independent FDS.
- The index finger often has a separate FDP which cannot be inactivated by the usual mass action manoeuvre.

Instead, for these two fingers FDS is tested by asking the patient to pinch hard with the DIP joint in full extension and the PIP joint in full flexion; this position can be maintained only if the superficialis tendon is active and intact.

LONG EXTENSORS

The *long extensors* are tested by asking the patient to extend the MCP joints. However, inability to do this does not necessarily signify paralysis or tendon rupture: the long extensor tendon may have slipped off the knuckle into the interdigital gutter (a common occurrence in RA).

FLEXOR POLLICIS LONGUS

Flexor pollicis longus is tested by immobilizing the thumb MCP joint and asking the patient to bend the single IP joint.

Grip strength

Grip strength is assessed (rather crudely) by asking the patient to squeeze the examiner's fingers; it may be diminished because of muscle weakness, tendon damage, finger stiffness or wrist instability. Strength can be measured more accurately with a mechanical dynamometer. Pinch grip should also be measured.

Neurological assessment

If symptoms such as numbness, tingling or weakness exist – and in all cases of trauma – a full neurological examination of the upper limbs should be carried out, testing power, reflexes and sensation. Further refinement is achieved by testing two-point discrimination, sensitivity to heat and cold (e16.1), stereognosis and fine pressure (see Chapter 11).

Functional tests

Function can be measured subjectively using patient-completed scales, but objective tests are more reliable. There are several types of grip (16.4), which can be tested by giving the patient a variety of tasks to perform.

FUNCTIONAL GRIP TESTS	
Precision grip	Picking up a pin
Pinch	Holding a sheet of paper
Sideways pinch	Holding a key
Chuck grip	Holding a pen
Hook grip	Holding a bag handle
Span	Holding a glass
Power grip	Gripping a hammer handle

Stereognosis is evaluated using Moberg's pickup test.

MOBERG'S PICKUP TEST FOR STEREOGNOSIS
Ask the patient to pick up and identify, with eyes closed, a number of objects from the desktop; the procedure is timed and the affected hand is compared with the 'good' hand.

Each finger has its special task: the thumb and index finger are used for pinch, but the index finger is also a sensory organ; slight loss of movement matters little, but if sensation is abnormal, the patient may not want to use the finger at all. The middle finger controls the position of objects in the palm. The ring and little fingers are used essentially for power grip (e.g. wielding a hammer or a wrench); stiffness is a real handicap.

Dexterity is important in all these functions; it may be lost in any type of nerve lesion, for example in a severe carpal tunnel syndrome (median nerve compression) because of the combination of thenar weakness, reduced sensation and diminished stereognosis and proprioception.

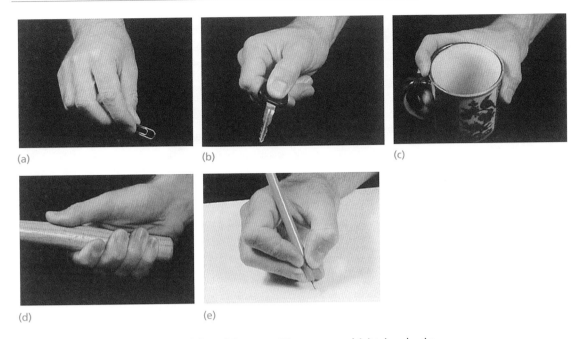

16.4 Hand function **(a)** Pinch, **(b)** key, **(c)** grasp, **(d)** power and **(e)** tripod grip.

CONGENITAL VARIATIONS

The hand and foot are much the most common sites of congenital deformities of the locomotor system; the incidence is about 1 : 1000 live births (16.5–16.7). Early recognition is important, and definitive treatment should be timed to fit in with the functional demands of the child.

There are seven types of malformation.

> **TYPES OF CONGENITAL HAND MALFORMATION**
>
> *Failure of formation* Total or partial absence of parts may be transverse ('congenital amputations') or axial (missing rays).
> *Failure of differentiation* Fingers may be partly or wholly joined together (syndactyly). This may be corrected by separating the fingers and repairing the defects with skin grafts.
> *Duplication* Polydactyly (extra digits) is the most common hand malformation. The extra finger should be amputated, if only for cosmetic reasons.

> *Undergrowth* The thumb can be very small or even absent.
> *Overgrowth* A giant finger is unsightly, but attempts at operative reduction are fraught with complications.
> *Constriction bands* These have the appearance of an elastic band constricting the finger. In the worst cases, this may lead to amputation.
> *Generalized malformations* The hand may be involved in generalized disorders such as Marfan's syndrome ('spider hands') or achondroplasia ('trident hand') (see Chapter 8).

Treatment may be relatively simple (e.g. removing an accessory small finger) but may be exceedingly complex.

ACQUIRED DEFORMITIES

Deformity may be due to disorders of:

- skin
- subcutaneous tissues

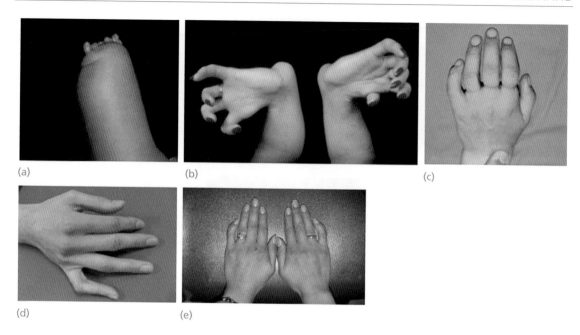

16.5 Congenital variations 1 (a) Transverse failure; **(b)** radial club hand and absent thumb; **(c)** constriction rings; **(d)** camptodactyly; **(e)** clinodactyly of both little fingers.

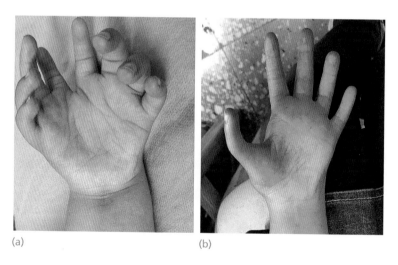

16.6 Congenital variations 2 (a) Mirror hand (also known as ulnar dimelia), with postoperative appearance **(b)** following removal of three rays and pollicization (where a thumb is created from an existing finger) of the fourth additional ray.

- muscles
- tendons
- joints
- bones
- neuromuscular function.

SKIN CONTRACTURE

Cuts and burns of the palmar skin are liable to heal with contracture; this may cause puckering of the palm or fixed flexion of the fingers.

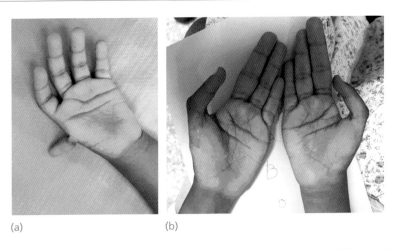

(a)   (b)

16.7 Congenital variations 3 (a) Hypoplastic thumb. **(b)** Two years following bilateral hypoplastic thumb amputation and index finger pollicization.

> ⚠ Surgical incisions should never cross flexor creases.

Established contractures may require excision of the scar and Z-plasty of the overlying skin.

DUPUYTREN'S CONTRACTURE

This is a nodular hypertrophy and contracture of the collagen within the fatty pulp of the hand. The condition is usually familial, but there is a higher than usual incidence in people with diabetes and epilepsy. Smoking and heavy alcohol consumption are also risk factors.

Clinical features

The patient – usually a middle-aged man – complains of a nodular thickening in the palm or a finger. This progresses gradually to pull down the MCP or the PIP joint. Pain is unusual (**16.8**).

 Similar nodules may be seen on the back of the finger joints (*Garrod's pads*), the soles of the feet (Ledderhose's disease) (**e16.2**) and the penis (*Peyronie's disease*).

Diagnosis

Dupuytren's contracture must be distinguished from skin contracture (where a previous laceration is usually obvious) and tendon contracture (where the 'cord' moves on passive flexion of the finger).

Treatment

If the deformity is static and there is no loss of function, no treatment is needed.

If the condition is causing symptoms (usually when the contracture is more than 30 degrees or the hand cannot go flat on a table), then treatment is considered (**16.9**). If the cord is very narrow and well defined, division with multiple perforations using a hypodermic needle ('percutaneous needle fasciotomy') is safe, quick and effective although the recurrence rate is very high. Broader cords can be treated with collagenase injections which dissolve the collagen. This avoids the risks and longer recovery of surgery but recurrence is high.

Surgery is more thorough and thus has a lower recurrence and usually a better correction; however there is a higher risk than a needle technique, and infection, nerve damage and hand stiffness can all occur. The aim is reasonable, not complete, correction; a satisfactory outcome is more predictable at the MCP joint than the PIP joint, but there is still a risk of recurrence or extension. For very dense disease or recurrent disease, a skin graft gives the most durable correction.

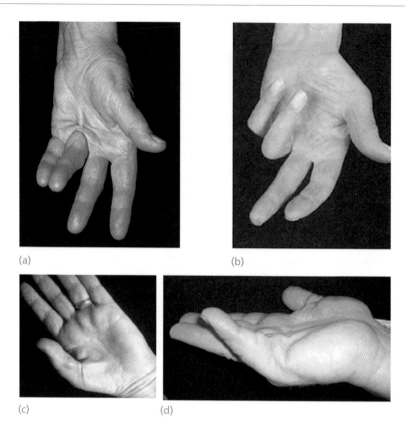

(a) (b)

(c) (d)

16.8 Dupuytren's disease Contractures may occur at **(a)** palmar crease, **(b)** PIP joint, **(c)** thumb web, **(d)** little finger.

NEUROMUSCULAR DISORDERS

Ulnar 'claw hand' (intrinsic-minus deformity)

Ulnar nerve lesions characteristically cause hyperextension at the MCP joints and flexion at the IP joints. This is due to paralysis of the intrinsic muscles which normally activate MCP flexion and IP extension. Thus it is sometimes called an *intrinsic-minus deformity* (**16.10**).

Shortening of intrinsic muscles (intrinsic-plus deformity)

Intrinsic muscle shortening produces flexion at the MCP joints with extension of the IP joints and adduction of the thumb – an *intrinsic-plus deformity*. Anatomically, this is the opposite of the intrinsic-minus deformity described above.

The main causes are muscle scarring or shortening after trauma or infection. Moderate contracture can be treated by releasing the intrinsic muscles where they cross the MCP joints.

Ischaemic contracture of the forearm muscles

This follows circulatory insufficiency due to injuries at or below the elbow. There is shortening of the long flexors; the fingers are held in flexion and can be straightened only when the wrist is flexed (**16.11**). Sometimes the picture is complicated by associated damage to the ulnar or median nerve (or both). If disability is marked, some improvement may be obtained by releasing the shortened muscles at their origin above the elbow, or else by excising the dead muscles and restoring finger movement with tendon transfers.

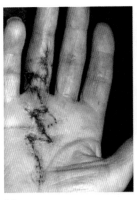
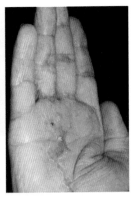

(a)

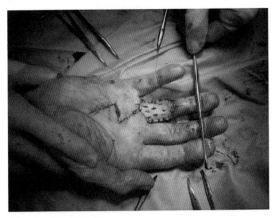

(b)

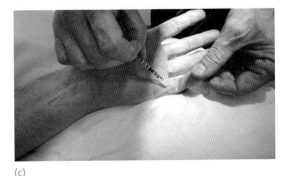

(c)

16.9 Dupuytren's disease – treatment (a) Z-plasty in the hand shortly after operation and 2 weeks later when healing is almost complete; **(b)** skin graft in theatre; **(c)** collagenase injection.

Spastic paresis

Cerebral palsy, head injury and stroke may result in typical deformities of the hand (**16.12**). The 'intrinsic-plus' posture is easily recognized.

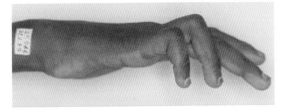

(a)

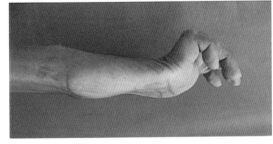

(b)

16.10 Ulnar 'claw-hand' (a) *High ulnar nerve paralysis* causing a *partial claw-hand deformity*: the paralysed intrinsic muscles cause the loss of flexion at the MCP joints and loss of extension at the IP joints, but because FDP is also partially paralysed the index and middle fingers are straight. **(b)** *Low ulnar nerve paralysis* (lower than the innervation of FDP), causing a *total claw-hand deformity* in which all the long flexors are still active.

Another common disability is 'thumb-in-palm'; the tendency to adduct and flex the thumb into the palm is increased by activity, especially finger flexion. Releasing the adductor pollicis from the third metacarpal may improve the appearance, but normal thumb pinch is rarely restored.

Tendon lesions

'Mallet' finger

The patient suddenly cannot straighten the terminal joint, but passive movement is normal (**16.13**). This is due to injury at the attachment of the extensor tendon to the terminal phalanx. The DIP joint should be splinted for 8 weeks, with the proximal joint free.

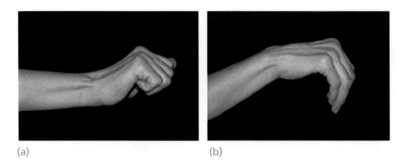

(a)   (b)

16.11 Contracture of the long flexors (a) When the wrist is extended, the fingers involuntarily curl into tight flexion. **(b)** When the wrist is flexed, tension on the long flexor muscles is relaxed and the fingers can uncurl to a certain extent.

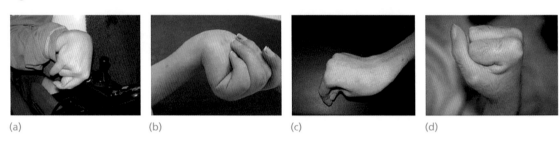

(a)   (b)   (c)   (d)

16.12 Spastic contracture – hand deformities (a–c) cerebral palsy, and **(d)** head injury with brain damage.

Ruptured extensor pollicis longus

The long thumb extensor may rupture after fraying where it crosses the wrist (e.g. after a Colles' fracture, or in RA). Direct repair is unsatisfactory and a tendon transfer, using the extensor indicis, is needed.

Dropped fingers

The patient is unable to hold the fingers in extension at the MCP joints. The cause usually lies not at the MCP joint but at the wrist, where the extensor tendons have ruptured (typically in RA).

If only one finger is affected, direct repair may be possible; otherwise the distal portion of the tendon can be attached to an adjacent finger extensor.

Boutonnière deformity

This is a flexion deformity of the PIP joint, due to interruption of the central slip of the extensor tendon. The lateral slips separate and the head of the proximal phalanx pops through the gap like a finger through a buttonhole. It is seen after trauma or in rheumatoid disease.

Post-traumatic rupture can sometimes be repaired; the chronic deformity in rheumatoid disease usually defies correction (e16.3).

Swan-neck deformity

This is the reverse of boutonnière: the PIP joint is hyperextended and the DIP joint flexed. It is due to imbalance of extensor versus flexor action in the finger, and is often seen in RA.

The deformity may be corrected by tendon rebalancing.

'Trigger finger'

This common condition presents as an intermittent 'deformity', usually of the ring or middle finger, sometimes of the thumb. The patient complains that, when the hand is clenched and then opened, the finger (or thumb) gets stuck in

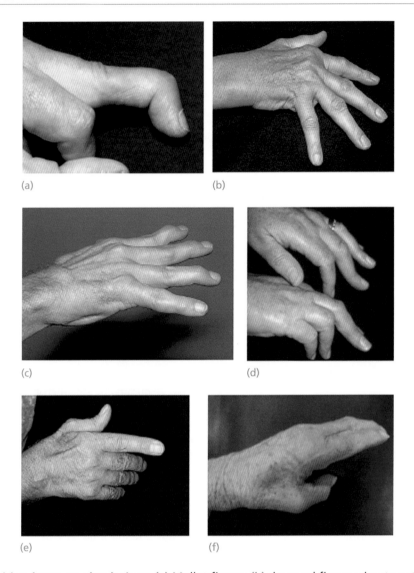

16.13 Deformities due to tendon lesions (a) Mallet finger; (b) dropped fingers due to extensor tendon ruptures at the wrist; (c) swan-neck deformities; (d) boutonnière deformities; (e) rupture of extensor pollicis brevis; (f) rupture of extensor pollicis longus.

flexion; with a little more effort, it suddenly snaps into full extension. The usual cause is thickening of the fibrous tendon sheath: the flexor tendon becomes temporarily trapped at the entrance to its sheath and then, on forced extension, it passes the constriction with a snap. A similar entrapment may occur due to a bulky tenosynovitis (e.g. in rheumatic disorders). A tender nodule or thickened tendon can usually be felt at the distal palmar crease. The condition is more common in diabetes.

Infantile trigger thumb ('snapping thumb) is usually misdiagnosed as a 'dislocating thumb'; sometimes it goes completely undiagnosed and the child grows up with the thumb permanently bent or the distal phalanx underdeveloped. Feel for the tell-tale thickening on the palmar aspect at the base of the thumb.

SECTION 2 REGIONAL ORTHOPAEDICS

Treatment

The condition often improves spontaneously, so there is no urgency about treatment. However, if it persists, or is particularly annoying, it can usually be cured by an injection of corticosteroid carefully placed at the entrance of the tendon sheath (e16.4).

Refractory cases need operation: the fibrous sheath is incised, allowing the tendon to move freely. In the case of the thumb, take particular care to avoid injuring the digital nerve, which runs close to the sheath.

For children, treatment can be deferred until the child is 3 years old, as spontaneous recovery is quite common.

BONE LESIONS

Malunited fractures may cause metacarpal or phalangeal deformity. This occasionally needs correction by osteotomy and internal fixation.

ACUTE INFECTIONS OF THE HAND

Infection of the hand is frequently limited to one of several well-defined compartments:

- under the nailfold (paronychia)
- the pulp space (whitlow)
- subcutaneous tissues elsewhere
- a tendon sheath
- one of the deep fascial spaces
- a joint.

The cause is almost invariably a *Staphylococcus* which has been implanted by trivial or unobserved injury.

Pathology

Acute inflammation and suppuration in small closed compartments (e.g. the pulp space or tendon sheath) may cause an increase in pressure to levels at which the local blood supply is threatened.

In neglected cases of infection, *tissue necrosis* is an imminent risk. Even if this does not occur, the patient may end up with a stiff and useless hand unless the infection is rapidly brought under control.

Clinical features

Usually there is a history of trauma, but it may have been so trivial as to pass unnoticed. A thorn prick can be as dangerous as a cut. Within a day or two, the finger (or hand) becomes painful and tensely swollen. The patient may feel ill and feverish and the pain becomes throbbing. There is obvious redness and tension in the tissues, and exquisite tenderness over the site of infection. Finger movements may be markedly restricted.

Principles of treatment

ANTIBIOTICS

As soon as the diagnosis is made and specimens have been taken for microbiological investigation, antibiotic treatment is started – usually with flucloxacillin and, in severe cases, with fusidic acid or a cephalosporin as well. This may later be changed when bacterial sensitivity is known.

REST AND ELEVATION

- *In a mild case*, the hand is rested in a sling.
- *In a severe case*, the arm is elevated in a roller towel while the patient is kept in hospital under observation.

Analgesics are given for pain.

DRAINAGE

If there are signs of an abscess (throbbing pain, marked tenderness and toxaemia), the pus should be drained (16.14). A tourniquet and either general or regional block anaesthesia are essential. The incision should be made at the site of maximal tenderness, *but never across a skin crease*. Necrotic tissue is excised and the area thoroughly washed and cleansed. The wound is either left open or lightly sutured and then covered with non-stick dressings. A pus specimen is sent for microbiological investigation.

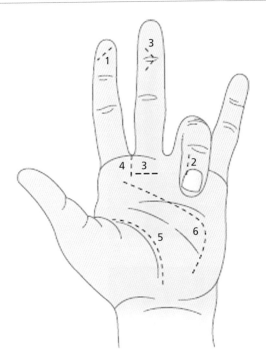

16.14 Incisions for infection The incisions for surgical drainage are illustrated here: (1), pulp space (directly over the abscess); (2), nailfold (it may also be necessary to excise the edge of the nail); (3), tendon sheath (two incisions, one distal and one proximal); (4), web space; (5), thenar space; 6, midpalmar space.

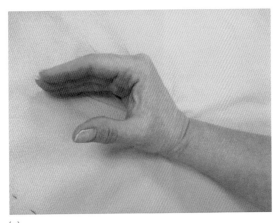

(a)

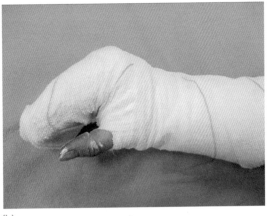

(b)

16.15 Position of safe immobilization (a,b) The MCP joints are 70° flexed, the finger joints extended and the thumb abducted. This is the position in which the ligaments are at their longest and splintage is least likely to result in stiffness.

SPLINTAGE

After draining tendon sheath or fascial space infections or if conservative treatment is likely to be prolonged, a removable splint should be applied, always with the joints in the position of safe immobilization (16.15).

POSITION OF SAFE IMMOBILIZATION
Wrist slightly extended MCP joints in 70° flexion IP joints extended Thumb in abduction

PHYSIOTHERAPY

Once the acute inflammation subsides, movements are encouraged. Ideally, this should be done under the direction of a physiotherapist specialized in 'hand therapy'. The splint is reapplied between exercise sessions.

SPECIFIC TYPES OF INFECTION

Paronychia

Infection under the nailfold is common (16.16). The area is swollen, red and tender.

At the first sign of infection, antibiotic treatment alone may be effective. If pus is present, it can often be released simply by lifting the

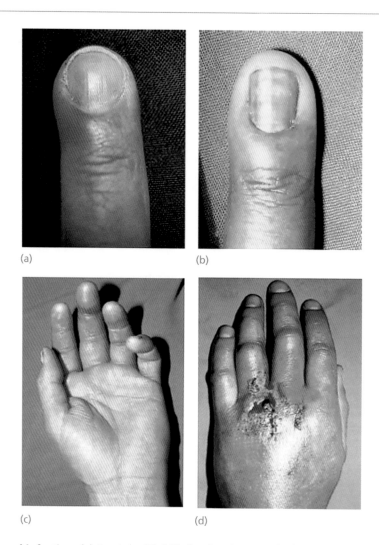

(a)   (b)

(c)   (d)

16.16 Types of hand infection (a) Acute nailfold infection (paronychia); **(b)** chronic paronychia; **(c)** flexor tenosynovitis of the middle finger following a cortisone injection; **(d)** septic human bite resulting in acute infection of the fourth MCP joint.

nailfold from the nail; otherwise the nailfold must be incised. Occasionally, a portion of the nail needs to be removed.

Pulp-space infection (felon)

Pulp-space infection (usually due to a prick or splinter) causes throbbing pain. The fingertip is swollen, red and acutely tender.

Antibiotic treatment is started immediately. However, if pus has formed, it must be released

through a small incision over the site of maximal tenderness.

Other subcutaneous infection

Anywhere in the hand, a blister or superficial cut may become infected, causing redness, swelling and tenderness.

A local collection of pus should be drained through a small incision over the site of maximal tenderness. It is important to exclude a deeper pocket of pus in a nearby tendon sheath or in one of the deep fascial spaces.

Tendon-sheath infection

Suppurative tenosynovitis is uncommon but dangerous (e16.5). The affected digit is painful and swollen; it is held bent, is very tender and the patient will not move it or permit it to be moved.

> ⚠ Unless treatment is swift and effective, there is a risk of *tendon necrosis* and the patient may end up with a useless finger.

KANAVEL'S SIGNS OF FLEXOR SHEATH INFECTION

Flexed posture of digit
Tenderness along the course of the tendon
Pain on passive finger extension
Pain on active flexion

TREATMENT

Treatment must be started as soon as the diagnosis is suspected. The hand is splinted and elevated and antibiotics are administered intravenously – initially a broad-spectrum penicillin or a systemic cephalosporin, to be modified if necessary once the organism has been cultured and tested for antibiotic sensitivity.

If there is no improvement after 24 hours, surgical drainage is essential. Two incisions are needed, one at the proximal end of the sheath and one at the distal end; using a fine catheter, the sheath is then irrigated with saline or Ringer's lactate solution (always from proximal to distal). The catheter is left in place for postoperative irrigation during the next 2 days.

> ⚠ A flexor tendon sheath infection needs immediate washout.

Tendon-sheath infection in the thumb or little finger may spread proximally to the synovial bursa. This has to be drained through a further incision just above the wrist.

At the end of the operation, the hand is swathed in absorbent dressings and splinted in the position of safe immobilization (see 16.15).

Deep fascial space infection

Infection from a web space or from an infected tendon sheath may spread to either of the deep fascial spaces of the palm. The palm is ballooned, so its normal concavity is lost. There is extensive tenderness and the whole hand is held still.

For drainage, an incision is made directly over the abscess and sinus forceps inserted; if the web space is also infected, it too should be incised. Postoperatively the hand is dressed and splinted as described above.

Joint infection

Any of the joints may be infected, either directly by a penetrating injury on injection, or indirectly from adjacent structures. At the onset, the clinical features may be hard to distinguish from those of acute gout. Joint aspiration will provide the answer.

Intravenous antibiotics are administered and the hand is splinted. If symptoms and signs do not improve within 24 hours, open drainage is needed.

Bites

Animal bites are usually inflicted by cats, dogs or farm animals. Many become infected and, although the common pathogens are staphylococci and streptococci, unusual organisms are also encountered.

Human bites and lacerations sustained during fist-fights are generally thought to be even more prone to infection. A variety of organisms (including anaerobes) are encountered, the commonest being *Staphylococcus aureus*, *Streptococcus* group A and *Eikenella corrodens*. All such wounds should be assumed to be infected. *X-rays* should be obtained, to exclude a fracture or foreign body.

TREATMENT

Treatment should be started immediately. Fresh wounds are carefully examined in the operating

SECTION 2 REGIONAL ORTHOPAEDICS

theatre and swab samples are taken for bacterial culture and sensitivity. If necessary, the wound should be extended and debrided; search for a fragment of tooth or a divit of articular cartilage from the joint. The hand is then splinted and elevated and antibiotics are given prophylactically until the laboratory results are obtained.

Established infection in bite wounds will need debridement, washouts and intravenous antibiotic treatment. The common organisms are all sensitive to broad-spectrum penicillins and cephalosporins. With animal bites, one should also consider the possibility of rabies.

Postoperative treatment consists, as usual, of copious wound dressings, splintage in the 'safe' position and encouragement of movement once the infection has resolved. Tendon lacerations can be dealt with when the tissues are completely healed.

> A human bite over the back of the knuckle – 'fight bite' – needs immediate and thorough washout.

RHEUMATOID ARTHRITIS

The hand, more than any other part of the body, is where RA displays its story.

PROGRESSION OF RA IN THE HAND

1 *Early on*, there is synovitis of the proximal joints and tendon sheaths.
2 *Later*, joint and tendon erosions prepare the ground for mechanical derangement.
3 *In the final stage*, joint instability and tendon rupture cause progressive deformity and loss of function.

Clinical features

Pain and stiffness of the fingers are early symptoms; often the wrist also is affected. Examination may show swelling of the MCP and PIP joints; both hands are affected, more or less symmetrically. Joint mobility and grip strength are diminished.

As the disease progresses, deformities begin to appear (and are increasingly difficult to correct) (**16.17**). In the late stage, one sees the characteristic ulnar deviation of the fingers and subluxation of the MCP joints, often associated with swan-neck or boutonnière deformities. When these abnormalities become fixed, functional loss may be so severe that the patient needs help with washing, dressing and feeding.

X-rays

- *During the initial stages*, X-rays show only soft-tissue swelling and osteoporosis around the joints (**16.18a**).
- *Later*, there is narrowing of the joint spaces and small periarticular erosions appear (**16.18b**).
- *In the last stage*, articular destruction may be marked, with joint deformity and dislocation (**16.18c**).

Treatment

In early cases, treatment is directed at controlling the systemic disease and the local synovitis. In addition to general measures, splints may reduce pain and swelling.

Persistent synovitis may benefit from local injections of methylprednisolone, but sometimes surgical synovectomy is needed.

As the disease progresses, it becomes important to prevent deformity. Splinting is useful (**e16.6**). Uncontrolled synovitis requires synovectomy (**e16.7**) followed by physiotherapy. Isolated tendon ruptures are repaired or bypassed by appropriate tendon transfers. Joint instability may require stabilization or arthroplasty.

In late cases with established deformities, reconstructive surgery may be needed (**16.19**), but treatment should be directed at restoring function rather than merely correcting deformity.

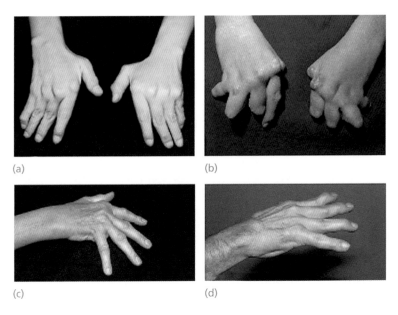

(a)

(b)

(c)

(d)

16.17 Rheumatoid arthritis **(a)** Typical deformities in established RA. The proximal joints are the ones most severely affected; there is subluxation of the MCP joints and the fingers are deviated ulnar-wards. **(b)** Severe rheumatoid deformities with dislocation of the MCP joints and ulceration of the skin over the knuckles. **(c)** 'Dropped fingers' due to rupture of extensor tendons where they cross the back of the wrist. **(d)** Swan-neck deformities of the fingers.

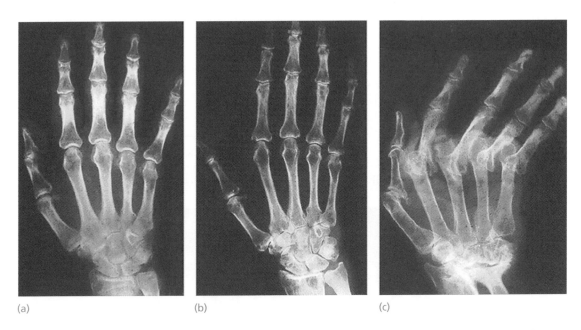

(a)

(b)

(c)

16.18 Rheumatoid arthritis – X-ray changes **(a)** Early on, the X-rays may show no more than soft-tissue swelling and juxta-articular osteoporosis. **(b)** A later stage showing characteristic tiny punched-out juxta-articular erosions at the second and third MCP joints. The wrist is now also involved. **(c)** In the most advanced stage, the MCP joints are dislocated and the hand is severely deformed.

SECTION 2 REGIONAL ORTHOPAEDICS

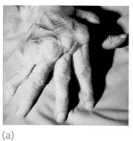
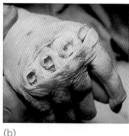
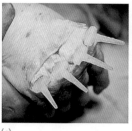
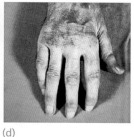

(a)   (b)   (c)   (d)

16.19 Rheumatoid arthritis – joint replacement (a) Before operation there is subluxation and deformity of all the finger MCP joints. **(b,c)** The eroded metacarpal heads are excised and flexible spacers inserted. **(d)** Postoperative result.

OSTEOARTHRITIS

OA of the DIP joints is very common in post-menopausal women and is usually a manifestation of polyarticular OA. It often starts with pain in one or two fingers; the distal joints become swollen and tender, the condition usually spreading to all the fingers of both hands. On examination, there is bony thickening around the DIP joints (Heberden's nodes) and some restriction of movement (**16.20**). Not infrequently, some of the PIP joints are involved (Bouchard's nodes) (**e16.8**) and the CMC joint of the thumb may show similar changes.

The distinction from RA is very important. In both conditions, the finger joints are swollen and stiff. However, whereas RA affects the proximal joints (particularly the MCP joints), OA affects mainly the terminal IP joints.

Treatment is symptomatic; pain and tenderness gradually subside and the patient is left with painless, knobbly fingers. Occasionally (if pain or

deformity is particularly marked), fusion of the DIP joint may be called for. If the PIP joint or the MCP joint are involved they can be replaced (**16.21**).

VASCULAR DISORDERS OF THE HAND

EMBOLI

Arising from the heart or from aneurysms in the arteries of the upper limb, emboli can lodge in distal vessels causing splinter haemorrhages, or in larger, more proximal vessels, causing ischaemia of the arm. A large embolus leads to the classic signs of pain, pulselessness, paraesthesia, pallor and paralysis. Untreated, gangrene or ischaemic contracture ensues.

> ⚠ If emboli are suspected, urgent assessment and treatment are required.

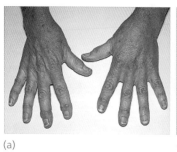

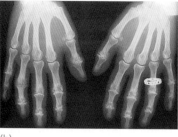
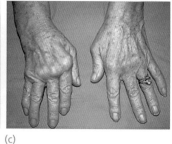

(a)   (b)   (c)

16.20 Osteoarthritis (a,b) OA affects mainly the DIP joints. The knobbly joints are called Heberden's nodes. **(c)** RA can look similar, but here it is mainly the proximal joints that are affected.

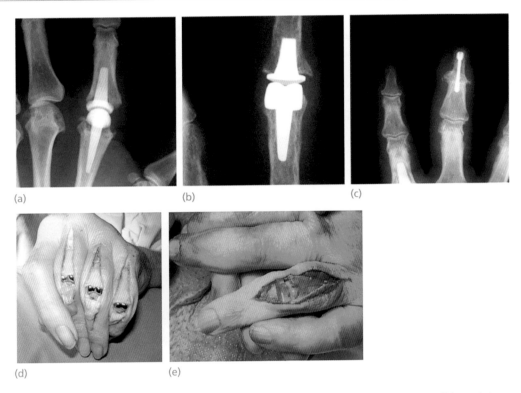

16.21 Osteoarthritis – operative treatment **(a)** Pyrocarbon MCP joint replacement; **(b)** PIP joint replacement; **(c)** arthrodesis of the DIP joint; **(d)** cobalt-chrome on polythene PIP replacement; **(e)** silastic PIP replacement.

RAYNAUD'S DISEASE

Raynaud's syndrome

Raynaud's syndrome is produced by a vasospastic disorder which affects mainly the hands and fingers. Attacks are usually precipitated by cold; the fingers go pale and icy, then dusky blue (or cyanotic) and finally red. Between attacks the hands look normal. The condition is most commonly seen in young women who have no underlying or predisposing disease.

Raynaud's phenomenon

This is the term applied when these changes are associated with an underlying disease such as scleroderma or arteriosclerosis. Similar, though milder, changes are also seen in thoracic outlet syndrome. The hands must be kept warm. Calcium channel blockade, iloprost infusions, botulinum toxin or digital sympathectomy (surgical removal of the sympathetic plexus around the digital arteries) may be needed.

GLOMUS TUMOUR

A glomus tumour is a rare but very troublesome condition (e16.9). Formed of small neural and vascular elements, it is very painful, especially in colder weather. On examination. there is a very localized and exquisitely tender spot, usually under or just alongside the nail bed.

Treatment is by removal under local anaesthetic after very careful pinpoint marking before surgery.

HAND–ARM VIBRATION SYNDROME

Excessive use of vibrating tools can damage the nerves and vessels in the fingers. There are two components: vascular and neurological.

- The *vascular component* is similar to Raynaud's phenomenon, with the fingertips turning white in cold weather, then changing through blue and red as the circulation is restored.
- The *neurological component* involves numbness and tingling in the fingertips. In advanced cases, there can be reduced dexterity.

Treatment is generally unsatisfactory, but includes avoidance of cold weather and smoking as well as, of course, vibrating tools.

OTHER GENERAL DISORDERS

A number of generalized disorders should always be borne in mind when considering the diagnosis of any unusual lesion that appears to be confined to the hand. It is beyond the scope of this text to enlarge on these conditions. The few examples shown in **16.22** serve merely as a reminder that a general history and examination are as important as focused attention on the hand.

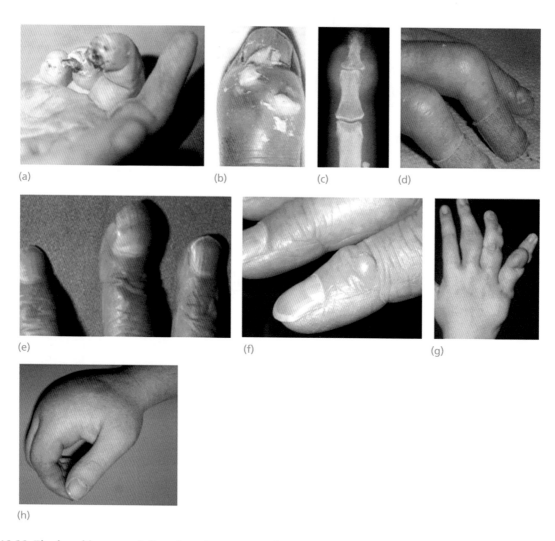

(a)   (b)   (c)   (d)

(e)   (f)   (g)

(h)

16.22 The hand in general disorders Some general conditions that may manifest with lesions in the hand: **(a)** scleroderma; **(b,c)** gouty tophi; **(d)** psoriasis; **(e)** implantation dermoid; **(f)** dermatofibroma; **(g)** Maffucci's syndrome; **(h)** Secretan's syndrome (hand oedema due to repetitive trauma, self-inflicted).

The neck

17

- Anatomy   345
- Clinical assessment   346
- Deformities of the neck   349
- Vertebral anomalies   349
- Acute intervertebral disc prolapse   350
- Chronic disc degeneration (Cervical spondylosis)   352
- Pyogenic infection   354
- Tuberculosis   354
- Rheumatoid arthritis   355
- Ankylosing spondylitis   357

ANATOMY

The cervical spine consists of seven vertebrae with a lordosis of 16 to 25 degrees. Palpable neck landmarks include:

- *hyoid bone*, which is at the level of C3
- *thyroid cartilage*, which lies at C4
- *cricoid cartilage*, which lies at C6.

The atlas (C1) is ring-shaped with no vertebral body or spinous process. It has large lateral masses that support the occipital condyles. The axis (C2) has a characteristic peg projecting proximally (the dens) which articulates with the atlas. The joint between C1 and C2 accounts for approximately 50% of cervical spine rotation. C3 to C7 are similar in shape.

The cervical articular facets lie at 0 degrees in the coronal plane and 40–55 degrees in the sagittal plane. The spinous processes are often bifid from C2 to C6 and C7 is longer (the vertebra prominens) (17.1).

The cervical spine contains eight pairs of nerve roots, exiting above the similarly numbered vertebrae through relatively narrow neural

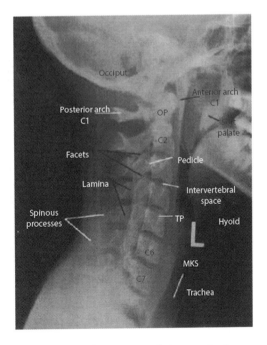

17.1 Radiological anatomy of the cervical region (Reproduced with permission from: Todd, M.M. Cervical spine anatomy and function for the anesthesiologist. *Can J Anaesth* 2001; 48 (Suppl 1): R1–R5.)

SECTION 2 REGIONAL ORTHOPAEDICS

foramina, making them vulnerable to compression from herniated disc material.

HISTORY

The common symptoms of neck disorder are pain and stiffness.

- *Pain* is felt in the neck itself, but it can be referred to the suprascapular areas, the shoulders or the upper arms. It may start suddenly (as with an acute intervertebral disc prolapse) or gradually (as in chronic disc degeneration). Always ask if it is associated with arm or hand paraesthesia.
- *Stiffness* may be either intermittent or continuous. Very restricted movement is often caused by muscle spasm as a protective reflex.
- *Deformity* usually appears as a wry neck, due to muscle spasm; think of a disc prolapse or a previously undiagnosed fracture.
- *Numbness, tingling and weakness* in the upper limbs may be due to pressure on a nerve root; weakness in the lower limbs may result from cord compression in the neck.
- *Headache* sometimes emanates from the neck, but if this is the only symptom, other causes are more likely.

 Always ask about previous neck injuries.

EXAMINATION

With the patient standing, look for unsteadiness and ask the patient to walk assessing the gait pattern. The upper trunk and upper limbs should be exposed (**17.2**). Start with the patient standing to observe neck posture, movements and shoulders. The anterior structures (trachea, thyroid and oesophagus) are best felt with the patient seated and the examiner standing behind the chair. The third part of the examination is carried out with the patient lying down; it is easier (and more reliable) to feel for muscle spasm

and point tenderness with the patient lying prone with their neck supported over a pillow. Neurological examination is performed with the patient lying supine.

Look

Any deformity is noted. From the back, skin blemishes, scapular abnormalities or muscular asymmetry can be seen. One shoulder may be higher and there may be muscle wasting in the arm or hand. Note any asymmetry of the pupils, drooping eye lids and dry skin, characteristics of Horner syndrome.

Feel

The neck and shoulders should be carefully palpated for tender areas, lumps and muscle spasm. Feel the neck in the four quadrants – anterior, posterior and lateral (left and right).

Move

Flexion, extension, lateral flexion and rotation are tested and the range of movements noted (**17.3**). Shoulder movements, likewise, should be recorded.

SPURLING'S TEST OF NECK MOVEMENT

The patient is instructed to rotate the neck to one side with the chin elevated: if this reproduces ipsilateral upper limb pain and paraesthesiae, it would increase the suspicion of a disc prolapse with cervical nerve root compression. Pain may be relieved by having the patient place the arm overhead (the abduction relief sign).

Neurological examination

Neurological examination of the upper limbs is mandatory in all cases; in some, the lower limbs also should be examined. Muscle power, reflexes and sensation should be carefully tested; even small degrees of abnormality may be significant.

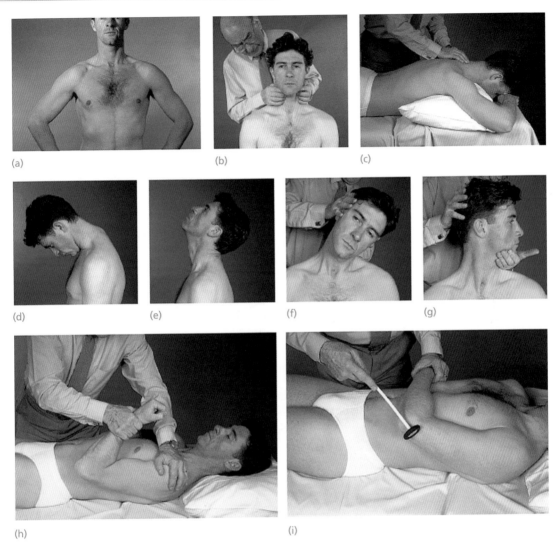

17.2 Examination (a) Look for any deformity or superficial blemish which might suggest a disorder affecting the cervical spine. **(b)** The front of the neck is felt with the patient seated and the examiner standing behind him. **(c)** The back of the neck is most easily and reliably felt with the patient lying prone over a pillow; this way muscle spasm is reduced and the neck is relaxed. **(d–g)** Movement: flexion ('chin on chest'); extension ('look up at the ceiling'); lateral flexion ('tilt your ear towards your shoulder'); and rotation ('look over your shoulder'). **(h,i)** Neurological examination is mandatory.

INVESTIGATION

Imaging

X-RAYS

X-ray examination should include all levels from the base of the occiput to T1. The standard series includes anteroposterior, lateral and open-mouth views (**17.4**).

- The *anteroposterior view* should show the outlines of the lateral masses; symmetry may be disturbed by destructive lesions or fractures.
- The *open-mouth view* shows the upper two vertebrae. The lateral margin of the atlas should align with the lateral margin of the axis and the space on each side of the dens should be equal.

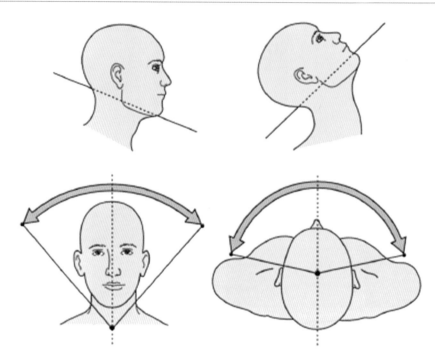

17.3 Normal range of motion Flexion and extension of the neck are best gauged by observing the angle of the occipitomental line, an imaginary line joining the tip of the chin and the occipital protuberance. In full flexion, the chin normally touches the chest; in full extension, the occipitomental line forms an angle of at least 45° with the horizontal, and more than 60° in young people. Lateral flexion is usually achieved up to 45° and rotation to 80° each way.

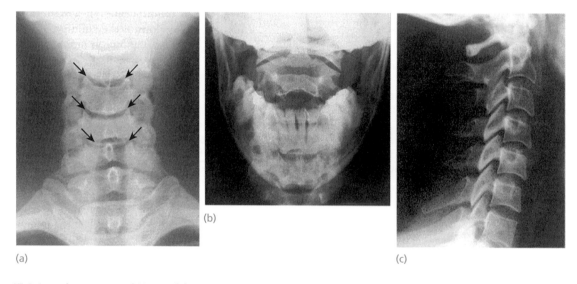

(a)

(b)

(c)

17.4 Imaging – normal X-rays (a) Anteroposterior view – note the smooth, symmetrical outlines and the clear, wide uncovertebral joints (arrows). **(b)** Open-mouth view – to show the odontoid process and atlantoaxial joints. **(c)** Lateral view – showing all seven cervical vertebrae.

- The *lateral view* should always include the base of the skull and the cervicothoracic junction, especially in trauma. If this is not achieved, additional oblique or lateral dynamic views in flexion and extension can be obtained in the cooperative and neurologically intact patient guided by the physician. The normal cervical curve shows four parallel lines: one along the anterior surfaces of the vertebral bodies, one along their posterior surfaces, one along the posterior borders of the lateral masses and one along the bases of the spinous processes; any malalignment suggests subluxation.

Inspect the disc spaces: loss of disc height and the presence of osteophytic spurs at the margins of adjacent vertebral bodies are features of chronic intervertebral disc degeneration, a common finding in elderly people and not necessarily the cause of neck pain. Also compare the posterior interspinous spaces: if one is wider than the rest, this may signify chronic instability of that segment, possibly due to a previously undiagnosed subluxation. An increase in the prevertebral cervical space in the context of trauma should raise a red flag and demands further investigation.

COMPUTED TOMOGRAPHY AND MAGNETIC RESONANCE IMAGING

Computed tomography (CT) and *magnetic resonance imaging (MRI)* are essential for defining detailed osseous anatomy, the intervertebral discs, the neural structures and the outlines of the spinal canal and intervertebral foramina. Remember, though, that 20% of asymptomatic people show radiological abnormalities and the scans must therefore be interpreted alongside the clinical assessment.

DEFORMITIES OF THE NECK

TORTICOLLIS ('WRY NECK', 'SKEW NECK')

In torticollis the chin is twisted upwards and towards one side. It may be either *congenital* or *secondary* to other local disorders.

Infantile (congenital) torticollis

Skew neck is sometimes seen in an infant or very young child. The sternocleidomastoid muscle on one side is fibrous and fails to elongate as the child grows. In some cases, a well-defined lump is felt in the muscle during the first few weeks of life, but deformity may not become apparent until the child is 2–3 years old. As the neck grows, the contracted sternocleidomastoid tethers the skull on one side, thus twisting the chin towards the opposite side (17.5). Secondary facial deformities may occur.

TREATMENT

If a child has a sternocleidomastoid 'tumour', subsequent deformity may be prevented by gentle, daily manipulation of the neck. Non-operative treatment is successful in most cases, but if the condition persists beyond 1 year, operative treatment is required to prevent progressive facial deformity. The contracted muscle is divided (usually at its lower end but sometimes at the upper end or at both ends) and the head is manipulated into the neutral position. After operation, correction is maintained with a temporary orthosis followed by stretching exercises.

Secondary torticollis

Wry neck, due to muscle spasm, may develop as a result of acute disc prolapse (the most common cause in adults), inflamed neck glands, vertebral infection, injuries of the cervical spine or ocular disorders.

VERTEBRAL ANOMALIES

Cervical vertebral anomalies are dealt with in Chapter 8. Odontoid dysplasia is particularly important and the subject warrants repetition in this section.

ODONTOID ANOMALIES

The odontoid may be absent or hypoplastic, an anomaly that should be suspected (and looked for even if the patient does not complain) in any case of

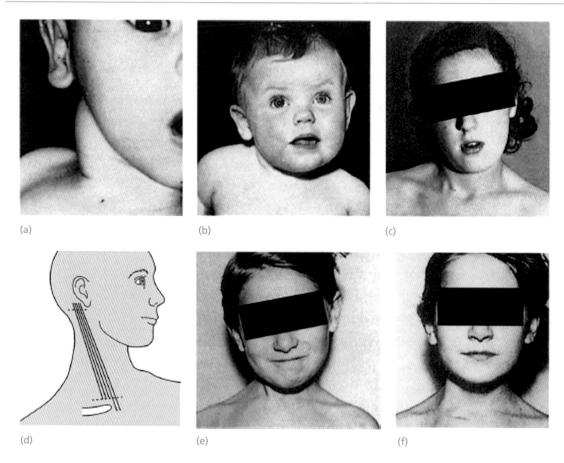

17.5 Torticollis Natural history: **(a)** sternocleidomastoid tumour in a child; **(b)** early wry neck; **(c)** deformity with facial hemiatrophy in the adolescent. Surgical treatment: **(d)** two sites at which the sternomastoid may be divided; **(e,f)** before and a few months after operation.

skeletal dysplasia involving the spine. This is especially important in patients undergoing operation; there is a risk that the atlantoaxial joint may subluxate under anaesthesia. Some patients present with pain or torticollis, or neurological complications such as transient paralysis or sphincter disturbances. In the majority of cases, the anomaly is discovered by chance in a routine cervical spine X-ray following trauma. Patients with symptoms should have surgical stabilization.

ACUTE INTERVERTEBRAL DISC PROLAPSE

Cervical disc prolapse may be precipitated by local strain or injury, especially sudden unguarded

flexion and rotation. It usually occurs immediately above or below the sixth cervical vertebra; in many cases (perhaps in all), there is a predisposing abnormality of the disc with increased nuclear tension.

The disc protrusion may press on the posterior longitudinal ligament, causing neck pain and stiffness as well as pain referred to the upper arm. Even more suggestive are associated symptoms of pain and paraesthesia in one or both arms.

Clinical features

The onset of symptoms may be related to a definite and severe strain. Subsequent attacks may be sudden or gradual in onset, and with trivial cause. The patient may complain of:

- pain and stiffness of the neck, the pain often radiating to the scapular region and sometimes to the occiput
- pain and paraesthesia in one upper limb (rarely both), often radiating to the outer elbow, back of the wrist and to the index and middle fingers.

Weakness is rare. Between attacks the patient feels well, although the neck may feel a bit stiff.

The neck may be tilted forwards and sideways. The muscles are tender and movements are restricted. The arms should be examined for neurological signs suggestive of nerve root irritation or compression.

Imaging

X-rays may reveal loss of the normal cervical lordosis (due to muscle spasm) or show narrowing of the disc space. However, the diagnosis should be confirmed by *MRI*, which will show whether the disc protrusion is pressing on the adjacent nerve root (17.6).

Differential diagnosis

Acute soft-tissue strain Acute strains of the neck can cause pain and stiffness which may last for weeks or months. The absence of neurological symptoms and signs is significant.

Neuralgic amyotrophy (acute brachial neuritis) Pain is sudden and severe, and situated over the shoulder, or the back of the shoulder, rather than in the neck itself. Multiple neurological levels are affected (extremely rare in disc prolapse). Look for signs of serratus anterior weakness (winging of the scapula).

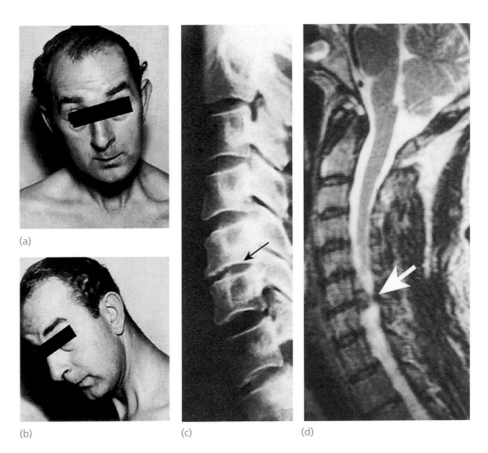

(a)

(b)   (c)   (d)

17.6 Acute disc prolapse (a,b) Acute wry neck due to a prolapsed disc. **(c)** The intervertebral disc space at C5/6 is reduced. **(d)** MRI in another case showing a large disc prolapse at C6/7.

Cervical spine infections Pain is unrelenting and local spasm severe. X-rays show erosion of the vertebral end plates.

Cervical tumours Neurological signs are progressive and X-rays or MRI may show bone destruction.

Treatment

Patient education and information should be provided. Heat and analgesics are soothing but, as with lumbar disc prolapse, there are only three satisfactory ways of treating the prolapse itself:

- rest
- reduction
- removal.

Rest A collar will prevent unguarded movement; it may be made of felt, sponge-rubber or polythene.

Reduction Traction may enlarge the disc space, permitting the prolapse to subside. The head of the couch is raised and weights (up to 8 kg) are tied to a harness fitting under the chin and occiput. Traction is applied intermittently for no more than 30 minutes at a time.

Removal If symptoms are refractory and severe enough or include motor deficit and myelopathy, the disc may be removed through an anterior approach; bone grafts are inserted to fuse the affected area and to restore the normal intervertebral height. The operation can also be performed using endoscopic techniques. The main purpose is to relieve pain and stop progression of the neurological deficit.

CHRONIC DISC DEGENERATION (CERVICAL SPONDYLOSIS)

Intervertebral disc degeneration is common from middle age onwards, even in people who have not been aware of any previous acute episode. With time, the discs collapse and flatten, and bony spurs appear at the anterior and posterior margins of the vertebral bodies on either side of the affected discs; those that develop posteriorly may encroach upon the intervertebral foramina, causing pressure on the nerve roots. Several levels may be affected and the condition is then usually referred to as 'spondylosis'. The condition is not always symptomatic, and many people go throughout life without experiencing anything more than slight stiffness.

Clinical features

Degenerative changes at the cervical spine are asymptomatic in the majority. When they do occur, symptoms usually have gradual onset. The patient, usually aged over 40 years, complains of neck pain and stiffness. The pain may radiate widely: to the occiput, the scapular muscles and down one or both arms. Paraesthesia, weakness and clumsiness are occasional symptoms. Typically, there are exacerbations of more acute discomfort, and long periods of relative quiescence.

The clinical appearance is usually normal. There may be tenderness in the soft tissues at the back of the neck and above the scapulae; neck movements are limited and painful at the extremes.

Careful neurological examination may show abnormal signs in one or both upper limbs.

Imaging

Typical *X-ray* features are narrowing of several disc spaces, bony spur formation at the anterior and posterior edges of the vertebral bodies and (in the anteroposterior view) osteoarthritic changes in the uncovertebral joints (17.7). Oblique views may show bony encroachment on the intervertebral foramina. *MRI* will show whether there is nerve root compression.

Differential diagnosis

Around two-thirds of the adult population experience neck pain during their lifetime, it is commonly non-specific. Other disorders associated with neck or arm pain and sensory symptoms must be excluded. *Cervical vertebral spur formation* is very common in older people and this can be misleading in patients with other disorders.

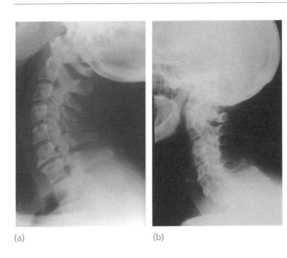

(a) (b)

17.7 Cervical spondylosis – X-rays (a) Degenerative features at one level, C6/7. Note the prominent 'osteophytes' at the anterior and posterior borders of these two vertebral bodies. **(b)** Marked degenerative changes at multiple levels.

Rotator cuff lesions   Pain around the shoulder may resemble the referred pain of cervical spondylosis. However, features such as specific pain or weakness on treating muscles of the rotator cuff and restricted shoulder movements should suggest a local problem.

Nerve entrapment syndromes   Median or ulnar nerve entrapment may give rise to intermittent symptoms of pain and paraesthesia in the hand. Characteristically, the symptoms are worse at night or are related to posture. In doubtful cases, nerve conduction studies and electromyography will help to establish the diagnosis. Remember, though, that the patient may have symptoms from both a peripheral and a central abnormality.

Cervical tumours   With tumours of the vertebrae, spinal cord, nerve roots or lymph nodes, the symptoms are unremitting. Imaging studies should reveal the diagnosis.

Treatment

CONSERVATIVE TREATMENT
Conservative treatment is the mainstay. During painful episodes, heat and massage are soothing; some patients benefit from a period in a restraining collar. Analgesics, anti-inflammatory medication and physiotherapy are the 'backbone' of treatment, patients usually being maintained in relative comfort by various measures including exercises, gentle passive manipulation and intermittent traction.

OPERATIVE TREATMENT
Surgical treatment is indicated if severe symptoms are relieved only by a rigid and irksome support, particularly if there are neurological changes due to nerve root compression.

Foraminotomy   If the main problems are referred pain in the upper limb and/or neurological symptoms and signs, and the MRI shows foraminal narrowing and nerve root compression at one or two levels, foraminotomy (through a posterior approach) may be indicated. Only part of the facet joint is removed so this segment should not become unstable. However, patients should be warned that pre-existing neck pain may not be eliminated.

Anterior discectomy and fusion   This operation is particularly suitable if the problem is primarily one of unrelieved neck pain and stiffness. Through a transverse incision at the front of the neck, the intervertebral disc is removed without disturbing the posteriorly situated neurological structures. After preparation of the intervertebral space, a suitably shaped autogenous bone graft (usually taken from the iliac crest) is inserted firmly between the adjacent vertebral bodies. An anterior plate is added if there is uncertainty about stability or if several levels are being fused.

Operative *complications* such as injury to the recurrent laryngeal nerve or (worse) the vertebral artery are unusual if sufficient care is exercised. Graft dislodgement and failed fusion are less likely with intervertebral plating.

Intervertebral disc replacement   Disc replacement operations have the (theoretical) advantage of removing the offending disc and preserving movement at the affected site. Short-term results appear to be as good as those achieved with anterior spinal fusion, with added benefits of lesser morbidity and shorter hospital stay. However, it is too early to assess the long-term outcome of these procedures.

Laminoplasty This procedure involves enlarging the spinal canal by lifting up the posterior elements of the vertebra. It is indicated for spinal cord compression secondary to developmental spinal canal stenosis, ossified posterior longitudinal ligament, multisegmental spondylosis associated with a narrow spinal canal and distal cervical spondylotic amyotrophy with canal stenosis. It is preferable to laminectomy because it can lessen postoperative kyphosis, instability and pain. The incidence of neck pain after laminoplasty, however, is reported to be high.

PYOGENIC INFECTION

Pyogenic infection of the cervical spine is uncommon, and therefore often misdiagnosed in the early stages when antibiotic treatment is most effective. The organism – usually *Staphylococcus aureus* – spreads haematogenously. Initially, destructive changes are limited to the intervertebral disc space and the adjacent parts of the vertebral bodies. Later, abscess formation occurs and pus may extend into the spinal canal or into the soft-tissue planes of the neck.

Clinical features

Vertebral infection may occur at any age. The patient complains of pain in the neck, often associated with muscle spasm and stiffness. Neck movements are severely restricted. Systemic symptoms are often mild but blood tests may show a leucocytosis and an elevated C-reactive protein (CRP) of erythrocyte sedimentation rate (ESR).

X-rays at first show either no abnormality or only slight narrowing of the disc space; later more obvious signs of bone destruction appear (17.8).

Treatment

Treatment is by antibiotics and rest. The cervical spine is 'immobilized' by traction; once the acute phase subsides, a collar may suffice. Operation is seldom necessary; if there is abscess formation, this will require drainage. As the infection subsides the intervertebral space is obliterated and the adjacent vertebrae usually fuse.

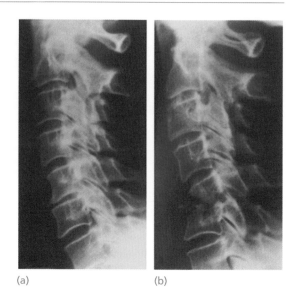

(a)   (b)

17.8 Pyogenic infection (a) The first X-ray, taken soon after the onset of symptoms, shows narrowing of the C5/6 disc space. **(b)** Three weeks later, there is destruction and collapse of the adjacent vertebral bodies.

TUBERCULOSIS

Cervical spine tuberculosis is rare. The organism is blood-borne and the infection localizes in the intervertebral disc and the anterior parts of the adjacent vertebral bodies. As the bone crumbles, the cervical spine collapses into kyphosis. A retropharyngeal abscess forms and points behind the sternocleidomastoid muscle at the side of the neck. In late cases, cord damage may cause neurological signs varying from mild weakness to tetraplegia.

Clinical features

The patient – usually a child – complains of neck pain and stiffness. Fever occurs in less than 20% of cases. In neglected cases, a retropharyngeal abscess may cause difficulty in swallowing or swelling in the posterior triangle of the neck. The neck is extremely tender and all movements are restricted. In late cases, there may be obvious kyphosis, a fluctuant abscess in the neck or a retropharyngeal swelling (17.9). The limbs should be examined for neurological defects.

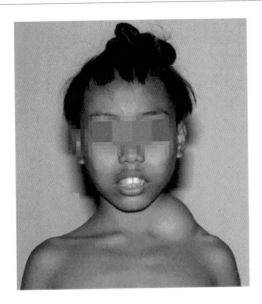

17.9 Tuberculosis This child had been complaining of neck pain and stiffness for several months. When she was brought to the clinic, she had a large lump at the side of her neck – a typical tuberculous abscess.

X-rays show narrowing of the disc space and erosion of the adjacent vertebral bodies.

Treatment

Treatment is initially by antituberculous drugs and 'immobilization' of the neck in a cervical brace or plaster cast for 6–18 months. Operative debridement of necrotic bone and anterior cervical vertebral fusion with bone grafts may be offered as an alternative to such prolonged immobilization.

URGENT INDICATIONS FOR OPERATION

To drain a retropharyngeal abscess
To decompress a threatened spinal cord
To fuse an unstable spine

RHEUMATOID ARTHRITIS

The cervical spine is severely affected in 30% of patients with rheumatoid arthritis (RA). Three sites of lesion are common.

COMMONEST SITES OF EROSION IN RA LESIONS

Atlantoaxial joints and the transverse ligament, with resulting instability
Atlanto-occipital articulations, allowing the odontoid peg to ride up into the foramen magnum
Facet joints in the midcervical region, sometimes ending in fusion but more often leading to subluxation.

Considering the amount of atlantoaxial displacement that occurs (often greater than 1 cm), neurological complications are uncommon.

Clinical features

The patient is usually a woman with advanced RA. She has neck pain and movements are markedly restricted. Symptoms and signs of root compression may be present in the upper limbs; less often there are upper motor neuron signs and lower limb weakness due to cord compression. However, there may be symptoms of vertebrobasilar insufficiency, such as vertigo, tinnitus and visual disturbance. Some patients, though completely unaware of any neurological deficit, are found on careful examination to have mild sensory or motor disturbance. Bear in mind that peripheral joint involvement and general debility can mask the signs of myelopathy.

Imaging

X-RAYS

X-rays show the features of an erosive arthritis, usually at several levels. Atlantoaxial instability is visible in lateral films taken in flexion and extension.

- *In flexion*, the anterior arch of the atlas rides forwards, leaving a gap of 5 mm or more between the back of the anterior arch and the odontoid process.
- *On extension*, the subluxation is reduced.

Atlanto-occipital erosion is more difficult to see, but a lateral tomograph shows the relationship of the odontoid to the foramen magnum. The

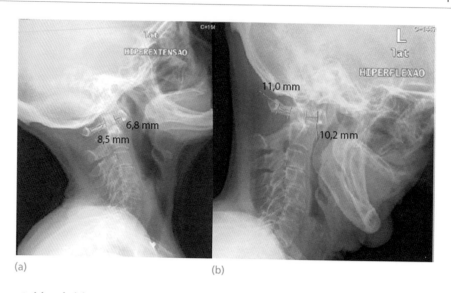

(a)　　　　　　　　　　(b)

17.10 Rheumatoid arthritis – X-rays Lateral dynamic X-ray views of an 82-year-old female patient with RA with C1–C2 instability. Note the change in the measured atlanto-dens interval (ADI) and space available for the cord (SAC) from hyperextension **(a)** to hyperflexion **(b)**.

odontoid tip is normally less than 5 mm above McGregor's line (a line from the posterior edge of the hard palate to the lowest point on the occiput); in erosive arthritis, the odontoid tip may be 10–12 mm above this line (**17.10**).

CT AND MRI

CT and *MRI* are useful for imaging 'difficult' areas such as the atlanto-dens and atlanto-occipital articulations, and for viewing the soft-tissue structures (especially the cord).

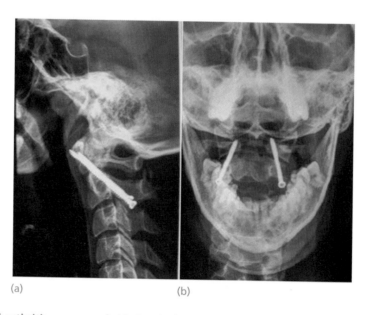

(a)　　　　　　　　　　(b)

17.11 Rheumatoid arthritis – surgery (a,b) Cervical C1–C2 fusion with atlantoaxial transarticular screw fixation (Magerl technique).

Treatment

Despite the startling X-ray appearances, serious neurological complications are uncommon. Effective control of inflammation by conventional disease-modifying antirheumatic drugs (DMARDs), glucocorticoids, methotrexate, sulfasalazine and leflunomide retards structural damage in RA. Wearing a collar can usually relieve pain.

INDICATIONS FOR OPERATIVE STABILIZATION OF THE CERVICAL SPINE

Severe and unremitting pain
Neurological signs of root or cord
   compression

Atlantoaxial surgical stabilization is usually accomplished using one of two techniques:

* a posterior approach by transarticular screw fixation (*Magerl technique* – **17.11**)
* a C1 lateral mass–C2 pedicle screw fixation construct (*Harms technique*).

Postoperatively, a cervical brace can be worn. However, if instability is marked and operative fixation insecure, a halo jacket may be necessary. In patients with very advanced disease and severe erosive changes, postoperative morbidity and mortality are high.

ANKYLOSING SPONDYLITIS

Ankylosing spondylitis can affect the cervical spine, causing neck pain and stiffness some years after the onset of backache. The neck gradually becomes rigid and kyphotic, although some movement is usually preserved at the atlanto-occipital and atlantoaxial joints.

An unacceptable 'chin-on-chest' deformity, and inability to lift the head high enough to see more than ten paces ahead, are indications for cervical spine osteotomy. The patient should be told that surgery carries a high complication rate.

■ Clinical assessment	359	■ Ankylosing spondylitis	
■ Scoliosis	365	(spondyloarthropathy)	381
■ Idiopathic scoliosis	367	■ Intervertebral disc lesions	381
■ Kyphosis	373	■ Low back pain	384
■ Spinal Infection	375	■ Spondylolisthesis	387
■ Pyogenic discitis/osteomyelitis	376	■ Spinal stenosis	389
■ Tuberculosis	378	■ Approach to diagnosis in patients	
■ Fungal infections	380	with low back pain	390
■ Parasitic infestations	381	■ Chronic back pain syndrome	391

CLINICAL ASSESSMENT

HISTORY

The usual symptoms of back disorders are pain, stiffness and deformity in the back, and pain, paraesthesia or weakness in the legs. The mode of onset is very important: Did it start suddenly (perhaps after lifting) or gradually? Are the symptoms constant, or are there periods of remission? Are they related to any particular posture?

- *Pain* is the commonest presenting symptom. It is usually felt low down and on either side of the midline, but it may extend into the upper buttock or thighs. It may originate from the disc, facets, ligamentous structures or nerve roots.
- *Sciatica* or pain radiating from the buttock into the thigh and calf secondary to nerve root compression or irritation may be mimicked by *referred pain* from other structures radiating into the lower limbs. True sciatica, most commonly due to a prolapsed intervertebral disc pressing on a nerve root, is characteristically more intense than referred low back pain (LBP), is aggravated by coughing and straining and is often accompanied by symptoms of root pressure such as numbness and paraesthesia.
- *Stiffness* may be sudden and almost complete (after a disc prolapse) secondary to muscle spasm or continuous and predictably worse in the mornings (suggesting arthritis or ankylosing spondylitis).
- *Deformity* is usually noticed by others, but the patient may become aware of shoulder asymmetry or of clothes not fitting well.
- *Numbness or paraesthesia* is felt anywhere in the lower limb, but can usually be mapped fairly accurately to one of the dermatomes. It is important to ask if it is aggravated by standing or walking and relieved by sitting down or bending forward – the classic symptom of spinal stenosis.

SECTION 2 REGIONAL ORTHOPAEDICS

• *Urinary retention or incontinence* can be due to pressure on the cauda equina. *Faecal incontinence or urgency, and impotence*, may also occur.

SIGNS WITH THE PATIENT STANDING

Adequate exposure is essential; patients must strip to their underclothes.

Look

1 Begin by standing face to face with the patient and note the general physique and posture (**18.1**).
2 View the patient from behind:
   • Does the patient stand upright or lean over to one side?
   • Is the pelvis level or is one leg shorter than the other?
   • Does the spine look straight or curved (*scoliosis*)?
   • Are there scars or other skin markings that may suggest a spinal disorder?
3 View the patient from the side:
   • Does the thoracic spine have a normal gentle forward curve (*kyphosis*)? An unduly prominent kyphotic curve is sometimes called *hyperkyphosis*; sharp angulation is called a *kyphos* or *gibbus*.
   • Does the lumbar spine have a normal bend slightly backwards (*lordosis*)? Note if it is unusually flat or excessively lordosed.
4 If the patient stands with one knee bent despite equal leg lengths, this suggests nerve root tension; flexing the knee relaxes the sciatic nerve and reduces the pull on the nerve root.

Feel

Palpate the spinous processes and the interspinous ligaments, noting any prominence or a 'step'. Localize any tenderness at each level.

Move

Flexion Ask the patient to bend forwards and try to touch the floor. Even with a stiff back, they may be able to do this by flexing the hips; so, watch the lumbar spine closely or measure spinal excursion (**18.2**). The mode of flexion is also important; hesitant movements, especially on regaining the upright position, may signify pain or segmental instability.

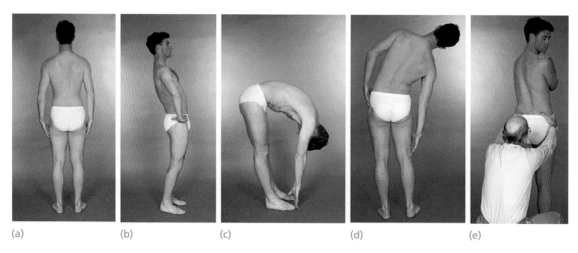

(a)   (b)   (c)   (d)   (e)

18.1 Examination **(a)** With the patient standing upright, look at the general posture and note particularly the presence of any asymmetry or frank deformity of the spine. Then ask them to **(b)** lean backwards (extension), **(c)** bend forwards to touch the toes (flexion) and then **(d)** lean sideways as far as possible, comparing the level of reach on the two sides. **(e)** Finally, hold the pelvis stable and ask the patient to twist first to one side and then to the other (rotation). Note that rotation occurs almost entirely in the thoracic spine and not in the lumbar spine.

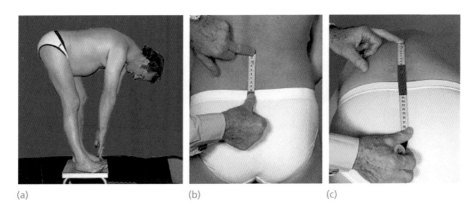

(a)   (b)   (c)

18.2 Measuring the range of flexion Bending down and touching the toes may look like lumbar flexion but this is not always the case. The patient in **(a)** has ankylosing spondylitis and a rigid lumbar spine, but he is able to reach his toes because he has good flexibility at the hips. Compare his flat back with the rounded back of the model in **18.1c**. You can measure the lumbar excursion. With the patient upright, select two bony points 10 cm apart and mark the skin **(b)**; as the patient bends forward, the two points should separate by a least a further 5 cm **(c)**.

Extension   Ask the patient to lean backwards; with a stiff spine they may cheat by bending the knees. The 'wall test' will unmask a disguised loss of extension: standing with the back flush against a wall, the heels, buttocks, shoulders and occiput normally all make contact with the surface.

Lateral flexion   Ask the patient to bend first to one side and then to the other; compare the range of movement to right and left.

Rotation   Ask the patient to twist the trunk to each side in turn while the pelvis is anchored by the examiner's hands; this is essentially a thoracic movement and should not be limited in lumbosacral disease.

Chest expansion   Assess rib excursion by measuring the chest circumference in full expiration and then full inspiration; the normal excursion is about 7 cm.

Muscle power   Distal muscle power is conveniently tested and compared by asking the patient to stand up on their toes (plantar flexion) and then to rock back on the heels (dorsiflexion); small differences between the two sides are easily spotted.

SIGNS WITH THE PATIENT PRONE

Examine the patient when they are lying prone (**18.3**).

- *Bony outlines* and small lumps can be felt more easily with the patient lying face down.
- *Deep tenderness* is easy to localize, but difficult to ascribe to a particular structure.
- *Some neurological features* are ideally elicited with the patient lying prone. *Hamstring power* is tested by having the patient flex the knee against resistance (the *femoral stretch test*). Pain felt in the front of the thigh and back suggests lumbar root tension.
- *Popliteal and posterior tibial pulses* are conveniently felt in this position.

FEMORAL STRETCH TEST OF HAMSTRING POWER

With the patient lying prone, bend the patient's knee with the hip flat against the couch. A positive sign is pain felt in the front of the thigh and the back, suggesting lumbar root tension.

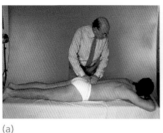
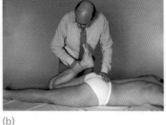
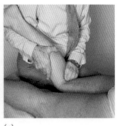

(a)   (b)   (c)

18.3 Examination with the patient prone (a) Feel for tenderness, watching the patient's face for any reaction. (b) Performing the femoral stretch test. You can test for lumbar root sensitivity either by hyperextending the hip or by acutely flexing the knee with the patient lying prone. Note the point at which the patient feels pain and compare the two sides. (c) While the patient is lying prone, take the opportunity to feel the pulses. The popliteal pulse is easily felt if the tissues at the back of the knee are relaxed by slightly flexing the knee.

SIGNS WITH THE PATIENT SUPINE

Observe the patient for pain and stiffness as they turn over. Examine hip and knee mobility before testing for cord or nerve root involvement. Also check the femoral and pedal pulses.

Straight leg raise test

This is the classic test for lumbosacral root tension (**18.4a,b**).

> **STRAIGHT-LEG RAISE TEST FOR LUMBOSACRAL ROOT TENSION**
>
> Holding the patient's knee straight, lift the leg from the couch until the patient experiences pain – not only in the lower back (common and not significant) but also in the buttock, thigh and calf (Lasègue's test). Note the angle at which this occurs; normally, it should be possible to raise the leg to 90° without causing undue discomfort. At the point where the patient experiences discomfort, passive dorsiflexion of the foot may cause an additional stab of pain. You can also ask the patient to raise the leg with the knee straight and rigid – and to stop when he or she feels pain.

Bowstring sign

The bowstring sign is more specific than the straight-leg raise test (**18.4c,d**).

> **BOWSTRING SIGN**
>
> Raise the patient's leg gently to the point where they experience sciatic pain; without reducing the amount of lift, bend the knee so as to relax the sciatic nerve. Buttock pain is immediately relieved; pain can be re-induced without extending the knee by pressing on the common peroneal nerve behind the posterolateral side of the knee, to tighten the nerve like a bowstring.

Crossed straight-leg raise test

Occasionally, straight-leg raising on the unaffected side produces pain on the affected side. This crossed straight-leg raise test is highly specific for a disc prolapse, often a large central prolapse. Cauda equina syndrome should be excluded.

Neurological examination

A full neurological examination of the lower limbs is essential.

- An absent ankle jerk on the side with sciatica, combined with paraesthesiae along the lateral border of the foot, suggests compression of the S1 nerve root.

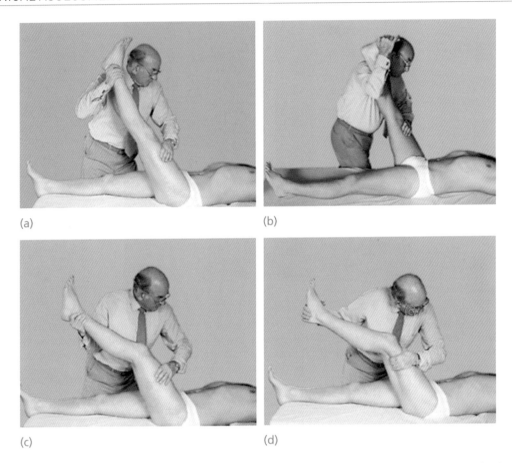

(a)   (b)

(c)   (d)

18.4 Sciatic stretch tests (a) Straight-leg raising. The knee is kept absolutely straight while the leg is slowly lifted; note where the patient complains of tightness and pain in the buttock – normally around 80–90° – and compare the two sides. **(b)** At that point, passive dorsiflexion of the foot causes an additional stab of pain. **(c)** Sciatic tension can also be shown by the bowstring sign. At the point where the patient experiences pain during straight leg raising, relax the tension by bending the knee slightly; the pain should disappear. Then apply firm pressure behind the lateral hamstrings **(d)**; this tightens the common peroneal nerve and the pain recurs with renewed intensity.

- Normal reflexes combined with paraesthesia on the dorsum of the foot suggest compression of the L5 nerve root.

INVESTIGATION

Imaging

X-RAYS

For the lower back, standing anteroposterior (AP) and lateral X-rays of the lumbar spine (18.5) and AP pelvis X-rays are required; occasionally, lumbar oblique and sacroiliac joint views are useful.

In the *AP view*, the spine should be straight and the soft-tissue shadows should outline the normal muscle planes. Curvature (scoliosis) is obvious, and best shown in standing views. Check the outlines of the pedicles, regular ovals near the lateral edges of the vertebral body: a missing or misshapen pedicle could be due to erosion by infection, a neurofibroma or metastatic disease. Individual vertebrae may show asymmetry or collapse. The sacroiliac

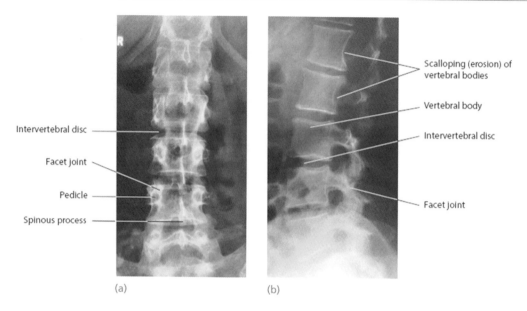

Intervertebral disc

Facet joint

Pedicle

Spinous process

Scalloping (erosion) of vertebral bodies

Vertebral body

Intervertebral disc

Facet joint

(a)   (b)

18.5 Lumbar spine X-rays (a,b) The most important normal features are demonstrated in the lower lumbar spine. **(b)** In this particular case, there are also signs of marked posterior vertebral body and facet joint erosions at L1 and L2, features that are strongly suggestive of an expanding neurofibroma.

joints may show erosion or ankylosis, as in tuberculosis (TB) or ankylosing spondylitis, and the hip joints may show features of osteoarthritis (OA). Don't forget the soft tissues: bulging of the psoas muscle or loss of the psoas 'shadow' may indicate a paravertebral abscess.

In the *lateral view* the normal thoracic kyphosis (up to 40 degrees) and lumbar lordosis should be regular and uninterrupted. Anterior shift of an upper segment upon a lower (spondylolisthesis) may be associated with defects of the posterior arch, shown best in oblique views. Vertebral bodies may be wedged or biconcave, deformities typical of osteoporosis or old injury. The intervertebral spaces may be edged by bony spurs (suggesting long-standing disc degeneration) or outlined by fine bony bridges (syndesmophytes – a cardinal feature of ankylosing spondylitis).

RADIOISOTOPE SCANNING

Isotope scans may pick up areas of increased activity, suggesting a fracture, a local inflammatory lesion or a 'silent' metastasis. Bone scans may include whole-body, three-phase, or regional imaging and single-photon emission computed tomography (SPECT).

COMPUTED TOMOGRAPHY

Computed tomography (CT) is helpful in the diagnosis of structural bone changes (e.g. a vertebral fracture) and intervertebral disc prolapse. When combined with myelography, it gives valuable information about the contents of the spinal canal.

MAGNETIC RESONANCE IMAGING

Magnetic resonance imaging (MRI) has virtually done away with the need for myelography, discography, facet arthrography and much of CT scanning. The spinal canal and disc spaces are clearly outlined in various planes (**18.6**).

Scans can reveal the physiological state of the disc as regards dehydration, as well as the effect of disc degeneration on bone marrow in adjacent vertebral bodies.

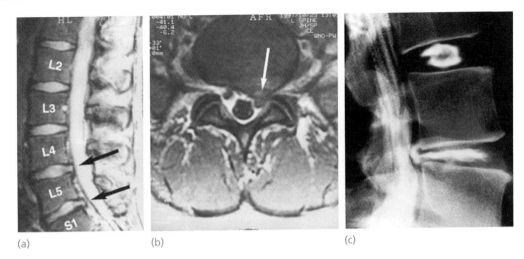

(a)   (b)   (c)

18.6 MRI and discography (a) The lateral T2-weighted MRI shows a small posterior disc bulge (arrow) at L4/5 and a larger protrusion at L5/S1. **(b)** The axial MRI shows the disc prolapse encroaching on the intervertebral canal and the nerve root on the left side. **(c)** Discography, showing normal appearance at the upper level and a degenerate disc with prolapse at the level below.

SCOLIOSIS

Scoliosis is a complex rotational deformity which may manifest with a thoracic or lumbar prominence, shoulder imbalance, coronal shift and infrequently pain.

POSTURAL SCOLIOSIS

In postural scoliosis, the deformity is secondary to some condition outside the spine, such as a short leg or a pelvic tilt. When the patient sits (thereby cancelling asymmetry), the curve disappears. Local muscle spasm associated with a prolapsed lumbar disc may also cause a skew back.

STRUCTURAL SCOLIOSIS

In structural scoliosis, there is a non-correctable deformity of the affected spinal segment, an essential component of which is vertebral rotation. The spinous processes swing round towards the concavity of the curve and the transverse processes on the convexity rotate posteriorly. In the thoracic region, the ribs on the convex side stand out prominently, producing the classical rib hump. Secondary (compensatory) curves nearly always develop to counterbalance the primary deformity; they too may become fixed.

Once established, the deformity is liable to increase throughout the growth period (and sometimes even afterwards).

Most cases have no obvious cause (*idiopathic scoliosis*); other varieties are *congenital* (due to bony anomalies), *neuropathic*, *myopathic* (associated with some muscle dystrophies) or a miscellaneous group of *connective-tissue disorders*.

Clinical features

Deformity is usually the presenting symptom: an obvious skew back or a rib hump in thoracic curves, and asymmetrical prominence of one hip in thoracolumbar curves. Balanced curves may go unnoticed until an adult presents with backache. *Pain* is a rare complaint and should alert the clinician to the possibility of a neural tumour and the need for MRI. *A family history* of scoliosis is not uncommon.

The spine may be obviously deviated from the midline, but if not, forward flexion demonstrates it (18.7). The level and direction of the major curve convexity should be noted: e.g. 'right thoracic' means a curve in the thoracic spine and convex to

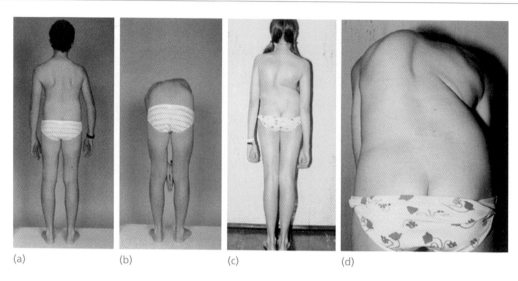

(a)   (b)   (c)   (d)

18.7 Structural scoliosis (a) Slight curves are often missed on casual inspection but the deformity becomes apparent when the spine is flexed **(b)**. **(c)** This young girl has a much more obvious scoliosis and asymmetry of the hips but what really worries her is the prominent rib hump, seen best when she bends over **(d)**.

the right; the hip juts out on the concave side and the scapula on the convex. With thoracic scoliosis, rotation causes the rib angles to protrude, producing a rib hump on the convex side. In balanced deformities, the occiput is over the midline; in unbalanced (or decompensated) curves, it is not. Side-on posture should also be observed; there may appear to be excessive kyphosis or lordosis.

The diagnostic feature of fixed (as distinct from postural or mobile) scoliosis is that forward bending makes the curve more obvious. Spinal mobility should be assessed and the effect of lateral bending on the curve noted. Is there some flexibility in the curve and can it be passively corrected?

Neurological examination is important. Any abnormality suggesting a spinal cord lesion calls for CT and/or MRI.

General examination includes a search for the possible cause and an assessment of cardiopulmonary function (which is reduced in severe curves). Skin pigmentation and congenital anomalies such as sacral dimples or hair tufts are sought.

Imaging

X-RAYS

Full-length posteroanterior (PA) and lateral X-rays of the spine and iliac crests must be taken

with the patient erect (**18.8a,b**). Structural curves show vertebral rotation: in the PA X-ray, vertebrae towards the apex of the curve appear to be asymmetrical and the spinous processes are deviated towards the concavity.

The upper and lower ends of the curve are identified as the levels where vertebrae start to angle away from the curve. The degree of curvature is measured by drawing lines on the X-ray at the upper border of the uppermost vertebra and the lower border of the lowermost vertebra of the curve; the angle subtended by these lines is the angle of curvature (*Cobb's angle*) (**18.8c**).

The site of the curve apex should be noted. Right thoracic curves are the commonest, the majority in girls due to adolescent idiopathic scoliosis. The primary structural curve is usually balanced by smaller, compensatory curves above and below. Lateral bending views are taken to assess the degree of curve correctability.

A view of the upper part of the pelvis will show whether the iliac apophysis has fully ossified and fused (*Risser sign* of skeletal maturity – **18.8d,e**), after which progression of the curve is minimal.

CT AND MRI

CT and MRI may be necessary to define a vertebral abnormality or cord compression.

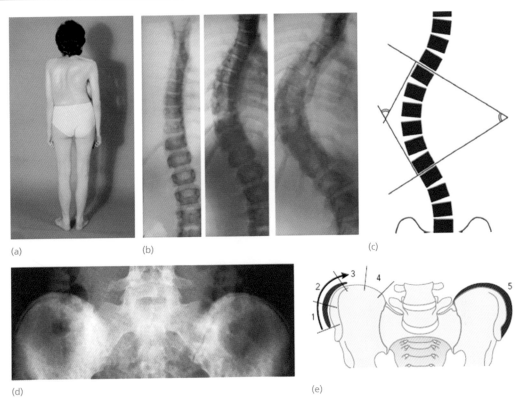

(a)   (b)   (c)

(d)   (e)

18.8 Adolescent idiopathic scoliosis (a) Typical thoracic deformity. **(b)** Serial X-rays show how this curve increased over a period of 4 years. **(c)** The angle of curvature is measured on the X-ray by Cobb's method: lines projected from the top of the uppermost and the bottom of the lowermost vertebral bodies in the primary curve define *Cobb's angle*. An AP view of the pelvis is needed to assess the *Risser sign* **(d,e)**. The iliac apophyses normally ossify progressively from lateral to medial; when fusion is complete, we know that spinal maturity has been reached and further increase in the angle of curvature is likely to be negligible.

Special investigations

- *Patients with severe chest deformities* should undergo pulmonary function tests. A marked reduction in vital capacity is associated with diminished life expectancy and carries risks for surgery.
- *Patients with muscular dystrophies or connective tissue disorders* require full biochemical and neuromuscular investigation.

Treatment

Prognosis is key: the aim is to prevent severe deformity. The younger the child and the higher the curve, the worse the prognosis. Management differs for the different types of scoliosis.

IDIOPATHIC SCOLIOSIS

This group constitutes about 80% of all cases of scoliosis and the deformity is often familial. The population incidence of serious curves (over 30 degrees and therefore needing treatment) is 3 per 1000. The age at onset defines three subgroups: adolescent, juvenile and infantile (**18.9**). A simpler division now in general use is *early-onset* (before puberty) and *late-onset* (after puberty).

LATE-ONSET (ADOLESCENT) IDIOPATHIC SCOLIOSIS (AGED 10 YEARS OR OVER)

This is the commonest type, making up 90% of cases, mostly in girls. Primary thoracic curves are

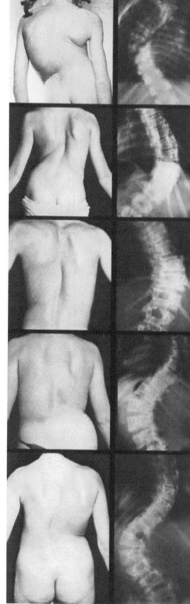

Infantile thoracic

60% male.
90% convex to left.
Associated with ipsilateral plagiocephaly.
May be resolving or progressive.
Progressive variety becomes severe.

Adolescent thoracic

90% female.
90% convex to right.
Rib rotation exaggerates the deformity.
50% develop curves of greater than 70°.

Thoracolumbar

Slightly more common in females.
Slightly more common to right.
Features mid-way between adolescent thoracic and lumbar.

Lumbar

More common in females.
80% convex to left.
One hip prominent but no ribs to accentuate deformity.
Therefore not noticed early, but backache in adult life.

Combined

Two primary curves, one in each direction.
Even when radiologically severe, clinical deformity relatively slight because always well balanced.

18.9 Patterns of idiopathic scoliosis Bracing is used far less than previously because of serious doubts as to its effectiveness beyond natural history.

usually convex to the right, lumbar curves to the left. Progression is not inevitable; most curves of less than 20 degrees either resolve spontaneously or remain unchanged. If a curve starts to progress, it usually goes on doing so until skeletal maturity (and, to a much lesser degree, beyond that). Reliable predictors of progression are:

- very young age at onset
- marked curvature
- incomplete Risser sign.

In prepubertal children, rapid progression is liable to occur during the growth spurt.

Treatment

The aims of treatment are:

- to prevent a mild deformity from becoming severe
- to correct an existing deformity that is unacceptable to the patient.

A period of observation may be needed before deciding between conservative and operative treatment. At 4- to 9-monthly intervals, the patient is examined, photographed and X-rayed to measure curves and check for progression.

NON-OPERATIVE TREATMENT

If the patient is approaching skeletal maturity and the deformity is acceptable (less than 30 degrees and well balanced), surgery is probably unnecessary unless X-rays show definite progression.

- *Exercises* have no effect on the curve but they do maintain muscle tone and may inspire confidence in a favourable outcome.
- *Bracing* has been used for many years in treating progressive curves of 20–30 degrees.
  - The *Milwaukee brace* is a pelvic corset connected by adjustable steel supports to a cervical ring carrying occipital and chin pads; it reduces the lumbar lordosis and encourages active stretching and straightening of the thoracic spine.
  - The *Boston brace* is an underarm brace that provides lumbar or low thoracolumbar support. Pads may be added to these devices to apply pressure at a particular site. Well-fitting braces allow participation in full daily activities, including sport and exercises.

Although bracing is still used, it does not actually improve the curve – at best it merely stops progression. Many surgeons no longer use braces due to lack of evidence of benefits, preferring to wait to see if the curve progresses

to the stage when corrective surgery would be justified.

OPERATIVE TREATMENT

> **INDICATIONS FOR SURGERY**
>
> Curves of more than 30° that are cosmetically unacceptable, especially in high-risk (prepubertal) patients.
> Milder curves with rapid progression.
> Balanced, double primary curves require operation only if they are greater than 40° and progressing.

The objectives are to:

- halt progression
- straighten the curve (including the rotational component)
- arthrodese the entire primary curve.

There are a number of surgical options.

Posterior instrumentation   In this approach, the spine is instrumented segmentally from posterior with pedicle screws and/or hooks which are connected to pre-contoured rods to correct the deformity via the mobile discs (**18.10**). Older sub-laminar wiring techniques may still be used if pedicles are too small for screws or to reduce cost in long neuromuscular scoliosis. If the deformity is rigid, it may require resection of the facets (Ponte osteotomies) and even concave rib resections to allow correction.

Anterior instrumentation   This is another option where the discs are resected and screws placed into the vertebral bodies, straightened with the addition of the rod (**18.11**). The advantage may be a shorter construct but it has the disadvantage of increased morbidity of a transthoracic approach. It is useful in thoracolumbar curves where excellent rotational correction can be induced with the disc release.

During correction, *spinal cord injury* may occur due to cord traction with column lengthening. Spinal cord electrophysiological monitoring should be performed, ideally both somatosensory and motor-evoked potential monitoring, during spinal correction.

If these facilities are not available or there is an electrophysiological alert, the 'wake-up test' is used. Anaesthesia is reduced to bring the patient to a semi-awake state and they are then instructed to move their feet. If there are signs of cord compromise, the instrumentation is relaxed or removed and reapplied with a lesser degree of correction.

Rib hump None of the instrumentation systems can completely eliminate the rib hump and it is often this that troubles the patient most of all. If the deformity is marked, it can be reduced significantly by performing a costoplasty, where short sections of rib are excised at multiple levels on the convex side.

Complications of surgery

Neurological compromise With modern techniques, the incidence of permanent paralysis has been reduced to less than 1%.

Spinal decompensation Overcorrection may produce an unbalanced spine. This should be avoided by careful preoperative planning.

Pseudarthrosis Incomplete fusion occurs in about 2% of cases and may require revision surgery.

Implant failure Implants may dislodge and rods fracture, especially in delayed/non-union.

EARLY-ONSET (JUVENILE) IDIOPATHIC SCOLIOSIS (AGED 4–9 YEARS)

This type is uncommon. The characteristics are similar to those of the adolescent group but the

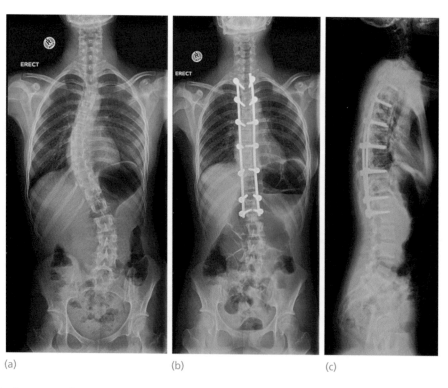

(a)   (b)   (c)

18.10 Scoliosis – posterior instrumentation (a) Preoperative AP X-ray; (b) postoperative AP X-ray; (c) postoperative lateral X-ray.

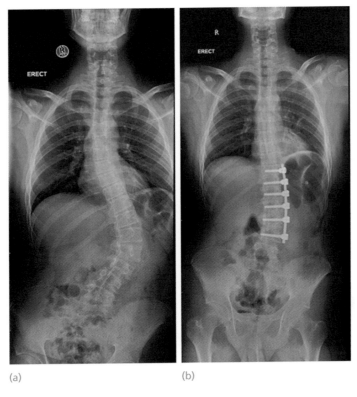

18.11 Scoliosis – anterior instrumentation (a) Preoperative AP X-ray; **(b)** postoperative AP X-ray.

prognosis is worse and surgical correction may be necessary before puberty. However, if the child is very young, a brace may hold the curve stationary until the age of 10 years, when fusion is more likely to succeed.

EARLY-ONSET (INFANTILE) IDIOPATHIC SCOLIOSIS (AGED 3 YEARS OR UNDER)

This variety is rare. Boys predominate and most curves are thoracic with convexity to the left. Around 90% of infantile curves resolve spontaneously, but progressive curves can become very severe and may lead to cardiopulmonary dysfunction.

Curves assessed as being potentially progressive should be treated by applying serial elongation–derotation–flexion (EDF) plaster casts under general anaesthesia, until the deformity resolves or until the child is big enough for a brace. From about the age of 4 years, curve

progression slows down or ceases and the child may not need further treatment. If the deformity continues to deteriorate, surgical correction may be required using growth rods.

CONGENITAL SCOLIOSIS

This includes the more common *failure of formation* (hemivertebrae) (18.12) and less common *failure of segmentation* (bar). Clinically, there may be hair, dimples or a pad of fat over the spine. There is a common association with renal, cardiac and neurological anomalies requiring investigation by abdominal ultrasound and MRI. It is often mild, but some cases progress to severe deformity, particularly those with unilateral fusion of vertebrae with contralateral hemivertebrae. Before any operation is undertaken, imaging is needed to exclude an associated dysraphism, particularly diastematomyelia and cord tethering, which must be dealt with prior to curve correction.

SECTION 2 REGIONAL ORTHOPAEDICS

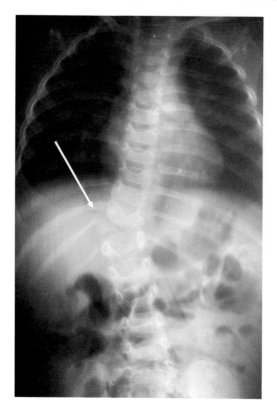

18.12 Congenital scoliosis The arrow indicates a hemivertebra at T11/T12. Note the additional articulating rib.

Treatment

Progressive deformities (usually involving rigid curves) will not respond to bracing and surgical correction is technically challenging. Management involves recognizing the progression potential and impairing growth with fusion over the small involved segment. If there is an existing deformity, hemivertebral resection and fusion may be required.

NEUROPATHIC AND MYOPATHIC SCOLIOSIS

NEUROMUSCULAR CONDITIONS ASSOCIATED WITH SCOLIOSIS
Poliomyelitis Cerebral palsy Syringomyelia Friedreich's ataxia Rarer lower motor neuron disorders and muscle dystrophies

The typical paralytic curve is a long, C-shaped curve (**18.13a,b**); initially, it is flexible but it becomes rigid with time. As the curve progresses, pelvic obliquity will ensue with sitting balance problems and

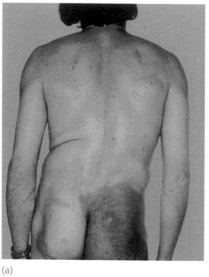

(a)

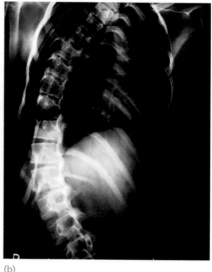

(b)

18.13 Other types of scoliosis (a) This patient has a short structural curve plus multiple skin lesions – features suggesting neurofibromatosis. **(b)** By contrast, the typical postpoliomyelitis 'paralytic' scoliosis shown in this X-ray is characterized by a long C-shaped curve.

pressure areas. *X-ray* with traction applied shows the extent to which the deformity is correctable.

Treatment

Treatment depends upon the degree of functional disability.

- *Mild curves* often require no treatment.
- *Moderate curves* with spinal stability are managed as for idiopathic scoliosis.
- *Severe curves*, associated with pelvic obliquity and loss of sitting balance, can often be managed by fitting a suitable sitting support; if this does not suffice, a long instrumented fusion of the spine to the pelvis may be required.

SCOLIOSIS AND NEUROFIBROMATOSIS

About one-third of patients with neurofibromatosis develop spinal deformity, varying from very mild to the most marked manifestations accompanied by skin lesions (**18.13a**), multiple neurofibromata and bony dystrophy affecting the vertebrae and ribs. The scoliotic curve is typically 'short and sharp'.

Treatment

Mild cases are treated as for idiopathic scoliosis. More severe deformities will usually need combined anterior and posterior instrumentation and fusion. Graft dissolution and pseudarthrosis are not uncommon.

KYPHOSIS

The term 'kyphosis' is used to describe both normal contour and abnormal (excessive dorsal curvature). The latter may be progressive; some people prefer the term *hyperkyphosis*. A *kyphos* (or *gibbus*) is a sharp posterior angulation due to localized collapse or wedging of one or more vertebrae. This may be the result of:

- a congenital anomaly
- a fracture (sometimes pathological)
- spinal TB.

POSTURAL KYPHOSIS

Postural kyphosis is common and may be associated with other postural defects such as flat feet. It is voluntarily correctable and treatment, if needed, consists of postural exercises.

STRUCTURAL KYPHOSIS

Structural kyphosis is fixed and associated with changes in the shape of the vertebrae (**18.14**).

- *In young children*, this may be due to congenital vertebral defects; it is also seen in skeletal dysplasias such as achondroplasia and in osteogenesis imperfecta.

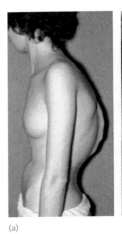
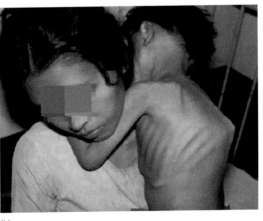

(a)   (b)

18.14 Kyphosis and kyphos (a) *Kyphosis* – a generalized exaggeration of the normal thoracic 'rounding' of the back, in this case due to Scheuermann's disease. **(b)** *Kyphos* – a localized spinal angulation, or gibbus, due to collapse of one or two spinal segments (here following tuberculous spondylitis).

- *Older children* may develop severe deformity secondary to tuberculous spondylitis.
- *In adolescents*, the commonest cause is Scheuermann's disease (adolescent kyphosis).
- *In adults*, kyphosis could be due to an old childhood disorder, e.g. tuberculous spondylitis, ankylosing spondylitis or spinal trauma.
- *In elderly people*, osteoporosis may result in vertebral compression and an increase in a previously mild, asymptomatic deformity.

CONGENITAL KYPHOSIS

Vertebral anomalies leading to kyphosis may be due to failure of formation (Type I), failure of segmentation (Type II) or a combination.

Type I kyphosis (failure of formation)

Type I is the commoner and worse type. Progressive deformity and posterior displacement of the residual vertebral segment may lead to cord compression. In children younger than 6 years with curves of less than 40 degrees, posterior spinal fusion alone may prevent further progression. Older children or more severe curves may need combined anterior and posterior fusion, and those with neurological complications will require cord decompression.

Type II kyphosis (failure of segmentation)

Type II usually takes the form of an anterior intervertebral bar; as the posterior elements continue to grow, that segment of the spine gradually becomes kyphotic. The risk of neurological compression is much less but, if the curve is progressive, a posterior fusion will be needed.

ADOLESCENT KYPHOSIS (SCHEUERMANN'S DISEASE)

This is a 'developmental' disorder in which there is abnormal ossification (and possibly some fragmentation) of the ring epiphyses at the upper and lower surfaces of each vertebral body. These cartilaginous end plates are weaker than normal and the affected vertebrae in the thoracic spine (which is normally mildly kyphotic) may become wedge shaped leading to an exaggerated *kyphosis*. Similar changes may occur in the lumbar spine, but here wedging is unusual.

Clinical features

The condition starts at puberty and affects boys more often than girls. An increasingly round-shouldered appearance may be noted and there may be backache and fatigue, sometimes increasing after the end of growth and it may become severe.

There is a smooth thoracic kyphosis but it may produce a marked hump and a compensatory lumbar lordosis. The deformity cannot be corrected by changes in posture. Movements are normal but tight hamstrings often limit straight leg raising. A mild scoliosis is not uncommon. Rare complications are spastic paresis of the lower limbs and – with severe deformity of the thorax – cardiopulmonary dysfunction.

In later life, patients with thoracic kyphosis may develop low back pain. This has been attributed to chronic low back strain or facet joint dysfunction due to compensatory hyperextension of the lumbar spine. In some cases, however, lumbar Scheuermann's disease itself may cause pain.

Imaging

X-ray features include irregular or fragmented vertebral end plates of several adjacent vertebrae on lateral radiographs (**18.15**). The changes are more marked anteriorly and may lead to wedging. There may also be small radiolucent defects in the subchondral bone (Schmorl's nodes), which are thought to be due to central (axial) disc protrusions. The angle of deformity is measured in the same way as for scoliosis, except that here the lateral X-ray is used and the lines mark the uppermost and lowermost affected vertebrae. Wedging of more than 5 degrees in three adjacent vertebrae and an overall kyphosis angle of more than 40 degrees are abnormal.

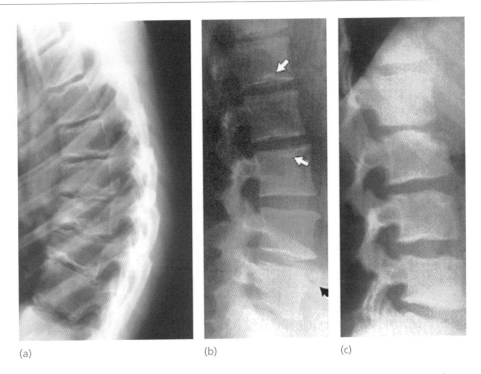

18.15 Scheuermann's disease – X-rays (a) X-rays of the young girl in **18.14a. (b,c)** In lumbar Scheuermann's, there is less wedging than in the thoracic region. End-plate fragmentation can be mistaken for a fracture of the vertebral body. Arrows show typical Schmorl's nodes.

Treatment

Treatment is usually not needed but the curvature may be painful during adolescence. Curves of less than 40 degrees require back-strengthening exercises and postural training. More severe curvature when the child is still growing benefits from 12–24 months in a brace. Older patients with a rigid curve of more than 60 degrees may need operative release, correction and instrumented fusion.

KYPHOSIS IN THE ELDERLY

Degeneration of intervertebral discs probably produces the gradually increasing stoop characteristic of the aged. The disc spaces become narrowed and the vertebrae slightly wedged. There is little pain unless OA of the facet joints is also present.

Postmenopausal osteoporosis may result in one or more compression fractures of the thoracic spine. Kyphosis is seldom marked and often the main complaint is of lumbosacral pain, which results from the compensatory lumbar lordosis in an ageing, osteoarthritic spine.

Treatment

Treatment is directed at the underlying osteoporosis. Fresh compression fractures may be treated by the transpedicular injection of methacrylate or bone graft substitute paste in order to stop further deformity and control pain ('vertebroplasty') or to correct the wedge deformity and maintain correction ('kyphoplasty'). The long-term outcomes and potential complications are, however, not yet fully understood.

SPINAL INFECTION

The axial skeleton accounts for 2–7% of all cases of osteomyelitis.

FACTORS PREDISPOSING TO SPINAL INFECTION

Diabetes mellitus
Malnutrition
Substance abuse
Human immunodeficiency virus (HIV) infection
Malignancy
Long-term use of steroids
Renal failure
Septicaemia

PYOGENIC DISCITIS/ OSTEOMYELITIS

Acute pyogenic infection of the spine is uncommon; elderly, chronically ill and immunodeficient patients are at greatest risk.

Pathology

Staphylococcus aureus is responsible in 50–60% of all cases, but in immunosuppressed patients Gram-negative organisms such as *Escherichia coli* and *Pseudomonas* are the most common. The usual sources of infection are:

- haematogenous spread from a distant focus of infection
- inoculation during invasive procedures (spinal injections and disc operations).

The infection usually begins in the vertebral end plates with secondary spread to the disc and adjacent vertebra. It may also spread along the anterior longitudinal ligament or outwards into the paravertebral soft tissues.

The spinal canal is rarely involved but, when it is (in the form of an epidural abscess), that is a surgical emergency. Despite rapid surgical decompression, the patient is often left with some degree of permanent paralysis.

Clinical features

Localized pain – the cardinal symptom – is often intense, unremitting and associated with muscle spasm and restricted movement. There may be point tenderness over the affected vertebra. Enquire about any invasive spinal procedure or a distant infection during the preceding few weeks. Systemic signs such as pyrexia and tachycardia are often present but not marked. In children, the diagnosis can be particularly difficult; however, restricted back movement is suspicious.

Imaging

- *X-rays* may show no change for several weeks. Early signs are loss of disc height, irregularity of the disc space, erosion of the vertebral end plate and reactive new bone formation (18.16). The early loss of disc height distinguishes vertebral osteomyelitis from metastatic disease, where the disc can remain intact despite advanced bone destruction.
- *Radionuclide scanning* will reveal increased activity at the site but this is non-specific.
- *MRI* may show characteristic changes in the vertebral end plates, intervertebral disc and paravertebral tissues. This investigation is highly sensitive but not specific.

Other investigations

The white blood cell (WBC) count, C-reactive protein (CRP) level and erythrocyte sedimentation rate (ESR) are usually elevated, and anti-staphylococcal antibodies may be present in high titres. Agglutination tests for *Salmonella* and *Brucella* should be performed, especially in endemic regions and in patients who have recently visited these areas. Blood culture may be positive; however, if it is negative, a closed needle biopsy is performed for bacteriological culture and tests for antibiotic sensitivity.

Treatment

With prompt and effective treatment, the outcome is usually favourable. Spontaneous fusion of infected vertebrae is a common feature of healed staphylococcal osteomyelitis.

NON-OPERATIVE TREATMENT
Treatment is started on the basis of a clinical diagnosis of infection and includes bed rest, pain relief and intravenous antibiotic administration

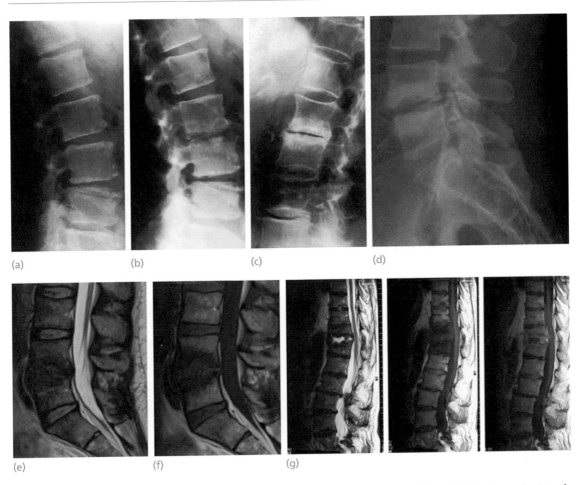

(a)   (b)   (c)   (d)

(e)   (f)   (g)

18.16 Pyogenic osteomyelitis and discitis Typical X-ray features are loss of disc height, irregularity of the disc 'space', end-plate erosion and reactive sclerosis. Progressive changes are shown in **(a)** and **(b)**. Reactive bone changes, shown in **(c)**, may end with ankylosis at the affected level. **(d)** X-ray shows L4/5 loss of disc height, endplate erosion and sclerosis. **(e–f)** MRI shows the disc and end-plate involvement without pus collection, typical of a low-grade discitis commonly from skin commensals such as *Propionibacterium acnes*. **(g)** MRI of T12/L1 spondylodiscitis with T2, T1 and with gadolinium contrast enhancement showing pus in the disc space.

using a 'best guess' regime that can be changed once the laboratory results and sensitivities are known. Intravenous antibiotics are continued for 1–2 weeks. If there is a good response (clinical improvement, a falling CRP and ESR and a normal WBC count), oral antibiotics can be used for a total treatment period of 6 weeks. Some centres treat for 12 weeks but with little evidence for this increased period. During this period nutritional support and management of comorbidities are essential in ensuring a successful outcome.

OPERATIVE TREATMENT

Surgery is seldom needed. Should the CRP or pain not be settled, surgical debridement may be indicated. An anterior approach is preferred; necrotic and infected material is removed and, if necessary, the cord is decompressed. The anterior column defect is reconstructed with bone grafts. If the spine is unstable, posterior instrumentation may be necessary. For a primary epidural abscess with neurological symptoms, laminectomy and drainage is indicated.

SECTION 2 REGIONAL ORTHOPAEDICS

TUBERCULOSIS

The spine is the most common site of skeletal TB, accounting for 50% of all musculoskeletal TB.

Pathology

Spread is haematogenous and the infection usually settles in a vertebral body adjacent to the intervertebral disc. Bone destruction and caseation follow, with infection spreading to the disc space and the adjacent vertebrae. In the lumbar area, the paravertebral abscess may track along muscle planes to involve the sacroiliac or hip joint, or along the psoas muscle to the thigh. As the vertebral bodies collapse, a sharp angulation (gibbus or kyphos) develops. There is a major risk of cord damage due to pressure by the abscess, granulation tissue, sequestra or displaced bone, or (occasionally) ischaemia from spinal artery thrombosis.

Spontaneous bony fusion of the involved levels may occur with healing but the persistent infection may cause spinal cord attenuation and late-onset paraplegia. Reactivation of healed disease may also occur.

Clinical features

There is usually a long history of ill health and backache; in late cases a gibbus deformity is the dominant feature. Concurrent pulmonary TB is a feature in most children under 10 years with thoracic spine involvement. Occasionally, the patient may present with a cold abscess pointing in the groin, or with paraesthesiae and weakness of the legs. There is local tenderness in the back and spinal movements are restricted. Neurological examination may show motor and/or sensory changes in the lower limbs. As spinal TB is found mostly in the thoracic spine, spastic paraparesis is a common presentation in adults.

In regions where TB is no longer common, the infection may be confined to a single vertebral body, symptoms may be mild and deformity can be slight. It is important to be alert to the possibility of this diagnosis, especially in patients who are HIV-positive.

Imaging

X-RAYS

The entire spine should be X-rayed, because vertebrae distant from the obvious site may also be affected. The earliest signs of infection are local osteoporosis of two adjacent vertebrae and narrowing of the intervertebral disc space, with fuzziness of the end plates. Progressive disease is associated with signs of bone destruction and collapse of adjacent vertebral bodies into each other. Paraspinal soft-tissue shadows may be due to either oedema or a paravertebral abscess. A chest X-ray is essential (18.17). With healing,

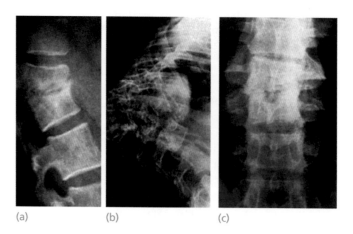

(a) (b) (c)

18.17 Spinal tuberculosis (a) Early X-ray changes with loss of disc space. **(b,c)** X-rays before and after operative debridement and spinal fusion using a rib strut graft.

bone density increases, the ragged appearance disappears and paravertebral abscesses may undergo resolution, fibrosis or calcification.

MRI AND CT

MRI and CT are invaluable to assess neurological compression, posterior vertebral element involvement, paravertebral abscesses, an epidural abscess and cord compression (18.18).

Special investigations

- *Skin tests* with attenuated mycobacterium (Mantoux and Tine) are sensitive but non-specific as they will react in vaccinated patients.
- *ESR* can also be useful but it is a non-specific marker.
- *WBC count* is usually normal but the differential may have a lymphocytosis and platelets raised.
- *HIV status* should be confirmed due to the association with TB.
- *Biopsy* is necessary to confirm the diagnosis and exclude drug-resistant strains, which are increasingly common.
- *Microscopy, culture and histological investigation* should be requested.
- *Polymerase chain reaction* (PCR) is both sensitive and specific and provides a result in 1–2 days as opposed to culture which takes up to 6 weeks.

Differential diagnosis

Spinal TB must be distinguished from other causes of vertebral pathology.

> **OTHER POSSIBLE CAUSES OF VERTEBRAL PATHOLOGY**
>
> Pyogenic infections
> Fungal infections
> Malignant disease
> Parasitic infestations, e.g. hydatid disease
> Disc space collapse, which is typical of infection
> Metastatic lesions, which may cause vertebral body collapse similar to that seen in TB but the disc space is usually preserved

Treatment

The objectives of treatment are to:

- eradicate or arrest the infection
- prevent or correct deformity
- prevent or treat associated neurological deficit.

MEDICAL THERAPY

In patients with minimal deformity and normal or mild neurological impairment, medical therapy is

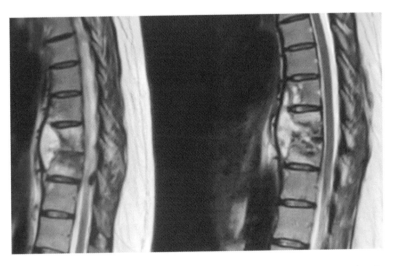

18.18 Spinal tuberculosis – MRI Sagittal MR images of advanced tuberculous infection with abscess formation beneath the anterior longitudinal ligament.

adequate. There is little consensus on antituberculous chemotherapy in terms of either drugs or duration. Most high-incidence regions use a combination of drugs, usually three or four (rifampicin, isoniazid, etham-butol and pyrazinamide), to minimize resistance and act against both the easily accessible mycobacteria and the latent intracellular group. They are available in a combination single tablet. Many use full drug treatment for the full duration of 9–12 months, whereas others follow the pulmonary strategy of a two-drug continuation phase after 2 months of three- or four-drug therapy. Dosages are weight-dependent and need to be adjusted as the patient improves in health status and gains weight.

Treatment is continued for the time period above, or until the X-ray shows resolution of the bone changes, the patient is constitutionally well and ESR has returned to normal. The patient must be monitored for the drugs' side effects of hepatitis, depression and loss of visual acuity. If resistant mycobacteria are confirmed on PCR or culture, second-line agents are required, usually involving a fluoroquinolone and aminoglycoside.

OPERATIVE TREATMENT

With progressive neurological deficit or marked kyphosis, surgical debridement and corrective instrumented fusion should be considered.

- *Anterior resection* of diseased tissue and *anterior spinal fusion* with a strut graft offers the double advantage of early and complete eradication of the infection and prevention of spinal deformity.
- *Posterior instrumentation* may be required for increased stability. Children who are growing and are seen to be at risk of developing severe kyphosis may need fusion of the posterior elements to minimize the expected deformity.

Antituberculous chemotherapy is still necessary, of course.

POTT'S PARAPLEGIA

Early-onset paresis

Early-onset paresis is usually within 2 years of disease onset and is due to pressure by inflammatory oedema, an abscess, caseous material,

granulation tissue or sequestra. The patient presents with lower-limb weakness, upper motor neuron signs, sensory dysfunction and incontinence. *CT and MRI* may reveal cord compression. In these cases, the prognosis for neurological recovery following surgery is good.

Late-onset paresis

Late-onset paresis is due to direct cord compression from increasing deformity, or (occasionally) vascular insufficiency of the cord; recovery following decompression is poor.

HUMAN IMMUNODEFICIENCY VIRUS AND SPINAL TB

HIV is one of the main reasons for the resurgence of TB, especially in the developing world. Initially, spinal TB, which is an extrapulmonary focus, was considered as AIDS-defining but, due to the high incidence of both diseases in some regions, this is not always the case. HIV patients are not homogeneous in their immune state. Patients with significantly impaired immunity are prone to developing opportunistic infections and atypical mycobacterial infections (*Mycobacterium intracellulare*, *M. avium*, *M. fortuitum*). There may be increasing atypical TB presentation in HIV patients.

Medical and surgical management are essentially the same but, in those patients with advanced disease, the patient's ability to survive a surgical insult must be considered. Often, they have large paraspinal abscesses with little kyphosis, and a simple procedure such as a costotransversectomy is all that is required. Initiation of antiretrovirals should be considered but it may result in increased TB disease due to a recovering immune system.

 Spinal TB in an HIV-positive patient can be life-threatening and needs to be managed by an infectious diseases specialist.

FUNGAL INFECTIONS

These are typically opportunistic infections occurring in an immunocompromised host or patient with extensive burns. *Aspergillosis* and

Cryptococcus are airborne fungi that initially affect the lungs; the spine is involved by haematogenous spread. The presentation, clinical findings and radiographic features may mimic those of TB. The *chest X-ray* may show a fungal ball or pneumonia. The diagnosis is made by sputum examination and bronchoscopy. The immunodiffusion test is specific for *Aspergillosis* and the latex agglutination test for *Cryptococcus*. A biopsy is performed to confirm the diagnosis.

Treatment

Neurological deficit is an indication for operative decompression. Specific treatment includes 5-flucytosine and amphotericin B, which act synergistically. Concurrent treatment of the underlying immunocompromised state is essential.

PARASITIC INFESTATIONS

The commonest parasitic infestation affecting the spine is due to the cestode worm *Echinococcus granulosis*, which causes hydatid disease. It is encountered mainly in areas where sheep are raised. Infestation occurs through ingestion of faecal contamination or by inhalation of desiccated particles in dust. Hydatid cysts in bone develop in about 1% of cases. It is usually detected in childhood but diagnosis may be delayed. The presentation and clinical features are similar to those of other forms of spondylitis. *X-rays* may reveal a translucent area with a sclerotic margin in the affected vertebral body.

Systemic treatment is with albendazole, usually three cycles of 25 days each. Operative treatment to achieve spinal decompression may be called for.

 Spillage of cyst contents must be avoided.

ANKYLOSING SPONDYLITIS (SPONDYLOARTHROPATHY)

This group of disorders is discussed in Chapter 3.

INTERVERTEBRAL DISC LESIONS

Low back pain is one of the most common causes of chronic disability in Western societies, and in the majority of cases the backache is associated with degeneration of the intervertebral discs in the lower lumbar spine. This is an age-related phenomenon that occurs in over 80% of people who live for more than 50 years and in most cases it is asymptomatic.

Pathology

With normal ageing, glycosaminoglycan production diminishes, leading to gradual desiccation of the disc. The annulus fibrosus develops fissures and disc nuclear material may prolapse through. The discs lose height and bulge beyond the margins of the vertebral bodies (**18.19**). Disc

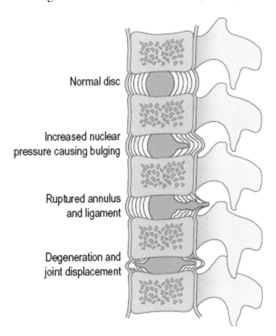

Normal disc

Increased nuclear pressure causing bulging

Ruptured annulus and ligament

Degeneration and joint displacement

18.19 Intervertebral disc prolapse and degeneration Diagrammatic representation of progressive stages in the development of *disc prolapse*. At first there is only bulging of the posterior part of the disc; the annulus fibrosus may go on to rupture and the nucleus pulposus is extruded posteriorly to one or other side. In disc degeneration (lowest figure), the disc becomes desiccated and collapses, causing displacement of the posterior facet joints.

protrusion against the ligaments causes formation of marginal osteophytes. Adjacent vertebral end plates ossify and become sclerotic while fatty change occurs in the subchondral bone marrow. This process is termed *spondylosis*.

Disc degeneration results in altered biomechanics and increased loading forces on the facet joints (which are intrinsically linked). Facet joint OA may lead to osteophyte encroachment into the canal causing spinal lateral recess stenosis. The ligamentum flavum thickens, which contributes to the stenosis, while the disc bulges from anteriorly into the spinal canal.

Imaging

X-RAYS

X-ray features of intervertebral disc degeneration have little correlation with symptoms. More than 50% of asymptomatic individuals of 30–39 years of age have disc degeneration.

MRI

MRI findings include annular fissures, Modic changes, disc degeneration and disc herniation. Modic changes are found in 46% of patients with non-specific LBP and 6% in the asymptomatic general population. Type 1 Modic changes have been linked to *Propionibacterium acnes* and *Corynebacterium propinquum* low-grade infections. This remains contentious and research continues into the condition. Most patients with proven disc pathology will not have Modic changes. As diagnostic markers, Modic signs have relatively low sensitivity.

Treatment

Asymptomatic lumbar disc degeneration does not require any treatment besides reassuring the patient that they are normal. Symptomatic conditions related to disc degeneration are discussed below.

ACUTE INTERVERTEBRAL DISC HERNIATION

Acute disc herniation (prolapse, rupture) is a result of underlying disc degeneration. It occurs most commonly in the fourth to fifth decades of life, is more common in men than women (3 : 1 ratio) and occurs mostly at L4/5 and L5/S1 disc levels.

RISK FACTORS FOR DISC PROLAPSE
Smoking
Heavy lifting, especially with torsional stress
Strenuous physical activity
Occupational driving

A '*protrusion*' is a posteriorly bulging disc with the outer annulus intact. When *rupture* occurs, fibrocartilaginous disc material is extruded posteriorly through the posterior longitudinal ligament; when disc material breaks free to lie in the canal, it is termed *sequestration*. A large central rupture may cause compression of the cauda equina. A posterolateral rupture presses on the nerve root proximal to its point of exit through the intervertebral foramen; thus, a herniation at L4/5 will compress the fifth lumbar nerve root, and a herniation at L5/S1, the first sacral root. Local inflammatory response with oedema aggravates the symptoms.

Acute back pain at the onset of disc herniation probably arises from disruption of the outermost layers of the annulus fibrosus and stretching or tearing of the posterior longitudinal ligament. Nerve root irritation causes pain in the buttock which may be referred or radiate down the posterior thigh and calf (*sciatica*). Pressure on the nerve root itself causes *paraesthesia* and/or *numbness* in the corresponding dermatome, as well as *weakness* and *depressed reflexes* in the muscles supplied by that nerve root.

Clinical features

Acute disc prolapse may occur at any age but it is uncommon in the very young and the very old. A common presentation is acute severe back pain which improves, followed by the development of buttock and leg pain (sciatica) a few days later. Both backache and sciatica are made worse by coughing or straining. Paraesthesia or numbness in the leg or foot, and occasionally muscle weakness may occur.

Cauda equina compression is rare but may cause urinary retention and perineal numbness and is an emergency.

The patient usually stands with a slight list to one side ('sciatic scoliosis'). Sometimes the knee on the painful side is held slightly flexed to relax tension on the sciatic nerve. All back movements are severely limited, and during forward bending the list may increase.

TESTS FOR DISC PROLAPSE

Palpation may find tenderness in the midline and paravertebral muscle spasm.

Straight-leg raising is restricted and painful on the affected side.

Dorsiflexion of the foot and bowstringing of the lateral popliteal nerve may accentuate the pain.

A crossed straight-leg raise test, if positive, is highly specific for a disc prolapse.

The femoral stretch test may be positive with a high or mid-lumbar prolapse.

Neurological examination

This may show muscle weakness (and, later, wasting), diminished reflexes and sensory loss corresponding to the affected level. L5 impairment causes weakness of big toe extension and knee flexion, with sensory loss on the outer side of the leg and the dorsum of the foot. S1 impairment causes weak plantarflexion and eversion of the foot, a depressed ankle jerk and sensory loss along the lateral border of the foot. With cauda equina compression, urinary retention is accompanied by loss of sensation over the sacrum.

Imaging

- *X-rays* are essential, not to show the disc space but to exclude bone disease. However, after several attacks the disc space may indeed be flattened.
- *MRI* is the default investigation for spinal pathology and has replaced other imaging modalities (18.20).
- Where there are contraindications to MRI (such as MRI incompatible pacemaker), a *CT myelogram* is indicated.

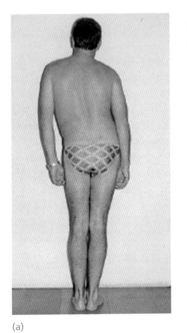

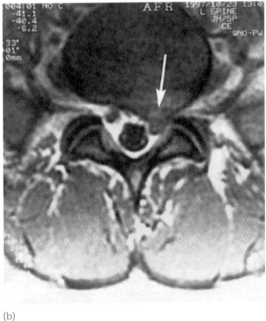

(a)   (b)

18.20 Prolapsed disc – clinical and MRI (a) This patient presented with acute LBP and sciatica. He has the characteristic sideways list (or tilt) due to paravertebral muscle spasm. **(b)** MRI showing the disc prolapse, with posterolateral protrusion towards the intervertebral foramen at L5/S1 (arrow).

Differential diagnosis

Space-occupying lesions, epidural abscess, tumours, epidural haematoma, stenosis and intradural pathology may present with sciatic symptoms. 'Red flags' (see 'Low back pain' below) require further investigation.

Direct sciatic nerve compression in the pelvis and upper thigh may occur with piriformis syndrome (compression neuropathy).

Treatment

Around 90% of symptomatic lumbar disc herniations will improve over 6 weeks irrespective of the advice or treatment given. All the usual conservative treatment modalities are symptomatic and have not been shown to change the natural history.

There are four elements in the treatment of acute disc herniation:

- rest
- reduction
- removal
- rehabilitation.

Rest   During an acute attack, the patient should be kept in bed, with hips and knees slightly flexed. An anti-inflammatory medication is useful.

Reduction   Continuous bed rest and traction for 2 weeks may allow the herniation to reduce. If the symptoms and signs do not improve significantly by then, *an epidural injection* of corticosteroid and local anaesthetic may help. If conservative measures fail, then discectomy is the treatment of choice.

Removal   Operative removal of a disc is indicated in some circumstances. The presence of a herniated disc, and the level, must be confirmed by CT or MRI before operating.

 A cauda equina compression syndrome which does not clear up within 6 hours of starting bed rest and traction must be treated as a surgical emergency.

INDICATIONS FOR OPERATIVE REMOVAL OF A DISC

A cauda equina compression syndrome which does not respond within 6 hours of starting bed rest and traction (see above)

Persistent pain and severely limited straight-leg raising after 2 weeks of conservative treatment

Neurological deterioration while under conservative treatment

Frequently recurring attacks

Surgical terms used are *laminectomy, laminotomy, discectomy* and *microdiscectomy.* These are largely historical divisions and most procedures are now done with magnification through a unilateral hemi-laminotomy approach.

Rehabilitation   After recovery from an acute disc rupture, or disc removal, the patient is mobilized and needs to limit physical exertion for 6–8 weeks to allow the annular defect to scar up and minimize re-prolapse. Non-impact exercises are usually safe.

LOW BACK PAIN

An estimated 80% of the normal population will experience LBP in their lifetime and this has enormous socioeconomic consequences. It is the leading cause of occupational disability worldwide. It is defined as pain and discomfort between the costal margin and inferior gluteal folds with or without leg pain. Pain may be acute (lasting less than 6 weeks), subacute (6–12 weeks) and chronic (more than 12 weeks).

CAUSES OF LBP

Mechanical (80%)

- *Muscular strains or from ligamentous injury*
- *Degenerative disc disease*
- *Facet joint disease (facet joint dysfunction)*

- *Spondylolysis*
- *Osteoporotic compression fractures*
- *Instability*
- *Sacroiliac joint pathology*

Neurogenic (15%)

- Herniated disc
- Spinal stenosis
- Foraminal stenosis
- Disc annular tear and neuritis

Non-mechanical back pain (1–2%)

- Infections
- Neoplasms
- Inflammatory conditions

Referred pain (1–2%)

- Gastrointestinal disease
- Renal disease
- Aortic aneurysm

Other (2–4%)

- Somatization disorder
- Fibromyalgia

Malingering

LOW BACK PAIN: RED AND YELLOW FLAGS

Red flags

- Age of onset less than 20 years or more than 55 years
- Recent history of violent trauma
- Constant progressive, non-mechanical pain (no relief with bed rest)
- Thoracic pain
- Past medical history of malignant tumour
- Prolonged use of corticosteroids
- Drug abuse, immunosuppression, HIV
- Systemically unwell
- Unexplained weight loss
- Widespread neurological symptoms (including cauda equina syndrome)
- Structural deformity
- Fever

Yellow flags

- Belief that back pain is harmful or potentially severely disabling
- Fear and avoidance of activity or movement
- Tendency to low mood and withdrawal from social interaction
- Expectation of passive treatment(s) rather than a belief that active participation will help

---

Mechanical pain is aggravated with movement, relieved by rest and is not radicular. An acute flare-up of pain often occurs on a background of chronic back pain. Patients with pain radiating down to the buttocks and posterior thigh may have neurogenic pain such as *spinal stenosis*. Poor walking distance is a typical feature, stenotic symptoms are typically relieved by flexion and the 'shopping-cart sign' is almost pathognmonic of spinal stenosis. When other symptoms occur, such as pins and needles, sensation changes and weakness, a radiculopathy is likely.

- *Red flags* are conditions in addition to back pain and warrant investigation to exclude serious pathology.
- *Yellow flags* are psychosocial factors that increase the risk of chronicity and disability from back pain.

Examination

- *Spine examination* may reveal muscle spasm, local tenderness and restriction of back movements. Pain on flexion may indicate disc pathology and with extension facet joint pain and spinal stenosis may predominate, but these tests have low specificity.
- The *hips* should be examined to exclude hip joint pathology and the *sacroiliac joints* are routinely assessed (e.g. with the FABER (Flexion, ABduction, and External Rotation)/Patrick's test).
- *Neurological assessment* includes eliciting nerve root irritation with the straight-leg raise test (L4–S1) and the femoral stretch test (L2–L4 nerve roots). Motor power, sensation and reflexes should be documented.

Imaging

X-RAYS

X-rays may be normal. However, in many cases, there are mild to moderately severe features of intervertebral disc degeneration, mainly flattening of the 'disc space' and marginal osteophytes. In the lateral view, there may be slight displacement of one vertebra upon another, either forwards (spondylolisthesis) or backwards (retrolisthesis); this may become apparent only during flexion or extension. X-rays of the pelvis help assess the hip joints and sacroiliac joints for pathology.

CT AND MRI

CT and MRI may reveal signs of disc degeneration as well as early features of OA in the facet joints. MRI findings of high intensity zones (annular tear), disc degeneration and Modic end-plate changes are suggestive as causes of low back pain but many asymptomatic individuals have similar findings.

Other tests

Full blood count, CRP and ESR help screen for non-mechanical causes of LBP such as infections, inflammatory conditions and neoplasms. In elderly patients, a serum protein electrophoresis and prostate-specific antigen in males should be part of the workup.

Treatment

CONSERVATIVE TREATMENT

Conservative treatment should be encouraged for as long as possible if the symptoms are neither severe nor disabling. Reassurance is often key to allay fears. Patients can be reassured that most cases of acute back pain are self-limiting and resolve over a few weeks. Treatment includes paracetamol and non-steroidal anti-inflammatory drugs (NSAIDs), short courses of opioids, or non-benzodiazepine muscle relaxants. Tricyclic antidepressants are more useful for chronic LBP and gabapentin tends to be used in radiculopathy.

Activity modification to avoid provoking activities is very important and the patient may need to change the nature of their work. Conventional physiotherapy and spinal manipulation for patients may be of benefit. In the longer term, weight control and strengthening of the vertebral and abdominal muscles (core muscles) may prevent recurrences. Counselling and support are often welcomed by the patient. In chronic radiculopathy, nerve root blocks may give short-term symptomatic relief and diagnostic information. Epidural steroids can be considered for spinal stenosis with some short-term benefit. Injections are ineffective in non-specific LBP.

OPERATIVE TREATMENT

 Only after all of the above measures have been tried and found to be ineffectual should a spinal fusion be considered. Strict guidelines need to be followed.

GUIDELINES FOR SPINAL FUSION

1 Ensure there is no other treatable pathology.
2 There should have been at least some response to conservative treatment.
3 Unequivocal evidence of pathology at a specific level.
4 The patient should be emotionally stable and should not exaggerate their symptoms or display inappropriate physical signs.
5 Patient and surgeon expectations need to align.
6 Surgery is effective for relief of pain and deformity in infections, tumours and fractures. Surgery is also cost-effective and superior to non-operative treatment for degenerative conditions with neural pain (prolapsed disc, spinal stenosis and spondylolisthesis).
7 Surgery for non-specific back pain is far less effective.

Surgery is traditionally aimed at stabilizing the painful segment with fusion; instrumentation increases the fusion rates but does not correlate with clinical outcomes. Options are posterior fusion, anterior fusion or combinations of both (18.21). Adjacent level degeneration is occasionally noted alongside fusion segments. Non-fusion stabilization technologies such as total disc replacement (TDR) were developed to address this. Although these initially held great promise, a high revision rate and devastating approach-related complications resulted in loss of favour of these implants for use in the lumbar spine.

SPONDYLOLISTHESIS

'Spondylolisthesis' means forward translation of one segment of the spine upon another. The shift is nearly always between L4 and L5, or between L5 and the sacrum (11% occur at L4/5 and 82% occur at L5/S1). Normal discs, laminae and facets constitute a locking mechanism that prevents each vertebra from moving forwards on the one below.

The *Wiltse–Newman classification of spondylolisthesis* is most commonly used.

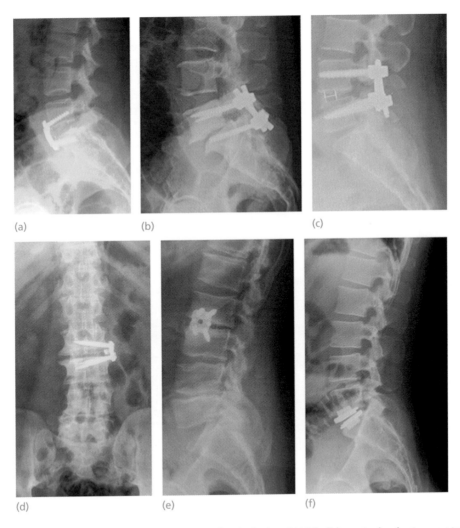

(a)　　　　　　(b)　　　　　　(c)

(d)　　　　　　(e)　　　　　　(f)

18.21 Surgical options (a) Anterior lumbar interbody fusion (ALIF); (b) posterior instrumented fusion; (c) transforaminal lumbar interbody fusion (TLIF); (d,e) direct lateral interbody fusion (DLIF); (f) TDR.

WILTSE–NEWMAN CLASSIFICATION OF SPONDYLOLISTHESIS

- I Dysplastic
- II Isthmic
  - IIA Disruption of pars as a result of stress fracture
  - IIB Elongation of pars without disruption related to repeated, healed microfractures
  - IIC Acute fracture through pars
- III Degenerative
- IV Traumatic
- V Pathologic
- VI Iatrogenic

Clinical features

DYSPLASTIC SPONDYLOLISTHESIS

Dysplastic spondylolisthesis (type I) is seen in children. It is usually painless but the mother may notice the unduly protruding abdomen. There may be an associated scoliosis. They will progress in around a third and are more likely to become high-grade slips with significant chance of neurological injury and more commonly require surgery. High-grade slips have more than 50% translation.

LYTIC OR ISTHMIC SPONDYLOLISTHESIS

This is the commonest variety. It occurs in adults and intermittent backache is the usual presenting symptom. Pain may be initiated or exacerbated by exercise or strain. On examination, the buttocks look curiously flat, the sacrum appears to extend to the waist and transverse loin creases may be prominent. A 'step' can often be felt when the fingers are run down the spine. Movements are usually normal in younger patients but may be restricted in older people. Healing can occur with immobilization especially with unilateral defects. When non-union occurs, the fracture becomes corticalized and filled with fibrous tissue. A 'lytic' defect is visible on X-ray.

DEGENERATIVE SPONDYLOLISTHESIS

This usually occurs in patients over 40 years with long-standing backache due to facet joint arthritis. Sometimes the presenting symptom is spinal 'claudication' due to narrowing of the spinal canal (see 'Spinal stenosis' below).

Imaging

X-rays show the forward shift of the upper part of the spinal column on the stable vertebra below; elongation of the arch or defective facets may be seen. The gap in the pars interarticularis is more easily seen in oblique X-ray views (**18.22**), and best of all in *CT scans*.

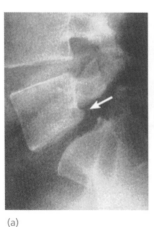 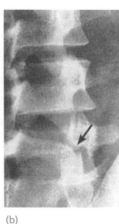 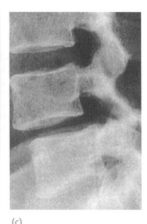

(a)   (b)   (c)

18.22 Spondylolisthesis – X-rays (a) There is a break in the pars interarticularis of L5, allowing the anterior part of the vertebra to slip forwards. In this case, the gap is easily seen in the lateral X-ray, but usually it is better seen in the oblique view **(b)**. In degenerative spondylolisthesis, there is no break in the pars – the degenerate disc and eroded facet joints permit one vertebra to slide forwards on the other **(c)**.

Treatment

CONSERVATIVE TREATMENT

Conservative treatment, similar to that for other types of back pain, is suitable for most patients.

OPERATIVE TREATMENT

> **INDICATIONS FOR OPERATIVE TREATMENT OF SPONDYLOLISTHESIS**
>
> Symptoms are disabling and interfere significantly with work and recreational activities.
> The upper vertebra has slipped forwards over more than 50% of the vertebral body below.
> Neurological compression is significant.

- *For children*, posterior intertransverse fusion *in situ* was previously favoured; if neurological signs appear, decompression can be carried out later. Instrumented reduction and circumferential fusion improves fusion rates and the posture, but the surgery is technically demanding and has a higher complication rate.
- *For adults*, either posterior or anterior fusion is suitable. However, in the 'degenerative' group, where neurological symptoms predominate, decompression without fusion may suffice.

SPINAL STENOSIS

Spinal stenosis refers to reduced spinal canal dimensions and neural compression and may be congenital or acquired.

- *Congenital* vertebral dysplasia occurs in achondroplasia or hypochondroplasia.
- *Acquired* stenosis occurs mostly with degeneration, and is the most common, but also in spondylolysis and spondylolisthesis, iatrogenic, post-traumatic, local infection and metabolic stenosis. It is categorized as central, lateral or foraminal.

Clinical features

Typically, a patient with backache complains of aching and/or numbness and paraesthesia in the thighs, legs or feet. The symptoms come on after standing upright or walking for 5–10 minutes and are consistently relieved by sitting or squatting with the spine somewhat flexed (hence the term '*spinal claudication*').

Examination, especially after getting the patient to reproduce the symptoms by walking, may show neurological defects in the lower limbs.

> Always check the upper limbs for signs of polyneuropathy and the lower limbs for evidence of peripheral vascular disease.

Nerve conduction studies and electromyography are helpful in establishing the diagnosis and severity of neurological change.

Symptoms are sometimes unilateral, suggesting an asymmetrical stenosis or intervertebral root canal stenosis. The distribution of pain and sensory abnormality will indicate which levels are affected.

Imaging

Lateral view X-rays may show degenerative spondylolisthesis or advanced disc degeneration and OA. Measurement of the spinal canal may be carried out on plain films, but more reliable information is obtained from *CT and MRI* (**18.23**).

Absolute stenosis is usually defined when the mid-sagittal diameter of the canal is less than 10 mm and *elative stenosis* with a mid-sagittal canal diameter of 10–13 mm. These are useful guidelines but they do not have reliable clinical correlation.

Treatment

CONSERVATIVE TREATMENT

Conservative measures, including instruction in spinal posture, may suffice. Localized symptoms due to root canal stenosis often respond to injection of a long-acting local anaesthetic and corticosteroid injection, which can be repeated two or three times at 3- or 6-monthly intervals.

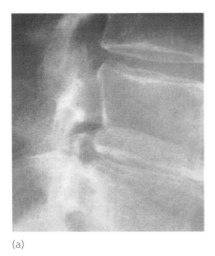 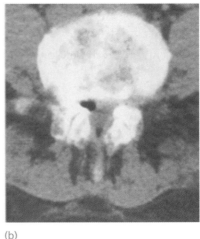

(a)   (b)

18.23 Spinal stenosis (a) A lateral X-ray shows marked narrowing of the spinal canal, but the CT scan **(b)** provides even more convincing evidence.

OPERATIVE TREATMENT

If conservative measures fail to provide sufficient relief, operative decompression will be needed. Posterior decompression is the mainstay of surgical treatment. For central stenosis, laminectomy is performed. The lateral recess stenosis is decompressed with undercutting facetectomies and removal of ligamentum flavum. Care should be taken to excise less than 50% of the facet joints and avoid damage to the pars interarticularis to prevent iatrogenic instability, which would necessitate fusion. Foraminal stenosis requires fusion to decompress and maintain foraminal patency. However, patients must be warned that the operation will not improve their backache. If there are clear-cut signs of spinal instability, segmental fusion may also be needed.

APPROACH TO DIAGNOSIS IN PATIENTS WITH LOW BACK PAIN

Chronic backache is a frequent cause of disability in the community. The following is a suggested approach to more specific diagnosis. Careful history-taking and examination will uncover one of five pain patterns.

THE FIVE PATTERNS OF LBP

Transient backache following muscular activity
Sudden, acute pain and sciatica
Intermittent LBP after exertion
Back pain plus pseudoclaudication
Severe and constant pain localized to a particular site

Transient backache following muscular activity This suggests a simple back strain that will respond to a short period of rest followed by gradually increasing exercise.

Sudden, acute pain and sciatica

- *In young people*, it is important to exclude infection and spondylolisthesis.
- *Patients aged 20–40 years* are more likely to have an acute disc prolapse. Diagnostic features are:
  - a history of a lifting strain
  - unequivocal sciatic tension
  - neurological symptoms and signs.
- *Elderly patients* may have osteoporotic compression fractures, but metastatic disease and myeloma must be excluded.

Intermittent LBP after exertion Patients of almost any age may complain of recurrent back-ache following exertion or lifting activities and this is relieved by rest. Features of disc prolapse are absent but there may be a history of acute sciatica in the past. In early cases, X-rays usually show no abnormality; later there may be signs of lumbar spondylosis in those over 50 years and OA of the facet joints is common.

These patients need painstaking examination to:

- uncover any features of radiological segmental instability or facet joint OA
- determine whether those features are incidental or are likely to account for the patient's symptoms.

In the process, disorders such as ankylosing spondylitis, chronic infection, myelomatosis and other bone diseases must be excluded by appropriate imaging and blood investigations.

Back pain plus pseudoclaudication These patients are usually aged over 50 and may give a history of previous, long-standing back trouble. The diagnosis of spinal stenosis should be confirmed by CT and/or MRI.

Severe and constant pain localized to a particular site This suggests local bone pathology, such as a compression fracture, Paget's disease, a tumour or infection. Spinal osteoporosis in middle-aged men is pathological.

CHRONIC BACK PAIN SYNDROME

Patients with chronic backache may despair of finding a cure for their trouble (or, indeed, even a diagnosis that everyone agrees on), and they often develop affective and psychosomatic ailments that subsequently become the chief focus of attention. This 'illness behaviour' is both self-perpetuating and self-justifying. It is usually accompanied by *'non-organic' (inappropriate) physical signs.*

'NON-ORGANIC' PHYSICAL SIGNS OF CHRONIC BACK PAIN SYNDROME

Pain and tenderness of bizarre degree or distribution

Pain on performing impressive but non-stressful manoeuvres such as pressing vertically on the spine or passively rotating the entire trunk

Variations in response to tests such as straight-leg raising while distracting the patient's attention

Sensory and/or motor abnormalities that do not fit the known anatomical and physiological patterns

Overdetermined behaviour during physical examination (trembling, sweating, hyper-ventilating, inability to move, a tendency to fall and exaggerated withdrawal) – usually accompanied by loud groaning and exclamations of discomfort

---

Patients with these features are unlikely to respond to surgery and they may require prolonged support and management in a special pain clinic – but only after every effort has been made to exclude organic pathology.

The immature hip	**393**	■ Intra-articular hip pathology –	
■ Developmental dysplasia of the hip	393	osteoarthritis of the hip joint	409
■ Developmental coxa vara	397	■ Mechanical causes of hip osteoarthritis	410
■ Irritable hip (transient synovitis)	397	■ Non-mechanical causes of hip	
■ Legg–Calvé–Perthes disease	399	osteoarthritis	413
■ Slipped capital femoral epiphysis	401	■ Non-operative treatment of hip	
The adult hip	**404**	osteoarthritis	415
■ Clinical assessment	404	■ Total hip arthroplasty	415

THE IMMATURE HIP

DEVELOPMENTAL DYSPLASIA OF THE HIP

Developmental dysplasia of the hip (DDH) is a spectrum of abnormalities ranging from mild acetabular dysplasia to irreducible dislocation. There is probably some, at least transient, abnormality in up to 10% of females but most are amenable to reassurance alone.

DDH is classed into four groups on the basis of clinical and sonographic examination.

- *Reduced and stable but dysplastic* The hip may be clinically normal or have subtle laxity. There is a shallow acetabular cup.
- *Reduced but dislocatable* The hip can be dislocated by the *Barlow manoeuvre* (**19.1**).
- *Dislocated but reducible* The femoral head is dislocated but can be reduced with gentle manipulation using the *Ortolani manoeuvre* (**19.2**).
- *Dislocated and irreducible* This is the most severe type. In unilateral cases there is asymmetrical abduction of the hip. The hip may be stiff, with tightness of the adductor longus tendon, and the femoral head cannot be reduced.

Pathophysiology

The femoral head and acetabulum develop from a single cleft of primitive mesenchymal cells. The femoral head begins to separate between 7 and 8 weeks' gestation. At 12 weeks, separation is complete with the femoral head almost completely contained within the acetabulum. Relative growth results in least coverage around term. The labrum develops postnatally, deepening the

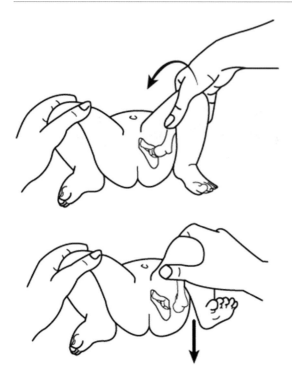

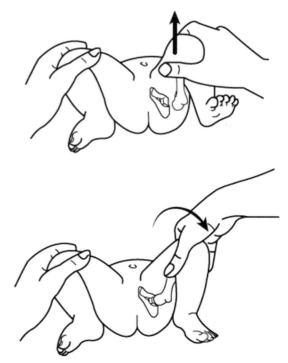

19.1 Barlow manoeuvre This manoeuvre pushes the femoral head superior and posterior out of the acetabulum.

19.2 Ortolani manoeuvre The dislocated femoral head is reduced by abduction and anterior translation.

socket. Walking is a potent stimulus to further acetabular development.

Dislocation of the hip can occur:

- at 10 weeks when the lower extremity limb bud rotates medially
- at 18 weeks when neuromuscular disorders may cause muscular imbalance, leading to dislocation around 18 weeks' gestation
- during the final 4 weeks of gestation, due to mechanical forces (e.g. in the left occiput anterior position, the left hip is adducted against the maternal sacrum), breech position, oligohydramnios, multiple fetuses, circulating maternal relaxin combined with the relatively low percentage acetabular coverage of the femoral head.

Postnatally, swaddling of the lower extremities holds the hips in extension and adduction.

Teratological dislocation leads to abnormal development of all parts of the hip joint, is associated with other disorders and treatment differs from other types of DDH.

In the subluxed position, the labrum is flattened by the femoral head. The acetabulum develops non-concentrically and does not deepen. Dislocation of the femoral head leads to stretching of the inferior capsule and adductors.

MAIN RISK FACTORS FOR DDH
Female gender
Firstborn child
Oligohydramnios
Breech positioning
Family history

Three percent of births are breech and of these 23% will have some degree of DDH. Other skeletal abnormalities commonly associated with DDH include torticollis and postural foot abnormality such as metatarsus adductus.

SECTION 2 REGIONAL ORTHOPAEDICS

Diagnosis

All neonates should undergo clinical hip examination. The role of ultrasound screening is debated.

The Barlow and Ortolani tests are the mainstays in examination. At a later stage, findings may include asymmetrical skin folds, although these are common in normal hips. In established dislocation, there is a leg length discrepancy (LLD), positive *Galeazzi* test and reduced range of abduction. Bilateral DDH is always more difficult to diagnose as symmetrical changes are more difficult to pick up.

Imaging

The use of multiplanar and dynamic ultrasound enables visualization of the femoral head within the acetabulum and assessment of the shape and depth of the acetabular cup (19.3). It is used for children under 6 months of age, after which plain X-ray is generally more helpful.

The shape of the acetabulum is assessed by measuring the alpha angle (angle between the straight edge of the ilium and the acetabular roof), a normal measurement is 60 degrees or greater. The beta angle is less helpful in clinical practice (Table 19.1).

Assessment is improved by adding a transverse stress image to the static coronal image.

Management and treatment

Early intervention leads to less complicated treatment and more favourable outcomes.

There is good evidence to support *management in the neonate*. The treatment of Ortolani-positive

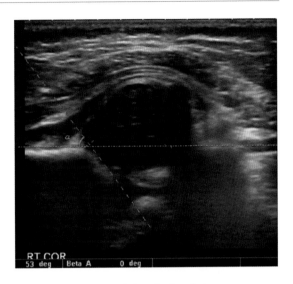

19.3 Developmental dysplasia of the hip Coronal static ultrasound of moderately dysplastic right hip with alpha angle of 53°.

hips, dislocated at rest but reducible, should begin as soon as practical. Conversely, it is reasonable to delay treatment of Barlow-positive hips for up to 2 weeks without compromising the final outcome, as a large percentage will stabilize. At 2 weeks, failure to improve either clinically or on the basis of an ultrasound is an indication to commence treatment.

Treatment involves maintaining hip abduction through the use of a brace; the most commonly used is the *Pavlik harness (PH)*. Poor positioning, prolonged treatment and lack of parental compliance are associated with treatment failure. Significant potential complications include avascular necrosis (AVN), femoral nerve and brachial plexus palsy. If these occur, PH therapy should

Table 19.1 Classification of ultrasonographic hip types (Graf)

Type	α angle (degrees)	β angle (degrees)	Age (months)	Acetabular roof (shape)	Femoral head (location)
I	>60	<55	Any	Normal	Central
IIa	43–60	55–77	0–3	Normal	Central
IIb	43–60	55–77	>3	Normal, delayed ossification	Central
IIIa	<43	>77	Any	Upward displacement	Lateralized
IIIb	<43	>77	Any	Upward displacement and bending	Lateralized
IV			Any	Stretched	Dislocated

be discontinued until resolution and often is abandoned. If PH fails to reduce the hip within 3–4 weeks, it should be discontinued.

The PH is worn 24 hours per day. Total treatment duration varies between clinicians but is generally agreed to be around 12 weeks for most and should not exceed 20 weeks.

Success rates following PH are excellent if treatment is commenced before 8 weeks of age.

The management of hips that are clinically stable but dysplastic or unstable on dynamic ultrasound is complex and controversial.

CLOSED REDUCTION

If the above fails, the next step is examination under anaesthetia and a *hip arthrogram* with a view to a closed reduction. *Preoperative traction* is controversial.

Closed reduction is performed by longitudinal traction, flexion and abduction of the hip with anterior translation. Reduction is confirmed with dynamic arthrogram. Medial dye pooling between the femoral head and acetabulum indicates inadequate reduction.

Following reduction, the hip is immobilized in a *hip spica cast* within the '*safe zone of Ramsey*'. This is the arc of motion through which the hip remains reduced without forced abduction. Adductor tenotomy is often performed.

Postoperatively, hip position is confirmed by 3D imaging, and the hip is immobilized for 12 weeks.

Closed reduction may fail due to a block to reduction or inability to hold the femoral head contained within a shallow acetabulum. Extra-articular blocks include tight adductors and iliopsoas tendon. Medial contraction of the joint capsule can also impede reduction. The transverse acetabular ligament may also hypertrophy, further limiting reduction.

OPEN REDUCTION

The timing of open reduction is controversial. Some feel that the hip should be allowed to 'loosen' before proceeding to open reduction, even if the ossific nucleus has not appeared; others feel that the presence of an ossific nucleus is protective and surgery should be deferred until it appears.

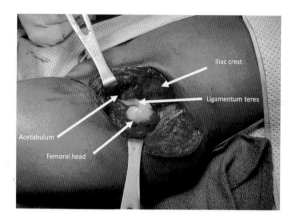

19.4 Open reduction of a dislocated left hip The cartilaginous iliac crest apophysis has been split, exposing the lateral aspect of the ilium. The femoral head, elongated ligamentum teres and empty acetabulum can be visualized.

The medial approach is preferred by some in patients under 1 year of age, but this may be associated with higher rates of late AVN.

Open reduction is usually performed through a transverse skin crease incision, between tensor fascia lata and sartorius with splitting of the iliac apophysis (**19.4**). The conjoined head of rectus femoris is divided, psoas tenotomy and a T-shaped capsulotomy performed. The ligamentum teres and transverse acetabular ligament are generally excised but the acetabular labrum is preserved if possible. In younger children, a capsulorraphy may suffice but with increasing age, pelvic and/or femoral osteotomies may be required. Following reduction and stabilization, the capsule is repaired.

Postoperatively the hip is immobilized in a spica cast for up to 12 weeks. 3D imaging should be performed postoperatively to confirm reduction.

OSTEOTOMIES

Osteotomies can be used to correct residual acetabular dysplasia (rarely before 18 months) and on the femoral side to correct femoral version or reduce wound tension.

Salter osteotomy The pubic symphysis is used as a rotational hinge to rotate the acetabulum leading to increased joint stability as well as the load-bearing portion of the acetabulum.

Pemberton osteotomy Pericapsular pelvic osteotomy achieves acetabular rotation by exploiting the plasticity of the horizontal arms of the triradiate cartilage, which need to be open. This is a volume-changing osteotomy commonly used in a shallow acetabulum with anterolateral wall deficiency.

Proximal femoral varus derotation osteotomy The proximal femur is typically valgus and anteverted. If the hip is stable in internal rotation and abduction but subluxes in flexion, increasing the varus angle and reducing excessive anteversion may help.

Femoral shortening osteotomy In long-standing high hip dislocation, reduction may place increased pressure on the femoral head within the acetabulum and femoral shortening osteotomy may be required to reduce the risk of AVN (**19.5**).

Periacetabular osteotomy (PAO) In teenagers with closed growth plates and young adults who present with dysplastic hips it is reasonable to offer corrective surgery to relieve symptoms and reduce the rate of progression to degenerative change, such as the Ganz periacetabular osteotomy.

DEVELOPMENTAL COXA VARA

This condition presents in childhood with a painless limp and LLD. Radiographs show a loss of the normal neck-shaft angle (coxa vara) and a triangular ossification defect in the inferior femoral neck.

Surgical treatment is often indicated to correct the neck shaft angle with a valgus osteotomy (**19.6**). If left untreated, the vertical shear forces through the physis (growth plate) of the femoral neck can result in worsening of the varus deformity and even dissociation of the femoral epiphysis from the neck (**19.7**).

IRRITABLE HIP (TRANSIENT SYNOVITIS)

Aetiology

Irritable hip is a common childhood condition affecting up to 1 in 1000.

- *Systemic infection* is one of the most common sources.
- *Allergic reaction* is also well described, with hypersensitivity of the synovial membrane in children with atopy.
- *Trauma* can cause hip capsule irritation or bony contusion.

The pathophysiology includes non-pyogenic inflammation and synovial membrane hypertrophy.

It usually occurs in children between 3 and 9 years of age. This is the same time as the peak in Legg–Calvé–Perthes disease (LCPD) presentation. It is twice as common in boys as girls and more common in Caucasians. The left and right hips are equally affected, but bilateral disease

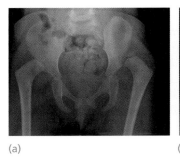 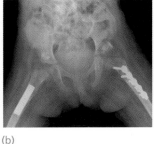 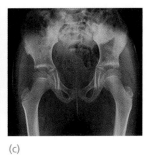

(a)   (b)   (c)

19.5 Bilateral DDH **(a)** X-ray of a 3-year-old female, managed by sequential hip open reduction, femoral shortening and acetabuloplasty **(b)**. **(c)** Postoperative radiograph 4 years following the surgeries showing normal hip development.

SECTION 2 REGIONAL ORTHOPAEDICS

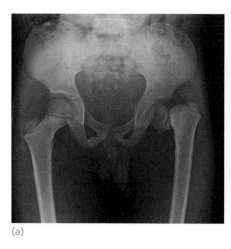 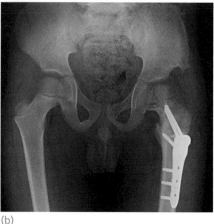

(a)   (b)

19.6 Coxa vara (a) Coxa vara of the left hip. Note the triangular ossification defect in the inferior femoral neck. **(b)** Postoperative appearance following valgus osteotomy.

is rare. Around a tenth of children will have a recurrent episode.

Presentation and examination

PRESENTATION

The most common presentation is an acute painful limp. Pain may be referred to the thigh, knee or buttock. The natural history is a 5- to 10-day

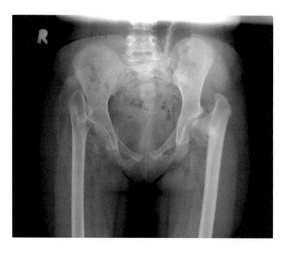

19.7 Coxa vara Untreated case of bilateral coxa vara with severe varus of the left hip and dissociation of the right femoral head epiphysis due to excessive vertical shear forces through the physis.

course of self-limiting symptoms although mild symptoms may persist.

PHYSICAL EXAMINATION

Examination often demonstrates refusal or limitations to weight-bearing on the affected limb. The hip is held in flexion and external rotation to maximize capsular volume. Range of motion is reduced. Children remain systemically well but may have a low-grade fever.

Investigation

Transient synovitis is a diagnosis of exclusion. *Blood tests* include full blood count (FBC), erythrocyte sedimentation rate (ESR) and C-reactive protein (CRP). Initial *X-rays* should be anteroposterior (AP) and frog-lateral images of both hips. *Ultrasound* (with or without guided needle aspiration) or *MRI* may be required.

Septic hip arthritis is the most important diagnosis to rule out. Diagnostic criteria are as described by Kocher (Table 19.2). The presence of two criteria indicates a 40% risk of septic arthritis, increasing to 99.6% when all four criteria are present. Ultrasound-guided needle aspiration of the hip joint is the gold-standard of diagnosis in equivocal cases. Treatment includes thorough irrigation and debridement of the joint followed by antibiotics until normalization of

Table 19.2 Modified Kocher criteria for septic hip arthritis

Criterion	Value
Fever	>38.5°C
FBC	>12.0 × 10⁹ cells/L
ESR	>40 mm/h
CRP	>2.0 mg/L
Weight-bearing	Complete inability

inflammatory markers and return of ability to weight-bear.

Osteomyelitis of the proximal femur may present with symptoms similar to the irritable hip but with raised inflammatory markers. MRI can be helpful in identifying bony changes and subperiosteal collections.

Approximately 1.5% of children who present with transient synovitis will later be diagnosed with LCPD.

Treatment

Treatment is focused on *symptom management* of this self-limiting condition once other conditions are excluded. Bed rest is helpful but poorly tolerated. Non-steroidal anti-inflammatory drugs (NSAIDs) are helpful for symptom control. Weight-bearing aids, such as crutches, may be necessary. Symptoms should resolve by 2–3 weeks.

Complications

Temporary local over-stimulation of growth may lead to coxa magna and over-lengthening.

LEGG–CALVÉ–PERTHES DISEASE

LCPD is idiopathic AVN of the proximal femoral epiphysis that affects approximately 1 in 1000 children. It commonly presents between 4 and 8 years of age with higher incidence in northern regions. Boys are five times more commonly affected. Bilateral cases are seen in approximately 10%.

LCPD is associated with other congenital conditions including:

- genitourinary malformations
- undescended testes
- inguinal hernia
- Down's syndrome
- thrombophilic conditions.

MAIN RISK FACTORS FOR LCPD

Low birth weight
Exposure to cigarette smoke
Short body length
Family history
Low socioeconomic status
Attention deficit hyperactivity disorder type 1

Pathophysiology

The pathophysiology may include a vascular insult and uncoupling of the bone metabolic process. Bony destruction is exacerbated by repetitive loading. Bone age often lags behind chronological age. Venous stasis may contribute to the vascular insult. Abduction and internal rotation stretch the posterior circumflex artery and may interrupt flow to the lateral epiphyseal artery as it traverses the capsule.

Following initial insult, increased osteoclast activity driving bony resorption is followed by persistent fibroblastic proliferation and fibrovascular replacement of trabeculae.

Presentation and examination

PRESENTATION

Presentation ranges from a painless limp to acute transient synovitis. Pain is often referred to the knee. Pain is worse on activity. Children aged 4–9 years with a persistent limp lasting longer than 10 days warrant investigation including AP and frog-lateral X-rays of both hips, FBC, ESR and CRP.

PHYSICAL EXAMINATION

Examination often demonstrates hip pain. Range of motion may be reduced, especially abduction and internal rotation. Prolonged disease can present with Trendelenburg gait and LLD.

SECTION 2 REGIONAL ORTHOPAEDICS

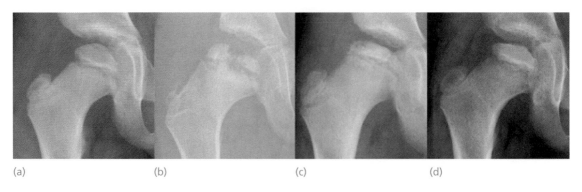

(a)   (b)   (c)   (d)

19.8 Waldenström staging of LCPD **(a)** Initial (up to 6 months); **(b)** fragmentation (6–12 months); **(c)** reossification (12–18 months); **(d)** remodelling.

Imaging

The disease follows distinct radiographic stages described by Waldenström (**19.8**). Radiographic changes can be seen after 3–6 months. The ossific nucleus is typically small and dense with lateral subluxation. There is often a subchondral fracture line within the femoral head. The physis becomes increasingly horizontal. Severe disease may progress to acetabular changes, early closure of the triradiate cartilage, and bicompartmentalization of the acetabulum and ischium varum (**19.9**).

HERRING CLASSIFICATION

This is the *most commonly used classification system* and is applied *early in the fragmentation stage*. It is based on involvement of the lateral pillar of the epiphysis.

HERRING CLASSIFICATION OF LCPD	
Group A	No lateral pillar involvement
Group B	>50% of lateral pillar height is maintained
Group B/C	50% loss of height
• *B/C-1*: the lateral pillar is less than 2–3 mm wide	
• *B/C-2*: minimal ossification	
• *B/C-3*: lateral pillar is depression	
Group C	Loss of over 50% of lateral pillar height.

This classification has demonstrated strong prognostic value and inter-observer reliability.

- Group A is associated with universally good outcomes.

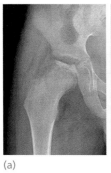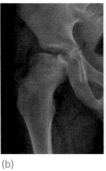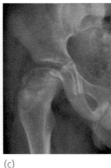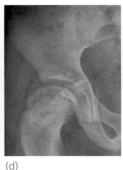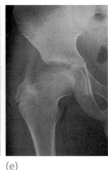

(a)   (b)   (c)   (d)   (e)

19.9 Legg–Calvé–Perthes disease A more severe case than in **19.8** that presented in the late fragmentation phase **(a,b)**. Resultant reossification **(c,d)** with final remodelling **(e)** demonstrating residual deformity with a shortened femoral neck (coxa breva) and an ovoid femoral head.

- Group B hips generally have poor outcomes in children older than 6 years.
- Group C hips have universally poor outcomes.

Treatment

The LCPD disease process is defined by destruction followed by regeneration. The primary aim is to prevent deformity before the remodelling phase. Containment alters joint mechanics to distribute forces more evenly across the epiphysis thereby protecting the weak and fragmented femoral head until reossification can occur.

NON-OPERATIVE TREATMENT

Non-operative treatment is generally reserved for children under 6 years of age with Herring A or B hips. Therapies include protected weight-bearing and activity restriction. Physiotherapy is also beneficial. Ultimate shape of the femoral head after reossification will dictate long-term outcomes. Routine use of bisphosphonates and bone morphogenetic proteins (BMPs) remains controversial.

OPERATIVE TREATMENT

Operative intervention may be indicated in children with persistent symptoms or reduced range of motion. Surgery is most beneficial if performed early in the fragmentation stage. Prerequisites for surgical containment include near-normal abduction under general anaesthetic and arthrogram demonstrating a containable congruent hip joint.

- *Under the age of 8 years*, the most common procedure is *proximal femoral varus osteotomy* correcting lateral subluxation, increasing head coverage and correcting excessive anteversion.
- *Over the age of 8 years*, or in children with more advanced disease, *pelvic osteotomy* is often required for adequate containment (e.g. shelf, Dega and Salter-innominate osteotomies).

Failure of containment and significant head collapse can result in hinged abduction due to a short femoral neck and high greater trochanter. Hip joint salvage may be achieved through a *valgus subtrochanteric osteotomy*.

SLIPPED CAPITAL FEMORAL EPIPHYSIS

Slipped capital femoral epiphysis (SCFE) (also known as slipped upper femoral epiphysis, SUFE) is the most common hip condition among adolescents from age 10 to 15 with an incidence of 1:10 000.

Pathophysiology

Mechanical overload leads to displacement of the proximal femoral physis through the hypertrophic zone. During adolescence, prior to growth-plate closure the extracapsular arterial ring supplying the metaphysis increases substantially and invests the subphyseal region, terminating at the hypertrophic zone. The physis is reinforced by a thick periosteal ring. During adolescence, the periosteum begins to thin and the force required for displacement to occur is reduced.

Histologically, the physis of hips that undergo SCFE is likely to demonstrate:

- physeal widening of up to 12 mm (normal is 2–6 mm)
- larger chondrocytes
- altered physeal column height and organization
- disruption of chondrocyte differentiation and ossification.

Several factors predispose to SCFE.

FACTORS PREDISPOSING TO SCFE

Increased proximal femoral retroversion increases torsional stress.
During the growth spurt, significant lengthening of the femoral neck leads to increased varus leading to a more vertically oriented physis, with increased shear.
Larger body habitus and additional weight further increase shear forces.

Hypothyroidism, osteodystrophy of chronic renal failure and *excessive growth hormone* are associated with SCFE. These children usually present under the age of 10 or over 16 with immature bone development. Children who present under the age of 10 or with weight below the 50th percentile should have an endocrine workup beginning with thyroid-stimulating hormone (TSH), blood urea nitrogen (BUN) and creatinine.

Presentation and examination

PRESENTATION

Children typically present in early adolescence with thigh, groin or knee pain (which may be isolated). Patients often present following an acute traumatic event, but may report prodromal symptoms preceding the event.

The average age of diagnosis is 12 years. Race plays a significant role, with highest incidences seen in the black, Hispanic and Pacific Island populations. Bilateral symptoms are seen in 20% of patients and this is higher in endocrine disorders. Between 15% and 35% of patients will develop a slip of the contralateral side within 18 months (metachronous slip).

PHYSICAL EXAMINATION

Examination will often demonstrate a short leg held in external rotation. Range of motion is often painful with limitations to abduction, flexion and internal rotation. Hip flexion often leads to obligate external rotation and abduction (*Drehmann's sign*). Weight-bearing patients often have an *antalgic* or *Trendelenburg gait*.

Imaging

X-RAYS

Plain X-rays should include AP and frog-lateral images of both hips. Lateral views are more sensitive for *early signs*, including:

- widening or irregularity of the physis
- loss of anterior head-neck concavity
- sharpening of the metaphyseal border
- loss of epiphyseal height.

Klein's line   Drawn along the superior border of the neck, this line should intersect the epiphysis; failure to do so results in a positive *Trethowan sign* (19.10).

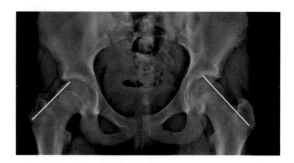

19.10 SCFE – Klein's line Line drawn bilaterally, with positive Trethowan sign in the left hip.

Steel sign   This is a double-density or metaphyseal blanch sign seen on the AP view due to overlapping of the epiphysis and metaphysis.

Capener's sign   This is seen as a reduction in the double-density crescent created by overlap of the posterior acetabulum and proximal metaphysis.

Southwick angle   This is the angle created by a line drawn perpendicular to the physis and a line parallel to the femoral shaft on the frog-lateral view.

MRI

MRI is useful in cases of high clinical suspicion with negative radiographic findings as it is more sensitive and may identify pre-slips.

Classification

A hip is considered to have a *stable slip* (10% risk of AVN) if the child is able to bear weight with or without the use of aids. It is *unstable* (47% risk of AVN) if the child is unable to bear weight.

RADIOGRAPHIC CLASSIFICATION: SOUTHWICK	
The difference in Southwick angle between the pathological and normal hip:	
Mild slip	<30° difference
Moderate slip	30–50° difference
Severe slip	>50° difference

RADIOGRAPHIC CLASSIFICATION: LATERAL SLIP GRADE	
Grade I	<33% slippage
Grade II	33–50% slippage
Grade III	>50% slippage off the metaphysis

Treatment

IN-SITU PINNING

Treatment focuses on stabilization of the epiphysis with induction of physeal fusion and growth arrest. This is usually achieved with *in-situ fixation* (19.11). Forced closed reduction increases the risk of AVN.

Stabilization is usually achieved with cannulated screws into the centre of the epiphysis and traversing perpendicular to the physis. Five screw threads should be contained within the epiphysis but it is critical that the joint is not penetrated.

Prophylactic fixation of an asymptomatic contralateral hip has been advocated in high risk including those who are under 10 years, have endocrine disorders or are obese. Sliding screw devices may allow continued growth in the young.

OPEN REDUCTION

Patients with highly displaced, unstable slips are at increased risk of developing femoroacetabular impingement (FAI) as well as AVN. In these cases, surgical hip dislocation, reduction and confirmation of femoral head vascularity may be beneficial.

PROXIMAL FEMORAL OSTEOTOMY

Traditionally, proximal femoral osteotomy has been performed in cases of severe slip. The closer to the joint the osteotomy is performed, the less correction is required, but at increased risk of AVN. They are usually performed through a Watson–Jones approach, or Southwick intertrochanteric osteotomy.

Dunn osteotomy This is performed at the proximal metaphysis to allow reduction of the epiphysis back onto the metaphysis. The femoral neck may be shortened slightly to reduce tension of the posterior vessels and thereby reduce risk of AVN. Reduction is held with smooth pins.

Kramer osteotomy This is an anterosuperior-based wedge osteotomy at the base of the femoral neck. Osteotomy at this location has a lower risk of AVN and is beneficial in children with a Trendelenburg gait preoperatively. However, correction is limited to 35–55 degrees and there is a higher risk of LLD.

Southwick osteotomy If significant deformity remains within the proximal femur following remodelling of SCFE, an intertrochanteric wedge osteotomy can be performed at the level of the lesser trochanter.

Late osteotomy Chronic proximal femoral deformity with extension, external rotation and

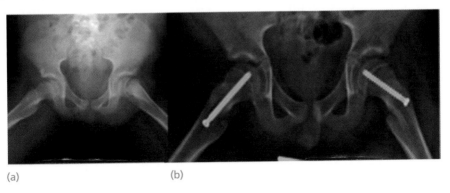

(a)   (b)

19.11 SCFE – in-situ pinning (a) Preoperative frog-lateral X-ray of child with left-sided SCFE. **(b)** Frog-lateral X-ray following in-situ pinning of left hip and prophylactic pinning for right hip in the same child.

shortening may benefit from correction with subtrochanteric osteotomy to produce flexion, internal rotation and valgus.

COMPLICATIONS

The most significant risk associated with SCFE is AVN. Surgical complications include chondrolysis and early osteoarthritis secondary to screw penetration.

THE ADULT HIP

CLINICAL ASSESSMENT

SYMPTOMS

Hip girdle pain

This can arise intra-articularly, extra-articularly or be referred from elsewhere.

- *Intra-articular pain* is generally felt in the groin and radiates down the front of the thigh into the knee. It also radiates around the hip girdle in a 'C-sign' distribution.
- *Extra-articular hip pathology* can also be felt around the hip girdle particularly laterally (e.g. trochanteric pain, abductor tendonitis).
- *Referred pain* may come from a variety of areas, commonly the lumbar–sacral spine radiating to the buttock. If there is radiculopathy, consider nerve root entrapment.

DIFFERENTIAL DIAGNOSIS OF PAIN AROUND THE HIP GIRDLE OUTSIDE THE HIP JOINT
Within the musculoskeletal system
• Trochanteric bursa
• Gluteus medius tendinitis
• Stress fracture
• Osteitis pubis
• Iliopsoas tendinitis or bursitis
• Iliopsoas abscess
• Adductor longus strain or tendinitis
• Referred from the spine
• Metastatic disease
Outside the musculosketetal system
• Inguinal hernia
• Inguinal lymphadenopathy
• Gastrointestinal
• Genitourinary
• Gynaecological

A structured approach to the assessment of pain helps with differentiation and to guide subsequent investigations.

SOCRATES: A STRUCTURED APPROACH TO PAIN ASSESSMENT	
Site	Where is the pain or the maximal site of the pain?
Onset	When did the pain start, and was it sudden or gradual?
Character	What is the pain like? An ache? Stabbing? Burning?
Radiation	Does the pain radiate anywhere?
Associations	Are any other symptoms associated with the pain?
Time course	Does the pain follow any pattern?
Exacerbating/ relieving factors	Does anything change the pain?
Severity	How bad is the pain?

Stiffness

The earliest and most reliable marker of intra-articular pathology is the loss of internal rotation.

As loss of movement progresses, patients with stiffness of the hip commonly report difficulties with pedicure and putting on their shoes and socks. The difficulties that patients report with the activities of daily living may be secondary to pain but also commonly these are a result of joint stiffness. Stiffness is most marked after inactivity.

Limp (gait disturbance)

The hip joint plays a fundamental role in locomotion. Limping may simply be a way of coping with pain, or it may be due to a change in limb length, hip abductor weakness or instability. An antalgic gait is characterized by pain leading to an uneven cadence whereby the patient spends less time with the painful leg loaded in the gait cycle. Patients also report a reduction in walking distance and stride length.

Snapping or clicking

Patients may report an audible sound or sensation from their hip. This may be associated with pain and may arise from intra-articular (e.g. labral tear or loose body) or extra-articular pathology (e.g. snapping tendon). The site of the sensation is informative.

SIGNS WITH THE PATIENT UPRIGHT

The fundamental principles of *look*, *feel* and *move* are applied to clinical examination of the hip joint. As the hip is a weight-bearing joint, it is critical to assess the patient both standing and lying in a suitable state of undress.

With the patient standing, posture and gait are examined and the Trendelenburg test is performed. The patient should also be inspected for scars, sinuses, muscle wasting or swelling.

Gait

TYPES OF GAIT

Antalgic gait   The patient spends less time on the painful limb so that stance phase is reduced.

Stiff leg gait   Restricted flexion and extension lead to circumduction and swinging of their leg.

Short leg gait   The patient dips down on the affected side.

Trendelenburg gait   This is the dynamic representation of the Trendelenberg test. Put simply,

with each step forward that the patient takes with the affected limb (abductor weakness) they lurch towards the unaffected limb in order to avoid overbalancing.

TRENDELENBURG TEST

In normal single-legged stance, the centre of gravity moves from the midline so that it lies over the weight-bearing leg. The abductors on the side of the weight-bearing leg contract to stop the pelvis dipping and the weight transferring back over the unsupported side. In clinical examination this is revealed by localizing and placing a finger on each anterior superior iliac spine (ASIS). As the patient stands on one leg, the finger on the ASIS of the unsupported leg will rise. This is a normal response and would be recorded as Trendelenburg negative. In a Trendelenberg-positive patient, the finger on the ASIS of the unsupported leg will fall.

SIGNS WITH THE PATIENT LYING

Look

Check that the pelvis is horizontal and the legs placed in a symmetrical position. Apparent limb length can be measured from the ASIS to the medial malleolus on each side. True LLD is determined by measurement from a fixed midline bony landmark (such as the xiphisternum) to the medial malleoli. A patient can have an apparent LLD without a true LLD, the most common causes being a scoliosis, pelvic obliquity and adductor contracture. Where the fixed posture of the limb makes one leg appear shorter, this may cause a functional LLD with no actual measurable LLD and needs to be considered when planning total hip arthroplasty (THA).

Feel

The hip joint lies deep so the joint line cannot be palpated. Other structures, such as the greater trochanter and abductor insertions, are palpated.

Move

The loss of internal rotation of the hip joint is the most reliable early clinical sign of intra-articular

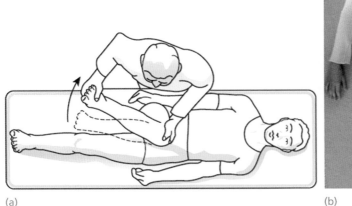

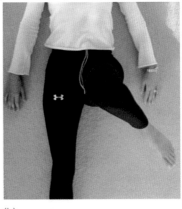

(a)

(b)

19.12 Clinical examination – internal rotation (a) How to assess internal rotation of the hip with the joint flexed. (b) A patient with normal 40° of internal rotation.

hip pathology (19.12). This may well be revealed on passive hip flexion, when there may be a tendency to fall into external rotation. With progress of joint stiffness, the development of a fixed external rotation contracture is common and thereafter fixed flexion.

Hip movement that causes pain which reproduces a patient's symptoms can be very helpful in discriminating between intra-articular and other causes.

IMAGING

X-rays

AP pelvis views together with a lateral projection of the affected side are required (19.13).

Computed tomography and magnetic resonance imaging

The pelvis is a complex 3D shape and the principal benefit of computed tomography (CT) and magnetic resonance imaging (MRI) is the multiplanar evaluation of the hip joint and surrounding structures.

- *CT* is widely available and accessible with no compatibility issues with metallic prostheses or devices such as pacemakers, but it does, of course, expose the patient to ionizing

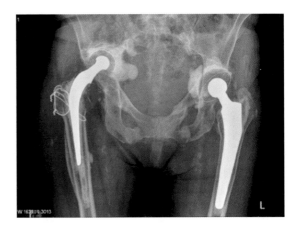

19.13 Imaging – X-ray Radiograph of a failed right THA with severe migration of the cemented acetabular socket. While it is clear that there is a major problem with the right socket, more detailed assessment is required to investigate the effect on surrounding structures. CT scans are extremely helpful to decide upon reconstruction technique and plan surgery.

radiation. It offers excellent definition of osseous anatomy and also has an increasing role in surgical planning (19.14).
- *MRI* produces excellent soft-tissue imaging and evaluation of bony integrity. It typically takes up to 45 minutes to perform and is degraded by movement. It is typically contraindicated in patients with pacemakers and

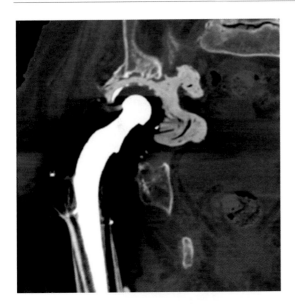

19.14 Imaging – CT Reformatted image obtained from multiplanar CT scan. This coronal slice demonstrates the enhanced detail available and allows accurate assessment of the amount and site of bone stock loss.

some other implantable devices. *Metal artifact reduction sequences (MARS)* MRI have led to a major improvement in images obtained around implants.

Ultrasound scanning

Ultrasound scanning can be very useful in soft-tissue assessment, and it has the major advantage that it is dynamic and the patient can interact with the operator to localize sites of tenderness. In addition, the patient can move the joint such that the dynamic behaviour of structures (e.g. snapping tendon) can be demonstrated. Ultrasound is also a helpful modality to deliver image-guided injections.

Arthrogram +/− local anaesthetic

The addition of contrast (e.g. gadolinium) in conjunction with CT and MRI has been shown to increase the diagnostic yield principally in the detection of labral lesions. In patients where clinical history and examination fail to confirm the diagnosis, an 'anaesthetic arthrogram' is helpful as a diagnostic test.

Following the injection of local anaesthetic, patients are requested to keep a pain diary. Significant improvement is a very helpful indicator of intra-articular pathology.

Modern surgical planning tools and 3D printing

CT planning and the production of 3D printed models allow the surgeon to perform a simulated procedure before entering the operating theatre (**19.15**). Models are particularly helpful in complex cases. This technology is currently expensive, but it is easy to envisage the future applications.

Arthroscopy of the hip

Hip arthroscopy can be considered as either diagnostic or therapeutic. Improvements in cross-sectional imaging have made purely diagnostic hip arthroscopy rare and improved instrumentation and techniques has seen growth in therapeutic procedures.

Modern hip arthroscopy has evolved to become a much more reproducible procedure. Specific traction tables aid controlled joint distraction. Pressure-controlled irrigation systems allow distention of the joint, and improvements in optics and scope technology result in significantly improved visualization (**19.16**).

INDICATIONS FOR HIP ARTHROSCOPY

Intra-articular

- Femoroacetabular impingement (e.g. osteochondroplasty)
- Labral tears
- Loose/foreign bodies
- Cartilage lesions
- Osteochondritis dissecans
- Ligamentum teres injuries
- Total hip replacement assessment

Extra-articular

- Iliopsoas tendinopathy
- Snapping iliotibial band
- Greater trochanteric pain syndrome

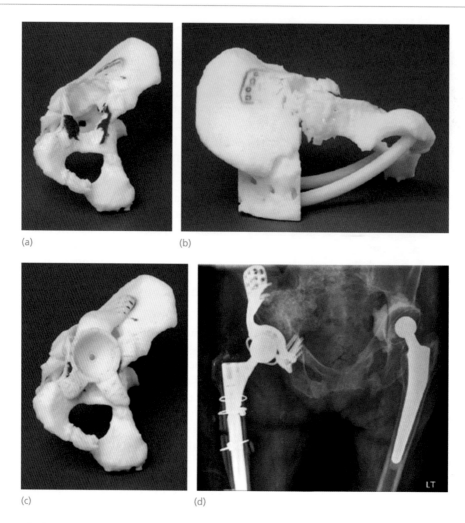

(a)   (b)

(c)   (d)

19.15 3D modelling (a,b) This is a 3D model of the case presented in **19.14**. It enabled the feasibility of revision THA to be confirmed and significantly aided preoperative planning. In this instance, due to the massive bone loss, a custom-made implant was used **(c,d)**.

COMPLICATIONS OF HIP ARTHROSCOPY
Anaesthetic complications – procedure performed under general anaesthetic
Traction-related injury – either from pressure (e.g. pudendal nerve in groin) or, less commonly, directly from over-stretch
Neurovascular injury – most commonly lateral cutaneous nerve of the thigh from portal placement
Extravasation of irrigation fluid
Infection

The central compartment of the hip comprises the articulating hyaline cartilage surfaces of the acetabulum and femoral head together with the ligamentum teres. The peripheral compartment comprises the intra-capsular recess outside the hip articulation.

Patients who are candidates for hip arthroscopy typically present with mechanical symptoms as well as groin pain. These mechanical symptoms can also compromise function and include:

• clicking
• catching

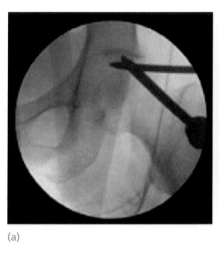
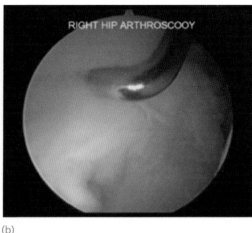

(a)　　　　　　　　　　　　　　(b)

19.16 Arthroscopy **(a)** Intraoperative image intensifier view of portal establishment set for hip arthroscopy. Note the distraction of the hip joint. **(b)** View obtained of the hip joint central compartment with probe demonstrating labral tear.

- locking
- buckling.

INTRA-ARTICULAR HIP PATHOLOGY – OSTEOARTHRITIS OF THE HIP JOINT

The hip joint is one of the commonest sites of osteoarthritis (OA). The classification of hip OA as primary or secondary is outdated, as is the use of the term 'wear-and-tear' arthritis. Over the past two decades there has been major progress in our understanding of the pathoanatomy that leads some patients to develop OA while others develop no problems. Causes are better considered as *mechanical* or *non-mechanical*.

MECHANICAL AND NON-MECHANICAL CAUSES OF HIP OA

Mechanical

- Developmental dysplasia of the hip (under-coverage)
- Femoroacetabular impingement (over-coverage)
- Legg–Calvé–Perthes disease, slipped capital femoral epiphysis (loss of sphericity)
- Post-traumatic (loss of congruency)

Non-mechanical

- Avascular necrosis of the femoral head
- Ankylosing spondylitis
- Inflammatory arthritis (e.g. rheumatoid arthritis, psoriatic arthritis and systemic lupus erythematosus)
- Primary disorders of cartilage and the synovium (e.g. synovial chondromatosis)

Mechanical causes

When there is loss of sphericity in the ball-and-socket joint, the articular surface is exposed to abnormal loads and contact forces leading to hyaline cartilage damage. The common mechanical causes include DDH (under-coverage), FAI (over-coverage), and as a long-term consequence of LCPD and SCFE. In post-traumatic OA, there is loss of congruency of the articulating surface.

Non-mechanical causes

These are conditions or processes that can only the hip joint or be part of a more widespread musculoskeletal disorder. Non-mechanical causes of hip OA include:

- AVN of the femoral head
- ankylosing spondylitis
- primary disorders of cartilage and the synovium (e.g. synovial chondromatosis)
- inflammatory arthropathies.

Clinical features

The classic presentation of hip OA is groin pain, stiffness and limp. Initially, this may be activity-related but later it occurs at rest and disturbs sleep. Loss of internal rotation of the hip is one of the most consistent clinical findings before other limitations develop.

Investigations

Plain X-rays of OA demonstrate four cardinal radiographic features (**19.17**):

- joint space narrowing
- subchondral sclerosis
- osteophyte formation
- subchondral cysts.

Superior joint space narrowing in the weight-bearing zone is the most common (e.g. cam FAI) or it can also occur more centrally, when it is termed *medial pole hip OA* (e.g. protrusio).

It is common for the first presentation of a mechanical precipitating cause to be end-stage OA. In younger women, it is common to find the hallmarks of more subtle dysplasia that did not present earlier in life whereas in men in particular radiological hallmarks of FAI are often present.

MECHANICAL CAUSES OF HIP OSTEOARTHRITIS

FEMOROACETABULAR IMPINGEMENT AND OSTEOARTHRITIS

FAI is considered a mechanical cause of hip OA due to loss of sphericity and essentially

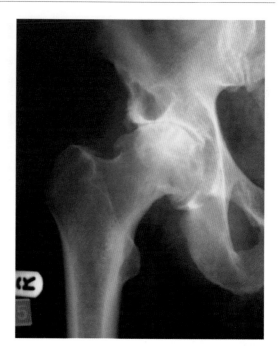

19.17 Hip OA The four cardinal radiographic features of OA are demonstrated. Note the loss of joint space due to hyaline cartilage loss and osteophyte formation, and subchondral sclerosis and subchondral cysts. In this example there is a large acetabular subchondral cyst that is termed a geode.

over-coverage of the ball-and-socket joint broadly divided into *pincer* and *cam* types.

- *In the pincer type*, there is either global over-coverage of the femoral head (circumferentially as in coxa profunda or protrusio) or focal anterior over-coverage (by the anterior part of the acetabular rim or by acetabular retroversion) (**19.18, 19.19**).
- *In the cam type*, there is loss of sphericity at the femoral head neck junction.

The common pathway of these FAI types is the pathological impact of bone against cartilage leading to damage to the labrum followed by abrasion or delamination of the hyaline cartilage. It is common to see a mixed picture.

Clinical features

Groin pain and *decreased range of movement* are typical. At first, these are only on provoking

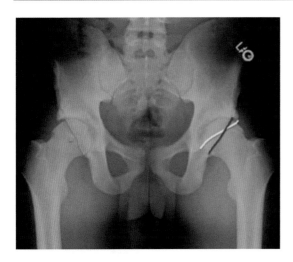

19.18 Pincer-type FAI due to focal anterior acetabular over-coverage As is common in FAI, the same abnormalities are present bilaterally. In the left hip the radiological crossover sign is demonstrated by tracing the overlap of the anterior (yellow line) and posterior (red line) acetabular walls. On the right hip it is possible to see how the centre of rotation is lateral to the posterior wall (blue line).

activities, but eventually the patient presents with the classical symptoms of established hip OA.

The typical patient with pincer-type FAI is female and over 40 years of age while the typical patient with cam-type FAI is a male and about 10–15 years younger. There is restricted internal rotation in flexion and adduction (often referred to as an impingement test).

Investigation

A well-centred AP *X-ray* of the hips (centred on the symphysis pubis) and a cross-table lateral radiograph of the hip are required. Abnormal signs related to anterior acetabular over-coverage include a cross-over sign and ischial spine sign. In cam-type FAI there is a characteristic 'bump' at the superior head-neck junction that may be accompanied by a 'pistol-grip' deformity of the proximal femur. Global acetabular over-coverage is associated with coxa profunda or protrusio.

MRI scans allow a more detailed assessment of hip morphology, the labrum and articular cartilage. *MRI arthrograms* are more sensitive and specific for detecting labral and some chondral lesions. 3-Tesla and delayed gadolinium-enhanced MRI of cartilage (dGEMRIC) may help detect early cartilage lesions.

Treatment

NON-OPERATIVE TREATMENT

Non-operative management of FAI involves symptom management, activity modification, physiotherapy and intra-articular injections. The state of the hyaline cartilage has a profound effect on treatment and outcome.

OPERATIVE TREATMENT

Impingement can be addressed by open or arthroscopic surgery. The principle is to resect the

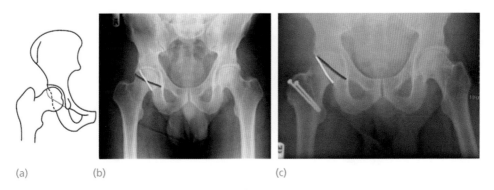

(a)   (b)   (c)

19.19 Pincer-type FAI secondary to focal anterior over-coverage (a) A positive crossover sign is demonstrated. (b) Following open surgical dislocation of the left hip via a Ganz osteotomy acetabular rim resection has been performed and labral refixation. (c) Note correction of the crossover sign and screw fixation of osteotomy.

'impingement lesion' by recontouring the head-neck junction (cam) or rim resection (pincer). Labral tears are repaired if possible. Realignment osteotomies may be considered.

HIP DYSPLASIA AND OSTEOARTHRITIS

DDH in the adult presents a spectrum of challenges. The pelvis and femur may be hypoplastic and there may be pronounced LLD (19.20). Scarring and retained metalwork from previous surgery is common. The key principle of joint replacement is restoration of the hip centre of rotation which can be challenging due to bone stock deficiency, small acetabulum and femur, excessive femoral anteversion and residual deformity.

The level of the degenerative 'false acetabulum' largely determines the complexity of the surgery. The Hartofilakidis classification provides useful context when planning surgery. Outcome after THA and implant survivorship are influenced by the extent of the dysplasia. In severe cases (>4 cm LLD) a subtrochanteric shortening osteotomy may be required to permit reduction and prevent nerve injury. Small modular implants are required.

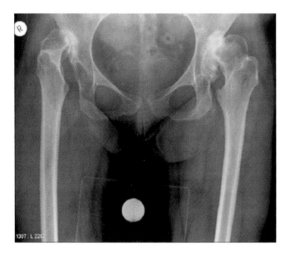

19.20 Hip dysplasia and OA Bilateral DDH with resulting mechanical OA.

THE HARTOFILAKIDIS CLASSIFICATION	
Dysplasia	Femoral head subluxated but still contained in the original acetabulum
Low	Femoral head articulates with the false acetabulum that partially overlaps the true acetabulum
High	Femoral head articulates with a hollow in the acetabular wing

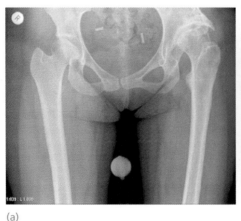

(a)

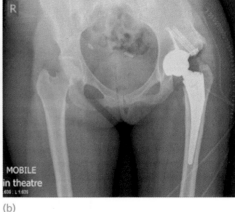

(b)

19.21 Mechanical OA as a result of DDH (a) Preoperative X-ray of a 32-year-old female patient who has had a previous shelf procedure. **(b)** Complex primary THA with bulk allograft.

POST-TRAUMATIC HIP OSTEOARTHRITIS

Trauma can disrupt joint surface congruity by direct injury, intra-articular fracture or dislocation, leading to mechanical OA. Extra-articular trauma can result in proximal femoral deformity, altering hip biomechanics and joint loading. AVN may also occur following trauma, particularly if femoral head blood supply is disrupted.

THA is the most frequent treatment for end-stage post-traumatic OA. These are often complex cases and require careful planning (19.21).

NON-MECHANICAL CAUSES OF HIP OSTEOARTHRITIS

AVASCULAR NECROSIS OF THE FEMORAL HEAD

The femoral head is the commonest site of AVN due to its vulnerable blood supply. AVN may develop due to ischaemia, direct cellular toxicity or altered differentiation of mesenchymal stem cells.

CAUSES OF FEMORAL HEAD AVN
Idiopathic
Excess alcohol consumption
Use of corticosteroids
Trauma, in particular displaced intracapsular hip fractures and traumatic hip dislocations
Sickle-cell anaemia
Gaucher's disease
Thrombophilia
Primary Cushing's disease
Chemo- and radiotherapy
Decompression sickness

The true incidence of hip AVN is difficult to determine; it eventually results in the collapse of subchondral bone causing joint incongruity (19.22).

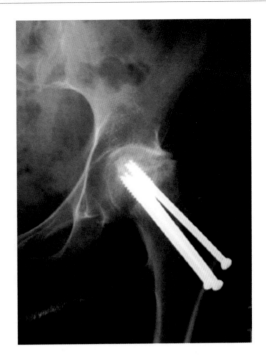

19.22 Avascular necrosis Post-traumatic post-collapse AVN following intracapsular hip fracture.

Diagnosis

Plain X-rays are often normal; the first signs usually appear after 6 months. At first, increased density/sclerosis is seen and the hip is *pre-collapse*. The classic appearance of a thin subchondral fracture line ('*crescent sign*') then develops, at which point the hip is *post-collapse*. Structural deformity then progresses (19.23).

MRI scans show characteristic changes in the marrow long before any abnormality is visible on plain radiographs. There is a band of altered signal intensity that represents the reactive zone between living and dead bone.

There are many proposed classifications. A key watershed that unifies all the proposed systems is the differentiation of the AVN into pre-collapse and post-collapse as this has very significant implications for successful treatment.

Treatment

PRE-COLLAPSE AVN

Pre-collapse AVN offers the opportunity for joint preservation. Protected weight-bearing,

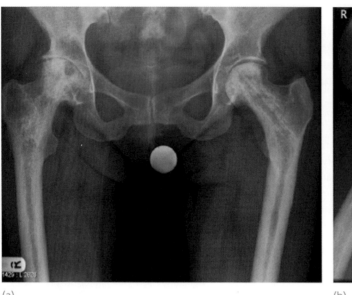
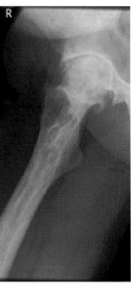

(a)   (b)

19.23 AVN secondary to sickle-cell anaemia (a,b) Note on the lateral view the classic bone-within-a-bone appearance. The right hip demonstrates established non-mechanical OA and in the left hip the tract from previous core decompression is visible in the femoral neck.

bisphosphonates and anticoagulation have been investigated with variable success. Larger areas of AVN (>25% of the femoral head) located in the weight-bearing zone will tend to progress.

The *surgical management* of pre-collapse AVN typically involves percutaneous decompression with bone grafting; stem cells, BMP and platelet-rich plasma (PRP) may also be added but the evidence base is poor. Vascularized bone grafts and femoral osteotomies are used less frequently than previously.

POST-COLLAPSE AVN

Hip preservation procedures are not recommended in post-collapse AVN. *THA* should be considered for symptom management but may have higher failure rates than THA for other indications such as OA.

ANKYLOSING SPONDYLITIS AND HIP OSTEOARTHRITIS

The hip joint is the most common site of peripheral joint involvement in ankylosing spondylitis (AS). With progressive hip involvement, the compensation for spinal stiffness is lost, profoundly affecting the patient's balance. Soft-tissue contractures, especially fixed flexion contracture develop.

The indications for THA in non-mechanical hip OA due to AS are as for other causes of OA based on an individualized patient assessment. Some complications, such as the formation of heterotopic ossification, are more frequent after total hip replacement for AS.

INFLAMMATORY ARTHRITIS OF THE HIP

In inflammatory arthritis there is progressive hyaline cartilage destruction via the synovium. Examples include rheumatoid arthritis (RA) and systemic lupus erythematosus (SLE). RA has an incidence of around 1–3% in the population, affects the hip joints in 15–20% of patients, and often affects both hips.

Disease-modifying antirheumatic drugs (DMARDs) have revolutionized the treatment of RA. They decrease pain and inflammation, reduce joint damage, and help preserve joint structure and function. Some of these drugs are also used in treating other conditions such as AS, psoriatic arthritis and SLE.

SECTION 2 REGIONAL ORTHOPAEDICS

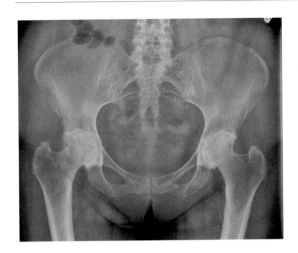

19.24 Inflammatory arthritis Note severe loss of joint space and periarticular cysts.

Initial X-ray findings may be minimal as the pain is arising from synovitis. Progressive hyaline cartilage destruction leads to joint space narrowing. Other common radiographic findings include cyst formation and acetabular protrusion (**19.24**).

Failure of non-surgical management is an indication for THA. Poor bone stock and osteopenia as a result of disuse and osteoporosis from long-term steroid use is common, increasing the risk of fracture. There is immunosuppression due to the underlying condition and medications which increases the risk of prosthetic joint infection. Multidisciplinary management helps optimize perioperative care. Anti-tumour necrosis factor (anti-TNF) agents should be stopped in the perioperative period as they inhibit wound healing, but cessation of other DMARDs such as methotrexate is controversial, as it often results in a generalized flare-up of symptoms and is not stopped for long enough to counter the immunomodulatory effect. Other joint involvement can affect postoperative rehabilitation.

NON-OPERATIVE TREATMENT OF HIP OSTEOARTHRITIS

The cornerstone of non-operative management of hip OA focuses on effective *pain management*. Simple oral pharmacological agents such as NSAIDs are initiated and opioid-based drugs are typically avoided. If they are required, other interventions should be considered. Paracetamol has been shown to be no more effective than placebo, but the placebo effect of drugs should not be underestimated.

Life-style modification and also weight reduction for overweight patients is important. The use of a walking stick or walking aids assists in maintaining mobility and reducing pain.

The most common course is that of steady decline with increasing pain and decreasing function, although some patients can have a rapidly progressive or relapsing and remitting course.

TOTAL HIP ARTHROPLASTY

THA is one of the most successful operations performed across all surgical specialties and the definitive treatment of end-stage hip OA. Oteotomy and arthrodesis are now performed very rarely, and excision hip arthroplasty is a salvage procedure only in the setting of persistent hip infection. The success of THA is in major part due to there being no trade-off in function as with these previously popular techniques. In worldwide joint registries OA is the leading indication for THA and accounts for over 90% of THA in Europe.

Indications

When non-operative management has failed to adequately control symptoms, THA should be considered. Although THA is generally highly successful, its risks must be weighed against the indications for the procedure and functional limitations facing the patient as complications, such as prosthetic joint infection, can be devastating. Matching the expectations of the patient and surgeon is also critical.

MOST COMMON INDICATIONS FOR THA
Severe pain on movement
Disturbed sleep due to pain
Pain at rest
Functional limitations during activities of daily living
Reduced walking distance

Table 19.3 Surgical approaches to the hip used to perform THA

Approach	Eponymous name	Intermuscular plane	Internervous plane
Direct anterior	Smith–Petersen	Sartorius and tensor fascia lata	Femoral nerve and superior gluteal nerve
Anterolateral	Watson–Jones	Tensor fascia lata and gluteus medius	Both supplied by superior gluteal nerve
Direct lateral/ Transgluteal	Hardinge / Omega	Muscle-splitting approach: gluteus medius	Superior gluteal nerve
Posterolateral	Moore / Southern	Reflection of short external rotators	*No internervous plane*

Preoperative assessment needs to consider comorbidities, which may preclude THA or have a significant effect on perioperative risk of both mortality and morbidity.

Age is an important factor to consider as the younger the patient when they undergo THA, the higher the lifetime risk of revision, although more than half of THAs will last for 25 years or more.

Surgical approach

A summary of the commonly used surgical approaches to perform THA is shown in Table 19.3. The surgeon most commonly decides on the choice of approach based on their training and competence. Other factors include previous incisions, obesity, risk of dislocation and deformity.

Implant types

THA comprises acetabular and femoral components that articulate at a bearing surface. These are broadly classified according to the type of fixation to bone.

- *Cemented fixation* provides mechanical fixation by interlocking with bone and
- *Uncemented fixation* relies on osseointegration, a biological bonding of the component to host bone.

A combination of fixation methods can be used. For example, a *hybrid THA* utilizes an uncemented acetabular component and a cemented femoral stem, while a *reverse hybrid THA* uses a cemented socket and uncemented stem.

The THA articulation or bearing can also be considered as two broad categories according to the materials used, i.e. hard-on-soft bearings (metal-on-polyethylene or ceramic-on-polyethylene) or hard-on-hard bearings (ceramic-on-ceramic or metal-on-metal (MoM)). Metal-on-polyethylene remains the most commonly used bearing surface in THA. Ceramic-on-ceramic bearings produce the lowest wear rates, but overall ceramic-on-polyethylene bearings are associated with the lowest risk of revision.

CEMENTED THA

The recent progress made in cemented THA has been in the evolution of surgical technique whereas in uncemented THA there has been much more significant progress in implant design. Polymethylmethacrylate (PMMA) cement acts not as a glue but as a grouting material filling the interstices.

Modern *cementing* involves several essential steps:

- vacuum-mixing in a sealed system
- lavage and brushing of the endosteal surface to remove loose cancellous bone and fat
- utilization of a distal plug and retrograde insertion of cement in the femur
- pressurization of the PMMA in both socket and femur, which is important to drive cement into the trabecular bone network and achieve interdigitation.

Hypotensive anaesthesia aids this process and care should be taken not to stress the prosthesis until the cement has hardened.

- *Cemented cup* design involves the insertion of a single-piece ultra-high molecular weight polyethylene (UHMWPE) implant.
- *Cemented stems* are generally made of either stainless steel or cobalt-chrome.

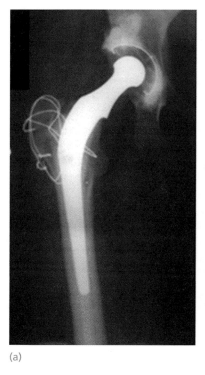
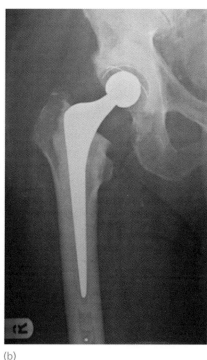

(a) (b)

19.25 Cemented THA **(a)** Charnley cemented THA 'sit-up and stay' philosophy stem design; **(b)** Exeter cemented THA 'slip and slide' philosophy stem design.

The majority of modern designs are modular, allowing exchange of the head and different materials to be used.

There are two schools of thought regarding the design of cemented stems (**19.25**). Both have demonstrated excellent longevity.

- The 'sit-up and stay' theory applies to the shape-closed implants popularized by *Charnley* that have historically been used in greater numbers.
- The 'slip and slide' force-closed or taper-slip designs are now the more commonly utilized cemented stem design, proposed initially by Robin Ling and Clive Lee in Exeter. The *Exeter* philosophy, as it is often termed, has demonstrated that a smooth, collarless, highly polished tapered femoral stem will continue settling within the cement mantle even after polymerization, thereby maintaining expansile pressure between cement and bone and thus maintaining fixation.

Antibiotic-loaded PMMA is used commonly in both the prevention and the treatment of prosthetic joint infection. In the revision setting, if the cement is well fixed to bone and there is only minimal damage to the cement mantle, 'cement-in-cement' revision can be performed, reducing morbidity.

UNCEMENTED THA

The success of modern uncemented THA owes much to the evolution of successful implant designs. The overwhelming majority of contemporary acetabular and femoral components are made of titanium alloy due to its favourable biomechanical and biological properties.

- *Ingrowth implants* have a porous surface that allows for the ingress of new bone formation.
- *Ongrowth implants* have a roughened surface that allows bone to grow onto but not into the implant.

SECTION 2 REGIONAL ORTHOPAEDICS

In both types, these surfaces can be coated, for example with calcium hydroxyapatite, to aid osseointegration.

Uncemented acetabular implants These comprise a modular titanium shell into which a liner is inserted. Shell designs differ in terms of its shape and geometry.

The acetabulum is prepared with hemispherical reamers. Hemispherical shells are inserted with a 1–2 mm press-fit, the strain energy created on impaction creates primary stability. Peripherally expanded socket designs are implanted line-to-line and it is the rim fit that provides maximal early stability. Supplemental screw fixation can aid primary stability. Secondary stability is achieved via bone ingrowth or ongrowth, which is generally achieved within 3 months. If initial implant stability is inadequate and there is significant micromotion, osseointegration will not occur. Both designs of uncemented socket have demonstrated excellent longevity.

Uncemented femoral stems These are subdivided according to the implant shape and extent of surface of the available for biological fixation. The most common contemporary designs are tapered (19.26); other designs include anatomical and cylindrical. The stem may be designed for proximal fixation only with surface transformation of the upper part of the prosthesis or the stem extensively coated throughout its length. More modern designs of titanium alloy femoral stems are associated with a reduction in thigh pain and stress-shielding, two complications commonly associated with historical cobalt-chrome stems.

HIP RESURFACING

Hip resurfacing (HR) involves the preservation of the femoral head and neck. Historically, HR failed due to poor implant materials that utilized a large femoral head on polyethylene which produced high volumetric wear and osteolysis. Modern resurfacing devices have large bearing MoM articulations (19.27). Other potential advantages include improved restoration of hip biomechanics with lower risk of limb-length discrepancy and low volumetric wear.

Unfortunately, MoM bearings were seen to be associated with adverse reactions to metal debris (ARMDs) and higher than expected revision rates leading to a decline in popularity and the recall or withdrawal of many MoM implants.

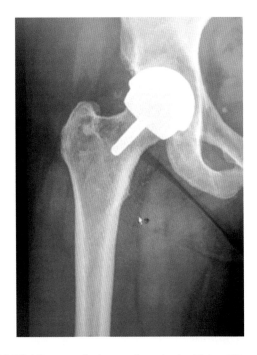

19.27 Hip resurfacing arthroplasty This utilizes an uncemented acetabular socket and a large diameter MoM bearing.

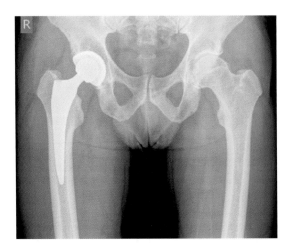

19.26 Uncemented THA Note the proximally coated tapered stem using a ceramic-on-polyethylene bearing.

The current indications for HR are restricted to young male patients with favourable anatomy and femoral heads large enough to allow a component size of 50 mm or over.

Rehabilitation following THA

Inpatient stay following THA has reduced dramatically. Enhanced recovery protocols are commonplace and day-case THA has become a reality in certain centres. The mean length of inpatient stay has been reduced to 3 days or less. Early mobilization aids discharge and reduces the risk of venous thromboembolism. Patients mobilize on crutches at time of discharge and will have negotiated stairs independently. In general, progress to full weight-bearing without support will usually take 4–6 weeks at the patient's own pace.

Complications

As for any surgical procedure, complications can be considered as immediate, early or late.

AGE AND COMORBIDITIES

THA is often performed on older patients with significant comorbidities. These may, of course, have a significant effect on perioperative risk, for example diabetes, where optimal blood sugar control is imperative to reduce perioperative morbidity and reduce the risk of early and late periprosthetic joint infection (PJI).

Examples of procedure-specific factors that increase the risk of complications include:

- previous hip operations
- severe deformity
- osteoporosis
- lack of preoperative planning.

POTENTIAL COMPLICATIONS FOLLOWING THA

Immediate

Anaesthetic-related (e.g. airway problems)

Anaphylaxis (e.g. to antibiotic prophylaxis or anaesthetic agents/drugs)
Blood loss and haemorrhage
Fracture and/or perforation
Nerve injury (e.g. sciatic)
Leg length discrepancy

Early

Venous thromboembolism (DVT and PE)
Urinary retention
Cardio/respiratory issues
Poor wound healing
Early periprosthetic joint infection
Dislocation
Fracture

Late

Wear and osteolysis
Aseptic implant loosening
Dislocation and recurrent instability
Late periprosthetic infection
Periprosthetic fracture
Heterotopic bone formation

OSTEOLYSIS

Osteolysis is the biological consequence of wear on the bearing surface. The wear particles that are produced interact with active macrophages, which results in cytokine release and the subsequent resorption of periprosthetic bone. This is associated with granuloma formation at the interface between implant and bone. Importantly, osteolysis can be asymptomatic and associated with or without aseptic loosening. Osteolysis is diagnosed on X-rays as lucent areas adjacent to implants. Modern bearing surfaces, in particular the widely used highly crosslinked UHMWPE, have reduced wear rates and osteolysis.

DISLOCATION AND SUBLUXATION

Dislocation and subluxation are related to implant design, patient factors such as cognitive impairment and neurological disease, and surgeon factors including surgical approach and component orientation. The integrity of the soft tissue, especially abductor muscle deficiency, can risk recurrent instability.

PERIPROSTHETIC FRACTURE

Fracture can occur immediately, early and later following THA. Treatment is dependent on the location of the fracture and its effect on implant fixation. When implant fixation is unaffected, internal fixation is most commonly performed; when the fracture compromises the implant fixation, revision THA is performed.

PJI

PJI represents the most serious complication of THA, other than mortality. Infection results in pain, poor quality of life and, if untreated, it can progress to cause major disability, amputation and death. The incidence of deep PJI requiring revision is currently 1–2%. PJI following THA can occur early or late, with late infection also associated with haematogenous spread to THA from a distant anatomical site.

Prevention of PJI starts at the time of pre-assessment where modifiable risk factors are improved. Preoperative screening of patients for methicillin-resistant *Staphylococcus aureus* (MRSA) is commonplace as well as a growing role for methicillin-sensitive *Staphylococcus aureus* (MSSA) screening in high-risk patients.

Intraoperative prevention of PJI is focused on trying to prevent bacterial contamination. Implant surgery is best performed in specific operating theatres with ultra-clean laminar airflow, strict aseptic technique and reduced operating room personnel and theatre traffic, along with the use of specific surgical hoods and gowns. Prophylactic antibiotics should be given prior to the induction and intraoperatively fluid balance should be optimized and patient-warming methods employed. Good surgical technique is also important, with blood management regimes that often include the use of tranexamic acid significantly reducing the risk of blood transfusion.

Postoperatively good wound care, pain management and nutrition together with standardized protocols to minimize postoperative complications such as chest infections can also help prevent PJI.

The *surgical treatment* of hip PJI involves debridement and implant exchange that can be accomplished in a single operation or more commonly as a two-stage procedure. These procedures are associated with significant patient morbidity and indeed mortality. Failure to eradicate infection is a contraindication to reimplantation of a hip prosthesis and in such circumstances an excision arthroplasty is a salvage procedure.

Contraindications

Active infection is an important contraindication to THA since it significantly increases the risk of PJI. Patients who are non-ambulant or have severe neurological problems such as post-neurological injury may not be good candidates. Similarly, patients with severe cognitive impairment or dementia need very careful consideration prior to THA as very marginal gains may well be outweighed by major risks.

Revision THA

Revision THA has changed dramatically over the past two decades and has evolved from a procedure that had a very limited armamentarium to a much more reproducible procedure with a wide range of strategies to deal with various degrees of surgical complexity. Nevertheless, an overriding rule of thumb is that, with each revision THA procedure that a patient undergoes, the functional outcome diminishes and the risk of complications increases.

The main reasons for revision surgery are:

- loosening
- infection
- dislocation.

Revision implants more commonly employ cementless fixation and specific techniques are employed to restore missing bone stock. This can involve the use of bone graft, which can be in the form of bone chips and impacted (impaction bone grafting) or structural bone grafts. Contemporary revision THA practice more commonly uses highly porous metal augments in cases of severe bone loss, and promising medium-term results over the past decade have been reported.

The knee

20

- Clinical assessment 421
- Swellings around the knee 430
- The diagnostic calendar 433
- Deformities of the knee in children 433
- Deformities of the knee in adults 435
- Lesions of the menisci 437
- Chronic ligamentous instability 440
- Patellofemoral disorders 441
- Tibial tubercle 'apophysitis' 445
- Patellar tendinopathy 445
- Osteochondritis dissecans 445
- Loose bodies 447
- Synovial chondromatosis 447
- Plica syndrome 448
- Tuberculosis 448
- Rheumatoid arthritis 449
- Osteoarthritis 450
- Osteonecrosis 452

CLINICAL ASSESSMENT

HISTORY

- *Pain* is the most common symptom. In inflammatory or degenerative disorders, it is usually diffuse and gradual in onset with osteoarthritis (OA) but typically sudden and severe with gout or infection. In mechanical disorders (especially after injury), it is usually localized and the patient can point to a painful spot.
- *Swelling*, too, may be diffuse or localized. When diffuse, it is suggestive of fluid within the joint or synovial thickening. If there was an injury, ask whether the swelling appeared immediately (injury to vascularized structure, e.g. anterior cruciate ligament (ACL), causing haemarthrosis) or gradually (injury to less vascular structure, e.g. meniscus). Different patterns suggest different likely diagnoses.

> **DIAGNOSTIC PATTERNS OF SWELLING IN THE KNEE**
>
> *Chronic diffuse swelling* – OA or synovitis
> *Intermittent swelling* – old meniscal tear or a loose body
> *Soft, well-defined, localized swelling* – inflamed bursa
> *Firm, fixed swelling along the lateral joint* – meniscal cyst; a loose body in the joint is also firm but it tends to move around on pressure
> *Bony hard swelling of distal end of the femur or the proximal end of the tibia* – sinister, needs workup to exclude a tumour

- *Stiffness* is a common complaint. It may fluctuate.
  - Early morning stiffness suggests an inflammatory disorder.
  - Stiffness after periods of inactivity is typical of OA.

- *Locking* is different from stiffness. The knee can still flex but it cannot extend fully; something has got jammed between the articular surfaces (usually a torn meniscus or a loose body). *Unlocking* is even more suggestive: the obstructing object has shifted and the joint can now move freely again. Do not be misled by 'pseudolocking'.
- *Deformity* is rarely the symptom that causes a patient to present unless rapidly progressive. It may be unilateral or bilateral: *valgus* or *varus*, *fixed flexion* or *hyperextension*. Knock knees and bandy legs are common in children and usually correct spontaneously during growth.
- *Giving way, instability or lack of trust in the knee* suggests a mechanical disorder caused by ligamentous, meniscal or capsular injury, or muscle weakness.
- *Limp* may be due to pain, instability or deformity. An antalgic gait may also be arising from the hip.
- *Loss of function* manifests as difficulty in standing from a low chair, diminishing walking distance, inability to run and difficulty going up and down steps. There may be gradual deterioration in the ability to perform everyday tasks, sports and work.

> ⚠ When a patient has a knee problem, always consider other sources of symptoms such as the back or hip.

SIGNS WITH THE PATIENT STANDING

For the examination, both lower limbs must be exposed from groin to toe or findings may be missed. It is easier to detect deformities with the patient standing up (**20.1**).

1. Look for asymmetry.
   - Is there muscle wasting?
   - Do the knees and ankles touch as is normal as the hips are wider and the knees in slight valgus?
   - Determine if any deformity is truly in the knee or in the distal femur or proximal tibia.

2. Then ask the patient to walk.
   - Is there a limp? If so, is it because the knee does not move freely as it swings through or because it does not straighten well when planted on the ground?
   - Is there an irregular rhythm with the patient trying to diminish weight-bearing on one or other side?

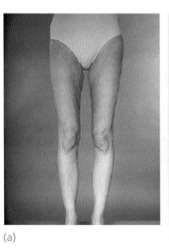
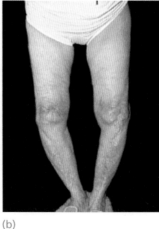
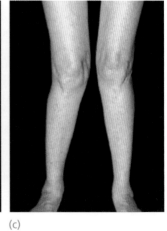

(a)   (b)   (c)

20.1 Examination standing **(a)** Look at the general shape and posture, first from in front and then from behind. Normally the knees are in slight valgus. **(b)** Varus deformity (osteoarthritis). **(c)** Valgus deformity (rheumatoid arthritis).

SIGNS WITH THE PATIENT SITTING

With the patient sitting on the edge of the examination couch, look at the position of the patella (20.2).

- Is it seated centrally or is it shifted to one side?
- Does it appear higher (*patella alta*) or lower (*patella baja/infera*) than usual?
- Ask the patient to straighten each knee in turn. Note the movement of the patella. Does it glide upwards in a smooth manner or does it momentarily veer sideways (maltracking or patellar instability)?

Patellar alignment can also be assessed by measuring the *Q-angle* (quadriceps angle). This is the angle subtended by a line drawn from the anterior superior iliac spine to the centre of the patella and another from the centre of the patella to the tibial tubercle (averages 14 degrees in men and 17 degrees in women). An increased Q-angle is regarded as a predisposing factor in the development of chondromalacia; however, small variations from the norm are not a reliable indicator of future pathology.

SIGNS WITH THE PATIENT LYING SUPINE

Subtle differences are easier to detect by comparing the abnormal with the normal side with the patient lying supine (20.3).

Look

- Is there any asymmetry?
- Look for fixed flexion.
- Are there scars from previous injuries or operations?
- Is there muscle wasting (if unsure, measure circumference)?
- Is there swelling and is it diffuse or localized?
- Is there bruising that may help localize the injury?

Feel

- Run the back of your hand down each limb from the thigh and across the knee. Does the knee feel warmer on one side, suggesting *inflammation*?

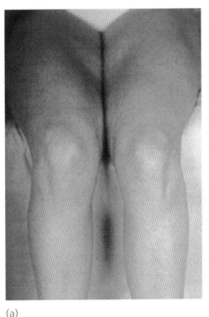
(a)

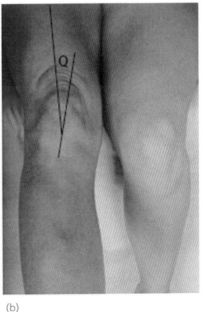
(b)

20.2 Examination with the patient sitting The two knees are compared for shape and symmetry. Note the position of the patellae **(a)** in relaxation; **(b)** in full extension and by measuring the Q-angle.

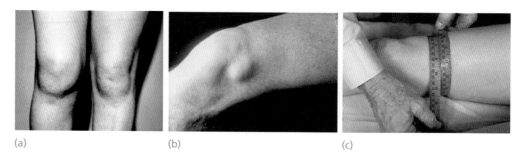

(a) (b) (c)

20.3 Examination with the patient supine Swelling may involve either the whole joint, as in (a), a patient with synovitis of the right knee, or may be due to a localized lesion, as in (b), a patient with a large loose body slipping around in the joint. Quadriceps wasting is common in all types of joint derangement; it can be accurately assessed by (c) measuring the thigh girth at a fixed distance above the joint line of each knee and comparing the two sides.

- Bend the patient's knee to about 70 degrees and sit on the edge of the couch facing the knee. Feel the bony contours around the joint, the attachments of ligaments and tendons, and the joint line. Note where there is *tenderness* (**20.4**).
- Feel for *synovial thickening*. Grasp the patella between the thumb and middle finger and try to lift it off the femoral groove: normally it can be gripped quite firmly but if the synovium is thickened, your fingers simply slip off the edges of the patella.
- Palpate the *patellofemoral joint* along its medial and lateral edges. Straighten the patient's knee and push the patella first towards the medial and then towards the lateral side, feeling with the fingers of your other hand for tenderness along the undersurface. Grind testing against the femoral trochlea may also elicit pain. This can be performed manually or by pressing gently against the proximal edge of the patella and ask the patient to contract the quadriceps muscles.

Move

- *Passive extension* can be tested by the examiner simply holding both legs by the ankles and lifting them off the couch. *Active extension* can be roughly tested by the examiner slipping a hand under each knee and then asking the patient to force the knees into the surface of the couch.
- *Passive* and *active flexion* are tested with the patient lying supine. Normally, the heel can be pulled up close to the buttock (0–150 degrees). The 'heel-to-buttock' distance is compared on the two sides (**20.5**).
- *Internal* and *external rotation*, though normally no more than about 10 degrees, should

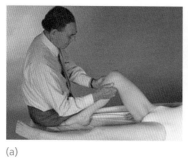

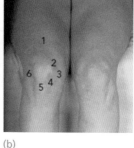

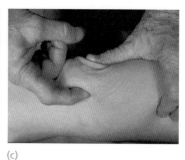

(a) (b) (c)

20.4 Feeling for tenderness (a) This is the best position for eliciting tenderness around the knee. (b) Landmarks are: (1), quadriceps tendon; (2), edge of patella; (3), medial collateral ligament; (4), the joint line; (5), patellar ligament; (6), lateral collateral ligament. (c) By pushing the patella to one or other side of the midline, you can feel under its edge.

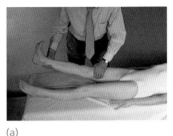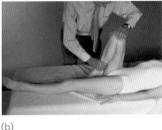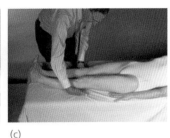

(a)   (b)   (c)

20.5 Movement The knee should move from full extension **(a)** through a range of 150° to full flexion **(b)**. Small degrees of flexion deformity (loss of full extension) can be detected by placing the hands under the knees while the patient forces the legs down on the couch **(c)**; if your hand can be extracted more easily on one side than the other, this indicates loss of the final few degrees of complete extension.

also be assessed. The patient's hip and knee are flexed to 90 degrees; one hand steadies and feels the knee, the other rotates the foot.

- *Crepitus* during movement may be felt with a hand placed on the front of the knee. It usually signifies patellofemoral roughness.
- The '*patellar apprehension test*', performed by pressing the patella laterally with the thumb while flexing the knee slowly, may induce anxiety and sharp resistance to further movement; it is diagnostic of recurrent patellar subluxation or dislocation.

Tests for intra-articular fluid

There are several ways to test for intra-articular fluid (**20.6**).

Cross-fluctuation This test is applicable only if there is a large effusion. The left hand is used to compress and empty the suprapatellar pouch while the right hand straddles the front of the joint below the patella; by squeezing with each hand alternately, a fluid impulse is transmitted across the joint.

Patellar tap The suprapatellar pouch is compressed with the left hand. With the other hand, the patella is then tapped sharply backwards onto the femoral condyles. In a positive test, the patella can be felt striking the femur and bouncing off again.

Bulge test This is a useful method of testing when there is a small effusion. Squeeze fluid out of the suprapatellar pouch, the medial compartment is emptied by pressing on the medial aspect

of the joint; that hand is then lifted away and the lateral side is sharply compressed – a distinct ripple is seen on the flattened medial surface as fluid is shunted across.

Juxtapatellar hollow If both knees are bent gradually and observed from below, a hollow appears lateral to the patellar ligament and disappears on further flexion; if there is fluid in the joint, this hollow fills quickly and disappears earlier or may not be seen at all.

Tests for ligamentous stability

COLLATERAL LIGAMENTS

The medial and lateral ligaments are tested by stressing the knee into valgus and varus: this is best done by tucking the patient's foot under your arm and holding the extended knee firmly with one hand on each side of the joint; the leg is then angulated alternately into varus and valgus. The test is performed at full extension and again at 30 degrees of flexion. There is normally some mediolateral movement at 30 degrees, but if this is excessive (compared to the normal side), it suggests a torn or stretched collateral ligament. Sideways movement in full extension is always abnormal; this may be due either to torn or stretched ligaments and capsule, or to loss of articular cartilage or bone on one side of the knee which allows the affected compartment to collapse (**20.7a–c**).

CRUCIATE LIGAMENTS

Routine examination for cruciate ligament stability involves testing for abnormal gliding movements in the anteroposterior (sagittal) plane.

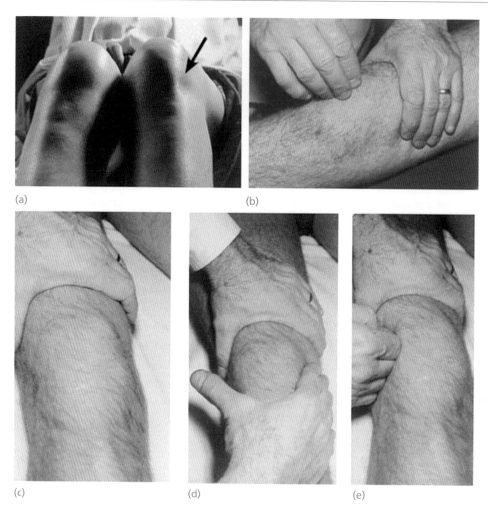

(a)   (b)

(c)   (d)   (e)

20.6 Testing for intra-articular fluid (a) The juxtapatellar hollow, which disappears in flexion if there is fluid in the knee. **(b)** Patellar tap test. **(c–e)** Doing the bulge test: compress the suprapatellar pouch **(c)**; empty the medial compartment **(d)**; push fluid back from the lateral compartment and watch for the bulge on the medial side **(e)**.

Posterior sag test With the patient's knees flexed 90 degrees and the feet resting on the couch, the upper tibia is inspected from the side; if its upper end has dropped back, or can be gently pushed back, this indicates a tear of the posterior cruciate ligament (PCL).

Anterior drawer test With the knee in the same position, the foot is anchored by the examiner sitting on it (provided this does not cause pain); then, using both hands, the upper end of the tibia is grasped firmly and rocked backwards and forwards to see if there is any anteroposterior glide (**20.7d**).

- Excessive anterior movement (a positive anterior drawer sign) denotes anterior cruciate laxity.
- Excessive posterior movement (a positive posterior drawer sign) signifies posterior cruciate laxity.

Lachman test More sensitive is the Lachman test, but this is difficult if the patient has big

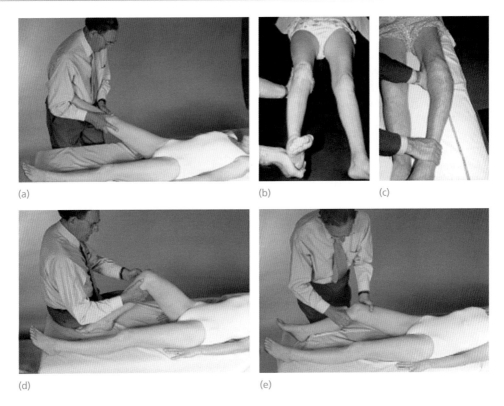

(a) (b) (c)

(d) (e)

20.7 Testing for instability There are two ways of testing the collateral ligaments (side-to-side stability): **(a)** by gripping the foot close to your body and guiding the knee alternately towards valgus and varus; **(b)** by gripping the femoral condyles (provided your hand is big enough) and then forcing the leg alternately into valgus and varus. **(c)** In this case, there was gross instability on the lateral side, allowing the knee to be pulled into marked varus. Cruciate ligament instability can be assessed by either the drawer test **(d)** or the Lachman test **(e)**, as described in the text.

thighs (or the examiner has small hands). The patient's knee is flexed 20 degrees; with one hand grasping the lower thigh and the other the upper part of the leg, the joint surfaces are shifted backwards and forwards upon each other (20.7e). If the knee is stable, there should be no gliding.

COMPLEX LIGAMENT INJURIES

When only a single ligament is damaged, the diagnosis is relatively easy. With combined injuries the direction of instability may be oblique or rotational. The *pivot shift test* may help to detect these. The patient lies supine with the lower limb completely relaxed. The examiner lifts the leg with the knee held in full extension and the tibia internally rotated (the position of slight rotational subluxation). A valgus force is then applied to the lateral side of the joint as the knee is flexed; a sudden posterior movement of the tibia is seen and felt as the joint is fully relocated. The test is sometimes quite painful and is generally best performed with the patient under anaesthesia.

Tests for meniscal injuries

McMurray's test This classic test for a torn meniscus is seldom used now that the diagnosis can easily be made by MRI. The test is based on trapping a loose meniscal tag between the articular surfaces and inducing it to snap free. The knee is flexed as far as possible; one hand steadies the joint and the other rotates the leg medially and laterally while the knee is slowly extended. The test is repeated several times, with the knee stressed in valgus or varus. It is not a sensitive or specific test.

SECTION 2 REGIONAL ORTHOPAEDICS

Thessaly test   This test is based on a dynamic reproduction of load transmission in the knee joint. With the affected knee flexed to 20 degrees and the foot placed flat on the ground, the patient takes their full weight on that leg while being supported (for balance) by the examiner. The patient is then instructed to twist their body to one side and then to the other three times (thus, with each turn, exerting a rotational force in the knee), keeping the knee flexed at 20 degrees. Patients with meniscal tears experience medial or lateral joint line pain and may have a sense of locking.

SIGNS WITH THE PATIENT LYING PRONE

Scars or lumps in the popliteal fossa are noted. If there is a swelling:

- Is it in the midline? – most likely a bulging capsule.
- Or is it to one side? – possibly a bursa. A semi-membranous bursa is usually just above the joint line, a Baker's cyst below it.

The popliteal fossa is carefully palpated. If there is a lump:

- Where does it originate?
- Does it pulsate?
- Can it be emptied into the joint?

Apley's test

- With the patient prone, the knee is flexed to 90 degrees and rotated while a compression force is applied; this, the *grinding test*, reproduces symptoms if a meniscus is torn.
- Rotation is then repeated while the leg is pulled upwards with the surgeon's knee holding the thigh down; this, the *distraction test*, produces increased pain only if there is ligament damage.

INVESTIGATION

Imaging

X-RAYS

Anteroposterior and lateral views are routine; it is often useful also to obtain tangential ('skyline') patellofemoral views and intercondylar (or tunnel) views.

The anteroposterior view should always be taken with the patient standing; unless the femorotibial compartment is loaded, joint space narrowing may be missed (20.8).

Both knees should be X-rayed, so as to compare the abnormal with the normal side. A Rosenberg

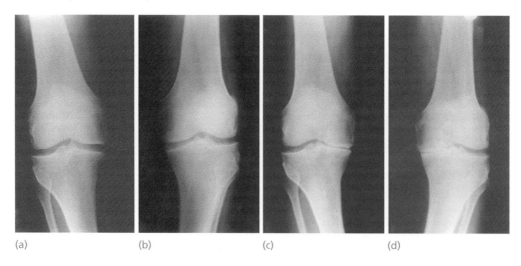

(a)   (b)   (c)   (d)

20.8 X-rays Anteroposterior views should always be taken with the patient standing. **(a,b)** Images obtained with the patient lying on the X-ray couch show only slight narrowing of the medial joint space on each side; but with weight-bearing **(c,d)** it is clear that the changes are much more marked than at first thought.

view is used to specifically assess the lateral compartment.

Tibiofemoral alignment can be measured on full-length standing views. Normal indices have also been established for patellar height and patellofemoral congruence. These features are discussed in the relevant sections of the chapter.

MAGNETIC RESONANCE IMAGING

Magnetic resonance imaging (MRI) has evolved to become the standard imaging method for diagnosing and grading the severity of many intra-articular and extra-articular problems (20.9). It is able to detect meniscal tears, ligament and capsular injuries, osteoarticular fractures and both benign and malignant tumours.

Arthroscopy

MRI has reduced the use of arthroscopy as a diagnostic tool but it remains useful (20.10).

USE OF ARTHROSCOPY AS A DIAGNOSTIC TOOL
To establish or refine the accuracy of diagnosis (e.g. to locate and perform excision biopsy of a pigmented villonodular synovitis (PVNS) lesion in the knee) To help in deciding a treatment strategy or to plan the operative approach (e.g. to determine the degree of articular cartilage damage in planning osteotomy around the knee)

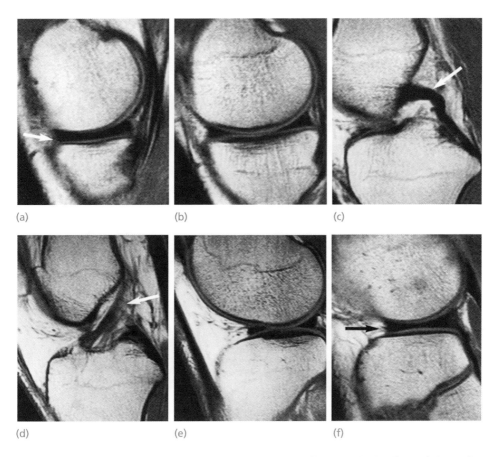

(a) (b) (c)

(d) (e) (f)

20.9 MRI A series of sagittal T1-weighted images proceeding from medial to lateral show the normal appearances of **(a,b)** the medial meniscus; **(c)** the PCL; **(d)** the somewhat fan-shaped ACL and **(e,f)** the lateral meniscus.

To confirm diagnosis and treat certain
joint conditions with specific operative
procedures (e.g. repair or excision of
a bucket-handle tear within a locked
knee joint or assessment and repair of
a rotator cuff tear)

There is increasing evidence to suggest that, in
certain conditions, arthroscopic intervention
is less effective than previously thought. For
example, washout of the osteoarthritic knee
and meniscectomy in the degenerate knee,
without the presence of mechanical symptoms,

are both procedures where surgery may not be
effective.

SWELLINGS AROUND THE KNEE

The knee is prone to a number of disorders which
present essentially as 'swelling'. The swelling is
often painless until the tissues become tense.
Malignancy must be excluded, although fortunately the majority of swellings are benign. They
can be divided into four groups:

- *swelling of the entire joint*
- *swellings in front of the joint*

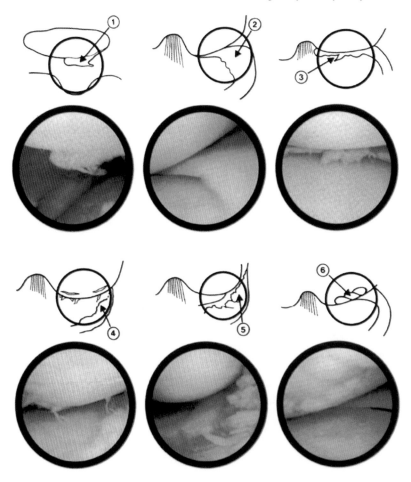

20.10 Arthroscopy Arthroscopic images of the interior of the right knee from the lateral side,
showing (1) chondromalacia patellae; (2) normal medial meniscus; (3) torn medial meniscus;
(4) degenerate medial meniscus and osteoarthritic femoral condyle; (5) rheumatoid synovium;
(6) osteochondritis dissecans of medial femoral condyle.

- *swellings behind the joint*
- *bony swellings.*

ACUTE SWELLING OF THE ENTIRE JOINT

Traumatic synovitis

Any moderately severe injury (including a torn or trapped meniscus or a torn cruciate ligament) can precipitate a reactive synovitis, but typically the swelling appears only after several hours. There is inhibition of quadriceps action and the thigh wastes. If the amount of fluid is considerable, its aspiration hastens muscle recovery.

Post-traumatic haemarthrosis

Tense swelling immediately after injury means blood in the joint. The knee is painful and it feels warm, tense and tender. Movements are restricted. *X-rays* are essential to see if there is a fracture; if there is not, then suspect a tear of the ACL.

Non-traumatic haemarthrosis

In patients with clotting disorders, the knee is a common site for acute bleeds. If the appropriate clotting factor is available, the joint should be aspirated and splinted. Bleeds can also occur from vascular lesions in the knee (e.g. PVNS).

Acute septic arthritis

 Acute pyogenic infection of the knee is an acute emergency and requires prompt treatment to prevent systemic spread of the infection and to prevent local damage to the knee. The organism is usually *Staphylococcus aureus*, but in adults gonococcal infection can occur.

The joint is swollen, painful and inflamed. The patient reports extreme pain on movement of the joint. Blood tests reveal an elevated white cell count, C-reactive protein (CRP) and erythrocyte sedimentation rate (ESR). Aspiration reveals pus in the joint; fluid should be sent for bacteriological investigation, including anaerobic culture.

Treatment consists of systemic antibiotics and drainage of the joint – ideally by arthroscopy, with irrigation and complete synovectomy; if fluid reaccumulates, it can be aspirated through a wide-bore needle. As the inflammation subsides, movement is begun, but weight-bearing may be deferred for 4–6 weeks.

Aseptic non-traumatic synovitis

Acute swelling, without a history of trauma or signs of infection, suggests *gout, pseudogout or inflammatory monoarthropathy.* Aspiration will provide fluid which may look turbid, resembling pus, but it is sterile and microscopy (using polarized light) reveals the crystals. *Treatment* with anti-inflammatory drugs is usually effective while investigation as to the cause of the swelling begins.

CHRONIC SWELLING OF THE ENTIRE JOINT

The diagnosis can usually be made on clinical and *X-ray* or *MRI* examination. The more elusive disorders should be fully investigated by joint aspiration, synovial fluid examination, arthroscopy and synovial biopsy.

Non-infective arthritis

The commonest causes of chronic swelling are *OA* and *rheumatoid arthritis (RA).* Other signs, such as deformity, loss of movement or instability, may be present and X-ray examination will usually show characteristic features.

Chronic infective arthritis

The most important condition to exclude is *tuberculosis*, of which there has been a resurgence of cases in the last two decades. Typically, the knee is swollen and the thigh muscles are wasted.

Other synovial disorders

Chronic swelling and synovial effusion without articular destruction should suggest conditions such as *synovial chondromatosis* and *PVNS*. The diagnosis will usually be obvious from an MRI scan and can be confirmed by arthroscopic synovial biopsy.

SWELLINGS IN FRONT OF THE KNEE

Prepatellar bursitis

This fluctuant swelling is confined to the front of the patella and the joint itself is normal. It is an uninfected bursitis due to constant friction between skin and bone. As such, it is seen mainly in workers who kneel, often without using protective knee pads. *Treatment* consists of firm bandaging, and kneeling is avoided; occasionally, aspiration is needed (perform this away from the midline). In chronic cases, the lump is best excised.

Secondary infection (possibly due to foreign body implantation) results in a warm, tender swelling.

Treatment is by rest, antibiotics and, if necessary, aspiration or excision.

Infrapatellar bursitis

The swelling is below the patella and superficial to the patellar ligament, being more distally placed than prepatellar bursitis. *Treatment* is similar to that for prepatellar bursitis.

Other bursae

Occasionally, a bursa deep to the patellar tendon or the pes anserinus becomes inflamed and painful. *Treatment* is non-operative.

SWELLINGS AT THE BACK OF THE KNEE

SEMIMEMBRANOSUS BURSA

The bursa between the semimembranosus and the medial head of gastrocnemius may become enlarged in children or adults. It presents usually as a painless lump behind the knee, slightly to the medial side of the midline and is most conspicuous with the knee straight. The lump is fluctuant and transilluminates. The knee joint is normal.

Recurrence is common if excision is attempted and, as the bursa normally disappears in time, a waiting policy is the treatment of choice.

Popliteal 'cyst'

Bulging of the posterior capsule and synovial herniation may produce a swelling in the popliteal fossa. It is usually caused by RA or OA, but it is still often called a 'Baker's cyst' (even though Baker's original description probably referred to an association with tuberculous arthritis). Occasionally, the 'cyst' ruptures and the synovial contents spill into the muscle planes causing pain and swelling in the calf – a combination which can easily be mistaken for deep vein thrombosis. The swelling may diminish following aspiration and injection of hydrocortisone; excision is not advised because recurrence is common unless the underlying condition is treated.

Popliteal aneurysm

This is the commonest limb aneurysm and is sometimes bilateral. Pain and stiffness of the knee may precede the symptoms of peripheral arterial disease, so it is essential to examine any lump behind the knee for pulsation. A thrombosed popliteal aneurysm does not pulsate, but it feels almost solid.

SWELLINGS AT THE SIDE OF THE JOINT

Meniscal cyst

This presents as a small, tense swelling, usually on the lateral side at or just below the joint line. Sometimes it is so tense that it can easily be mistaken for a bony lump. It is usually tender on pressure.

BONY SWELLINGS AROUND THE KNEE

The knee is a relatively superficial joint therefore bony swellings are often visible and almost always palpable. Common examples are cartilage-capped exostoses (osteochondromata) and the characteristic painful swelling of Osgood–Schlatter disease of the tibial tubercle.

> ⚠ *Malignancy,* although rare, must be excluded.

An *MRI scan* is mandatory in the investigation of bony swellings around the knee that display any concerning features. Features that suggest malignancy are often referred to as 'red flags'.

RED FLAGS FOR MALIGNANCY

Disproportionate pain
Sudden increase in size
History of previous malignancy

THE DIAGNOSTIC CALENDAR

Disorders of the knee can occur at any age but certain conditions are more common during specific periods of life:

- *Congenital knee disorders* may be present at birth or may become apparent only during the first or second decade of life.
- *Adolescents* with anterior knee pain are usually found to have one of the following:
  - chondromalacia patellae
  - patellar instability
  - osteochondritis
  - a plica syndrome (remember that pain may arise from the hip).
- *Young adults* engaged in sports are the most frequent victims of meniscal tears and ligament injuries. Examination should include a variety of tests for ligamentous instability that would be quite inappropriate in elderly patients.
- *Patients above middle age* with chronic pain and stiffness probably have OA. With primary OA of the knees, other joints also are often affected; polyarthritis does not necessarily (nor even most commonly) mean RA.

DEFORMITIES OF THE KNEE IN CHILDREN

By the end of growth, the knees are normally in 5–7 degrees of valgus, although there is significant normal variation. In some circumstances, excessive deformity is seen:

- bow leg (genu varum)
- knock knee (genu valgum)
- hyperextension (genu recurvatum).

PHYSIOLOGICAL BOW LEGS AND KNOCK KNEES

Bow legs (genu varum) in babies and knock knees (genu valgum) in 4-year-olds are so common that they are considered to be stages of normal development (**20.11**).

- Bilateral bow-legged appearance can be recorded by measuring the distance between the knees with the child standing and the heels touching; it should be less than 6 cm.

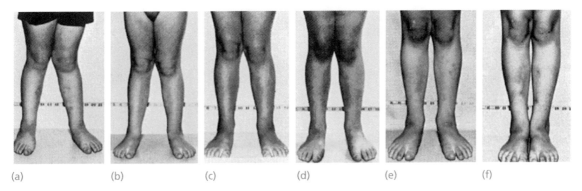

(a)   (b)   (c)   (d)   (e)   (f)

20.11 Physiological genu valgum 'Knock knees' in young children usually correct spontaneously. (a–f) These pictures of the same child were obtained at various ages between 3 and 7 years.

- Knock knee can be estimated by measuring the distance between the medial malleoli when the knees are touching with the patellae facing forwards; it is usually less than 8 cm.

Treatment

In the occasional case where, by the age of 10 years, the deformity is still marked, *operative correction* can be offered.

- *Stapling* or figure-of-eight plates ('8-plates') applied to either side of the physis can be used on the convex side of the deformity to temporarily slow growth (known as 'guided growth') (**20.12**), but there is a small risk that normal growth will not resume when removed.
- *Permanent hemi-epiphysiodesis* (fusion of one half of the physis) can achieve similar results but needs careful timing.
- *Corrective osteotomy* (supracondylar osteotomy for valgus knees and high tibial osteotomy for varus knees) can be used in later presentation once growth is complete, or for more severe deformities when guided growth is likely to be ineffective (**20.13**).

PATHOLOGICAL BOW LEGS AND KNOCK KNEES IN CHILDREN

Disorders which cause distorted epiphyseal and/or physeal growth may give rise to bow leg or knock knee; these include some of the skeletal dysplasias and the various types of rickets, as well as injuries of the epiphyseal and physeal growth cartilage (**20.14**). A unilateral deformity is likely to be pathological, but it is essential in all cases to look for signs of injury or generalized skeletal disorder. If angulation is severe, operative correction will be necessary.

Blount's disease is a progressive bow-legged deformity due to abnormal growth of the posteromedial part of the proximal tibia. The children are often overweight and start walking early; the condition is bilateral in 80% of cases. Children of Afro-Caribbean descent appear to be affected more frequently than others. Deformity is noticeably worse than in physiological bow legs and may include internal rotation of the tibia (**20.15**). The child walks with an outward thrust of the knee; in the worst cases there may be lateral subluxation of the

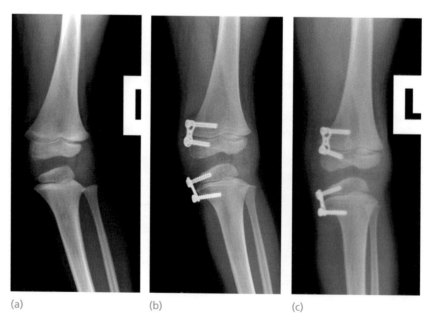

(a)   (b)   (c)

20.12 Significant genu valgum (a) Genu valgum in a 5-year-old boy that was worsening with time. **(b,c)** Operative management performed with guided growth using '8-plates' on the convex side of the deformity to temporarily slow the medial physeal growth. Plates are removed once alignment is restored.

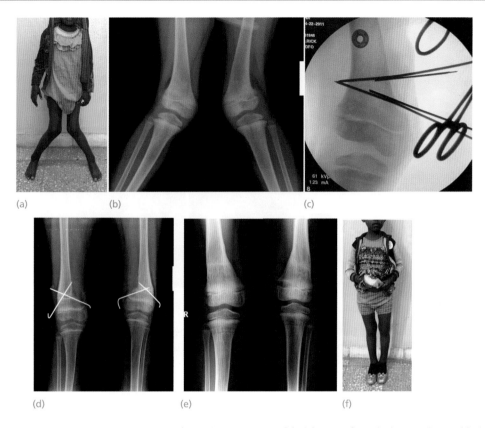

(a)   (b)   (c)

(d)   (e)   (f)

20.13 Severe genu valgum (a,b) Genu valgum in an 8-year-old girl. Use of guided growth was likely to be unsuccessful due to the severity. **(c–f)** Bilateral closing wedge supracondylar osteotomies were performed.

tibia. Spontaneous resolution is rare. On X-ray, the proximal tibial epiphysis is flattened medially and the adjacent metaphysis is beak-shaped. In older children (8–10 years old), there can be severe depression of the medial plateau of the tibia, requiring a 'hemiplateau elevation' in conjunction with a proximal tibial corrective osteotomy through the tibial metaphysis, needed to correct the varus and internal rotation. In established cases, hemi-epiphysiodesis is rarely successful.

RECURVATUM

Congenital genu recurvatum may be due to abnormal intrauterine posture and may recover spontaneously or with casting. Occasionally, there is dislocation of the knee that requires operative reduction if reduction is not achieved by serial flexion casting (**20.16**).

DEFORMITIES OF THE KNEE IN ADULTS

GENU VARUM AND GENU VALGUM

Angular deformities are common in adults (usually bow legs in men and knock knees in women). They may be the *sequel to childhood deformity* and, if so, usually cause no problems. However, if the deformity is associated with early OA, patients may present with significant symptoms. In the absence of overt OA, if there is persistent severe pain with radiological signs of early joint damage (usually seen on MRI), an osteotomy can be performed – above the knee for valgus deformity and below the knee for varus. Preoperative planning should include radiographic measurements to determine the mechanical and anatomical axes of both bones and the lower limb, as well as estimation of the centre of rotation of angulation.

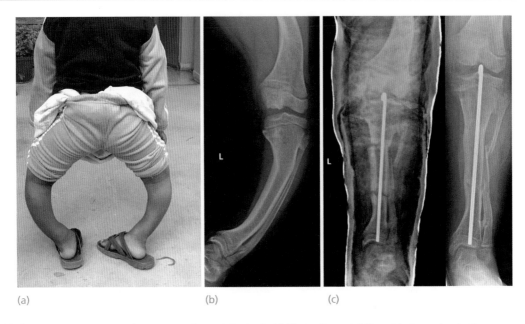

(a)   (b)   (c)

20.14 Severe genu varum due to previous rickets **(a,b)** Note the additional internal rotation deformity. **(c)** Operative management with an intramedullary rush rod (a smooth stainless-steel pin). A three-level osteotomy was required to restore alignment.

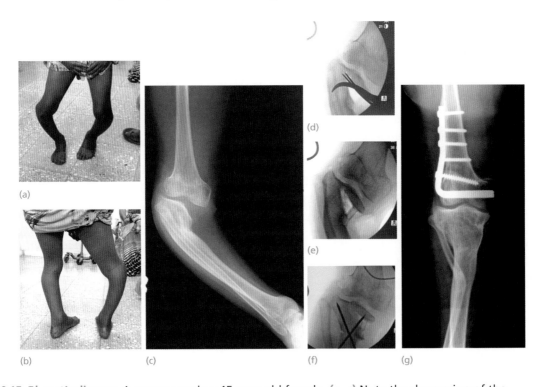

(a)

(b)   (c)   (d)

(e)

(f)   (g)

20.15 Blount's disease A severe case in a 15-year-old female. **(a–c)** Note the depression of the medial tibial plateau, as well as the marked proximal tibia varus deformity. **(d–g)** Operative correction required elevation of the plateau to restore the joint line, stabilized with fibula autograft (a 'hemiplateau elevation'), followed by a proximal tibia osteotomy and later distal femoral corrective osteotomy.

Deformity may be entirely *secondary to arthritis* – usually varus in OA and valgus in RA. Stress X-rays or MRI can be useful. Depending on the degree of joint damage, osteotomy or joint replacement may be considered.

Other causes of varus or valgus deformity are:

- *ligament injuries*
- *malunited fractures*
- *Paget's disease.*

Where possible, the underlying disorder should be dealt with; provided the joint is stable, corrective osteotomy may be all that is necessary.

GENU RECURVATUM (HYPEREXTENSION OF THE KNEE)

Normal people with generalized ligament laxity tend to stand with their knees back-set immitating a genu recurvatum deformity. In adults, acquired cases are more common, for example prolonged traction, especially on a frame, or holding the knee hyperextended in plaster, may overstretch ligaments, leading to permanent hyperextension deformity. Ligaments may become overstretched following chronic or recurrent synovitis (especially in RA), the hypotonia of rickets, the flailness of poliomyelitis or the insensitivity of Charcot's disease.

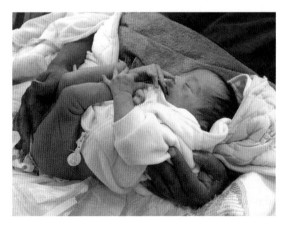

20.16 Congenital dislocation of the knees in an infant Serial flexion casting is initially performed. If unsuccessful, quadriceps lengthening or femoral shortening, combined with open reduction of the knee is required to reduce the dislocation.

In paralytic conditions such as poliomyelitis, recurvatum is often seen in association with fixed equinus of the ankle. In moderate degrees, this may actually be helpful (e.g. in stabilizing a knee with weak extensors). However, if excessive and prolonged, it may give rise to a permanent deformity. If bony correction is undertaken, the knee should be left with some hyperextension to preserve the stabilizing mechanism. If quadriceps power is poor, the patient may need a caliper. Severe paralytic hyperextension can be treated by fixing the patella into the tibial plateau, where it acts as a bone block.

Other causes of recurvatum are *growth plate injuries* and *malunited fractures.* These can be safely corrected by osteotomy.

IMPORTANT ROLES OF THE MENISCI
Improving articular congruency and stability of the knee Controlling rolling and gliding actions of the joint Distributing load during movement

LESIONS OF THE MENISCI

During weight-bearing, at least 50% of the contact stresses are taken by the menisci when the knee is loaded in extension, and 90% in flexion. Meniscectomy leads to marked increases in articular stresses.

The medial meniscus is less mobile than the lateral, and it cannot easily accommodate abnormal stresses.

Even in the absence of injury, there is gradual degeneration and change in the material properties of the menisci with age, making tears more likely with ageing, often in association with osteoarthritic changes. In younger people, meniscal tears are usually the result of a specific trauma.

MENISCAL TEARS

The meniscus consists mainly of circumferential collagen fibres held by a few radial strands. It is therefore more likely to tear along its length than

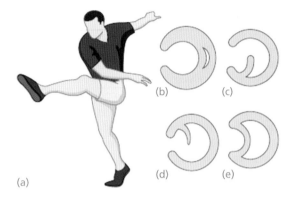

20.17 Torn medial meniscus (a) The meniscus is usually torn by a twisting force with the knee bent and taking weight; the initial split **(b)** may extend anteriorly **(c)**, posteriorly **(d)** or both ways to create a 'bucket-handle' tear **(e)**.

across its width (**20.17**). The split is usually initiated by a rotational and shearing force, which occurs when the knee is flexed and twisted under load; hence the frequency in footballers. In middle life, when fibrotic change has restricted mobility of the meniscus, tears can occur with relatively little force.

In some cases, tears are *vertical* along the length of the meniscus. If the separated fragment remains attached front and back, the lesion is called a *bucket-handle tear* (**20.17e**). The torn portion can sometimes displace towards the centre of the joint and becomes jammed between femur and tibia causing a block to movement or 'locked knee'. Other patterns include posterior or anterior horn tears and parrot beak tears where an oblique tear pattern creates a flap of meniscus that may be stable (unlikely to displace) or unstable (displaced or likely to displace).

Horizontal tears are usually 'degenerative' and stable. Some are associated with meniscal cysts or complex, with the tear pattern lying in many planes. These tears may be displaced or likely to displace and acts as an irritant, giving rise to recurrent synovial effusion and mechanical symptoms. All except the most peripheral part of the meniscus is avascular and spontaneous repair does not occur unless the tear is in the outer third, which is vascularized from the attached synovium and capsule.

Clinical features

The patient is usually a young person who sustains a twisting injury to the knee. Pain is often severe and further activity is avoided. Occasionally, the knee is 'locked' in partial flexion. Almost invariably swelling appears a few hours later, or perhaps the following day.

With rest, the initial symptoms subside, only to recur periodically after trivial twists or strains. Sometimes the knee gives way spontaneously and this is, again, followed by pain and swelling.

It is important to remember that in patients aged over 40 years the initial injury may be unremarkable and the main complaint is of recurrent 'giving way' or 'locking'.

'Locking' (the sudden inability to extend the knee fully) suggests a bucket-handle tear. The patient sometimes learns to 'unlock' the knee by bending it fully or by twisting it from side to side.

On examination, the joint may be held slightly flexed and there is often an effusion. In late presentations, the quadriceps will be wasted. Tenderness is localized to the joint line, in the vast majority of cases on the medial side. Flexion is usually full but extension is often slightly limited.

Between attacks of pain and effusion there is a disconcerting paucity of signs, but special tests may alert one to the diagnosis. The history is helpful, and McMurray's test, Apley's grinding test and the Thessaly test may be positive

Imaging

Plain X-rays are normal but *MRI* is a reliable method for confirming the diagnosis and may even reveal tears that are missed by arthroscopy.

Treatment

DEALING WITH THE LOCKED KNEE

Usually the knee 'unlocks' spontaneously; if not, gentle passive flexion and rotation may do the trick. Forceful manipulation is unwise; after a few days' rest, the knee may well unlock itself. If the knee does not unlock, arthroscopy is indicated. If symptoms are not marked, it may be better to wait a week or two and let the synovitis settle down, thus making the operation easier; if the tear is confirmed, the offending fragment is removed or repaired if possible.

CONSERVATIVE TREATMENT

If the joint is not locked, *MRI* plays a critical role in planning further treatment. If a peripheral tear has been identified and the lesion may be repairable, then arthroscopy and suture repair of the meniscus can be employed, particularly in the younger patient. However, in other unstable or potentially unstable tears non-operative care should be instigated as many patients will settle.

OPERATIVE TREATMENT

> ### INDICATIONS FOR SURGERY FOR MENISCAL TEARS
>
> If the joint cannot be unlocked
> If mechanical symptoms (locking or catching) are recurrent and non-operative treatment has failed

In most cases, if available, an *MRI scan* should be obtained to determine the pattern of tear and to plan treatment with the patient. Tears close to the periphery, which have the capacity to heal, can be sutured; at least one edge of the tear should be red (i.e. vascularized) (**20.18**). In appropriate cases, the success rate for both open and arthroscopic repair can be high.

Tears other than those in the peripheral third are dealt with by excising the torn portion. Total meniscectomy predisposes to late secondary OA and causes greater morbidity than partial meniscectomy.

Arthroscopic meniscectomy has distinct advantages over open meniscectomy:

- shorter hospital stay
- lower costs
- more rapid return to function.

However, it is by no means free of complications.

Postoperative pain and stiffness are reduced by prophylactic non-steroidal anti-inflammatory drugs (NSAIDs). In some patients, a flare of pain can occur, which can persist for a number of months. In some cases, there is a rapid progression of articular cartilage damage and the development of arthritis.

MENISCAL DEGENERATION

Patients over 45 years old may present with symptoms and signs of a meniscal tear often with no preceding injury. *MRI* reveals a horizontal cleavage tear – the characteristic 'degenerative'

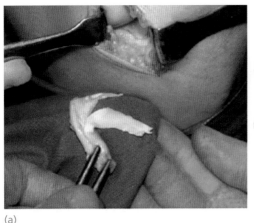

(a)

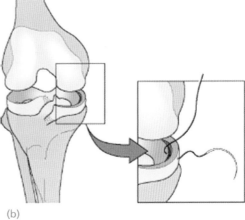

(b)

20.18 Torn meniscus – operation (a) Removal of a torn medial meniscus. (b) Repair is appropriate if at least one edge of the tear is vascularized. This can be done arthroscopically.

lesion – or detachment of the anterior or posterior horn without an obvious tear. Associated OA or chondrocalcinosis is common.

Meniscectomy is only indicated if mechanical symptoms are marked, such as a mechanical block to movement.

DISCOID LATERAL MENISCUS

In the foetus the meniscus is not semilunar but disc-like. If this disc-like shape persists postnatally, symptoms can occur if the whole meniscus is unstable or more typically where a tear occurs. Usually, a young patient complains that, without any history of injury, the knee gives way and 'thuds' loudly. A characteristic clunk may be felt at 110 degrees as the knee is bent and at 10 degrees as it is being straightened. The diagnosis is easily confirmed by *MRI*.

If there is only a clunk, *treatment* is not essential. If pain is intrusive, the meniscus may be partially excised, leaving a normally shaped meniscus.

MENISCAL CYSTS

Cysts of the menisci most often arise from horizontal cleavage tears (20.19). It is also suggested that synovial cells infiltrate into the vascular area between meniscus and capsule and multiply there. The multilocular cyst contains gelatinous fluid and is surrounded by thick fibrous tissue.

CHRONIC LIGAMENTOUS INSTABILITY

The knee is a complex hinge which depends heavily on its ligaments for mediolateral, anteroposterior and rotational stability. Ligament injuries, from minor strains through partial ruptures to complete tears, are common in sportsmen, athletes and dancers. Whatever the nature of the acute injury, the victim may be left with chronic instability of the knee – a sense of the joint wanting to give way, or actually giving way, during unguarded activity. This is sometimes

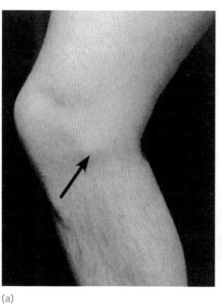
(a)

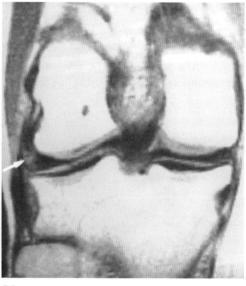
(b)

20.19 Meniscal cyst (a) Typical appearance of a small, firm swelling at or just below the joint line. (b) MRI showing the cyst arising from the edge of the meniscus (arrow). The patient presents with pain and a small lump can be seen and felt, usually on the lateral side of the joint; it may feel surprisingly firm (or tense), particularly when the knee is extended. If the symptoms are sufficiently troublesome, the cyst can be decompressed or removed arthroscopically (resecting the lower half of the cleavage tear decompresses the cyst); any meniscal lesion can be dealt with at the same time.

accompanied by pain and recurrent episodes of swelling. There may be a meniscal tear, but meniscectomy is likely to make matters worse; some patients present with meniscectomy scars on both sides of the knee.

Examination should include special tests for ligamentous instability as well as radiological investigation and arthroscopy.

> ⚠ It is important not only to establish the nature of the lesion but also to measure the level of functional impairment against the needs and demands of the individual patient before advocating treatment.

Injuries of the knee and leg are dealt with in detail in Chapter 31.

PATELLOFEMORAL DISORDERS

RECURRENT DISLOCATION OF THE PATELLA

Acute dislocation of the patella is dealt with in Chapter 31. In 15–20% of cases (mostly children) the first episode is followed by recurrent dislocation or subluxation after minimal stress. This is due, in some measure, to disruption or stretching of the medially based ligamentous structures (e.g. the medial patellofemoral ligament – MPFL) which normally stabilize the extensor mechanism. However, in a significant proportion of cases, there is no history of an acute strain and the initial episode is thought to have occurred 'spontaneously'. It is now recognized that in all cases of recurrent dislocation, but particularly in the latter group, one or more *predisposing factors* are often present.

FACTORS PREDISPOSING TO DISLOCATION OF THE PATELLA

Generalized ligamentous laxity
Underdevelopment of the lateral femoral condyle and flattening of the intercondylar groove

---

Maldevelopment of the patella (which may be unusually small or seated too high)
Valgus deformity of the knee
External tibial torsion
A primary muscle defect

Repeated dislocation damages the contiguous articular surfaces of the patella and femoral condyle; this may result in further flattening of the condyle, so facilitating further dislocations.

Dislocation is almost always towards the lateral side; medial dislocation is seen only in rare iatrogenic cases following overzealous lateral release or medial transposition of the patellar tendon.

Clinical features

Girls are affected more commonly than boys and the condition is often bilateral. The main (or only) complaint is that from time to time the knee suddenly gives way and the patient falls; this may be accompanied by pain and sometimes the knee gets stuck in flexion.

Although the patella always dislocates laterally, the patient may think it has displaced medially because the uncovered medial femoral condyle stands out prominently.

If the knee is seen while the patella is dislocated, the diagnosis is obvious (20.20). There is usually tenderness on the medial side of the joint. Later, the joint becomes swollen, and aspiration may reveal a blood-stained effusion.

Between attacks clinical signs are sparse; however, the *apprehension test* is positive and the patient should be carefully examined for features that are known to predispose to patellar instability.

Imaging

- *X-rays* may reveal loose bodies in the knee from new or old osteochondral fractures. A lateral view with the knee in slight flexion may show a high-riding patella and tangential views can be used to measure the sulcus angle and the congruence angle.

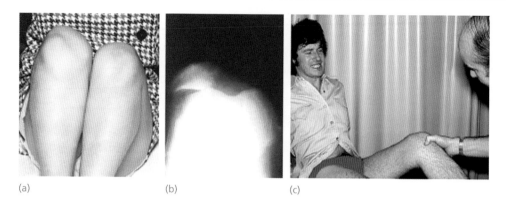

(a)   (b)   (c)

20.20 Patellofemoral instability (a,b) This young girl presented with recurrent subluxation of the right patella. The knee looks abnormal and the X-ray shows the patella riding on top of the lateral femoral condyle. **(c)** Performing the *apprehension test* – watch the patient's face.

- *MRI* is helpful and may show signs of the previous patellofemoral soft-tissue disruption on the medial side of the knee or trochlear dysplasia.

Treatment

If the patella is still dislocated, it is pushed back into place while the knee is gently extended.

INDICATIONS FOR IMMEDIATE SURGERY

Inability to reduce the patella (e.g. with a rare 'intra-articular' dislocation)
The presence of a large, displaced osteo-chondral fragment

Usually, a *knee brace* is applied and retained for 2–3 weeks to allow the soft tissues to heal; isometric quadriceps-strengthening exercises are encouraged and the patient is allowed to walk with the aid of crutches. *Exercises* are continued for at least 3 months, concentrating on strengthening vastus medialis. If recurrences are few and far between, conservative treatment may suffice; as the child grows older the patellar mechanism tends to stabilize.

About 15% of children with patellar instability suffer repeated and distressing episodes of dislocation, and for these patients surgical reconstruction is indicated. Several methods are employed (**20.21**).

PRINCIPLES OF OPERATIVE TREATMENT FOR DISLOCATION OF THE PATELLA

To repair or strengthen the medial patellofemoral ligaments
To realign the extensor mechanism so as to produce a mechanically more favourable angle of pull

---

PATELLOFEMORAL PAIN SYNDROME (CHONDROMALACIA OF THE PATELLA; PATELLOFEMORAL OVERLOAD SYNDROME)

There is no clear consensus concerning the terminology, aetiology and treatment of pain and tenderness in the anterior part of the knee. It is common among active adolescents and young adults. It is often associated with softening and fibrillation of the articular surface of the patella – *chondromalacia patellae*. Orthopaedic surgeons have tended to regard chondromalacia as the cause (rather than one of the effects) of the disorder, but chondromalacia is commonly found in those with no anterior knee pain and some patients with the typical clinical syndrome have no cartilage softening.

Pain over the anterior aspect of the knee occurs as one of the symptoms in a number of well-recognized disorders.

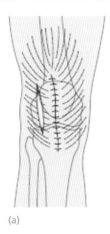
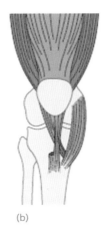
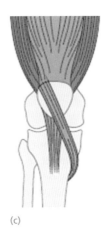
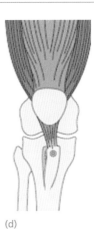

(a)   (b)   (c)   (d)

20.21 Patellar instability – operative treatment Several methods are employed. **(a)** Lateral release and vastus medialis tethering. **(b)** Transposition of lateral half of patellar ligament towards the medial side (Roux–Goldthwait). **(c)** Medial tethering by using semi-tendinosus tendon. **(d)** Medial transposition of patellar ligament insertion (Elmslie–Trillat).

CAUSES OF ANTERIOR KNEE PAIN

Referred from hip

Patellofemoral disorders

Patellar instability
Patellofemoral overload
Osteochondral injury
Patellofemoral OA

Knee joint disorders

Osteochondritis dissecans
Loose body in the joint
Synovial chondromatosis
Plica syndrome

Periarticular disorders

Patellar tendinitis
Patellar ligament strain
Bursitis
Osgood–Schlatter disease

When these are excluded and no other cause can be found, one is left with a clinically recognizable syndrome that has earned the unsatisfactory label of 'anterior knee pain' or 'patellofemoral pain syndrome'. The basic disorder is probably *mechanical overload*. Rarely, a single injury may damage the articular surfaces. Much more common is damage caused by *repetitive overload*.

POSSIBLE CAUSES OF REPETITIVE OVERLOAD

Malcongruence
Malalignment of the lower extremity and/
  or the patella
Muscular imbalance of the lower
  extremity
Overactivity

'Overload' means either direct stress on a load-bearing facet or sheer stresses in the depths of the articular cartilage at the boundary between high-contact and low-contact areas. This leads to changes in the articular cartilage and subchondral bone. The cartilage may look normal, while the underlying bone shows reactive vascular congestion. Alternatively, there may be obvious cartilage softening and fibrillation, with or without subarticular intraosseous hypertension.

Cartilage fibrillation usually occurs on the medial patellar facet or the median ridge, remains confined to the superficial zones and generally heals spontaneously. It is not a precursor of progressive OA in later life. Occasionally, the lateral facet is involved – Ficat's 'hyperpression zone' syndrome – and this may be progressive.

Clinical features

The patient, often a teenage girl or an athletic young adult, complains of pain over the front of the knee or 'under the knee-cap'. Often both knees are affected. Symptoms are aggravated by activity or climbing stairs, or when standing up after prolonged sitting.

At first sight, the knee looks normal, but careful examination may reveal malalignment or tilting of the patella. The quadriceps may be wasted and there may be a small effusion. Patellofemoral pain is elicited by pressing the patella against the femur and asking the patient to contract the quadriceps – first with central pressure, then compressing the medial facet and then the lateral. If, in addition, the apprehension test is positive, this suggests actual previous subluxation or dislocation. Patellar tracking, height and the quadriceps angle are assessed.

Imaging

- *X-ray* examination should include:
  - *skyline views* of the patella, which may show abnormal tilting or subluxation
  - *lateral view* with the knee partly flexed to see if the patella is riding high or is unusually small.
- The most accurate way of showing and measuring patellofemoral malposition is by *CT* or *MRI*, with the knees in full extension and varying degrees of flexion.

Arthroscopy

The findings at arthroscopy are usually of mild fibrillation and softening of the articular cartilage on the undersurface of the patella. Arthroscopy is also useful in excluding other possible causes of anterior knee pain (see box 'Causes of anterior knee pain', above).

Treatment

NON-OPERATIVE TREATMENT

In the vast majority of cases, the patient will be helped by adjustment of stressful activities and physiotherapy, combined with reassurance that most patients recover. Exercises are directed specifically at strengthening the medial quadriceps so as to counterbalance the tendency to lateral tilting or subluxation of the patella.

OPERATIVE TREATMENT

If symptoms persist, surgery can be considered, usually after at least 6 months of non-operative treatment.

Malalignment Extensor mechanism malalignment is treated with a realignment procedure:

- *proximal realignment* – a combined open release of the lateral retinaculum and reefing of the oblique part of the vastus medialis
- *distal realignment.*

 Realignment procedures improve the tracking angle but run the risk of increasing patellofemoral contact pressures and thus aggravating the patient's symptoms.

Articular damage When articular cartilage damage is identified, *chondroplasty* can be employed, where shaving of the patellar articular surface is performed arthroscopically using a power tool. Soft and fibrillated cartilage is removed, in severe cases down to the level of subchondral bone; the hope is that it will be replaced by fibrocartilage.

Lateral facet pressure syndrome This remains one of the few indications for performing *lateral release*, where the lateral knee capsule and extensor retinaculum are divided longitudinally, either open or arthroscopically. This sometimes succeeds on its own (particularly if significant patellar tilting can be demonstrated on X-ray or MRI), but more often patellofemoral realignment will be needed as well.

Tubercle

- In *Maquet's tibial tubercle advancement operation* the tubercle, with the attached patellar ligament, is hinged forwards and held there with a bone-block. This has the effect of reducing patellofemoral contact pressures. Some patients resent the bump on the front part of the tibia and the operation may substitute a new set of complaints for the old.

- Alternatively, the *Fulkerson anteromedial tibial tubercle transfer and elevation* can be used with satisfactory mid-term results.

These operations are now performed infrequently.

TIBIAL TUBERCLE 'APOPHYSITIS'

This condition (also called *Osgood–Schlatter disease*) is characterized by pain and swelling of the tibial tubercle. It is a fairly common complaint among adolescents, particularly those engaged in strenuous sports. It is, in fact, a traction injury of the incompletely fused apophysis into which part the patellar ligament is inserted.

On examination, the tibial tuberosity is unusually prominent and tender. Sometimes, active extension of the knee against resistance is also painful. *X-rays* show displacement or 'fragmentation' of the tibial apophysis (**20.22**). Spontaneous recovery is usual, but it takes time. During this period, activities such as football, cycling, strenuous walking and hill-climbing should be restricted.

PATELLAR TENDINOPATHY

A patellar ligament strain or partial rupture may lead to a traction 'tendinitis' causing repeated episodes of pain and local tenderness – usually close to its attachment at the lower pole of the patella. If persistent, it may lead to calcification within the ligament. The condition is fairly common in adolescent athletes and has acquired the eponym *Sinding-Larsen–Johansson syndrome*. It usually resolves spontaneously; if it does not, the painful area is carefully removed keeping the major part of the ligament in continuity.

OSTEOCHONDRITIS DISSECANS

The prevalence of osteochondritis dissecans (OCD) is between 15 and 30 per 100 000 with a male to female ratio of 5:3. An increase in its incidence has been observed in recent years, probably due to the growing participation of young children of both genders in competitive sports.

An area of subchondral bone becomes avascular and an osteocartilaginous segment becomes demarcated.

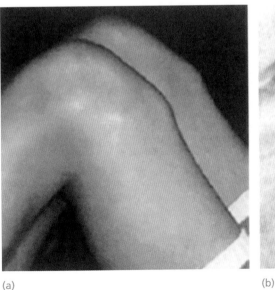

(a)

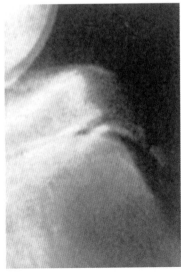

(b)

20.22 Osgood–Schlatter disease This boy complained of a painful bump below the knee **(a)**. **(b)** X-ray shows the traction injury of the tibial apophysis.

PROGRESSION OF OCD

1. At first, the overlying cartilage is intact and the fragment is stable.
2. Over a period of months, the fragment separates but remains in position ('OCD lesion *in situ*').
3. Finally, the fragment breaks free to become a loose body in the joint. The small crater is slowly filled with fibro-cartilage, leaving a depression on the articular surface.

The most likely cause is trauma. Over 80% of lesions occur on the lateral part of the medial femoral condyle and lesions are bilateral in 25% of cases.

Clinical features

The patient, usually a male aged 15–20 years, presents with intermittent ache or swelling. Later, there are attacks of giving way and the knee feels unreliable. From time to time, the knee may 'lock'.

The quadriceps muscle is wasted and there may be a small effusion. Two signs are almost diagnostic.

DIAGNOSTIC SIGNS OF OCD

Tenderness localized to one femoral condyle

Wilson's sign: if the knee is flexed to 90°, rotated medially and then gradually straightened, pain is felt; if the test is repeated with the knee rotated laterally, the patient feels no pain.

Imaging

- *Plain X-rays*, especially intercondylar (tunnel) views, may show a line of demarcation around a lesion, usually in the lateral part of the medial femoral condyle (**20.23**). Once the fragment has become detached, the empty hollow may be seen, as may a loose body elsewhere in the joint.
- *Radionuclide scans* show increased activity around the lesion, and *MRI* consistently shows an area of low signal intensity in the T1-weighted

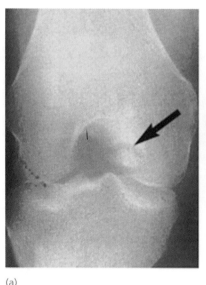
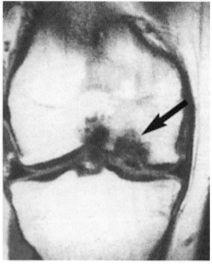

(a)   (b)

20.23 Osteochondritis dissecans – imaging The lesion is best seen in the 'tunnel view', usually along the lateral side of the medial femoral condyle **(a)**. Here, the osteochondral fragment has remained in place, but sometimes it appears as a separate body elsewhere in the joint. **(b)** MRI provides confirmatory evidence.

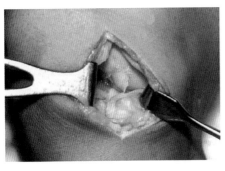

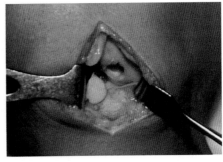

(a)

(b)

20.24 Osteochondritis dissecans Intraoperative pictures showing the articular lesion **(a)** and the defect left after removal of the osteochondral fragment **(b)**.

images. These investigations usually indicate whether the fragment is 'stable' or 'loose', based on the presence of fluid under the lesion.

Treatment

In the earliest stage, when the cartilage is intact and the lesion 'stable', no treatment is needed, but impact activities are curtailed for 6–12 months. Small lesions often heal spontaneously, but those in adults are more likely to be unstable.

If the fragment is 'unstable' – i.e. surrounded by a clear boundary with sclerosis of the underlying bone, or showing MRI features of separation, or even detached – treatment will depend on the size of the lesion. A small fragment can be removed by arthroscopy and the base drilled; the bed will eventually be covered by fibrocartilage. A large fragment (more than 1 cm in diameter, **20.24**) can be fixed *in situ* with pins or Herbert screws. In older patients, removal of the unstable fragment and cartilage repair techniques (e.g. microfracture or autologous cartilage implantation (ACI) are carried out.

LOOSE BODIES

CAUSES OF LOOSE BODIES
Injury
OCD
OA

Charcot's disease (large osteocartilaginous bodies)
Synovial chondromatosis

Clinical features

Loose bodies may be asymptomatic, but may cause sudden locking without injury. Sometimes the locking is only momentary and usually the patient can wriggle the knee until it suddenly unlocks. Sometimes, especially after the first attack, there is an effusion, due to synovitis. A pedunculated loose body may be felt; one that is truly loose tends to slip away during palpation (aptly named a 'joint mouse') (**20.25**). *X-rays* will usually confirm the diagnosis; most loose bodies are radio-opaque and the examination also shows an underlying joint abnormality.

A loose body causing symptoms should be removed, unless the joint is severely osteoarthritic. This can usually be done with the aid of arthroscopy.

SYNOVIAL CHONDROMATOSIS

This is a rare disorder resulting in multiple loose bodies, often in pearly clumps. Myriad tiny fronds undergo cartilage metaplasia at their tips; these tips break free and may ossify. It has, however, been suggested that chondrocytes may be cultured in the synovial fluid and that some of

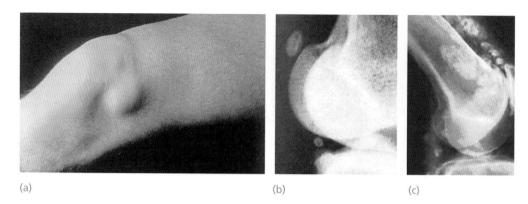

(a)

(b)

(c)

20.25 Loose bodies (a) This loose body slipped away from the fingers when touched; the term 'joint mouse' seems appropriate. **(b)** Which is the loose body here? Not the large one (which is a normal fabella), but the small lower one opposite the joint line. **(c)** Multiple loose bodies are seen in synovial chrondromatosis, a rare disorder of cartilage metaplasia in the synovium.

the products are then deposited onto previously normal synovium, so producing the familiar appearance. *X-rays* reveal multiple loose bodies; on arthrography they show as negative defects.

The loose bodies can be removed arthroscopically and a synovectomy performed.

PLICA SYNDROME

A plica is the remnant of an embryonic synovial partition. They are found in over 20% of people, usually as a *median infrapatellar fold* (the ligamentum mucosum), less often as a *suprapatellar curtain* draped across the opening of the suprapatellar pouch or a *mediopatellar plica*.

Plicas are not pathological but acute trauma or repetitive strain may cause the plica to become oedematous, thickened and eventually fibrosed. Once this occurs, it may impinge on other structures in the joint and causing synovial irritation.

Clinical features

Usually a young adult complains of an ache in the front of the knee, with intermittent episodes of clicking or 'giving way'. Symptoms are aggravated by exercise or climbing stairs. There may be muscle wasting and a small effusion. There is tenderness near the upper pole of the patella and over the femoral condyle. Occasionally, the thickened band can be felt. Movement of the knee may cause catching or snapping.

There is debate as to whether this is a real and distinct clinical entity. Distinct clinical features consistent with direct impingement of a plica should be present and a chondral lesion on the femoral condyle secondary to plica impingement at arthroscopy confirms the diagnosis.

Treatment

The first line of treatment is rest, NSAIDs and adjustment of activities. If symptoms persist, the plica can be divided or excised by arthroscopy.

TUBERCULOSIS

Tuberculosis of the knee may appear at any age, but it is more common in children than in adults.

Clinical features

Pain and limp are early symptoms, or the child may present with a swollen joint and a low-grade fever. The thigh muscles are wasted, thus accentuating the joint swelling. The knee feels warm and there is synovial thickening. Movements are restricted and often painful. The Mantoux test is often positive and the ESR may be increased.

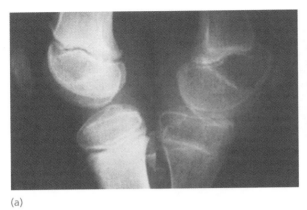
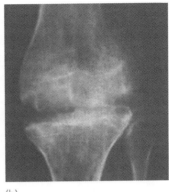

(a)   (b)

20.26 Tuberculosis – X-rays (a) Lateral views of the two knees. On one side the bones are porotic and the epiphyses enlarged, features suggestive of a severe inflammatory synovitis. (b) Later, the articular surfaces are eroded.

Imaging

Common features are periarticular osteoporosis and, in children, enlargement of the bony epiphyses. Joint space narrowing and progressive erosion of the articular surfaces are late signs (**20.26**).

Diagnosis

During the early stages the condition may resemble monoarticular rheumatoid synovitis, or juvenile chronic arthritis. A synovial biopsy may be necessary to establish the diagnosis.

Treatment

General antituberculous chemotherapy should be given for 12–18 months (see Chapter 2).

- *In the active stage* the knee is splinted. The synovitis usually subsides but may require debridement along with bone abscesses.
- *In the healing stage*, the patient is allowed up wearing a weight-relieving caliper which is gradually withdrawn. The patient is observed for any sign of recurrent inflammation. If the articular cartilage is maintained, movement is encouraged and weight-bearing slowly resumed. If the articular surface is destroyed, immobilization is continued until the joint stiffens.
- *In the aftermath*, the joint may be painful; it is then best arthrodesed, but in children this

is usually postponed until growth is almost completed. The ideal position for fusion is 10–15 degrees of flexion, 7 degrees of valgus and 5 degrees of external rotation.

In some cases, once it is certain that the disease is quiescent, joint replacement may be feasible.

RHEUMATOID ARTHRITIS

Occasionally, RA starts in the knee as a chronic monoarticular synovitis followed by polyarticular involvement.

Clinical features

- *During the early stage*, the patient complains of pain and chronic swelling. There may be a large effusion and wasting of the thigh muscles. The thickened synovium is often palpable.
- *With advancing articular erosion*, the joint becomes unstable, muscle wasting increases and there is some restriction of movement. X-rays may show loss of joint space, osteopenia and marginal erosions. There is a complete absence of osteophytes.
- *In the late stage*, the joint becomes increasingly deformed and painful; in some patients there is only a jog of painful movement. X-rays reveal the bone destruction characteristic of advanced disease (**20.27**).

SECTION 2 REGIONAL ORTHOPAEDICS

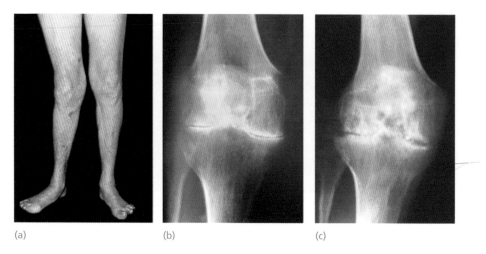

(a)　　　　　　　　　(b)　　　　　　　　　(c)

20.27 Rheumatoid arthritis **(a)** Patient with RA showing the typical valgus deformity of the knee; the feet and toes also are affected. **(b,c)** X-rays showing progressive erosive arthritis resulting in joint destruction and deformity.

Treatment

In addition to general treatment with anti-inflammatory and disease-modifying drugs, local splintage and injection of triamcinolone will usually reduce the synovitis. The introduction of anti-tumour necrosis factor (anti-TNF) medication has revolutionized the orthopaedic treatment of the condition by greatly reducing long-term joint destruction.

Synovectomy is now rarely required but can be performed arthroscopically.

Total joint replacement is useful in advanced joint destruction. However, it is less successful if the knee has been allowed to become very unstable or stiff. Care must be taken to preserve the collateral ligaments and extensor mechanism. Modification of antirheumatic drugs should be done in conjunction with a rheumatologist to minimize the risk of infection and wound issues while avoiding rheumatoid flares as much as possible.

OSTEOARTHRITIS

The knee is the commonest of the large joints to be affected by OA. There may be a predisposing factor: injury to the articular surface, a torn meniscus and ligamentous instability or pre-existing deformity of the knee but more commonly, no obvious cause can be found. There is a significant genetic predisposition. The male to female distribution is more or less equal in white (Caucasian) peoples, but black African women are affected far more frequently than men.

OA is a disease of the whole joint. Cartilage breakdown usually starts in an area of high load. Thus, with long-standing varus, the changes are most marked in the medial compartment. The characteristic features of cartilage fibrillation, sclerosis of the subchondral bone and peripheral osteophyte formation are usually present.

Clinical features

Patients are usually over 50 years old and are often overweight.

- *Pain* is the leading symptom, worse after use, or (if the patellofemoral joint is affected) on stairs.
- There is *stiffness* in the joint. After rest, the joint feels stiff and it hurts to 'get going' after sitting for any length of time.
- *Swelling* is common, and giving way or locking may occur.

On examination, there may be an obvious deformity (usually varus) or the scar of a previous operation. The earliest sign is often a fixed flexion deformity due to shortening of the posterior capsule. The quadriceps muscle is usually wasted.

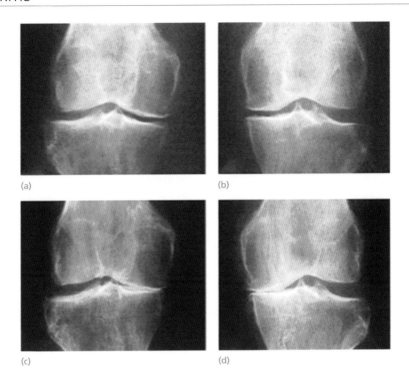

(a)　　　　　　　　　　　　　　(b)

(c)　　　　　　　　　　　　　　(d)

20.28 Knee X-rays X-rays taken with this patient lying down **(a,b)** suggest only minor cartilage loss on the medial side of each knee. Weight-bearing views **(c,d)** show the true position; there is severe loss of articular cartilage in the medial compartment of both knees.

Except during an exacerbation, there is little fluid and no warmth; nor is the synovial membrane thickened. Movement is somewhat limited and is often accompanied by patellofemoral crepitus. There is gradual deterioration of function, often with 'good days' and 'bad days'.

Imaging

 Always ask for weight-bearing X-ray views.

Standard X-rays of the knee to investigate OA include a weight-bearing anteroposterior view to demonstrate joint space narrowing, and a lateral view. Typically, the tibiofemoral joint space is diminished (often only in one compartment) and there is subchondral sclerosis (**20.28**). Osteophytes and subchondral cysts are usually present and sometimes there is soft-tissue calcification in the suprapatellar region or in the joint itself (chondrocalcinosis).

Treatment

CONSERVATIVE TREATMENT

If symptoms are not severe, treatment is conservative. Analgesics can be prescribed for pain. Local measures include quadriceps exercises and the application of warmth (e.g. radiant heat or shortwave diathermy). Joint loading is lessened by using a walking stick or using an off-loader brace. Intra-articular corticosteroid injections will often relieve pain and can be used repeatedly.

OPERATIVE TREATMENT

INDICATIONS FOR OPERATIVE TREATMENT OF OA
Persistent pain unresponsive to conservative treatment
Progressive deformity
Progressive instability

SECTION 2 REGIONAL ORTHOPAEDICS

Arthroscopic washouts are not effective in the treatment of OA.

Realignment osteotomy Typically an upper tibial valgus osteotomy for medial compartment disease in a young patient, this is often successful in relieving symptoms and staving off the need for 'end-stage' surgery.

Replacement arthroplasty This is indicated in patients with bone-on-bone OA changes within the knee who describe moderate to severe symptoms that have not been responsive to at least 3 months of non-operative measures. Total knee replacement (the most commonly used) is effectively a 'resurfacing' procedure; with modern techniques and meticulous attention to anatomical alignment of the knee, the results are excellent. If the disease is confined to one compartment, a unicompartmental replacement can be performed as an alternative to osteotomy or total joint replacement. The ACL must be intact for this approach.

Arthrodesis This is indicated only if there is a strong contraindication to arthroplasty (e.g. previous infection) or to salvage a failed arthroplasty.

OSTEONECROSIS

The usual site of knee osteonecrosis is the dome of one of the femoral condyles. Two main categories are identified.

- *Osteonecrosis associated with a definite background disorder.* Examples include:
  - corticosteroid therapy
  - alcohol abuse
  - sickle-cell disease
  - hyperbaric decompression sickness
  - systemic lupus erythematosus (SLE)
  - Gaucher's disease.
- *'Spontaneous' osteonecrosis* of the knee, popularly known by the acronym SONK. This is due to a small insufficiency fracture of a prominent part of the osteoarticular surface in osteoporotic bone; the vascular supply to the free fragment is compromised.

Clinical features

Patients are usually over 60 years old and women are affected three times more often than men.

There is sudden, acute pain on the medial side of the joint. Pain at rest also is common.

On examination, there is a small effusion, with tenderness on pressure upon the medial femoral or tibial condyle rather than along the joint line.

Imaging

- *X-ray* appearances are initially unimpressive, but a radionuclide scan may show increased activity. Later the classic radiographic features of osteonecrosis appear (see Chapter 6).
- *MRI* shows bone marrow and allows differentiation between necrotic and viable areas with a high level of specificity. It shows the area of reactive bone surrounding the osteonecrotic lesion and can demonstrate the integrity of the overlying cortical shell of bone and articular cartilage. Sequential MRI scans are helpful in determining the clinical course.

Prognosis

Symptoms and signs may stabilize and the patient may be left with no more than slight distortion of the articular surface; or one of the condyles may collapse, leading to OA. Lesions that are >40% of the condyle carry a worse prognosis.

Treatment

Treatment is conservative in the first instance and consists of measures to reduce loading of the joint and analgesics for pain. If symptoms or signs increase, operative treatment may be considered. Bisphosphonates may encourage healing.

SURGICAL OPTIONS FOR OSTEONECROSIS
Drilling
Bone grafting
Core decompression of the femoral condyle at a distance from the lesion
Osteotomy for patients with persistent symptoms and well-marked articular surface damage
Joint replacement if the femoral condyle collapses

The ankle and foot $\quad$ 21

- Clinical assessment — 453
- Congenital abnormalities — 457
- Pes planus and pes valgus (flat foot) — 462
- Pes cavus (high-arched foot) — 465
- Hallux valgus — 467
- Hallux rigidus — 470
- Deformities of the lesser toes — 471
- Tuberculous arthritis — 472
- Rheumatoid arthritis — 472
- Seronegative arthropathies — 473
- Gout — 474
- Ankle osteoarthritis — 474
- The diabetic foot — 475
- Disorders of the tendo Achillis — 476
- The painful ankle — 477
- The painful foot — 478
- Toenail disorders — 480
- Skin lesions — 480

CLINICAL ASSESSMENT

HISTORY

The most common presenting symptoms are pain, deformity, swelling and impaired function. It is helpful to know whether the symptoms are constant or provoked by standing or walking, or by shoe pressure.

- *Pain* over a bony prominence or a joint is probably due to a local disorder. Pain across the entire forefoot (*metatarsalgia*) is less specific and is often associated with uneven loading and muscle fatigue. Often the main complaint is of shoe pressure on a tender corn over a joint or a callosity.
  - Osteoarthritic pain at the first metatarsophalangeal (MTP) joint is often better in firm-soled shoes.
  - Hallux valgus/bunions will be exacerbated by close-fitting shoes.
  - A functionally or mechanically unstable ankle often feels better in boots.
  - Metatarsalgia is worse in shoes with a higher heel.
  - Morton's neuroma or a prominent metatarsal head feels like a marble or pebble in the shoe.

Always ask whether the pain started after some unusual activity; metatarsal stress fractures occur even in physically fit athletes, ballet dancers and soldiers on route marches.

- *Deformity* may be in the ankle, the foot or the toes. Parents often worry about their children who are 'flat-footed' or 'pigeon-toed'. Elderly patients may complain chiefly of having difficulty fitting shoes.
- *Instability* of the ankle or subtalar joint produces repeated episodes of the joint 'giving way'. Ask about any previous injury (e.g. a 'twisted ankle').
- *Corns and callosities* (thickened, often tender, plaques of skin on the toes or the soles of the

feet) are a frequent cause for complaints. They are usually produced by localized pressure and friction.

• *Numbness and paraesthesia* may be felt in a circumscribed field served by a single nerve, or more generally in all the toes and both feet, suggesting a peripheral neuropathy.

Signs with the patient standing and walking

Ask the patient's to expose their lower limbs from the knees down and examine them first from the front and then from behind (21.1). The heels are normally in slight valgus while standing and inverted when on tiptoes; the degree of diversion should be equal on the two sides, showing that the subtalar joints are mobile and the tibialis posterior muscles are functioning.

Deformities such as flat foot, cavus (high-arched) foot, hallux valgus and crooked toes are noted. Corns over the proximal toe joints and callosities on the soles are common in older people.

Ask the patient to walk. Note whether the gait is smooth or halting and whether the feet move through the walking cycle symmetrically. Concentrate on the sequence of movements that make up the walking cycle. It begins with heel-strike, then moves into stance, then push-off and finally swing-through before making the next heel-strike. Gait may be disturbed by pain, muscle weakness, deformity or stiffness. A fixed equinus deformity results in the heel failing to

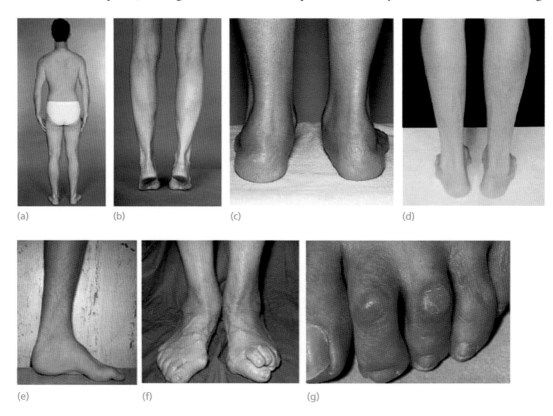

(a)   (b)   (c)   (d)

(e)   (f)   (g)

21.1 Examination with the patient standing Look at the patient as a whole, first from in front and then from behind. **(a,b)** The heels are normally in slight valgus and should invert equally when a patient stands on tiptoes. **(c)** This patient has flat feet (pes planovalgus), while the patient in **(d)** has the opposite deformity, varus heels and an abnormally high longitudinal arch – pes cavus **(e)**. From the front you can again notice **(f)** the dropped longitudinal arch in the patient with pes planovalgus, as well as the typical deformities of bilateral hallux valgus and over-riding toes. **(g)** Corns on the top of the toes are common.

strike the ground at the beginning of the walking cycle; sometimes the patient forces heel contact by hyperextending the knee. If the ankle dorsiflexors are weak, the forefoot may strike the ground prematurely, causing a 'slap'; this is called foot drop (or drop foot). In some cases, during swing-through the leg is lifted higher than usual so that the foot can clear the ground; this is known as a high-stepping gait.

SIGNS WITH THE PATIENT SITTING OR LYING

Each foot is examined in turn, so that the findings can be compared (21.2, 21.3).

Look

Holding the heel square, inspect the dorsum, sides and plantar aspects of the foot. Callosities (on the plantar aspect) or corns (on the dorsum) indicate where there is high pressure or friction. Look for swelling over joints or tendon sheaths. Atrophic changes in the skin and toenails are suggestive of a neurological disorder, vascular disorder or fungal infection.

Feel

Pain and tenderness localize well to the affected structures because the foot and ankle are not shielded by thick muscle layers. Feel along the bony prominences, joint lines and tendon sheaths. Feel also for pulses (about one in six individuals does not have a dorsalis pedis pulse) and check the sensation and skin temperature.

Move

Check each joint in turn for both active and passive movements. Muscle power can be tested at the same time.

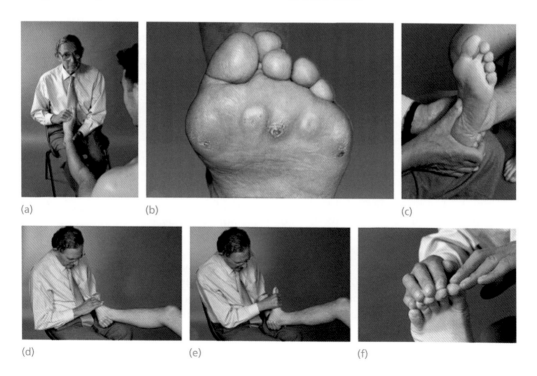

(a) (b) (c)

(d) (e) (f)

21.2 Examination with the patient sitting (a) The patient is seated with their foot on the examiner's lap. Keep an eye on the patient's face as well as the foot. **(b)** Look for skin lesions and deformities, especially of the toes; don't forget the sole where callosities go together with toe deformities. **(c)** Feel for tenderness over every joint and along the tendons and ligaments. Then test for movements in the ankle and the toes **(d–f)**.

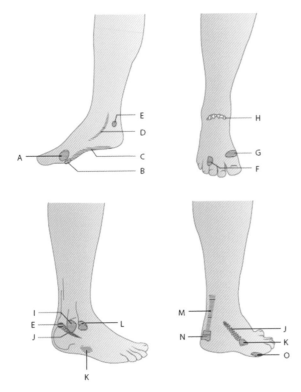

21.3 Where does it hurt? Where is it tender?

A Medial to first MTP joint – bunion
B Beneath first MTP joint – sesamoiditis
C Plantar fascia – plantar fasciitis
D Posterior to medial malleolus/line of tibialis posterior – tibialis posterior tendinitis or tear, and in planovalgus collapse of hindfoot
E Retrocalcaneal bursa – bursitis
F In third interspace – Morton's neuroma
G Dorsal to first MTP joint – osteoarthritis, hallux limitus/rigidus
H Anterior ankle joint line – impingement from osteophytes in osteoarthritis
I Bony tip/lateral malleolus – ankle fracture (Ottawa guidelines)
J Posterior/inferior to lateral malleolus – peroneal tenosynovitis or tear
K Base of fifth metatarsal – fracture or insertional problem with peroneus brevis
L Anterolateral angle of ankle joint – lateral gutter impingement in post-traumatic ankle with soft-tissue problems
M Achilles tendon – Achilles tendinitis/paratendinitis
N Achilles insertion – insertional tendinitis
O Beneath metatarsal heads – 'metatarsalgia'

Ankle joint With the heel grasped in the left hand and the midfoot in the right, the ranges of plantarflexion and dorsiflexion can be estimated.

Subtalar joint When assessing inversion and eversion, make sure that the ankle is fully plantigrade (at a right-angle to the leg); this prevents movement occurring at the ankle.

Midtarsal joint The heel is held still with one hand while the other moves the tarsus up and down and from side to side.

Toes The MTP and interphalangeal (IP) joints are tested separately. Extension (dorsiflexion) of the great toe at the MTP joint should normally exceed 70 degrees and flexion 10 degrees.

Tests for stability

Ankle stability should be tested in both coronal and sagittal planes, always comparing the two sides. The ankle is held in 10 degrees of plantarflexion and the joint stressed into valgus and then

varus. Anteroposterior (AP) stability is assessed by performing an anterior '*drawer test*'.

> **DRAWER TEST FOR AP STABILITY OF THE ANKLE**
>
> With the ankle held in 10 degrees of plantarflexion, grip the distal tibia with one hand and, with the other hand, grasp the heel and try to shift the hindfoot forwards and backwards.

Patients with recent ligament injury may have to be examined under anaesthesia. The same tests can be performed under X-ray and the positions of the two ankles measured and compared (see below under 'Imaging').

GENERAL EXAMINATION

If there are any symptoms or signs of vascular or neurological impairment, or if multiple joints are affected, a more general examination is essential.

IMAGING

- In the adult, the *standard X-ray* views of the ankle are AP, mortise (an AP view with the ankle internally rotated 15–20 degrees) and lateral. Medial and lateral oblique projections allow better assessment of the subtalar joint. The calcaneum is usually X-rayed in axial and lateral views. X-ray under load, weight-bearing, is helpful in showing the coronal relationship of heel to tibia in stance. The foot, toes and intertarsal joints are well displayed in standing dorsoplantar and lateral views.
- *Stress X-rays* complement the clinical tests for ankle stability; if stress manoeuvres are painful, they can be carried out under general anaesthesia.
- *Computed tomography (CT) scans* are important in assessing fractures and for congenital bony coalitions. *Radio-isotope scanning* is excellent for localizing areas of abnormal blood flow or bone remodelling activity, signs that suggest the presence of covert infection.
- *Magnetic resonance imaging (MRI)* and *ultrasound* are used to demonstrate soft-tissue problems, such as tendon and ligament injuries. They can be used to diagnose joint effusions and bone infections as well.

GLOSSARY OF FOOT POSTURES

Plantigrade is the normal neutral position of the foot – i.e. when the patient stands the sole is at right angles to the leg.

Talipes equinus refers to the shape of a horse's foot – i.e. the hindfoot is fixed in plantarflexion (pointing downwards).

Plantaris looks similar, but the ankle is neutral and only the forefoot is plantarflexed.

Equinovarus describes a foot that points both downwards and inwards.

Calcaneus is fixed dorsiflexion at the ankle. A dorsiflexion deformity in the midfoot produces a *rocker-bottom foot*.

The longitudinal arch forms the medial border of the foot. Even when weight-bearing, the medial border normally forms a slight arch.

The anterior or transverse arch is formed by the arrangement of the slightly splayed metatarsals in the forefoot.

Pes planovalgus (flat foot) describes a flattened longitudinal arch. A dropped metatarsal arch is called *anterior flat foot*.

Pes cavus is a foot with an excessively high arch.

Hallux valgus means lateral deviation of the big toe.

Hammer toe aptly describes a flexion deformity of the proximal IP joint of one of the lesser toes.

Claw toes denotes curled flexion of all the toes.

CONGENITAL ABNORMALITIES

TALIPES EQUINOVARUS (IDIOPATHIC CLUB FOOT)

In this deformity, the foot is curved downwards and inwards – the ankle in equinus, the heel in varus, and the forefoot adducted, flexed and supinated. The skin and soft tissues of the calf and the medial side of the foot are short and underdeveloped. If the condition is not corrected early, secondary growth changes occur in the bones and these are permanent. Even with treatment, the foot is liable to be short and the calf may remain thin.

The deformity is relatively common, with an incidence of 1–2 per 1000 births. Boys are affected twice as often as girls and it occurs bilaterally in nearly one-half of the cases. A family history increases the risk by 20–30 times.

The cause is unknown. There are theories, and some evidence in support, of a chromosomal defect, arrested development *in utero*, or an embryonic event such as a vascular injury. The abnormal distribution of types 1 and 2 muscle fibres in the affected leg and alteration of electromyography and nerve conduction velocities suggest a neuromuscular basis, but the true cause remains unknown. Club foot is occasionally associated with spina bifida or other neurological conditions, so spinal examination is mandatory. Similar deformities are seen in some infants with myelomeningocele and arthrogryposis.

Clinical features

The deformity is usually obvious at birth; the foot is both turned and twisted inwards so that the sole faces posteromedially (21.4). The main features can be remembered by the mnemonic CAVE.

CAVE: MAIN FEATURES OF CLUB FOOT	
Cavus	Plantar flexion of the medial ray of the forefoot
Adductus	Forefoot adduction deformity
Varus	Inward or varus deformity of the heel
Equinus	Fixed plantarflexion through the ankle

The clinical features have been classified by Pirani so that the severity can be assessed at birth and the progress of treatment can be monitored. The scoring system allocates 0, 0.5 or 1.0 for each of six clinical features with the foot held in the best position possible:

- medial crease
- lateral border of the foot
- lateral head of talus
- posterior crease
- empty heel
- ankle dorsiflexion.

In a normal baby, the foot can be dorsiflexed and everted until the toes almost touch the front of the leg. In club foot, this manoeuvre meets with varying degrees of resistance; in severe cases, the deformity is fixed.

The infant must always be examined for associated disorders such as congenital hip dislocation and spina bifida (21.4e).

Imaging

X-rays are used mainly to assess progress after treatment in the older child and are rarely used in initial assessment.

- The *anteroposterior film* is taken with the foot 30 degrees plantar flexed and the tube likewise angled 30 degrees perpendicular. Lines are drawn through the long axis of the talus parallel to its medial border and through that of the calcaneum parallel to its lateral border; they normally cross at an angle of 20–40 degrees (*Kite's angle*) but in club foot the two lines may be almost parallel.
- The *lateral film* is taken with the foot in forced dorsiflexion. Lines drawn through the mid-longitudinal axis of the talus and the lower border of the calcaneum should meet at an angle of about 40 degrees.

Treatment

The aim of treatment is to produce and maintain a plantigrade, supple foot that will function well. Treatment should begin early, preferably within a few days of birth.

PONSETI TECHNIQUE

The *Ponseti technique* is the international standard of care with a >90% success rate. It consists of careful manipulation of the foot with serial application of above-knee plaster of Paris casts to maintain the correction. This didactic technique typically requires four or five casts in the infant to correct the forefoot and midfoot deformity (21.5). Residual equinus at this stage is corrected by a percutaneous Achilles tenotomy, often performed in the outpatient clinic under local anaesthetic. After correction has been achieved, the child is placed in a foot abduction brace (FAB), initially full-time for 3 months and then during nap times and at night until they are 4 years old. Compliance is essential to minimize the risk of recurrence. If recurrence occurs in the older child, manipulation and casting are resumed and a tibialis anterior tendon transfer (to the lateral cuneiform) is performed. Relapse is most likely to occur in children with neuromuscular disorders.

OPERATIVE TREATMENT

Resistant cases may need surgery to achieve correction. This is now largely restricted to the syndromic club foot (e.g. secondary to arthrogryposis

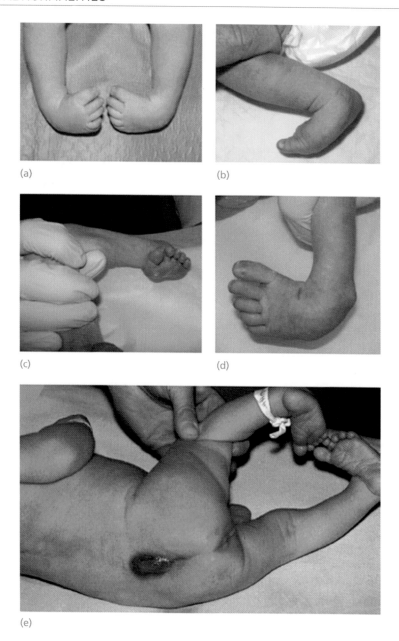

(a)

(b)

(c)

(d)

(e)

21.4 Talipes equinovarus (club foot) (a) True club foot is a fixed deformity, unlike **(b)** postural talipes, which is easily correctable by gentle passive movement. **(c,d)** With true club foot, the poorly developed heel is higher than the forefoot, which points downwards and inwards (varus). **(e)** Always examine the hips for congenital dislocation and the back for spina bifida (as in the case shown here).

and spina bifida). Ponseti management is still the preferred treatment but recalcitrant cases may require a posteromedial release (PMR). This involves a surgical release of the affected joints (talonavicular, calcaneocuboid and subtalar) and

certain ligaments, as well as lengthening of the long toe flexors and tibialis posterior.

After operative correction, the foot is immobilized in its corrected position in a plaster cast. Kirschner wires (K-wires) are sometimes inserted

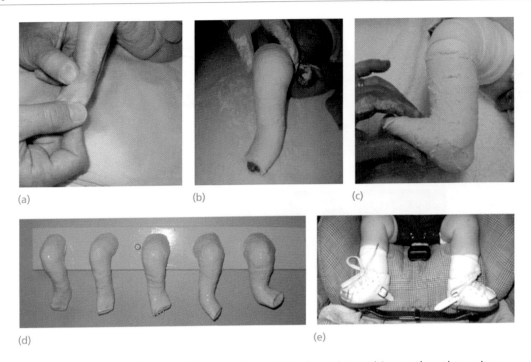

(a)   (b)   (c)

(d)   (e)

21.5 Congenital talipes equinovarus Treatment consists of serial stretching and casting using Ponseti's method. **(a)** The fulcrum of correction is rotation around the lateral talar head. **(b)** A plaster cast is applied to hold the position achieved by stretching until **(c)** at least 15° of dorsiflexion are achievable at the ankle. About 80% of feet will need a percutaneous Achilles tenotomy to achieve the corrected position. **(d)** A series of plaster casts showing the gradual correction from cast to cast. **(e)** To maintain the corrected position, boots on a bar (FAB) are worn full-time for 3 months and then only at nap times and at night until the fourth birthday.

across the talonavicular and subtalar joints to maintain the position. The wires and cast are removed at 6–8 weeks, after which a customized orthosis is used to maintain the correction.

In some older children who have had a severe, stiff recurrence of the deformity, or who have presented late, the Ilizarov technique may be used. This involves the use of tensioned wires mounted on rings that permit gradual repositioning of the foot and ankle.

Late presenters often have severe deformities with secondary bony changes (**21.6**), and the relapsed club foot is further complicated by scarring from previous surgery. A deformed, stiff and

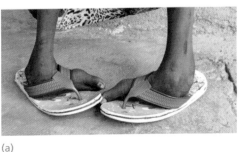
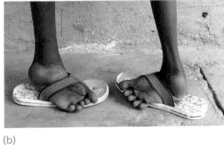

(a)   (b)

21.6 Talipes equinovarus (a,b) Bilateral untreated club foot in a 17-year-old female patient.

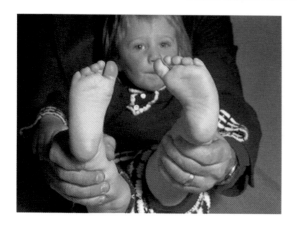

21.7 Metatarsus adductus In contrast to club foot, the deformity here is limited to the forefoot.

painful foot in an adolescent is best salvaged by corrective osteotomies and fusions. The mainstay of this is the 'triple arthrodesis' where correction is achieved through excising and fusing the talonavicular, calcaneocuboid and subtalar joints.

METATARSUS ADDUCTUS

Metatarsus adductus varies from a slightly curved forefoot to something resembling a mild club foot (21.7). The important difference is that, in metatarsus adductus, the deformity occurs across the tarsometatarsal joints whereas in the club foot, the adduction tends to happen at the midfoot (talonavicular joint).

The majority (90%) either improve spontaneously or can be managed non-operatively using serial corrective casts followed by straight-last shoes. Serial casts work well and may need to be supplemented, for the more resistant forms, by a release of the abductor hallucis muscle.

TALIPES CALCANEOVALGUS

Calcaneovalgus foot is a relatively common deformity with a dorsiflexed foot where the dorsum of the foot abuts the anterior border of the shin. There is a deep crease (or several wrinkles) on the front of the ankle, and the calcaneum juts out posteriorly. Unlike congenital vertical talus (which also presents as an acutely dorsiflexed foot), this deformity is flexible. It is sometimes bilateral, often corrects spontaneously or with stretching and rarely needing serial casting.

Posteromedial bowing of the tibia is associated with a calcaneovalgus foot (21.8). The foot also abuts the anterior shin and the distal tibia deformity can be seen clinically as well as on plain X-rays. This condition is usually unilateral and is associated with an initial leg length discrepancy of 1–2 cm that can become up to 5 cm at maturity. The posteromedial tibial bow typically remodels spontaneously over the first few years of life but some patients will require intervention closer to maturity to equalise the leg length discrepancy.

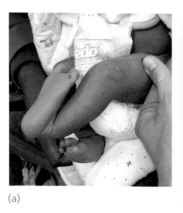
(a)

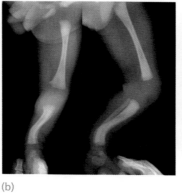
(b)

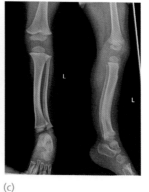
(c)

21.8 Talipes calcaneovalgus (a) Posteromedial bow of the tibia associated with a calcaneovalgus foot deformity; **(b)** X-ray at 2 months of age; **(c)** X-ray at 3 years of age showing how the deformity is remodelling.

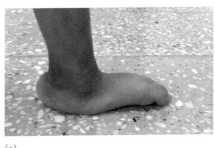
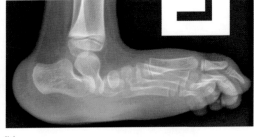

(a)   (b)

21.9 Congenital vertical talus in a 3-year-old child with myelomeningocele Note the rockerbottom deformity of the sole of the foot **(a)**. **(b)** The X-ray demonstrates a vertically orientated talus with dorsal dislocation of the navicular.

CONGENITAL VERTICAL TALUS

This rare congenital condition causes a rigid flat foot due to an irreducible dorsal dislocation of the talonavicular joint. It is usually unilateral. The hindfoot is in fixed equinus, the talus is vertically orientated and the dorsally dislocated navicular results in a rockerbottom deformity **(21.9)**. Passive correction is impossible. Around 50% of cases are associated with neuromuscular conditions such as spina bifida and arthrogryposis.

Management starts with serial casting using a so-called 'reverse Ponseti' technique followed by open reduction and stabilization of the talonavicular joint with a K-wire, together with an Achilles tenotomy.

MACRO- AND POLYDACTYLY OF THE FOOT

Polydactyly, a condition in which there are more than five toes on the foot, is the most common congenital anomaly of the forefoot **(21.10a,b)**. In *macrodactyly*, one or more toes are abnormally enlarged. Operative resection may be required if there are functional limitations in these cases **(21.10c,d)**.

PES PLANUS AND PES VALGUS (FLAT FOOT)

The term 'flat foot' applies when the apex of the longitudinal arch has collapsed and the medial

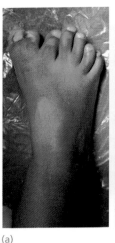
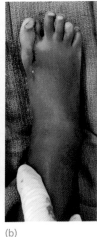
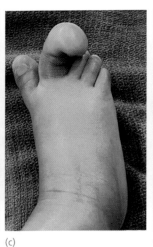
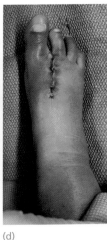

(a)   (b)   (c)   (d)

21.10 Other congenital foot conditions (a) Polydactyly of the foot with **(b)** postoperative image following resection of the second and third toes. **(c)** Macrodactyly of the second ray with **(d)** the postoperative appearance following ray resection.

border of the foot is in contact (or nearly in contact) with the ground; the heel becomes valgus and the foot pronates at the midfoot. The appearance of flat foot can be normal and without symptoms (the arch is not formed until 4–6 years of age and about 15% of the population have supple asymptomatic flat feet) but some conditions are characterized by flat feet that are stiff and painful.

FLAT FOOT IN CHILDREN AND ADOLESCENTS

Flat foot is a common complaint among children and teenagers, or rather their parents – the children themselves usually don't seem to mind!

Two forms of the condition are encountered: flexible (by far the more common) and rigid.

- *Mobile (or 'flexible') flat foot* often appears in toddlers as a normal stage in development, and it usually disappears after a few years when medial arch development is complete.
- *Stiff (or 'rigid') flat foot* which cannot be corrected passively should alert the examiner to an underlying abnormality such as:
  - tarsal coalition (often a bar of bone connecting the calcaneum to the talus or the navicular)
  - an inflammatory joint condition
  - a neurological disorder.

Clinical features

The deformity becomes noticeable when the youngster stands. The first test is to ask them to go up on their toes: if the heels invert and the medial arches form up, it is probably a flexible (or mobile) deformity (**21.11**). This can be checked by performing the *Jack test* (*great toe extension*).

> ### JACK TEST FOR FLEXIBLE FLAT FOOT
>
> When the great toe is lifted, the medial arch should reappear while the heel adopts a more neutral position and the tibia rotates externally.

Go on to examine the foot with the child sitting or lying. Feel for localized tenderness and test the range of movement in the ankle, the subtalar and midtarsal joints. A tight Achilles tendon may induce a *compensatory flat foot* deformity.

Teenagers sometimes present with a *painful, rigid flat foot*. On examination, the peroneal and extensor tendons appear to be in spasm (which is the reason the condition is sometimes called

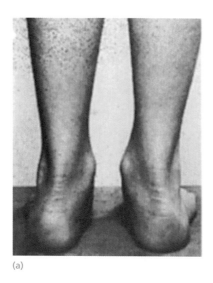
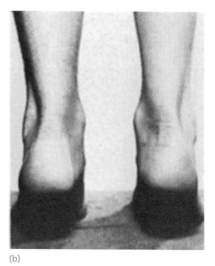

(a)   (b)

21.11 Flat foot (a) Standing with the feet flat on the floor, the medial arches are seen to have dropped and the heels are in valgus; but is it flexible or rigid? **(b)** When the patient goes up on his toes, the medial arches are restored, indicating that these are 'mobile' (flexible) flat feet. If this does not occur, look carefully for a tarsal coalition.

spasmodic flat foot). These patients should be further investigated for the presence of some underlying condition: a tarsal coalition, an inflammatory arthritis or a neuromuscular disorder. In many cases, however, no specific cause is identified.

The clinical assessment is completed by a general examination for joint hypermobility and signs of any other associated condition.

Imaging

- *X-rays* are unnecessary for asymptomatic, flexible flat feet. For painful or stiff flat feet, standing AP, lateral and oblique views may help to identify underlying disorders.
- *CT scanning* is the most reliable way of demonstrating tarsal coalitions (**21.12**).

Treatment

Children with flexible flat feet seldom require treatment; parents should be reassured and told that the 'deformity' will probably correct itself in time; even if it does not fully correct, function is unlikely to be impaired. Medial arch supports or heel cups can be tried but do not alter the growth of the foot.

If there is a tight tendo Achillis, stretching exercises help. Where the condition is obviously due to a neuromuscular disorder such as poliomyelitis, splintage or operative correction and muscle rebalancing may be needed.

Painful spasmodic flat foot can be temporarily relieved by rest in a cast or a splint. Tarsal coalitions can be excised successfully as long as they are not larger than 50% of the joint area.

FLAT FOOT IN ADULTS

When an adult presents with symptomatic flat feet (**21.13**), the first thing to ask is whether they have always had flat feet or whether it is of recent onset. Constitutional flat feet that have been more or less asymptomatic for many years may start causing nagging pain after a change in daily activities. More recent deformities may be due to an underlying disorder such as rheumatoid arthritis (RA) or generalized muscular weakness.

Where there is no underlying abnormality, little can be done apart from giving advice about sensible footwear and arch supports.

Patients with painful, rigid flat feet may require more robust splintage (and, of course, treatment for any generalized condition such as RA).

Unilateral flat foot should raise suspicion of tibialis posterior synovitis or rupture. Women in later midlife are predominantly affected. Onset is usually insidious, affecting one foot much more than the other. There may be systemic factors such as obesity, diabetes, corticosteroid medication or past surgery. Aching is felt in the line of the tendon and, as the tendon stretches out, the foot drifts into planovalgus, producing the

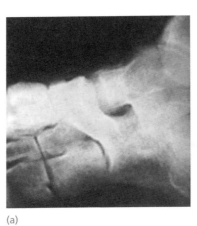
(a)

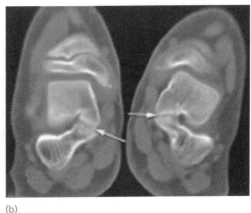
(b)

21.12 Tarsal coalition (a) X-ray appearance of a calcaneonavicular bar. (b) CT image showing incompletely ossified talocalcaneal bars bilaterally (arrows).

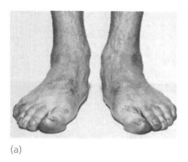
(a)

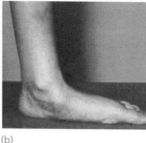
(b)

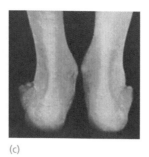
(c)

21.13 Flat foot in adults – clinical features (a) The medial arches have dropped and the feet appear to be pronated. (b) The medial border of the foot is flat and the tuberosity of the navicular looks prominent. (c) The heels are in valgus and the toes are visible lateral to the outer edge of the heel on the left side (the 'too-many-toes' sign).

typical deformity. If the tendon ruptures, the ache or pain will often improve, temporarily, but the foot deformity then worsens.

Treatment

Treatment should start before the tendon ruptures. Consider:

* rest
* anti-inflammatory medication
* support from an insole
* ultrasound-guided steroid injections into the tendon sheath.

Failure to improve may call for surgery: the tendon sheath can be decompressed and the synovium excised; the calcaneum may be osteotomized to shift the axis of weight-bearing more medially, so protecting the tendon. A ruptured tendon can sometimes be reconstructed with a tendon graft. As a last resort, a triple arthrodesis of the subtalar, talonavicular and calcaneocuboid joints may be needed to correct or prevent a worsening deformity.

PES CAVUS (HIGH-ARCHED FOOT)

In pes cavus, the foot is highly arched and the toes are drawn up into a 'clawed' position, forcing the metatarsal heads down into the sole (**21.14**). Often the heel is inverted and the soft tissues in the sole are tight. In the forefoot, under the prominent metatarsal heads, callosities may appear.

The close resemblance to deformities seen in neurological disorders, where the intrinsic muscles are weak or paralysed, suggests that all forms of pes cavus are due to some type of muscle imbalance.

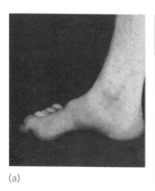
(a)

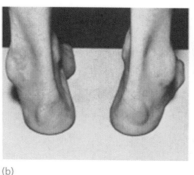
(b)

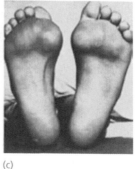
(c)

21.14 Pes cavus and claw toes (a) Typical appearance of 'idiopathic' pes cavus. Note the high arch and claw toes. (b) This is associated with varus heels. (c) Look for callosities under the metatarsal heads.

NEUROMUSCULAR CAUSES OF PES CAVUS	
Muscular dystrophies	**Cord lesions**
• Duchenne • Becker	• Poliomyelitis • Syringomyelia • Diastomatomyelia • Tethered cord
Neuropathies	**Cerebral disorders**
• HMSNI • HMSN II	• Cerebral palsy • Friedreich's ataxia

COLEMAN BLOCK TEST FOR PES CAVUS
The patient is helped to stand with the heel and lateral part of the foot resting on a 1 inch (2 cm) block and the medial part of the forefoot and great toe dipping over the edge of the block to touch the floor. If, in this position, the heel varus corrects, then mobility of the subtalar joint is demonstrated.

Clinical features

The condition often becomes noticeable by the age of 8–10 years, before there are any symptoms. As a rule, both feet are affected and, in some cases, there is a past history of a spinal disorder.

The overall deformity is usually obvious. At first, the position is mobile and the deformity can be corrected passively by pressure under the metatarsal heads; as the forefoot lifts, the toes flatten out automatically. Later, the deformities become fixed with the toes hyperextended at the MTP joints and flexed at the IP joints. Pain may then be felt under the metatarsal heads or over the toes where shoe pressure is most marked; callosities appear at the same sites. Walking tolerance is usually reduced.

The *Coleman block test* is used to check if the deformity is reversible (**21.15**).

Neurological examination is important, to identify causal disorders such as hereditary motor and sensory neuropathies and spinal cord abnormalities (tethered cord syndrome, syringomyelia). Poliomyelitis is also a significant cause in some parts of the world.

Imaging

 Weight-bearing films are essential for showing the components of foot deformities.

- *Lateral weight-bearing X-rays* of the foot will reveal the components of the high arch (**21.16**).
- *MRI scans* of the entire spine are important to rule out any structural problem in the spinal cord.

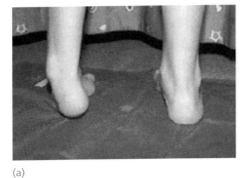 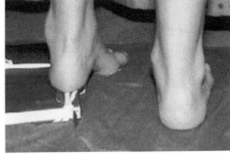

(a)   (b)

21.15 Coleman block test This simple test is used on a high-arched foot to see if the heel is flexible. **(a)** Normal stance showing the varus position of the heel. **(b)** With the patient standing on a low block to permit the depressed first metatarsal to hang free, the heel varus is automatically corrected if the subtalar joint is mobile.

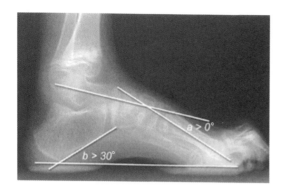

21.16 Pes cavus – weight-bearing X-rays In standing lateral views, some measurements are helpful in describing the type of high-arched foot: the axes of the talus and first metatarsal are parallel in normal feet but cross each other in a plantaris deformity (Meary's angle, *a*); the calcaneal pitch, *b*, is greater than 30° in calcaneus deformities.

Treatment

Often no treatment is required; apart from the difficulty of fitting shoes, the patient has no complaints. Patients with significant discomfort may benefit from fitting custom-made shoes with moulded supports, but this does not alter the deformity or influence its progression.

If symptoms persist and the deformities are still passively correctable, a tendon rebalancing operation may be worthwhile: the long toe flexors are released and transplanted into the extensor expansions to pull the toes straight. Unfortunately, even this may offer only temporary relief.

A painful foot with fixed deformities presents a more difficult problem. The aim of surgery is to provide a pain-free, plantigrade, supple but stable foot. This could involve release of contractures, corrective osteotomies and tendon transfers. In principle, the deformity should be corrected before tendon transfers can address the muscle imbalance around the foot.

If recurrence follows corrective surgery, arthrodesis to maintain a functional and stable foot is needed; this is usually an arthrodesis of the talonavicular, calcaneocuboid and subtalar joints – the triple arthrodesis. For the clawed toes, IP joint fusions may be necessary.

If an underlying neurological cause is identified, this must also be addressed.

HALLUX VALGUS

Hallux valgus is the commonest of the foot deformities. In people who have never worn shoes, the big toe is in line with the first metatarsal. In people who habitually wear shoes, the hallux assumes a valgus position; but only if the angulation is excessive is it referred to as 'hallux valgus' (**21.17**).

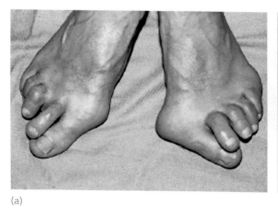
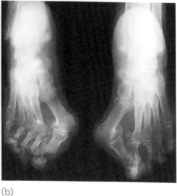

(a)   (b)

21.17 Hallux valgus This 58-year-old woman **(a)** complained of painful bunions and corns, unsightly feet and difficulties with fitting shoes. **(b)** Standing X-rays showed the abnormal first intermetatarsal angulation and the marked valgus angulation at the first MTP joint – worse in the left foot than the right.

Splaying of the forefoot, with varus angulation of the first metatarsal, predisposes to lateral angulation of the big toe in people who wear shoes. This *metatarsus primus varus* may be congenital, or it may result from loss of muscle tone in the forefoot in elderly people. Hallux valgus is also common in RA.

The elements of the deformity are lateral deviation and rotation of the hallux, together with a prominence of the medial side of the head of the first metatarsal (a *bunion*); there may also be an overlying bursa and thickened soft tissue. Lateral deviation of the hallux may lead to overcrowding of the lateral toes and sometimes over-riding.

Clinical features

Hallux valgus is most common in women between 50 and 70 years and is usually bilateral. An important subgroup, with a strong familial tendency, appears during late adolescence.

Often there are no symptoms apart from the deformity. Pain, if present, may be due to a number of causes.

CAUSES OF HALLUX VALGUS

Shoe pressure on a large or an inflamed bunion
Splaying of the forefoot and muscle strain (metatarsalgia)
Associated deformities of the lesser toes
Secondary osteoarthritis (OA) of the first MTP joint

Imaging

Standing views will show the degree of metatarsal adduction and hallux angulation. The first intermetatarsal angle is normally less than 9 degrees and the toe valgus angle at the MTP joint less than 15 degrees. Any greater degree of angulation should be regarded as abnormal. Three types of deformity can be identified (**21.18**).

TYPES OF HALLUX VALGUS DEFORMITY

Type 1 MTP joint normally centred but articular surfaces, though congruent, are tilted towards

---

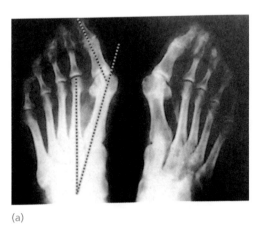

(a)

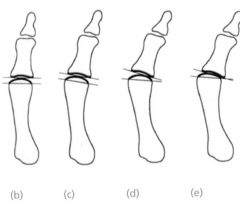

(b)   (c)   (d)   (e)

21.18 Hallux valgus – X-rays (a) The intermetatarsal angle (between the first and second metatarsals) as well as the MTP angle of the hallux are recorded. Piggott defined three types of hallux valgus, based on the position and tilt of the first MTP articular surfaces: in normal feet **(b)** the articular surfaces are parallel and centred upon each other. In congruent hallux valgus **(c)** the lines across the articular surfaces are still parallel and the joint is centred, but the articular surfaces are set more obliquely to the long axes of their respective bones. In **(d)** the deviated type of hallux valgus, the lines are not parallel and the articular surfaces are not congruent. In the subluxated type **(e)** the surfaces are neither parallel nor centred.

valgus. The joint is stable and any deformity is likely to progress very slowly or not at all.

Type 2 Articular surfaces are not congruent, the phalangeal surface being tilted towards valgus. The joint is somewhat unstable and likely to progress

Type 3 MTP joint both incongruent and slightly subluxated. The joint is even more unstable and almost certain to progress.

• *Type 1* is a stable joint and any deformity is likely to progress very slowly or not at all.
• *Type 2* is somewhat unstable and likely to progress.

• *Type 3* is even more unstable and almost certain to progress.

Treatment

ADOLESCENTS AND YOUNG ADULTS

Deformity is usually the only 'symptom', but the patient is anxious to prevent it becoming more severe and painful. Conservative treatment is justified as a first measure; operative correction (**21.19**) carries a 20–40% recurrence rate in this age group. The patient is encouraged to wear shoes with deep toe-boxes, soft uppers and low heels.

Mild deformity If the deformity is mild (less than 25 degrees at the MTP joint), it can be corrected by either a soft-tissue rebalancing operation or by a metatarsal osteotomy.

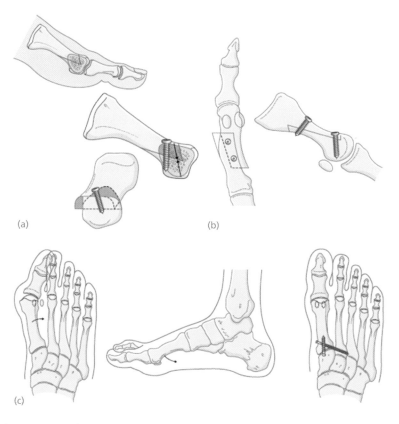

(a)   (b)

(c)

21.19 Hallux valgus – operative treatment **(a)** Distal metatarsal osteotomy – chevron; **(b)** double metatarsal osteotomy – scarf; **(c)** basal realignment and arthrodesis – Lapidus. These may be fixed in a variety of ways, and several modifications have been described.

- If the X-ray shows a *congruent* MTP articulation, the deformity is largely bony and therefore amenable to correction by a distal metatarsal osteotomy.
- If the MTP articulation is *incongruent*, the deformity is in the joint and soft-tissue realignment is indicated: tight structures on the lateral side (adductor hallucis, transverse metatarsal ligament and lateral joint capsule) are released, the prominent bone on the medial side of the metatarsal head is pared down, and the capsule on the medial side is tightened by reefing.

Moderate and severe deformities In moderate and severe deformities, the hallux valgus angle may be greater than 30 degrees and intermetatarsal angle wider than 15 degrees. If the MTP joint is *congruent*, a distal osteotomy combined with a corrective osteotomy of the base of the proximal phalanx is recommended. For greater deformities, if the joint is subluxed, a soft-tissue adjustment is needed as well as a metatarsal osteotomy to reduce the wide intermetatarsal angle.

ADULTS

Surgical treatment is more readily offered to older patients. This usually takes the form of excision of the bunion, metatarsal osteotomy and soft-tissue rebalancing. However, if the MTP joint is frankly osteoarthritic, arthrodesis of the joint may be a better option.

Hallux valgus in aged patients with limited mobility is best treated by shoe modifications. The classic Keller's operation (excision of the proximal third of the proximal phalanx, as well as the bunion prominence) has fallen into disuse because of the high rate of recurrent deformity and complications such as loss of control over great toe movement and recurrent metatarsalgia.

HALLUX RIGIDUS

'Rigidity' of the first MTP joint may be due to local trauma or osteochondritis dissecans of the first metatarsal head, but in older people it is usually caused by long-standing joint disorders such as gout, pseudogout or OA. In contrast to hallux valgus, men and women are affected with equal frequency.

Clinical features

Pain arises from the inability of the big toe to extend (dorsiflex), making push-off painful. Walking on slopes or rough ground becomes difficult. The hallux is straight and the MTP joint feels knobbly; a tender 'bunion' on the dorsum of the MTP joint (actually a large osteophyte) is characteristic (**21.20**).

X-ray changes are those of OA; the joint space is narrowed, there is bone sclerosis and, often, large osteophytes at the joint margins. In younger patients, there may be squaring of the

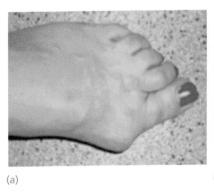
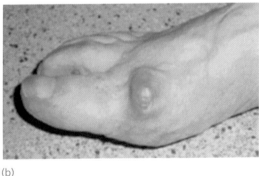

(a)   (b)

21.20 'Bunions' Compare the two types of 'bunion'. **(a)** Medial bunion in hallux valgus – what the surgeon will refer to as a bunion; **(b)** dorsal prominence of an osteophyte in hallux rigidus – what referral letters from GPs will often refer to as a bunion.

metatarsal head indicating previous osteochondritis dissecans.

Treatment

Non-steroidal anti-inflammatory drugs (NSAIDs) and intra-articular injection of corticosteroid and local anaesthetic help with intermittent symptoms. Stiff insoles that offload the first MTP joint may help but are bulky. A rocker-soled shoe may abolish pain by allowing the foot to 'roll' without the necessity for dorsiflexion at the MTP joint.

If symptoms warrant, in young patients the best procedure is a simple extension osteotomy of the proximal phalanx, to mimic dorsiflexion at the IP joint. In older patients, where the extent of the disease is limited, simply removing the osteophyte and a little of the metatarsal head dorsally (cheilectomy) might be effective and this can be combined with an extension osteotomy in the proximal phalanx to alter weight-bearing. If the joint is more arthritic, then a fusion offers a good chance of returning the patient to function and walking comfortably without a limp. Arthroplasty is controversial, often with poor long-term results.

DEFORMITIES OF THE LESSER TOES

Common deformities of the lesser digits are hammer toe, claw toe, mallet toe and overlapping toe (21.21).

HAMMER TOE

'Hammer toe' is an isolated flexion deformity of the proximal IP joint of one of the lesser toes, usually the second or third. The distal IP joint and the MTP joint are pulled into hyperextension. Shoe pressure may produce a painful corn on the dorsally projecting proximal IP.

Operative correction is indicated for pain or for difficulty with shoes. The toe is shortened and straightened by excising the proximal interphalangeal (PIP) joint and performing a fusion.

CLAW TOE

The IP joints are flexed and the MTP joints hyperextended. This is an 'intrinsic-minus' deformity that is seen in neurological disorders (e.g. peroneal muscular atrophy, poliomyelitis and peripheral neuropathies) and in RA. Usually, however, no cause is found. The condition may also be associated with pes cavus.

Clinical features

The patient complains of pain in the forefoot and under the metatarsal heads. The condition is usually bilateral and walking may be severely restricted.

At first, the joints are mobile and can be passively corrected; later, the deformities become fixed and the MTP joints subluxed or dislocated. Painful corns and callosities develop and, in the most severe cases, the skin ulcerates at the pressure sites.

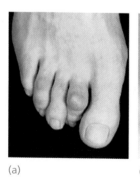
(a)

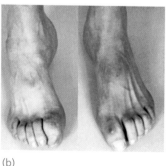
(b)

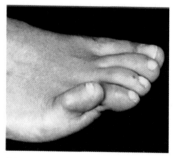
(c)

21.21 Disorders of the lesser toes (a) Hammer-toe deformity; (b) claw toes (weakness of the intrinsic muscles and cavus feet); (c) overlapping fifth toe.

Treatment

So long as the toes can be passively straightened, the patient may obtain relief by wearing a metatarsal support. A daily programme of intrinsic muscle exercises is important. If this fails to relieve discomfort, 'dynamic' correction is achieved by transferring the long toe flexors to the extensors which removes a powerful IP flexor and converts it to a MTP flexor and IP extensor.

When the deformity is fixed, it may either be accepted and accommodated by special footwear, or treated by IP arthrodesis (with or without extensor hallucis longus transfer), joint excision or amputation.

MALLET TOE

The distal IP joint is flexed. The toenail or the tip of the toe presses into the shoe, resulting in a painful callosity. If conservative treatment (chiropody and padding) does not help, the distal IP joint is exposed, the articular surfaces excised and the toe straightened; flexor tenotomy may be needed. A thin K-wire is inserted across the joint and left in position for 6 weeks to hold the joint until fusion is achieved.

OVERLAPPING TOE

This is a common congenital anomaly. If symptoms warrant, the toe may be straightened by a dorsal V/Y-plasty, reinforced by transferring the flexor to the extensor tendon. Tight dorsal and medial structures may have to be released. The toe is held in the overcorrected position with tape or K-wire for 6 weeks. Severe deformities or relapses may need a transfer of the long extensor tendon beneath the proximal phalanx to the abductor digiti minimi.

COCK-UP DEFORMITY

The MTP joint is dislocated and the little toe sits on the dorsum of the metatarsal head. Through a longitudinal plantar incision, the proximal phalanx is winkled out and removed; the wound is closed transversely, pulling the toe out of the hyperextended position.

TAILOR'S BUNION

An irritating bunionette may form over an abnormally prominent fifth metatarsal head. If the shoe cannot be adjusted to fit the bump, the bony prominence can be trimmed, preserving the tendon of the fifth toe abductor. If the metatarsal shaft is bowed laterally, it can be straightened by performing either a distal osteotomy or a metatarsal base varus correction.

TUBERCULOUS ARTHRITIS

Tuberculous infection of the ankle joint begins as a synovitis or as an osteomyelitis; because walking is painful, the patient may present before joint space narrowing develops. Sinus formation occurs early.

X-rays show regional osteoporosis, sometimes a bone abscess and, with late disease, narrowing and irregularity of the joint space.

Treatment

In addition to general treatment (see Chapter 2), a neutral removable splint is used.

If the disease is arrested early, the patient is allowed up non-weight-bearing in a calliper, gradually taking more and more weight and then discarding the calliper altogether.

In the long term, stiffness is inevitable and, if this is accompanied by pain, arthrodesis is the best treatment.

RHEUMATOID ARTHRITIS

The ankle and foot are commonly affected with RA. Early on, there is synovitis of the joints as well as of the sheathed tendons (usually the peronei and tibialis posterior). As the disease progresses, joint erosion and tendon dysfunction lead to increasingly severe deformities.

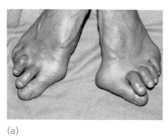 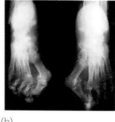 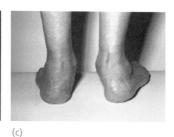

(a) (b) (c)

21.22 Rheumatoid arthritis (a,b) Forefoot deformities are like those in non-rheumatoid feet but more severe. **(c)** Swelling and deformity of the hindfoot due to a combination of arthritis and tenosynovitis. In this case, both the ankle and the subtalar joints are affected.

FOREFOOT

Pain and swelling of the MTP joints occur early. Tenderness is at first localized to the MTP joints before spreading to the rest of the foot. There is increasing weakness of the intrinsic muscles and, with joint destruction, the characteristic deformities appear: a flattened anterior arch, hallux valgus, claw toes and prominence of the metatarsal heads in the sole (patients say it feels like walking on pebbles) (**21.22a,b**).

Subcutaneous nodules, corns and callosities are common and may ulcerate. In the worst cases, the toes are dislocated, inflamed, ulcerated and useless.

X-rays show osteoporosis and periarticular erosion at the MTP joints. Curiously – in contrast to the situation in the hand – the smaller digits (fourth and fifth toes) are affected first.

Treatment

Corticosteroid injections and attention to footwear may relieve symptoms from synovitis. MTP joint synovectomy may slow progression.

Once deformity is advanced, treatment is that of the claw toes and hallux valgus. An effective operation is excision arthroplasty of the MTP joints of lesser toes in order to relieve pressure in the sole and to correct the toe deformities. For the hallux, an MTP fusion is preferred.

ANKLE AND HINDFOOT

The earliest symptoms are pain and swelling around the ankle (**21.22c**). Walking becomes increasingly difficult and, later, deformities appear. On examination, swelling and tenderness are usually localized to tenosynovitis of tibialis posterior or of the peronei. Less often, there is swelling of the ankle joint and its movements are restricted. Inversion and eversion may be painful and limited.

In the late stages, the tibialis posterior may rupture, or become ineffectual; with progressive erosion of the tarsal joints, the foot gradually drifts into severe valgus.

X-rays show osteoporosis and, later, erosion of the tarsal and ankle joints.

Treatment

Splintage helps with symptoms arising from synovitis while waiting for systemic treatment to control the disease. Initially, tendon sheaths and joints may be injected with corticosteroid, but this should not be repeated more than two or three times. A lightweight below-knee orthosis will restore stability and may be worn almost indefinitely.

If the synovitis does not subside, synovectomy may help. In late stages, arthrodesis of the ankle and tarsal joints can still restore modest function and abolish pain. The place of arthroplasty is not yet firmly established.

SERONEGATIVE ARTHROPATHIES

The seronegative arthropathies are dealt with in Chapter 3. These conditions are similar to RA but clinical features are often asymmetrical and the ankle and hindfoot tend to be more severely affected than the forefoot.

In psoriatic arthritis, the toe joints are sometimes completely destroyed. An inflammatory reaction around the insertions of tendons and ligaments is a feature of the spondyloarthropathies. This appears in the foot as plantar fasciitis and Achilles tendinitis. Splintage and local injection of triamcinolone are helpful.

GOUT

Swelling, redness, heat and exquisite tenderness of the MTP joint of the big toe ('podagra') is the epitome of gout (see also Chapter 4) (21.23). The ankle joint, or one of the lesser toes, may be similarly affected – especially following a minor injury. The condition may closely resemble septic arthritis, but the systemic features of infection are absent. The serum uric acid level may be raised.

Chronic tophaceous gout is not uncommon. Lumpy tophi may appear around any of the joints. The diagnosis is suggested by the characteristic X-ray features and confirmed by identifying the typical crystals in the tophus.

Treatment

Treatment with NSAIDs will abort the acute attack of gout; until the pain subsides, the foot should be rested and protected from injury. Painful or ulcerating tophi may require local curettage of the bone lesions.

ANKLE OSTEOARTHRITIS

OA of the ankle is almost always secondary to some underlying disorder: a malunited fracture, recurrent instability, osteochondritis dissecans of the talus, avascular necrosis of the talus or repeated bleeding with haemophilia. Sometimes the ankle is involved in generalized OA and crystal arthropathy.

Clinical features

Ankle OA causes pain, stiffness and an antalgic gait, particularly when first standing up from rest. Patients often indicate the site of pain as being transversely across the front of the ankle. The ankle is usually swollen, with palpable anterior osteophytes and tenderness along the anterior joint line. The foot may be turned outwards in the stance phase, to compensate for the loss of ankle movement.

X-rays show the typical features of OA:

- joint space narrowing
- subchondral sclerosis
- osteophyte formation.

The predisposing disorder is almost always easily detected.

Treatment

Painful exacerbations can be managed with analgesics or NSAIDs. Offloading the joint can be achieved with the use of a walking stick and weight loss helps. Arthrodesis is a good solution

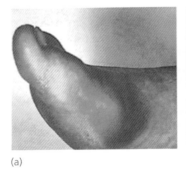 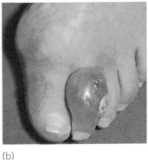 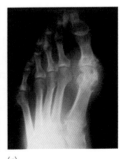

(a)   (b)   (c)

21.23 Gout (a) The classic picture: acute inflammation of the first MTP joint. **(b)** Tophaceous gout of the second toe. **(c)** X-ray of the first MTP joint; the large excavations are occupied by crystalline tophi.

for a painful stiff joint although arthroplasty of the ankle may have a place in the low-demand individual.

THE DIABETIC FOOT

The complications of long-standing diabetes mellitus often appear in the foot, causing chronic disability (21.24). About 40% of non-trauma related amputations in British hospitals are for complications of diabetes.

FACTORS AFFECTING THE DIABETIC FOOT
A predisposition to peripheral vascular disease Damage to peripheral nerves Reduced resistance to infection Osteoporosis

Problems are more common in those who have been diagnosed as diabetic for more than a decade or who have poor glycaemic control.

Peripheral vascular disease Atherosclerosis affects mainly the medium-sized vessels below the knee. The patient may complain of intermittent claudication or ischaemic changes and there may be ulceration or, worse still, gangrene in the foot.

Peripheral neuropathy Patients may complain of symmetrical numbness and paraesthesia, but they are usually unaware of the systemic abnormality. Motor loss may lead to claw toes with high arches and this, in turn, may predispose to plantar ulceration. Neuropathic joint disease (Charcot joints) occurs in less than 1% of diabetic patients, yet diabetes is the commonest cause of a neuropathic joint in Europe and North America. The midtarsal joints are the most commonly affected, followed by the MTP and ankle joints. A minor provocative incident, such as a twisting injury or a fracture, leads to a painless progressive collapse of the joint. *X-rays* show destruction of the joint.

Infection Uncontrolled diabetes reduces immunity and, in combination with peripheral neuropathy and ischaemia, increases the risk of infection after minor trauma.

Osteoporosis Loss of bone density in diabetes may be severe enough to result in insufficiency fractures around the ankle or in the metatarsals.

Management

PREVENTION OF FOOT-RELATED COMPLICATIONS OF DIABETES
Regular attendance at an appropriate clinic for management of diabetes Full compliance with the medication Checks for early signs of vascular or neurological abnormality

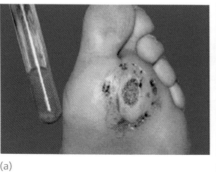 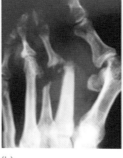 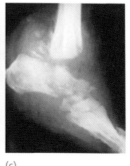

(a) (b) (c)

21.24 The diabetic foot **(a)** Ulceration in a patient with Type 1 diabetes. **(b)** Severe toe deformities in a patient with diabetic neuropathy. **(c)** Neuropathic destruction of the ankle and tarsal joints, following an undisplaced fracture in a poorly controlled diabetic patient.

SECTION 2 REGIONAL ORTHOPAEDICS

Taking heed of advice on foot care and
footwear
A high level of skin hygiene
Use of adaptive and supportive orthoses
if there is deformity or joint instability

Diabetic foot clinics are a multidisciplinary effort of physician, surgeon, podiatrist and orthotist. Regular examination for early signs of neuropathy should include the use of Semmes–Weinstein hairs (for testing skin sensibility) and a biothesiometer (for testing vibration sense). Peripheral vascular examination is enhanced by Doppler assessment.

The presence of ulcers calls for differentiation between vascular, neuropathic or combined causes. Ischaemic changes need the attention of a vascular surgeon who can advise on ways of improving the local blood supply. Neuropathic ulcers require total contact casts followed by custom-made shoes with total contact insoles to avoid recurrence.

Neuropathic joint disease is a major challenge. Arthrodesis has a very poor union rate; 'containment' of the problem in a weight-relieving orthosis may be the best option.

⚠ Careful attention is needed for signs of
gangrene.

• *Dry gangrene* of the toe can be left to demarcate before amputation.
• *Wet gangrene and infection* may call for immediate amputation.

DISORDERS OF THE TENDO ACHILLIS

ACHILLES TENDINITIS

Athletes, joggers and hikers often develop pain and swelling around the tendo Achillis, due to local irritation of the tendon sheath or the paratenon. Function is inhibited because of pain, especially at push-off.

The tendon feels thickened and tender in the watershed area about 4 cm above its insertion. An *ultrasound scan* may be helpful in confirming the diagnosis. If the onset is very sudden, suspect tendon rupture.

Treatment

If the condition starts acutely, it will often settle within about 6 weeks if treated appropriately. Advice on rest, ice, compression and elevation (RICE) and the use of an NSAID (oral or topical) are helpful. When symptoms improve, stretching exercises and muscle strengthening are introduced. A removable in-shoe heel-raise might be helpful.

Treatments such as radiofrequency coblation or extracorporeal shockwave lithotripsy are now showing some promise. Operative treatment is seldom necessary.

ACHILLES TENDON RUPTURE

A ripping or popping sensation is felt at the back of the heel. This most commonly occurs in sports requiring an explosive push-off: squash, badminton, football, tennis or netball.

The typical site for rupture is at the vascular watershed 5 cm above the tendon insertion. The condition is often associated with poor muscle strength and flexibility, failure to warm up and stretch before sport, previous injury or tendinitis and ill-advised corticosteroid injection.

Plantarflexion of the foot is usually inhibited and weak (although it may be possible, as the long flexors of the toes are also ankle flexors). There is often a palpable gap at the site of rupture; bruising comes out a day or two later. The calf squeeze test (Thompson's or Simmonds' test) is diagnostic of Achilles tendon rupture (**21.25**). *Ultrasound scans* can be used to confirm the diagnosis.

SIMMONDS' TEST FOR ACHILLES TENDON RUPTURE

With the patient lying prone with their feet overhanging the end of the bed, both calves are squeezed. If the foot fails to plantarflex, the Achilles tendon is likely to be ruptured.

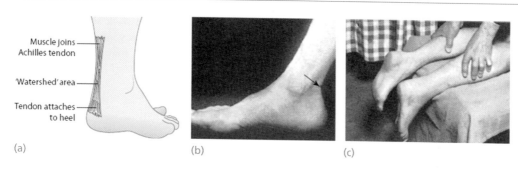

21.25 Rupture of tendo Achillis (a) The soleus may tear at its musculotendinous junction, but the tendo Achillis itself ruptures about 5 cm above its insertion in the 'watershed' area. **(b)** There is a visible and palpable depression at the site of rupture just above the heel. **(c)** Simmonds' test: both calves are being squeezed but only the left foot plantarflexes – the right tendon is ruptured.

Treatment

EARLY

If the patient is seen early, the ends of the tendon may approximate when the foot is passively plantarflexed. If so, a plaster cast or boot is applied with the foot in equinus; rehabilitation and physiotherapy regimes vary, but active rehabilitation with staged reduction of equinus and early physiotherapy starting at 4–6 weeks achieves low rates of re-rupture. *Operative repair* is associated with an earlier return to function and better push-off strength with equivalent re-rupture rates to modern rehabilitation regimes. There are, however, risks associated with operative tendon repair, including wound healing problems and sural nerve neuroma.

LATE

For ruptures that present late, reconstruction using local tendon substitutes (e.g. flexor halluces longus tendon) or strips of fascia lata is still possible.

THE PAINFUL ANKLE

Except after trauma or in RA, persistent pain around the ankle usually originates in one of the periarticular structures or in the talus rather than the joint itself.

Tenosynovitis

Tenderness and swelling are localized to the affected tendon, and pain is aggravated by active movement. Local injection of corticosteroid usually helps.

Rupture of tibialis posterior tendon

Pain starts suddenly and sometimes the patient reports having felt the tendon snap. The heel is in valgus during weight-bearing; the area around the medial malleolus is tender, and active inversion of the ankle is both painful and weak.

In active patients, operative repair or tendon transfer (flexor digitorum longus) is worthwhile. For poorly mobile patients, or indeed anyone who is prepared to put up with the inconvenience of an orthosis, splintage may be adequate.

Osteochondritis dissecans of the talus

Unexplained pain and slight limitation of movement in the ankle of a young person may be due to a small talar dome osteochondral fracture. *Tangential X-rays* will usually show the tiny fragment. *MRI* is also helpful. If the articular surface is intact, it is sufficient simply to restrict activities. If the fragment has separated, it may have to be removed arthroscopically.

Avascular necrosis of the talus

The talus is one of the preferred sites of 'idiopathic' necrosis. The causes are the same as for necrosis at other more common sites such as the femoral head (see Chapter 6). If pain is marked, arthrodesis of the ankle may be needed.

THE PAINFUL FOOT

Pain may be felt predominantly in the heel, the midfoot or the forefoot.

COMMON CAUSES OF FOOT PAIN

Mechanical pressure (which is more likely if the foot is deformed)
Joint inflammation or stiffness
A localized bone lesion
Peripheral ischaemia
Muscular strain

PAINFUL HEEL

Traction 'apophysitis' (Sever's disease)

This mild traction injury usually occurs in young boys. Pain and tenderness are localized to the tendo Achillis insertion (**21.26**). *X-rays* may show increased density or apophyseal irregularity, but often the painless heel looks similar. The heel of the shoe should be raised a little and strenuous activities restricted for a few weeks.

Calcaneal bursitis

Older girls and young women often complain of painful bumps on the backs of their heels. The posterolateral portion of the calcaneum is prominent and shoe friction causes a bursitis. *Treatment* is conservative: open-back shoes and padding of the heel. If symptoms warrant it, removal of the calcaneal prominence may help.

Plantar fasciitis

Pain under the ball of the heel, or slightly forwards of this, is a common complaint in people (mainly men) aged 30–60 years. It is worse on weight-bearing and there is marked tenderness along the distal edge of the heel contact area. A *lateral X-ray* of this site often shows a bone 'spur' extending distally on the undersurface of the calcaneum; this is an associated, not causative feature.

Plantar fasciitis is sometimes encountered in patients with inflammatory disorders such as gout, ankylosing spondylitis and Reiter's disease.

Treatment is conservative:

- NSAIDs
- fascial stretching exercises and massage
- local injection of corticosteroids
- a pad under the heel to offload the painful area.

The condition can take 18–36 months to resolve but it is generally self-limiting.

Bone lesions

Calcaneal lesions such as infection, tumours and Paget's disease can give rise to unremitting pain in the heel. The diagnosis is usually obvious on *X-ray* examination.

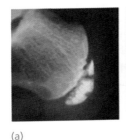
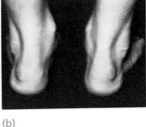
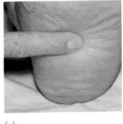
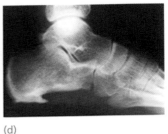

(a)   (b)   (c)   (d)

21.26 Painful heel (a) Sever's disease – the apophysis is dense and fragmented. **(b)** Bilateral 'heel bumps'. **(c)** The usual site of tenderness in plantar fasciitis. **(d)** X-ray in patients with plantar fasciitis often shows what looks like a spur on the undersurface of the calcaneum. In reality, this is a 2D view of a small ridge corresponding to the attachment of the plantar fascia. It is doubtful whether the 'spur' is responsible for the pain and local tenderness.

PAIN OVER THE MIDFOOT

CHILDREN

In children, pain in the midtarsal region is unusual. Two possible causes are:

- *Köhler's disease* ('osteochondritis' – flattening and increased density on X-ray of the navicular)
- a bony coalition across the midtarsal joints.

In both, a period of observation is wise; in Köhler's disease spontaneous resolution is likely and not all bony coalitions will need removal.

ADULTS

In adults, especially if the arch is high, a ridge of bone sometimes develops on the adjacent dorsal surfaces of the medial cuneiform and the first metatarsal (the *'overbone'*). A lump can be seen and it feels hard; it may become tender if the shoe presses on it. If shoe adjustment fails to provide relief, the lump may be bevelled off.

PAIN IN THE FOREFOOT

Any foot abnormality which results in faulty weight distribution may cause nagging pain in the forefoot – *metatarsalgia*. It is therefore a common complaint in patients with hallux valgus, claw toes, pes cavus or flat foot. However,

there are several specific disorders which cause localized pain in the forefoot (21.27).

Sesamoiditis

Pain and tenderness directly under the first metatarsal head, typically aggravated by walking or passive dorsiflexion of the great toe, may be due to sesamoiditis. Symptoms usually arise from irritation or inflammation of the peritendinous tissues around the sesamoids.

Treatment consists of reduced weight-bearing and a pressure pad in the shoe. In resistant cases, a local injection of methylprednisolone and local anaesthetic often helps.

Freiberg's disease

'Osteochondritis' (or 'osteochondrosis') of a metatarsal head is actually a type of traumatic osteonecrosis of the subarticular bone. It usually affects the second metatarsal head (rarely the third) in young adults. There is pain over the MTP joint and a bony lump (the enlarged metatarsal head) is palpable and tender. *X-rays* show the head to be flattened and wide, the neck thick and the joint space apparently increased.

A walking plaster or moulded sandal will help to reduce pressure on the metatarsal head. If symptoms persist, synovectomy, debridement and trimming of the metatarsal head (cheilectomy)

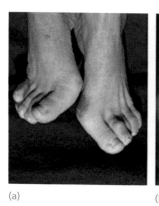 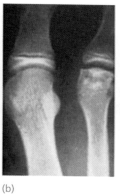 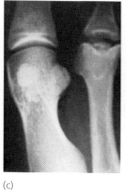 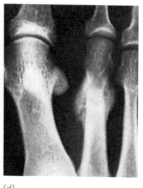

(a) (b) (c) (d)

21.27 Pain in the forefoot (a) Long-standing deformities such as dropped anterior arches, hallux valgus, hammer toe, curly toes and overlapping-toes (all of which are present in this patient) can cause metatarsalgia. Localized pain and tenderness suggest a more specific cause. **(b,c)** Stages in the development of Freiberg's disease. **(d)** Periosteal new bone formation along the shaft of the second metatarsal, the classical sign of a stress fracture.

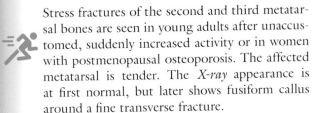

should be considered. Pain relief is usually good and the range of dorsiflexion is improved.

Stress fracture

Stress fractures of the second and third metatarsal bones are seen in young adults after unaccustomed, suddenly increased activity or in women with postmenopausal osteoporosis. The affected metatarsal is tender. The *X-ray* appearance is at first normal, but later shows fusiform callus around a fine transverse fracture.

Treatment usually consists of rest and reassurance.

Interdigital nerve compression (Morton's metatarsalgia)

The patient, usually a woman of around 50 years, complains of pain in the forefoot ('as if walking on a pebble in the shoe') with radiation to the toes. Tenderness is localized to one of the intermetatarsal spaces – usually the third – and pressure just proximal to the interdigital web may elicit both the pain and a tingling sensation distally. Squeezing the metatarsal heads together may produce a painful click (Mulder's click).

This is essentially an entrapment or compression syndrome affecting one of the digital nerves, but secondary thickening of the nerve creates the impression of a 'neuroma'.

If symptoms do not respond to the use of protective padding and wearing wider shoes, *treatment* with a steroid injection into the interspace will provide lasting relief in about 50% of cases. If this also fails, nerve compression can usually be relieved by operative division of the tight transverse intermetatarsal ligament. Intractable cases may need excision of the 'neuroma'.

Tarsal tunnel syndrome

Pain and sensory disturbance in the medial part of the forefoot, unrelated to weight-bearing and often worst at night, may be due to compression of the posterior tibial nerve behind and below the medial malleolus. This is sometimes due to a space-occupying lesion such as a ganglion, haemangioma or varicosity. Paraesthesia and

numbness may follow the characteristic sensory distribution. The diagnosis is difficult to establish but nerve conduction studies may show slowing of motor or sensory conduction.

Treatment to decompress the nerve involves exposing it behind the medial malleolus and following it into the sole; sometimes it is trapped by the belly of adductor halluces arising more proximally than usual.

TOENAIL DISORDERS

The toenail of the hallux may be ingrown, overgrown or undergrown (**21.28**).

Ingrown toenail

The nail grows into the nail groove; this ulcerates and its wall grows over the nail, so the term 'embedded toenail' would be better. The patient is taught to cut the nail square, to insert pledgets of wool under the ingrowing edges and always to keep the feet clean and dry. If these measures fail, the portion of germinal matrix which is responsible for the 'ingrow' should be ablated, either by operative excision or by chemical ablation with phenol. Rarely is it necessary to remove the entire nail or completely ablate the nail bed.

Overgrown toenail (onychogryphosis)

The nail is hard, thick and curved. A chiropodist can usually make the patient comfortable, but occasionally the nail may need excision.

Undergrown toenails

A subungual exostosis grows on the dorsum of the terminal phalanx and pushes the nail upwards. The exostosis should be removed if the nail deformity is causing problems, usually with footwear.

SKIN LESIONS

Typical skin lesions of the foot include corns, callouses, pressure ulcers and keratoderma (**21.29**).

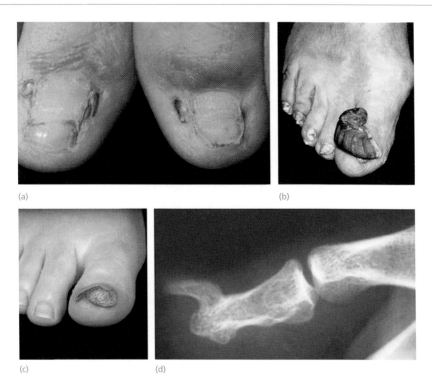

21.28 Toenail disorders (a) Ingrown toenails; (b) overgrown toenail (onychogryphosis); (c,d) exostosis from the distal phalanx, pushing the toenail up.

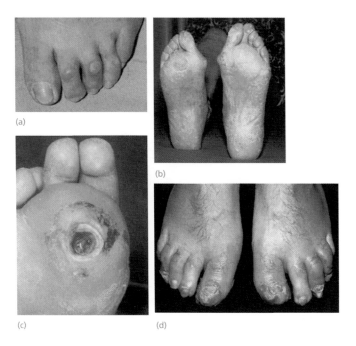

21.29 Skin lesions (a) Corns; (b) plantar callosities in a patient with claw toes and a 'dropped' anterior metatarsal arch; (c) a typical pressure ulcer in a patient with long-standing diabetic neuropathy; (d) keratoderma blennorrhagica, a complication of Reiter's disease.

Section 3

Trauma

22 The management of major injuries   485

23 Principles of fractures   513

24 Shoulder and upper arm injuries   551

25 Elbow and forearm injuries   565

26 Wrist injuries   589

27 Hand injuries   607

28 Spine and thorax injuries   625

29 Pelvic injuries   643

30 Hip and femur injuries   653

31 Knee and leg injuries   675

32 Ankle and foot injuries   697

The management of major injuries

22

- Management at the scene of the accident   486
- Management in hospital   487
- Airway and cervical spine   490
- Breathing and chest injuries   493
- Circulation – shock   497
- Head injuries   499

- Abdominal injuries   503
- Musculoskeletal injuries   504
- Burns   506
- Crush syndrome   509
- Multiple organ failure   510

Throughout the developed world trauma is the commonest cause of death in people under the age of 40 years, with the largest proportion resulting from road accidents. For every death, three victims suffer permanent disability, causing personal tragedy and a drain on a nation's healthcare economy.

These deaths follow a trimodal pattern:

- 50% of patients die on scene from unsurvivable injuries
- 30% survive but die between 1 and 3 hours after injury
- the remaining 20% die from complications during the 6 weeks after injury (**22.1**).

The second peak in the death rate is due mostly to hypoxia and loss of blood with hypovolaemic shock; these are potentially preventable and hence this period has been called '*the golden hour*'. The third peak is due largely to multisystem

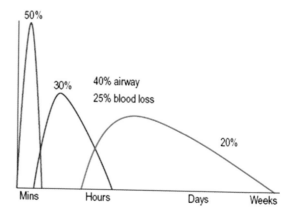

22.1 Death following trauma The trimodal distribution of mortality following severe trauma.

failure and sepsis needing high levels of intensive care, but it is reducible by early and effective management.

The management of severe injuries proceeds in five well-defined stages.

STAGES IN THE MANAGEMENT OF SEVERE INJURIES

1 Emergency treatment immediately after the accident
2 Resuscitation and evaluation in the hospital accident department
3 Early treatment of life-threatening injuries
4 Treatment of potentially life-threatening injuries
5 Long-term rehabilitation

MANAGEMENT AT THE SCENE OF THE ACCIDENT

IMMEDIATE ACTIONS AND TRIAGE

Trauma scenes are hazardous, and personal safety is essential (e22.1).

> Always ensure your own personal safety at the scene of an accident.

If there are multiple casualties, identify priorities by *triage*. This is a sorting system based on the injured person's ability to walk, breathe and maintain a pulse, followed by a scored, physiological assessment placing the individual in one of the following categories:

- *Priority 1*   Immediate
- *Priority 2*   Urgent
- *Priority 3*   Delayed
- *Priority 4*   Dead

ASSESSMENT AND INITIAL MANAGEMENT

The nature of the incident and pattern of vehicle damage help in predicting the likely injuries. Early recognition is based on a rapid and systematic questioning and examination of the casualty.

Access to an entrapped person may be limited, but an immediate examination can be made of the *airway, breathing* and *circulation* – the 'ABC'

of trauma assessment, which guides immediate management, extrication and transfer.

Management

> Life-threatening injuries in the ABC categories are treated first; the exception to this is *catastrophic external haemorrhage*, when bleeding must be controlled first.

The ABC system is then followed: C–ABC.

At all times the cervical spine must be immobilized, in case there is vertebral injury.

Control pain, if necessary.

AIRWAY

Casualties with airway obstruction can succumb within minutes.

1 Open the airway by pulling the jaw forward, *but do not extend the neck*, and remove all visible foreign bodies.
2 Use airway devices if the casualty's airway remains obstructed.
3 Intubation following rapid sequence induction of anaesthesia is the gold standard, but this should be performed by a doctor trained in anaesthesiology.
4 If intubation fails, a surgical airway will be required.

BREATHING

1 Administer high-flow oxygen with a non-rebreathing reservoir mask.
2 Support ventilation with a bag–valve–mask (BVM) assembly, and ventilate intubated casualties.
3 Examine the chest for signs of a *tension pneumothorax* which will need immediate decompression using a large-bore intravenous cannula inserted through the second intercostal space in the midclavicular line.
4 Follow this by thoracostomies if the patient is intubated.
5 Cover open chest wounds with an occlusive, three-sided dressing.

CIRCULATION

1. Control haemorrhage by pressure and, if needed, a temporary tourniquet.
2. Insert intravenous (IV) or intraosseous (IO) cannulas.
3. Limit IV fluids in haemorrhagic shock; titrate crystalloid fluid in 250 mL boluses to maintain a radial pulse only.
4. Consider bilateral thoracostomies and clamshell thoracotomy if post-traumatic cardiac arrest occurs.

An extended system (ABCDE) would also include:

- *Disability* – assess the neurological status using the Glasgow Coma Score (GCS), and note the pupil size.
- *Environmental situation* – keep the patient exposed but ensure that normothermia is maintained.

Extrication and immobilization

1. Managing an entrapped casualty is difficult and extrication is a priority.
2. Protect the spine using manual immobilization, cervical collars and rigid immobilization devices.
3. Analgesia may be required.
4. Splint limb fractures and dislocations. Use femoral traction splints for midshaft femur fractures if the pelvic ring is intact.
5. Stabilize pelvic fractures with compression devices.

 Always protect the spine when assessing and extricating a casualty.

Transfer to hospital

 Delayed or prolonged transfer to hospital is associated with poor outcomes, but *the ABCs must be addressed before transferring the patient.*

1. Match the destination hospital to injury severity, and make a 'trauma call' (e22.2).
2. Maintain the casualty's oxygen saturations above 95%, and end-tidal carbon dioxide

($EtOO_2$) at a low normal level (4.0–4.5 kPa) if ventilated.
3. Control haemorrhage.
4. Continue IV Hartmann's to maintain a radial pulse.

ON-SCENE PRIORITIES

1. Stay safe
2. Obtain access
3. Protect the cervical spine
4. Free the airway
5. Ensure ventilation
6. Arrest haemorrhage
7. Combat shock
8. Control pain
9. Splint fractures
10. Transfer to hospital

MANAGEMENT IN HOSPITAL

After reaching the hospital, the following factors are important:

- organization and trauma teams
- assessment and management (*the ATLS concept*)
- initial management
- definitive care.

ORGANIZATION AND TRAUMA TEAMS

'Get the right patient to the right hospital in the right amount of time.' (Trunkey)

In certain circumstances, it may be appropriate to bypass a smaller hospital in order to reach a facility which can manage more severe injuries.

Casualty patients need rapid assessment and resuscitation to avoid their dying during the 'golden hour'. Crucial for this requirement is *a multidisciplinary team led by a doctor with advanced trauma skills.*

THE ATLS CONCEPT

ATLS® (Advanced Trauma Life Support) is central to the internationally recognized training programme for the management of major injuries. The programme teaches a two-stage initial

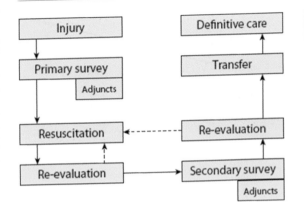

22.2 Algorithm of Advanced Trauma Life Support (ATLS) initial assessment and management

assessment and management followed by transfer to definitive care (**22.2**). This calls for:

- a *primary survey and simultaneous resuscitation* (rapid assessment and treatment of life-threatening injuries)
- followed by a *secondary survey* (head-to-toe re-evaluation to identify all other injuries).

Specialist skills such as anaesthesia are employed in addition to core basic ATLS® skills. Certain facilities should also be available.

FACILITIES REQUIRED

- Electrocardiographic (ECG) monitoring
- Pulse oximetry (arterial oxygen saturation)
- $EtCO_2$
- Arterial blood gas measurements (ABGs)
- Urethral catheters
- Nasogastric tubes
- X-rays (chest and pelvis)
- Focussed Assessment Sonography for Trauma (FAST)
- Computed tomography (CT)

PRIMARY SURVEY AND RESUSCITATION

Airway obstruction kills in minutes. In degrees of urgency, it is followed by respiratory failure, circulatory failure and expanding intracranial mass lesions. Hence the development of the 'ABC' sequence, the goal of which is to preserve perfusion of the brain with oxygenated blood (**e22.3**).

THE ABC(DE) SEQUENCE

1. **A**irway with cervical spine protection
2. **B**reathing
3. **C**irculation with haemorrhage control
4. **D**isability or neurological status
5. **E**xposure and **E**nvironment

Throughout, the cervical spine must be protected until a vertebral injury has been excluded. This is achieved by manual in-line immobilization or triple immobilization with a cervical collar, head supports and strapping.

 Never extend the neck or twist until a cervical spine injury has been excluded.

A – Airway with cervical spine protection

The sound of an obstructed airway (stridor) is unmistakable. Support the airway, suction secretions and blood and place OP or NP airways. Further options are the laryngeal mask airway, tracheal intubation or operative provision of an airway (cricothyrotomy). The airway must be checked frequently throughout the resuscitation phase; one that appears initially to be safe may not remain so.

B – Breathing

If, despite a clear airway, ventilation is inadequate the chest should be carefully examined for pneumothorax or a flail thoracic segment.

- *Tension pneumothorax* is a life-threatening complication and should be treated by immediate decompression.
- *Sucking chest wounds* must be covered.
- *A flail chest* may require endotracheal intubation and positive pressure ventilation. The BVM is a hand-held device that manually supplies positive pressure ventilation.

It is essential to give all severely injured patients supplemental oxygen and to take a blood sample for measurement of the arterial oxygen tension (PaO_2) and carbon dioxide tension ($PaCO_2$).

C – Circulation with haemorrhage control

Assess for bleeding and shock and control external haemorrhage. Feel the carotid, femoral and radial pulses (Table e22.1). Site IV or IO cannulas, and draw samples for diagnostic tests and cross-matching. If blood is available, initially treat shock with 2 L of warmed Hartmann's. Use FAST to identify body cavity haemorrhage.

D – Disability (level of consciousness)

Assess neurological status using the GCS (Table 22.1). Consider intoxication but assume a lowered GCS is secondary to a cerebral injury until proved otherwise. Examine pupils for equality.

E – Exposure and environment

Remove clothing and 'log-roll' the patient to examine the entire body. Maintain normothermia, warm fluids and ventilated gases.

Table 22.1 Glasgow Coma Score

Response	Score
Eye opening:	
Spontaneous	4
On command	3
On pain	2
Nil	1
Best motor response:	
Obeys	6
Localizes pain	5
Normal flexor	4
Abnormal flexor	3
Extensor	2
Nil	1
Verbal response:	
Orientated	5
Confused	4
Words	3
Sounds	2
Nil	1

SECONDARY SURVEY

Once the patient has been resuscitated, a 'head-to-toe survey' is carried out. The back can be examined by gently 'log-rolling' the patient onto their side.

Take a history if possible and establish whether trauma was subsequent to a medical collapse, and whether the patient is receiving long-term treatment.

Examination

Head and face   Examine for contusions, lacerations and fractures, and examine eyes and ears for bleeding. Reassess the GCS. The presence of facial or head injuries should raise suspicions about concomitant brain injury.

Neck   Examine for a step in the cervical spine indicative of fracture/dislocation, and contusions over the anterior neck indicative of laryngeal damage.

Chest   Inspect and auscultate to identify a pneumothorax. Palpate to detect fractured ribs, sternum, and subcutaneous emphysema and percuss to reveal a tension pneumothorax and haemothorax.

Abdomen   Examine for contusions and wounds; auscultate and palpate. Don't forget the perineum, rectum and vagina.

Pelvis   Check for unequal leg length and local tenderness.

Limbs   Examine for swelling, contusions, deformity, tenderness and pallor. Feel the pulses.

Neurological assessment   Examine for lateralizing signs, loss of sensation and motor power, and abnormality of reflexes. Document levels of sensory loss.

Imaging

* *CT scanning*, preferably with a fast spiral CT, is now the method of choice for patients with acute major trauma; it should be obtained at the earliest opportunity. Modern CT scanners can provide high-definition images within minutes while the patient is returned to the emergency department for continuing resuscitation (**22.3**).

SECTION 3 TRAUMA

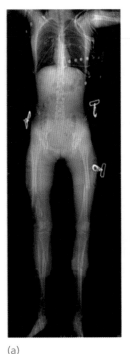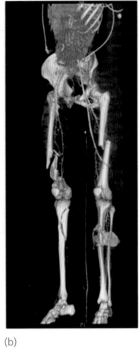

(a)   (b)

22.3 Imaging (a,b) CT scanning is the imaging mode of choice. Multiple injuries are rapidly displayed.

- *X-rays* of the chest, pelvis, spine and limbs are obtained as indicated or if the patient is not stable enough for CT.

> *Lateral cervical spine X-rays* do not exclude fractures or unstable necks and so do not alter management; if required, they can be performed as part of the secondary survey.

- *eFAST* (Extended focussed assessment with sonography in trauma) detects intraperitoneal fluid or blood, pericardial tamponade and pneumothorax.

GENERAL CARE

Pain management

Pain can be controlled in several ways, depending on the type of trauma.

- *Intravenous analgesia* – titrate morphine against response and administer an antiemetic.

- *Inhalational analgesia* – Entonox is good for short-term use but is contraindicated in patients with untreated pneumothorax. Disposable methoxyflurane inhalers can be used in place of Entonox and can be used safely in the presence of a suspected pneumothorax.
- *Nerve blocks* – discuss this with the orthopaedic surgeon to avoid masking possible compartment syndrome.

Re-evaluation

The vital signs should be checked repeatedly to assess the response to treatment. The patient should not leave the Emergency Department until their condition is stable, unless it is to be taken directly to the operating theatre for the control of haemorrhage or some other surgical emergency.

Intrahospital and interhospital transfer

Transfer is indicated when the patient's needs exceed local resources. Even the shortest transfer within a hospital is fraught with hazard as monitoring and resuscitation are difficult on the move, and so any transfer must be carefully planned.

DEFINITIVE CARE

Specialist care may be required to manage specific injuries identified during the initial assessment and investigation.

AIRWAY AND CERVICAL SPINE

Until the airway is secured and protected, the cervical spine should be stabilized by manual in-line immobilization as a cervical collar makes intubation difficult.

> Once the airway is securely protected, triple immobilization with a stiff collar, head blocks and tape should be used until an unstable injury is excluded.

Awareness

- *Head injury* is the most common cause of airway compromise. As consciousness and muscle tone decrease, the pharynx and tongue obstruct the glottis.
- *Maxillofacial trauma* can disrupt facial bones and this, with tissue swelling and bleeding, may obstruct the pharynx. These patients may need to sit up to open the airway (e22.4).
- *Neck trauma* causes haemorrhage and swelling, distorting and obstructing the airway. Tracheal intubation can be impossible and surgical alternatives are likely to be difficult.
- *Laryngeal trauma*, heralded by hoarseness and coughing of bright red blood, may cause surgical emphysema and sudden airway obstruction.
- *Inhalational burns* result in rapid swelling and airway obstruction, requiring early and expert intubation.

Recognition

Examine for signs of airway obstruction.

> ### EXAMINATION FOR SIGNS OF AIRWAY OBSTRUCTION
>
> **Look**
>
> - Agitation, aggression, anxiety
> - Depressed level of consciousness
> - Cyanosis
> - Sweating
> - Use of accessory muscles of ventilation (tracheal tug and intercostal recession)
>
> **Listen**
>
> - Noisy breathing
> - Stridor
> - Hoarse voice
> - Faint or absent sounds of breathing
>
> **Feel**
>
> - Reduced passage of air through mouth and nose

Management

Chin lift   Lift the mandible forwards with fingertips (22.4a).

Jaw thrust   Pull the mandible up and forwards, combined with BVM ventilation. Effective with small jaws, thick necks and in edentulous patients (22.4b,c).

Oropharyngeal (OP) airway   Slide the airway above the tongue until the flange rests on the teeth. Use only in obtunded patients with absent gag reflexes (22.5, e22.5, e22.6).

Nasopharyngeal (NP) airway   Insert along the floor of the nasal cavity, with caution if a basal skull fracture is suspected (e22.7).

Oropharyngeal suction   Clear secretions and blood.

Laryngeal mask airway and supra-glottic airway   These are passed over the tongue into the oropharynx and inflate the cuff. This is effective, and requires less training than tracheal intubation. However, it does not protect the airway so it should be replaced with a tracheal tube.

Tracheal intubation   Orotracheal intubation is the preferred method for securing and protecting the airway, but it is a difficult procedure in unanaesthetized casualties (e22.8).

Needle cricothyroidotomy   This is the insertion of a thin cannula through the cricothyroid membrane into the trachea to allow jet insufflation of the lungs with oxygen; it is used in 'can't intubate, can't ventilate' situations. Oxygenation is achievable, but ventilation limited. It should only be attempted if intubation has failed.

Complications include:

- misplacement
- surgical emphysema
- barotrauma.

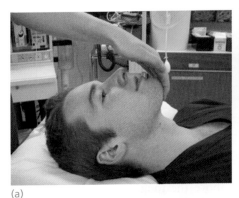

(a)

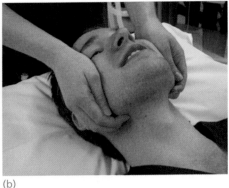

(b)

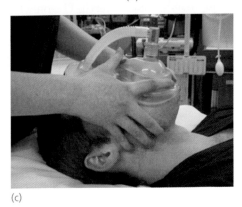

(c)

22.4 Chin lift and jaw thrust (a) In the chin lift, the chin is lifted forwards with the practitioner positioned at the casualty's head or side, using one hand. This pulls the jaw and pharyngeal structures forward off the posterior pharyngeal wall and glottis, and opens up the airway. **(b)** The jaw thrust is a more assertive manoeuvre that is effective in patients with small jaws or thick necks, or who are edentulous. From the casualty's head, the thenar eminences are rested on the casualty's maxillae (assuming no obvious fracture), and the four fingers positioned under the angles of the mandible. Using the thenar eminences to provide a counterpoint on the maxillae, the mandible is lifted up and forwards to open up the airway as with the chin lift. **(c)** Jaw thrust with oxygen mask.

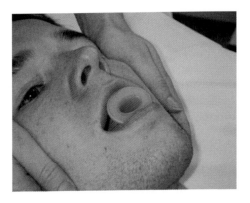

22.5 Oropharyngeal airway – correct position

Surgical cricothyroidotomy When orotracheal intubation fails, a tracheal tube can be inserted through the cricothyroid membrane into the trachea, thus enabling oxygenation and full ventilation.

Complications include:

- haemorrhage
- damage to laryngeal structures
- false passage formation
- misplacement of the tracheal tube
- surgical emphysema
- barotrauma.

Airway: Summary

Whatever the means of airway management used, the goal is to secure and protect the airway.

The focus should be on oxygenation and ventilation, not intubation.

Casualties die from hypoxia and hypercarbia, not failure of intubation.

BREATHING AND CHEST INJURIES

Awareness

Only 10% of blunt chest injuries and 20% of penetrating injuries require thoracotomy. Non-surgical management involves supportive treatment and the insertion of chest drains.

Six immediately life-threatening injuries are recognized and managed during the primary survey, and eight potentially life-threatening injuries are sought during the secondary survey (see boxes).

Recognition

If, despite a clear airway, ventilation is inadequate the chest and surrounding areas should be carefully examined for signs of respiratory dysfunction.

EXAMINATION FOR SIGNS OF RESPIRATORY DYSFUNCTION

Look

- Tachypnoea, laboured breathing and paradoxical respiration
- Cyanosis
- Plethora and petechiae
- Unequal chest inflation
- Bruising and contusions
- Penetrating chest injuries
- Distended neck veins

Listen

- Absent breath sounds
- Noisy breathing/crepitations/stridor/ wheeze
- Reduced air entry unilaterally

Feel

- Tracheal deviation
- Tenderness
- Crepitus/instability
- Surgical emphysema

Chest X-rays may be performed if the patient is not stable enough for *CT*. Severely injured patients are given supplemental oxygen and a blood sample is taken for measurement of the PaO_2 and $PaCO_2$.

Management of immediately life-threatening chest injuries

Administer high-flow oxygen and ventilate the lungs if breathing is absent or inadequate. Intubated trauma patients must be ventilated.

IMMEDIATELY LIFE-THREATENING CHEST INJURIES (PRIMARY SURVEY)

1. Tension pneumothorax
2. Open pneumothorax (sucking chest wound)
3. Massive haemothorax
4. Cardiac tamponade
5. Flail chest
6. Disruption of tracheobronchial tree

TENSION PNEUMOTHORAX

Air builds up under pressure in the pleural cavity, leading to collapse of the lung and shift of the mediastinum away from the affected side, obstructing venous return to the heart (**22.6**). This results in hypoxia and loss of cardiac output, and ultimately, pulseless electrical activity (PEA) cardiac arrest.

Diagnosis should be clinical, not radiological.

SECTION 3 TRAUMA

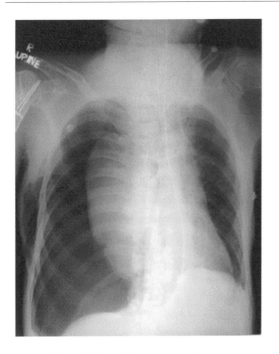

22.6 Right-sided tension pneumothorax

> **DIAGNOSTIC SIGNS OF TENSION PNEUMOTHORAX**
>
> Absent breath sounds (*on* the side of the pneumothorax)
> Hyper-resonance (*on* the side of the pneumothorax)
> Deviated trachea (*away* from the side of the tension pneumothorax)
> Surgical emphysema (chest and neck)

Immediately decompress the tension pneumothorax by inserting a large-bore cannula into the pleural cavity of the affected side, through the second intercostal space, in the midclavicular line. Follow with a wide-bore chest drain. If the expertise is immediately available, an open thoracostomy is the definitive treatment.

OPEN PNEUMOTHORAX

An open wound in the chest wall will result in a simple pneumothorax ('sucking chest wound'). With a large defect, air is drawn into the pleural cavity rather than the lung, leading to hypoxia

and hypercarbia. A flap valve effect can lead to a tension pneumothorax.

Apply an occlusive dressing, sealed on three sides, leaving the fourth side open to prevent tensioning.

MASSIVE PNEUMOTHORAX

Up to 1500 mL (one-third of the blood volume) can rapidly accumulate in the chest following blunt or penetrating chest injury, leading to hypoxia and shock. Massive bleeds are more likely to require surgical repair and pulmonary lobectomy.

> **DIAGNOSTIC SIGNS OF MASSIVE PNEUMOTHORAX**
>
> Hypoxia, reduced chest expansion
> Absent breath sounds
> Dullness to chest percussion
> Hypovolaemic shock

Treat by inserting a chest drain, correcting hypovolaemia and transfusing blood. If more than 1500 mL of blood is drained initially, or bleeding continues at >200 mL/hour or the patient remains haemodynamically unstable, surgical referral and thoracotomy are indicated.

CARDIAC TAMPONADE

This is accumulation of blood within the pericardium resulting in a loss of cardiac output leading to PEA cardiac arrest. It is more common with penetrating trauma between the nipple lines or scapulae.

> **DIAGNOSTIC SIGNS OF CARDIAC TAMPONADE**
>
> Distended neck veins
> Muffled heart sounds
> Fall in arterial blood pressure/paradoxical pulse

Investigate by eFAST, CT or transoesophageal echocardiogram.

Manage with aspiration using a large needle, although this is unreliable; clamshell thoracotomy is the preferred treatment if the skills are immediately available.

FLAIL CHEST

Multiple rib fractures damage the structural integrity of the chest wall; as the patient inspires, the flail segment is sucked in (paradoxical respiration). The injury causes a lung contusion resulting in hypoxia, further compromised by pain.

DIAGNOSTIC SIGNS OF FLAIL CHEST

Pain, tenderness and crepitus
Fractured ribs on chest X-ray
Hypoxia on estimating ABGs

Manage initially with oxygen and analgesia. Patients may require early intubation and IV fluid restriction. Fractured ribs or costochondral disruption rarely requires surgical stabilization.

DISRUPTION OF TRACHEOBRONCHIAL TREE

Disruption of the tracheobronchial tree can result in a bronchopleural fistula, causing air to leak into the pleura and preventing inflation of the lung, even with a chest drain *in situ*. Selective endobronchial intubation of the opposite lung may be required.

DIAGNOSTIC SIGNS OF DISRUPTION OF TRACHEOBRONCHIAL TREE

Persistent pneumothorax
Pneumomediastinum
Pneumopericardium
Surgical emphysema
Air below the deep fascia of the neck

Management of potentially life-threatening chest injuries

SIMPLE PNEUMOTHORAX

This results from air entering the pleural cavity, causing collapse of the lung and hypoxia. No mediastinal shift develops, and cardiac output is maintained. The cause is usually a lung laceration.

POTENTIALLY LIFE-THREATENING CHEST INJURIES (SECONDARY SURVEY)

1 Simple pneumothorax
2 Haemothorax
3 Pulmonary contusion
4 Tracheobronchial tree injury
5 Blunt cardiac injury
6 Traumatic aortic disruption
7 Traumatic diaphragmatic injury
8 Mediastinal traversing wounds

DIAGNOSTIC SIGNS OF DISRUPTION OF SIMPLE PNEUMOTHORAX

Absence or reduction of breath sounds
Absent lung markings on chest X-ray

A simple pneumothorax can develop into a tension pneumothorax, precipitated by intubation and ventilation, use of nitrous oxide and air transport.

A chest drain should be inserted. This carries the potential complication of visceral damage, and trochars should not be used. Make a horizontal skin incision in the fifth intercostal space, above the sixth rib, just anterior to the midaxillary line; then bluntly dissect down to and through the pleura with forceps. A finger sweep will confirm entry into the empty pleura, and the chest tube can be introduced with forceps and connected to a valve or underwater drain (**22.7**).

HAEMOTHORAX

Smaller haemothoraces are normally self-limiting, and rarely require operative intervention. The only diagnostic sign is dullness to percussion, and this is not very reliable. A *supine chest X-ray* may show opacification, but may not reveal moderate amounts of blood. FAST or CT is more reliable.

Treatment is placement of a large-calibre basal chest drain. If drainage continues at more than 200 mL/hour, thoracotomy should be considered.

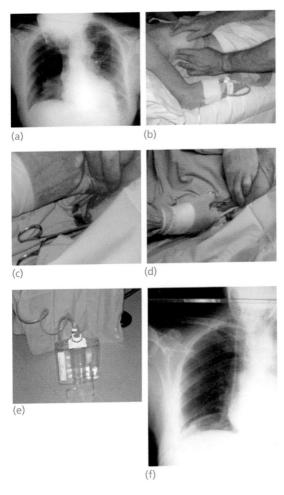

(a)   (b)
(c)   (d)
(e)
(f)

22.7 Chest drain insertion sequence **(a)** Chest X-ray to confirm the correct side. **(b)** Identify the fifth intercostal space, just anterior to the midaxillary line on the affected side. **(c)** Insert a gloved little finger through the incision into the chest cavity and finger-sweep to ensure the cavity is empty and the incision is above the diaphragm (no viscus is felt). **(d)** Grasp the tip of an appropriately sized thoracostomy tube between the tips of the forceps and introduce it through the incision into the chest cavity. Unclamp the forceps and slide the tube posteriorly along the inside of the chest wall. **(e)** Attach the tube to an underwater drain or Heimlich valve and observe for tube fogging and underwater bubbling. **(f)** Check lung reinflation with chest X-ray.

PULMONARY CONTUSION

This is the commonest potentially life-threatening chest injury. Hypoxia is dependent on the extent of the contusion and pain. Around 50% of patients will develop bilateral acute respiratory distress syndrome (ARDS).

Pulmonary contusion may not be associated with obvious rib fractures, particularly in the young. The initial *chest X-ray* may not reveal the extent of the contusion, which can develop over 48 hours, and diagnosis depends on the mechanism of injury and hypoxia. The condition is managed supportively with oxygen administration and ventilation.

TRACHEOBRONCHIAL TREE INJURY

This is a rare injury. Diagnostic signs are haemoptysis, surgical emphysema and persistent pneumothorax. *CT* may be diagnostic, but bronchoscopy may be required.

Treat initially with one or more large chest drains with or without a high-volume, low-pressure pump. Persistent bronchopleural fistulae may require operative intervention.

BLUNT CARDIAC INJURY

This follows a direct blow to the anterior chest wall, associated with a fractured sternum. Myocardial contusion, chamber rupture and valvular disruption can result in hypotension, dysrhythmias and ventricular fibrillation.

Manage supportively and monitor for 24 hours when risk of dysrhythmia diminishes.

AORTIC DISRUPTION

This occurs mostly in the proximal thoracic aorta. Specific clinical signs and symptoms are often absent, and the mechanism of injury should provoke suspicion. *Chest X-ray* shows a widened mediastinum with loss of the aortic knuckle and deviation of the trachea to the right, and *CT* is highly specific.

Manage supportively, and control blood pressure. Once the injury is confirmed, surgical repair is required (e22.9).

DIAPHRAGMATIC INJURY

This is associated with blunt and penetrating trauma to the abdomen. Rupture is more common on the left, and rarely found in isolation, being associated with other chest, abdominal and pelvic injuries. Diaphragmatic ruptures associated with penetrating trauma result in a smaller tear.

Signs and symptoms can be subtle. *Chest X-ray* may show an elevated but indistinct hemidiaphragm, requiring *CT*.

Manage supportively, and consider chest drain insertion. Definitive treatment is surgical.

MEDIASTINAL TRAVERSING WOUNDS

Penetrating objects that cross the mediastinum may damage the lungs and mediastinal structures. The diagnosis is made by examination of the chest and trauma imaging. The significant finding is an entrance wound in one hemithorax and an exit wound or radiologically visible missile in the other.

Haemodynamically unstable patients should be assumed to have a haemothorax, tension pneumothorax or cardiac tamponade until proved otherwise.

Manage with bilateral chest drains. Stable patients should undergo extensive investigation with ultrasound, CT, angiography, oesophagoscopy and bronchoscopy as indicated, and early consultation with a cardiothoracic surgeon.

BREATHING/CHEST INJURIES: SUMMARY

The primary goal in management of traumatic chest injuries is to rapidly identify and manage the six immediately life-threatening injuries within the primary survey.

The eight potentially life-threatening injuries should be sought within the primary and secondary surveys, and they may require sophisticated imaging to diagnose.

Only 15% of chest injuries require operative intervention.

CIRCULATION – SHOCK

Shock is circulatory failure and inadequate perfusion of tissues with oxygenated blood, which leads to organ damage and death from multi-organ failure. Management comes after attention to the airway and breathing – unless there is catastrophic external bleeding, the control of which takes precedence.

Awareness

There are five types of shock.

FIVE TYPES OF SHOCK

Vasoconstrictive

- Hypovolaemic
- Cardiogenic

Vasodilative

- Septic
- Neurogenic
- Anaphylactic

- *Hypovolaemic shock,* secondary to haemorrhage, is the most common. As the circulating blood volume decreases, compensatory mechanisms maintain systolic blood pressure up to around 30% blood loss in a fit patient. Above this, compensation increasingly fails until coma is followed by death at around 50% blood loss.
- *Cardiogenic shock* occurs in trauma patients who have suffered a myocardial infarction, or direct myocardial injury.
- *Neurogenic shock* is seen in high spinal cord transections.
- *Septic shock* and *anaphylactic shock* are unusual in acute trauma.

Recognition

Diagnosis depends on a rapid assessment of the patient and assessment of vital signs; blood pressure and pulse alone are not adequate.

The patient becomes apathetic and thirsty; breathing is shallow and rapid; the lips and skin are pale and the extremities feel cold and clammy. As compensation fails, the pulse becomes rapid and feeble, the blood pressure drops and the patient may become confused. Eventually, renal function is impaired and urinary output falls (Table e22.2).

If it is difficult to measure the blood pressure reliably and repeatedly, continuous intra-arterial pressure monitoring should be instituted. Manual sphygmomanometry with a cuff and stethoscope is considerably more accurate than automated noninvasive blood pressure machines.

Hypovolaemic shock unresponsive to treatment is commonly due to bleeding into body cavities or potential spaces and can be identified by eFAST or CT. Remember the epigram: 'Count *bleeding onto the floor and four more*' (chest; abdomen; pelvis/retroperitoneum; long bones). The patient loses more blood than you think in closed fractures (**22.8**).

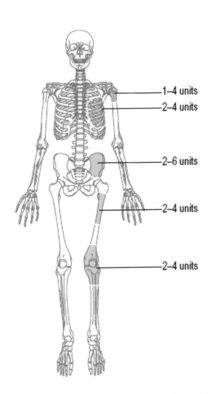

22.8 Severe injuries – blood loss in closed fractures The patient loses more blood than you think.

Management

Control bleeding   Several methods are available; the choice depends upon the severity of blood loss. Consider:

- elevation and direct pressure
- pelvic slings for unstable pelvic fractures
- use of tourniquet (e22.10)
- wound packing with haemostatic dressings
- circumferential pressure dressings
- intravenous administration of tranexamic acid (an antifibrinolytic agent).

 Maintain normothermia at all times.

Secure vascular access   Venous cannulation is usually appropriate. Site two large-bore cannulas.

- *Central venous cannulation* is associated with dangerous complications and should be avoided unless performed by an expert.
- *Femoral vein cannulation* is an option.
- *Intraosseous cannulation* has superseded cutdown. Cannulas can be inserted through bone cortex into the marrow cavity of the tibia or the humeral head using an EZ-IO® driver and needle set (**22.9**).

Administer intravascular fluids   If blood is immediately available, or haemorrhage controlled, give 2 L of warmed Hartmann's (20 mL/kg in children) followed by transfusion. If bleeding is persistent and blood unavailable, give fluids in 250 mL boluses, titrated against a palpable radial pulse; this minimizes dilutional anaemia and increased bleeding as the blood pressure is restored. There is little evidence to support the use of colloids, and the role of hypertonic solutions has yet to be determined.

Titrate fluids against response, gauged by blood pressure, pulse rate, peripheral perfusion, central venous pressure (CVP) and measurement of metabolic acidosis.

Monitor the response to a fluid challenge. Rapid responders respond quickly and remain stable; transient responders respond and then

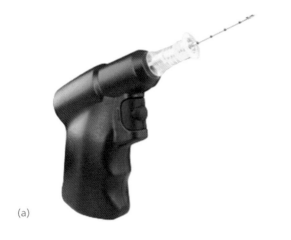

(a)

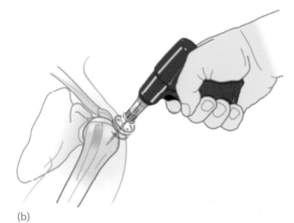

(b)

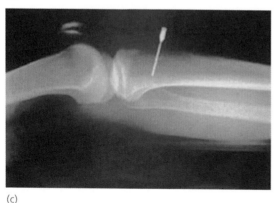

(c)

22.9 Intraosseous cannulation EZ-IO System (a) Intraosseous vascular access hand-held power driver. **(b)** Intraosseous needle insertion humeral head. **(c)** Intraosseous needle in place in the medial proximal tibia.

deteriorate, causing significant ongoing shock; non-responders show minimal or no response – suspect exsanguinating haemorrhage or other pathology (e.g. a tension pneumothorax).

Transfuse blood and blood products Transfuse blood, fresh frozen plasma and platelets in a ratio of $1:1:1$ to maintain the haemoglobin above 10 g/dL. Regularly check haemoglobin, platelet count and clotting times. Consider giving clotting factors as advised by a haematologist.

CIRCULATION – SHOCK: SUMMARY

In patients suffering from haemorrhagic, hypovolaemic shock, the source of the bleeding must be identified and surgically or radiologically controlled.

The priorities for restoring and maintaining adequate circulation are as follows:

- Control external and pelvic bleeding, give tranexamic acid and keep the patient warm.
- Administer restricted volume resuscitation with crystalloids until blood is available.
- Transfuse blood and plasma in a 1 : 1 ratio – replace blood with blood.
- Turn off the tap – call a surgeon to achieve definitive control early.

HEAD INJURIES

Most head injuries result from a blow that causes either direct damage or intracerebral movement due to rapid acceleration or deceleration.

DAMAGE CAUSED BY HEAD INJURIES

Minor contusion causing transient loss of consciousness or amnesia
Severe contusion or laceration, due either to direct injury or to shearing forces
Localized intracranial bleeding
Fractures of the skull

Diffuse oedema and a rise in intracranial pressure

High-velocity penetrating injuries (e.g. gunshot wounds) also cause diffuse and severe brain damage as the pressure wave moves across the brain

The primary brain injury occurs at the time of the initial trauma from sudden distortion and shearing of brain tissue. Swelling and raised intracerebral pressure (ICP) are compounded by hypoxia, hypercarbia and hypotension. Extradural, subdural and intracerebral bleeding may contribute further to the rise in ICP. If the ICP is sustained above 20 mmHg, permanent brain damage can result; this is *the secondary brain injury*, which accounts for a significant number of fatalities.

When pressure compensation reaches its limit, the ICP rises exponentially causing uncal herniation with pupillary dilatation on the side of the injury. Ultimately, the cerebellum herniates through the foramen magnum, leading to brainstem death.

Prompt management of the ABCs helps to prevent these secondary changes.

 It is often the *secondary* brain injury, rather than the primary brain injury, which kills or maims the patient. Maintain brain perfusion by meticulous management of ABC.

Awareness

In the UK, head injuries account for more than 50% of trauma deaths, following road traffic crashes, assaults and falls. These injuries can be classified into three groups based on the GCS.

GCS CLASSIFICATION OF HEAD INJURIES

Mild

- GCS 13–15 (80% of cases)
- 55% have mild disability at 1 year

Moderate

- GCS 9–12 (10% of cases)
- 63% have significant disability at 1 year

Severe

- GCS 3–8 (10% of cases)
- 85% have significant disability at 1 year

Recognition

During the primary survey:

- Assess the airway, cervical spine, breathing and circulation.
- *Commence resuscitation before neurological assessment in order to limit the secondary brain injury.*
- Assess the GCS; examine the pupils for equality, diameter and response to light. With increased intracranial pressure and tentorial herniation, compression of the third nerve results in dilatation of the pupil and a failure to react to light.

Reassess thoroughly *during the secondary survey*; look for lateralizing signs and motor and sensory deficits.

DIAGNOSTIC SIGNS OF A BASAL SKULL FRACTURE

Otorhinorrhoea (cerebrospinal fluid [CSF] leakage from ear or nose)

Periorbital haematomas ('raccoon eyes') (22.10)

Subconjunctival haemorrhage without a posterior margin

Retromastoid bruising (Battle's sign)

Open wounds should be gently explored with a gloved finger to exclude underlying skull fractures.

 Patients who have suffered a severe head injury or who have a suspected intracranial bleed require an *urgent CT*.

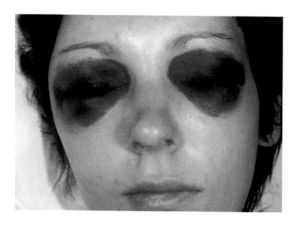

22.10 Head injury Periorbital haematomas ('racoon eyes') suggest the presence of a basal skull fracture.

SPECIFIC INDICATIONS OF A SEVERE HEAD INJURY REQUIRING CT

A drop in GCS
Suspected skull fracture
Seizures
Focal neurological signs
Vomiting
Amnesia

Management

Most head injuries are fairly trivial and require no more than careful examination and reassurance. There are several indications for admission to hospital for observation and reassessment.

INDICATIONS FOR ADMISSION TO HOSPITAL

Diminished level of consciousness
History of transient loss of consciousness or amnesia
Skull fracture
Abnormal neurological signs

In patients who appear to be comatose, drowsy, restless or merely confused, it may be difficult to distinguish the effects of a head injury from those of hypoglycaemia, alcohol or drugs. All such patients, as well as those whose cerebral dysfunction may be due to shock or hypoxia, should be graded on the GCS and kept under observation until the diagnosis is clear. If there is any chance that the patient has suffered an intracranial bleed, a CT scan is urgent.

HEAD INJURY: MANAGEMENT

Ensure exemplary oxygenation, normocapnia and normotension
For mild head injury (GCS 13–15): admission, monitoring and observation
CT and referral if deterioration is observed
For moderate head injury (GCS 9–12): CT and referral to neurosurgeon
For severe head injury (GCS 3–8): resuscitation, anaesthesia (rapid sequence induction) and intubation
Control of vascular filling pressures and CVP monitoring, and maintenance of arterial normotension
Early CT and referral to neurosurgeon; IV mannitol 0.5 mg/kg if advised
Urgent transfer to a specialist unit

CONCUSSION

Following a blow, there is a transient loss of consciousness, often associated with amnesia. However, brief the period of unconsciousness, the skull should be X-rayed (**22.11**). If the patient was unconscious for only a few minutes and is now fully conscious, and a skull fracture has been excluded, they can be allowed to go home in the care of a responsible adult who will look after them for the next 48 hours. If this cannot be arranged, they should be admitted for observation. Those with either a skull fracture or an impaired level of consciousness will also need a CT scan.

SCALP WOUNDS

After thorough cleaning, scalp wounds can be sutured, provided there is no underlying depressed fracture.

FRACTURES

- *A linear fracture* may be quite harmless, but a CT should be obtained to exclude intracranial damage or haematoma (**22.12**). If there is a CSF leak (otorrhoea or rhinorrhoea), the patient is given prophylactic benzyl penicillin.
- *A depressed fracture* requires exploration, elevation and clearance of damaged tissue.

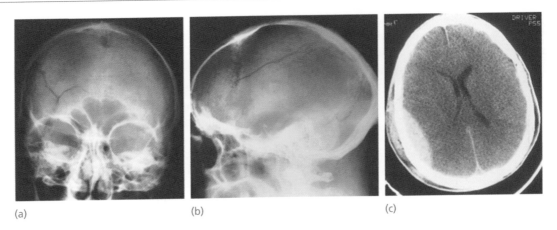

(a)   (b)   (c)

22.11 Head injuries – imaging **(a,b)** X-rays showing a fracture of the parietal bone. **(c)** The CT scan shows an extradural haematoma with distortion of the lateral ventricle on that side.

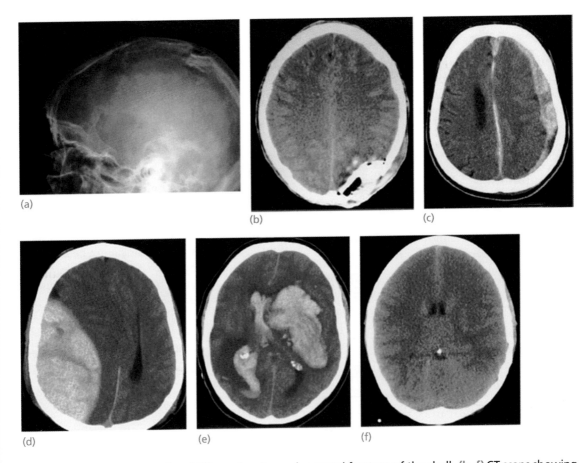

(a)

(b)   (c)

(d)   (e)   (f)

22.12 Fractured skull – imaging **(a)** X-ray showing a depressed fracture of the skull. **(b–f)** CT scans showing various injuries: **(b)** a fracture; **(c)** a subdural haematoma; **(d)** an extradural haematoma and compression of the left ventricle; **(e)** an intracerebral haematoma; **(f)** diffuse brain injury with loss of both ventricles.

EXTRADURAL HAEMATOMA

The classic scenario is of a patient who has a head injury but seems to be perfectly well, is allowed to go home and then rapidly becomes unconscious. There may be a minor fracture which causes bleeding and cerebral compression. Look for a fixed dilated pupil on the affected side. *CT* shows an extradural haematoma and a shift of the brain.

 Extradural haematoma requires urgent treatment: burr holes and evacuation of the haematoma; if necessary, the middle meningeal artery is ligated.

SIGNS FOR REFERRAL TO A NEUROSURGEON

Persistent coma after initial resuscitation (GCS <8)
Unexplained confusion >4 hours
Post-admission deterioration in GCS
Progressive, focal neurological signs
Seizure without full recovery
Definite or suspected penetrating injury
CSF leak

SEVERE BRAIN CONTUSION

Patients with severe head injuries (a GCS score of 8 or less) require early intubation and ventilation with management on an intensive care unit (ICU) until recovery or brain death. Operative treatment may be required. The main indication for craniotomy is the development of an intracranial haematoma.

HEAD INJURIES: SUMMARY

Head-injured patients require early assessment and recognition of their brain injury.
A severe blow to the head causes a primary brain injury.
Hypoxia and hypercarbia cause cerebral swelling and a secondary brain injury.
Secondary brain injury should be minimized by optimal oxygenation, ventilation and blood pressure management.

ABDOMINAL INJURIES

 The immediately life-threatening injury is bleeding into the peritoneal cavity.

Awareness

Blunt abdominal trauma is a cause of avoidable death but is difficult to detect. Visceral rupture and laceration cause internal bleeding.

Penetrating injuries between the nipples and the perineum produce unpredictable damage (e.g. from tumbling and fragmenting bullet fragments). High-velocity rounds transfer kinetic energy to the viscera, causing cavitation and tissue destruction despite deceptively small entrance wounds (22.13). Look carefully for stab wounds; they may also be very small but they can penetrate deeply

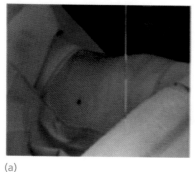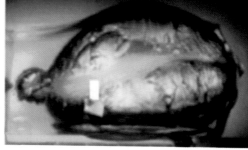

(a)   (b)

22.13 High-velocity gunshot injury (a) Entry wound; (b) tissue cavitation.

and damage several structures. Rapid deceleration can rupture internal organs (e22.11).

Recognition

During the primary survey, inspect the abdomen for wounds, abrasions and contusions. Examine flanks, posterior abdomen, back, perineum and genitalia, and perform rectal examination. eFAST has supplanted diagnostic peritoneal lavage. *Early CT* is indicated, but a shocked patient may need urgent transfer to surgery.

Management

Initial management of an abdominal injury is to manage shock as described in circulation management and control external bleeding. If unresponsive, administer further fluid and transfuse blood. Pass a gastric tube and a urinary catheter unless signs of urethral injury are present.

Bleeding into the abdomen is an indication for immediate laparotomy. The patient will require supportive critical care, and may require ventilation on an ICU.

ABDOMINAL INJURIES: SUMMARY

Abdominal injuries are difficult to assess in the multiply injured patient.
The immediate threat to life is bleeding into the peritoneal cavity.
Shock should be treated effectively.
Early imaging with eFAST and CT should be performed.
Early consultation with a surgeon should be facilitated – diagnostic or definitive laparotomy may be required.

MUSCULOSKELETAL INJURIES

 Pelvic fractures and femoral shaft fractures can cause death from haemorrhage; in the absence of catastrophic bleeding, musculoskeletal injuries are not immediately life-threatening, but they may nevertheless be limb-threatening.

PELVIC FRACTURES

Bleeding into the pelvis and retroperitoneum can result in non-responsive shock. Potential causes are road accidents, falls from a height and crush injuries.

The injury may be suspected during the primary survey as a cause of circulatory failure.

DIAGNOSTIC SIGNS OF PELVIC FRACTURE

Pelvic ring tenderness
Leg shortening
Swelling and bruising of the lower abdomen, the thighs, the perineum, the scrotum or vulva

---

Look for blood at urethral meatus. Obtain an anteroposterior (AP) *X-ray and/or CT* if the patient is stable. The CT will show the fracture and the extent of bleeding.

Management

Treat shock. Position a pelvic compression device such as the SAM Sling™ (22.14) around the pelvis at the level of the greater trochanters, and tighten as indicated. If these are not available, manual approximation can be used; this can be facilitated with a sheet wrapped around the pelvis and twisted anteriorly.

Once in place, do not remove this until surgical intervention is available. Developments in

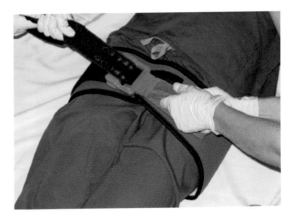

22.14 SAM Sling™ Ratcheted compression belt in use.

interventional radiology have enabled embolization to be used to control haemorrhage from a fractured pelvis.

> **PELVIC FRACTURES: SUMMARY**
>
> Pelvic fractures can result in life-threatening haemorrhage and should be recognized and managed as part of the circulation assessment during the primary survey.
> Pelvic compression devices should be used to minimize bleeding, and a rapid surgical referral should be made for definitive management.

SPINAL INJURIES

Indirect injuries are the most common, typically the result of falls or vehicular accidents. *Direct injuries* are usually associated with firearms and knives. There is an association between cervical and spinal damage with all injuries above the clavicles, and 5% of head-injured patients have an associated spinal injury; 10% of those with a cervical spine fracture have a second, non-contiguous spinal fracture.

A high spinal transection will cause vasodilatory, neurogenic shock.

> **DIAGNOSTIC SIGNS OF A HIGH SPINAL INJURY**
>
> Hypotension
> Low diastolic blood pressure
> Widened pulse pressure
> Bradycardia
> Warm, well-perfused extremities

Spinal injuries are usually recognized during the secondary survey. Be careful to maintain immobilization throughout the examination; log-roll the patient to examine the vertebral column from neck to sacrum. Perform a rectal examination to assess anal tone, and identify loss of somatic sensory and motor function.

If the casualty is conscious, has no neck pain, has no distracting painful injury, is not intoxicated and has not received any analgesia, the cervical spine can be examined and a fracture clinically excluded to enable immobilization to be dispensed with. Obtain *X-ray and/or CT* during the secondary survey.

Management

In high spinal transections, the patient's respiratory function may be compromised, leading to ventilatory failure. This may require rapid sequence induction and ventilation by an experienced anaesthetist.

Neurogenic shock may need circulatory support with vasoconstrictors and chronotropes.

Spinal fractures and neurological deficit are managed by immobilization and referral to a spinal surgeon.

> **SPINAL INJURIES: SUMMARY**
>
> Spinal injuries should be identified during the secondary survey and managed according to the ABCs.
> Immobilization is crucial throughout, and ventilatory and circulatory failure must be recognized and managed.
> Injuries should be excluded clinically, or with CT and MRI, as soon as possible.

LONG-BONE INJURIES

Musculoskeletal injuries occur in 85% of patients sustaining blunt trauma. Although not immediately life-threatening, they present a potential threat to life and threaten the integrity and survival of the limb. Crush injuries can lead to compartment syndrome, myoglobin release and renal failure.

Examine the patient from head to toe in all planes. Examine limbs but do not specifically elicit crepitus. Assess peripheral circulation and neurological status. Confirm the presence of pulses with Doppler ultrasound. Obtain *X-rays* as soon as the patient is stable.

Management

Ensure that the airway and ventilation are optimized, and then control limb haemorrhage with direct pressure, tourniquets, wound packing or haemostatic dressings as described previously. Large tissue deficits may need ongoing fluid and blood replacement as immediate haemorrhage control can be difficult.

Reduce fractures and dislocations and splint in the anatomical position.

LIMB INJURIES: SUMMARY

Limb injuries are not immediately life-threatening in the absence of catastrophic haemorrhage.

They should be recognized and initially managed in the secondary survey.

Fracture reduction, splinting and immobilization are instituted before prompt surgical consultation.

Antibiotics should be given early in open fractures.

BURNS

Risk is highest in the 18–35 year age group; serious burns occur most frequently in children under 5 years. The mortality is 4% in specialist burns hospitals, with a higher death rate in patients over 65 years.

THERMAL BURNS

The threat to life arises through compromise of the airway, breathing and circulation.

Inhalation of super-heated gases and toxic smoke causes inhalational burns, smoke intoxication and carbon monoxide poisoning. Direct thermal injury is usually limited to the upper airway and can result in rapid airway obstruction. Smoke inhalation initiates an inflammatory reaction in the bronchioles, leading to bronchospasm, oedema and respiratory failure.

Carbon monoxide poisoning causes cerebral hypoxia and coma, due to the tight binding of carbon monoxide to the haemoglobin, forming carboxyhaemoglobin. Hydrogen cyanide can also be present, leading to profound tissue hypoxia.

Depth of burn is classified according to the degree and extent of tissue damage.

Burns are diagnosed during the primary survey, to determine immediately life-threatening airway injuries, respiratory failure, shock and coma. Blood carboxyhaemoglobin levels are assayed to quantify carbon monoxide poisoning.

DIAGNOSTIC SIGNS OF THERMAL BURN AIRWAY INJURIES

Facial burns
Singed nasal hair
Soot in the mouth or nose
Hoarseness
Carbonaceous sputum
Expiratory wheezing
Stridor

Assess depth of the burn (Table 22.2) and the extent as a percentage of body surface area (BSA) using the 'rule of nines' (22.15). The palmar surface of the patient's hand, including the fingers, represents approximately 1% of the BSA. The values are different in infants since they have a disproportionately larger head and smaller lower limb surface areas.

Management

Secure the airway with anaesthetic support, and optimize oxygenation and ventilation. This

Table 22.2 Depth of burn

Depth of burn	Damage	Clinical features
First degree	Epidermal	Reddening and pain without blistering
Second degree	Dermal	Superficial or deep partial-thickness with pain, blistering and variable skin damage
Third degree	Full-thickness	Painless, charred, leathery with skin destruction
Fourth degree	Subcutaneous	Deep tissue destruction

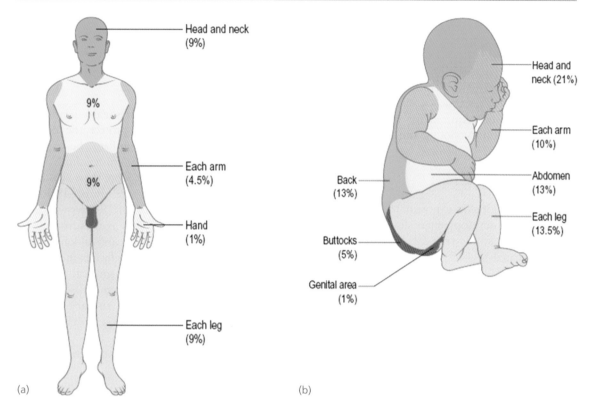

22.15 Burns (a) Extent of burns in adults – the 'rule of nines'. (Note that the back of the thorax and the back of the lower torso each carry another 9%; the back of each arm carries another 4.5% and the back of each leg carries another 9%). **(b)** Burn extents in infants differ markedly from those in adults, as they have a large surface area for the head.

can be very difficult if the airway is burnt by inhalation.

Carboxyhaemoglobin levels may indicate the need for hyperbaric therapy and ventilation with 100% oxygen. Circumferential neck and chest burns may need to be incised to allow effective breathing and ventilation.

The circulation should be supported in any burn patient with signs of shock or a burn greater than 20% BSA. Two large-bore intravenous cannulae are sited, preferably although not necessarily, through unburned skin. If intravenous cannulation or central venous cannulation is not possible, intraosseous or intravenous cut-down techniques should be used, as shock will develop rapidly in patients with large and deep burns. Calculate the volume and rate of fluid administration from the time of the burn according to the Parkland formula.

> **PARKLAND FORMULA: INTRAVENOUS FLUID REQUIREMENTS IN PARTIAL- AND FULL-THICKNESS BURN PATIENTS**
>
> **Adults**
>
> Hartmann's or Ringer's lactate:
> 4 mL × weight (kg) × % BSA over initial 24 hours
> Half over first 8 hours from the time of burn (other half over subsequent 16 hours)
>
> **Children**
>
> Hartmann's or Ringer's lactate:
> 3 mL × weight (kg) × % BSA over initial 24 hours plus maintenance
> Half over first 8 hours from the time of burn (other half over subsequent 16 hours)

SECTION 3 TRAUMA

Dress wounds with loose, clean, dry dressings, plastic sandwich wrap, specialized gel dressings or saline-moistened dressings. Patients with circumferential, deep burns of the limbs may develop eschars with compromise of the distal circulation requiring surgical escharotomy. Opioid analgesia will be required for partial-thickness burns in addition to cooling and dressing.

CHEMICAL BURNS

These occur with skin exposure to strong alkalis and acids. Full development is slower than that in thermal injury, so the true extent can initially be underestimated.

Management

Minimize irreversible damage and maximize salvage of reversible damage. If dry powder is present, brush it off before irrigating with tap water. Do not use neutralizing agents.

 Make an urgent referral to a burns unit. Involve a burns specialist for all patients with severe or unusual burns.

Determine the chemical involved and its concentration.

* *Alkali burns* are often full-thickness and look pale, leathery and slippery.
* *Acid burns* are frequently partial-thickness and result in erythema and erosion.

ELECTRICAL BURNS

These are caused by contact between an electrical source and earth. Severe electrical skin burns are associated with high-voltage shocks, whereas domestic low-voltage shocks may cause death from ventricular fibrillation without superficial burning. Electrical muscle damage can result in rhabdomyolysis and renal failure.

The airway may be obstructed if the victim is unconscious and prolonged apnoea may follow paralysis of the respiratory muscles. The heart may arrest in ventricular fibrillation or

asystole. Examine the entry and exit points, as the extent of underlying muscle damage may not be apparent.

Management

The immediate priority is personal safety of the rescuer. Secure the airway, protect the cervical spine and oxygenate and ventilate the casualty. Gain vascular access and administer fluids if the casualty is shocked or burnt more than 20% BSA. If cardiac arrest occurs, institute advanced life support (ALS). Monitor the heart for arrhythmias. There may be musculoskeletal injuries from associated trauma or muscle spasm and all long bones should be examined and *X-rayed* when indicated.

Tissue damage may need surgical debridement, and compartment syndrome may develop, requiring fasciotomies. Site a urinary catheter and test urine for myoglobinuria; treat with IV fluids and mannitol.

Consult early with burns and critical care specialists.

COLD INJURY BURNS

Cold injury can be systemic (hypothermia) or localized (tissue damage).

HYPOTHERMIA

Hypothermia is a core temperature of below 35 °C (95 °F). Systemic effects depend on the degree of heat loss: as the core temperature drops, conscious level deteriorates and the airway obstructs as coma ensues. Respiratory and cardiac functions deteriorate until respiratory and cardiac arrest result.

LOCALIZED COLD INJURY

Localized cold injury is seen in three forms: frostnip, frostbite and non-freezing injury.

Frostnip   This is reversible on warming.

Frostbite   causes freezing and tissue damage; four degrees are recognized:

* *first degree* – hyperaemia and oedema without skin necrosis

- *second degree* – vesicle formation with partial-thickness skin necrosis
- *third degree* – full-thickness and subcutaneous tissue necrosis, with haemorrhagic vesicle formation
- *fourth degree* – deep necrosis, including muscle and bone.

Non-freezing injury presents as trench or immersion foot, with microvascular endothelial damage, stasis and vascular occlusion.

- *At the primary survey*, the patient is cold to the touch, looks grey and is peripherally cyanosed. A temperature probe will gauge the degree of hypothermia.
- *During the secondary survey*, local injuries are assessed. The affected part of the body initially appears hard, cold, white and anaesthetic.

Management

HYPOTHERMIA

Hypothermia is treated by securing the airway, optimizing oxygenation and ventilation and treating shock with warmed IV fluids.

Rewarming depends on the degree of hypothermia.

- *For mild and moderate hypothermia*, use passive and active external rewarming.
- *For severe hypothermia and hypothermic cardiac arrest*, active internal (core) rewarming such as thoracic lavage or cardiopulmonary bypass is needed.

LOCALIZED COLD INJURY

Localized cold injury is managed by removing wet clothing, elevating and dressing the extremities. Rapid rewarming is the most effective therapy for frostbite. As soon as possible, the injured extremity should be placed in gently circulating water at a temperature of 40–42 °C (104–107.6 °F) for approximately 10–30 minutes, until the distal extremity is pliable and erythematous. Surgical debridement may be required.

> **BURNS: SUMMARY**
>
> *Thermal burns* are assessed by depth and extent, and managed by addressing the airway, breathing and circulation. Huge volumes of intravenous fluids may be required to maintain homeostasis.
> *Chemical burns* are treated primarily by copious irrigation with water.
> *Electrical burns* may be associated with severe tissue damage and systemic disturbance, and treatment is needed for the local burns and systemic cardiac, respiratory and renal complications.
> *Cold injury* can be systemic hypothermia, which is treated by active external and internal rewarming, depending on severity, or localized tissue damage. Localized tissue damage is treated by rapid rewarming and delayed surgical debridement.

CRUSH SYNDROME

This is seen when a limb is compressed for extended periods (e.g. following entrapment in a vehicle or rubble). The crushed limb is under-perfused and myonecrosis follows, leading to the release of toxic metabolites when the limb is freed and so generating a re-perfusion injury. Reactive oxygen metabolites create further tissue injury. Membrane damage and capillary fluid reabsorption failure result in swelling that may lead to a compartment syndrome, thus creating more tissue damage from escalating ischaemia. Tissue necrosis also causes systemic problems such as renal failure from free myoglobin, which is precipitated in the renal glomeruli. Myonecrosis may cause a metabolic acidosis with hyperkalaemia and hypocalcaemia.

Clinical features and treatment

The compromised limb is pulseless and becomes red, swollen and blistered; sensation and muscle power may be lost.

The most important measure is prevention. From an intensive care perspective, a high urine flow is encouraged with alkalization of the urine with sodium bicarbonate; this prevents myoglobin precipitating in the renal tubules. If oliguria or renal failure occurs, renal haemofiltration will be needed.

If a compartment syndrome develops, and is confirmed by pressure measurements, a fasciotomy is indicated. Excision of dead muscle must be radical to avoid sepsis. Similarly, if there is an open wound, this should be managed aggressively. If there is no open wound and the compartment pressures are not high, the risk of infection is probably lower if early surgery is avoided.

MULTIPLE ORGAN FAILURE

Multiple organ failure or dysfunction syndrome (MODS) is the clinical manifestation of a severe systemic inflammatory reaction, following a triggering event such as trauma, infection or inflammation. It develops in 5–15% of patients requiring ICU admission; it is now the commonest cause of long stays in surgical ICUs and the most frequent cause of death.

In its classical form (following severe sepsis), it manifests with pulmonary features of ARDS and is most likely to occur in elderly patients with poor health. Its pathogenesis is still unclear but it appears to be a disorder of the host defence system, involving an unregulated and exaggerated immune response which results in an excessive release of inflammatory mediators. It is these mediators that produce widespread microvascular damage leading to organ failure (e22.12).

MODS usually progresses through four clinical phases.

CLINICAL PHASES OF MODS

1 *Shock* (hypoperfusion)
2 *Active resuscitation*
3 *Stable hypermetabolism*
   (systemic inflammatory response)
4 *Organ failure*

In the majority of critically ill patients who develop MODS, the lungs are the first organs to fail; the other organs following in a sequential fashion. Dysfunction ranges from minor changes to massive alterations in pulmonary physiology – the hallmark of ARDS. Over a period of a few days the picture may change from pulmonary congestion to diffuse alveolar destruction. The early changes are reversible, but once diffuse alveolar damage occurs, there is usually an inexorable progression to severe hypoxaemia. In the worst cases, this is followed by multiple organ failure and death.

Clinical features

After a variable period following injury with hypovolaemic shock, the patient develops mild dyspnoea. Even before this, if blood gases are measured, they may show a diminished PaO_2. These changes are common after long-bone fractures, and 'fat embolism' is often suspected.

By the second or third day, the clinical features are more obvious: the patient is restless, with an increased pulse rate, oliguria, mild cyanosis and signs of respiratory distress. *X-rays* may now show diffuse pulmonary infiltrates (**22.16**). Special lung function tests are required to show the full extent of the condition.

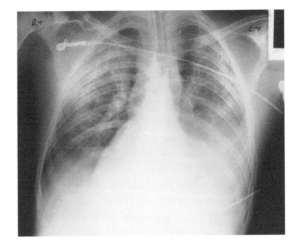

22.16 Adult respiratory distress syndrome X-ray showing diffuse pulmonary infiltrates in both lungs.

In the most severe cases, by about 10 days post injury, pulmonary deterioration is followed by liver failure and renal failure. The changes are irreversible and the outcome is fatal.

Treatment

 The most important aspect of management is the early and effective treatment of shock.

There is also evidence that the following measures will reduce the incidence of pulmonary dysfunction and organ failure, especially in patients with multiple injuries:

- early stabilization of fractures
- early excision of necrotic tissue
- prompt treatment of infection
- expert attention to nutritional requirements.

The treatment of established ARDS is supportive and aims to minimize further lung damage until recovery occurs, while optimizing oxygen delivery to the tissues. This requires highly specialized methods of artificial ventilation and continuous cardiopulmonary assessment in an intensive care facility.

FAT EMBOLISM SYNDROME

Circulating fat globules larger than 10 μm in diameter occur in most adults after closed fractures of long bones, and histological traces of fat can be found in the lungs and other internal organs. A small percentage of these patients develop clinical features similar to those of ARDS; this was recognized as *fat embolism syndrome* long before ARDS entered the medical literature. Whether fat embolism syndrome is an expression of the same condition or whether it is an entirely separate entity is still uncertain.

The source of the fat emboli is probably the bone marrow, and the condition is more common in patients with multiple fractures.

Clinical features

Early warning signs of fat embolism (usually within 72 hours of injury) are a slight rise of temperature and pulse rate. In more pronounced cases, there is breathlessness and mild mental confusion or restlessness. Pathognomonic signs are petechiae on the trunk, axillae and in the conjunctival folds and retinae. In more severe cases, there may be respiratory distress and coma, due to both brain emboli and hypoxia from involvement of the lungs. The features at this stage are essentially those of ARDS.

There is no infallible test for fat embolism; however, urinalysis may show fat globules in the urine and the blood PaO_2 should always be monitored; values below 8 kPa (60 mmHg or less) within the first 72 hours of any major injury must be regarded as suspicious. A *chest X-ray* may show classical changes in the lungs.

Management

Management of severe fat embolism is supportive. Symptoms can be reduced with the use of supplemental high inspired oxygen concentrations immediately after injury. Prompt stabilization of long-bone fractures also appears to reduce the likelihood of fat embolism occurring; this also allows the patient to be nursed in the sitting position, which optimizes the ventilation–perfusion match in the lungs. Intramedullary nailing is not thought to increase the risk of developing the syndrome.

Principles of fractures

23

■ How fractures occur	513	**Open fractures**	**528**
■ Types of fracture	514	■ Gunshot Injuries	532
■ Classification of fractures	514	**Complications of fractures**	**532**
■ How fractures heal	515	■ Early complications	533
■ Clinical features of fractures	518	■ Late complications	537
■ Secondary injuries	521	**Stress (fatigue) fractures**	**543**
Treatment of closed fractures	**521**	**Pathological fractures**	**544**
■ Reduction	521	**Injuries of the physis**	**546**
■ Holding reduction	522	**Injuries to joints**	**548**
■ Restoration of function	528		

A fracture is a break in the structural continuity of bone. It may be no more than a crack but more often the break is complete. The fragments may be displaced or undisplaced. If the overlying skin remains intact, it is a closed fracture; if the skin or one of the body cavities is breached, it is an open fracture (also known as a *compound fracture*), liable to contamination and infection.

HOW FRACTURES OCCUR

Fractures are caused by:

* injury
* repetitive stress
* abnormal weakening of the bone ('pathological' fracture).

FRACTURES DUE TO INJURY

Most fractures are caused by sudden and excessive force (overloading), which may be direct or indirect.

* With a *direct force (direct injury)*, the bone breaks at the point of impact causing a transverse fracture with or without a butterfly fragment; the soft tissues are also damaged.
* With an *indirect force (indirect injury)*, the bone breaks at a distance from where the force is applied; soft-tissue damage at the fracture site is not inevitable.

FATIGUE OR STRESS FRACTURES

These occur in normal bone which is subjected to repeated heavy loading, typically in high loading conditions or when the intensity of exercise is significantly increased from baseline. The heavy loading creates minute deformations that initiate the normal process of remodelling (*Wolff's law*). Repeated and prolonged loading causes bone resorption to occur faster than replacement, leaving the area liable to fracture. Similar conditions may occur if medication alters the normal balance of bone resorption and replacement.

PATHOLOGICAL FRACTURES

Fractures may occur even with normal stresses if the bone has been weakened (e.g. osteoporosis, Paget's disease, bisphosphonate therapy) or through a lytic lesion (bone cyst or metastasis).

TYPES OF FRACTURE

Fractures are variable in appearance but for practical reasons they are divided into a few well-defined groups.

COMPLETE FRACTURES

The bone is split into two or more fragments (23.1).

- In a *transverse fracture,* the fragments usually remain in place after reduction.
- In an *oblique or spiral,* they tend to shorten and redisplace even with splintage.
- In an *impacted fracture,* the fragments are jammed tightly together and the fracture line is indistinct.

- A *comminuted fracture* is one with more than two fragments that is often unstable.

INCOMPLETE FRACTURES

The bone is incompletely divided and the periosteum remains in continuity. In a *greenstick fracture* the bone is buckled or bent; this is seen in children. Children can also sustain injuries where the bone is only plastically deformed (misshapen). In contrast, *compression fractures* occur when cancellous bone is crumpled, such as in vertebral bodies, calcaneum and the tibial plateau.

CLASSIFICATION OF FRACTURES

Sorting fractures into groups with similar features brings advantages when done well: it allows information about a fracture to be applied to others in the group and facilitates a common dialogue.

A universal, anatomically based system facilitates communication and exchange of data from a variety of countries and populations, thus contributing to advances in research and treatment. An

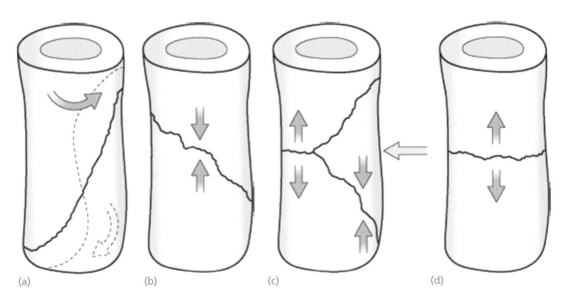

(a)   (b)   (c)   (d)

Figure 23.1 Mechanism of injury (a) Spiral pattern (twisting); (b) short oblique pattern (compression); (c) triangular 'butterfly' fragment (bending) and (d) transverse pattern (tension). Spiral and some (long) oblique patterns are usually due to low-energy indirect injuries; bending and transverse patterns are caused by high-energy direct trauma.

SECTION 3 TRAUMA

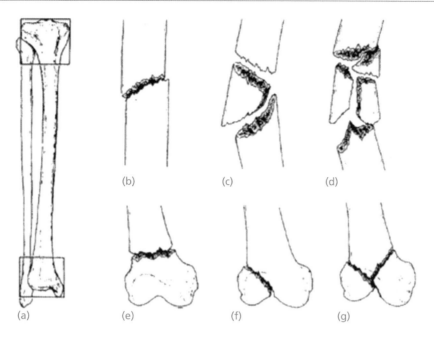

Figure 23.2 Müller's classification (a) Each long bone has three segments – proximal, diaphyseal and distal; the proximal and distal segments are defined by a square based on the widest part of the bone. **(b–d)** Diaphyseal fractures may be simple, wedge or complex. **(e–g)** Proximal and distal fractures may be extra-articular, partial articular or complete articular.

alphanumeric classification developed by Müller and colleagues, known as AO/OTA classification and fulfilling the objective of being comprehensive, has now been adapted and revised (**23.2**). In this system, the first digit specifies the bone (1 = humerus, 2 = radius/ulna, 3 = femur, 4 = tibia/fibula, 5 = spine, 6 = pelvis/acetabulum, 7 = hand, 8 = foot, 9 = craniomaxillofacial bones) and the second digit specifies the segment (1 = proximal, 2 = diaphyseal, 3 = distal, 4 = malleolar). A letter specifies the fracture pattern (for diaphysis: A = simple, B = wedge, C = complex; for metaphysis: A = extra-articular, B = partial articular, C = complete articular). Two further numbers specify the detailed morphology of the fracture.

HOW FRACTURES HEAL

Fracture healing is characterized by a process of new bone formation and fusion of the fragments. The bone heals by either primary (without callus formation) or secondary (with callus formation) fracture healing. The process varies according to the type of bone involved and the amount of movement at the fracture site. The mechanical strain applied across the fracture gap plays a major role in directing the healing response. Absolute stability and compression leads to primary bone healing, while relative stability leads to secondary bone healing. Excessive motion may lead to delayed or non-union.

Callus formation occurs in response to movement at the fracture site. It serves to stabilize the fragments as rapidly as possible. Most fractures are splinted in order to:

- alleviate pain
- ensure that union takes place in good position
- permit early movement of the limb and a return of function.

HEALING BY DIRECT UNION (PRIMARY BONE HEALING)

If the fracture site is absolutely stable (e.g. impacted or compressed with absolute stability), there is no stimulus for callus. Osteoblastic

SECTION 3 TRAUMA

new bone formation occurs directly between the fragments. Where the exposed fracture surfaces are in intimate contact, internal bridging may occasionally occur *(contact healing)*. Gaps are invaded by new capillaries and osteoprogenitor cells growing in from the edges with new bone laid down on the exposed surface *(gap healing)*. Where the gaps are narrow (>200 μm), osteogenesis produces lamellar bone; wider gaps are filled first by woven bone, which is then remodelled to lamellar bone. By 3–4 weeks, penetration and bridging of the area by bone remodelling units occurs (osteoclastic 'cutting cones' followed by osteoblasts). Rigid fixation may therefore mean there is a long period during which the bone depends entirely upon the metal implant for its integrity.

HEALING BY CALLUS (SECONDARY BONE HEALING)

Healing by callus, though indirect, has distinct advantages: it ensures mechanical strength while the bone ends heal, and with increasing stress the callus grows stronger.

Secondary bone healing is the most common form of healing in tubular bones; in the absence of rigid fixation, it proceeds in five stages (**23.3**):

1. haematoma
2. inflammation
3. soft callus formation
4. hard callus formation (**23.4**)
5. remodelling.

 The periosteum is an excellent source of local mesenchymal stem cells that can enhance bone repair. It is imperative that, as much as it is possible, the periosteum is left in place and remains viable.

UNION, DELAYED UNION AND NON-UNION

Time to union varies due to age, constitution, blood supply, type of fracture and other factors.

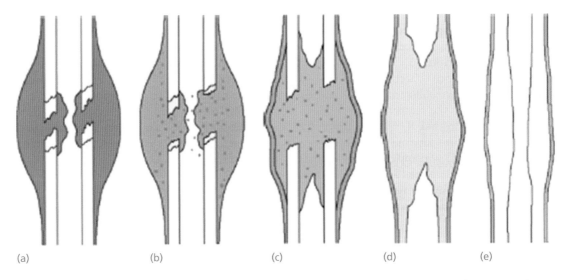

(a)   (b)   (c)   (d)   (e)

Figure 23.3 Fracture healing Five stages of healing. (**a**) *Haematoma:* there is tissue damage and bleeding at the fracture site. (**b**) *Inflammation:* inflammatory cells (cytokines) appear in the haematoma; the bone ends die back for a few millimetres. (**c**) *Soft callus formation:* the cell population changes to osteoblasts; over time, the callus calcifies and woven bone appears in the fracture callus. (**d**) *Hard callus formation:* the fracture is solidly united. (**e**) *Remodelling:* the newly formed bone is remodelled to resemble the normal structure. Woven bone is replaced by lamellar bone.

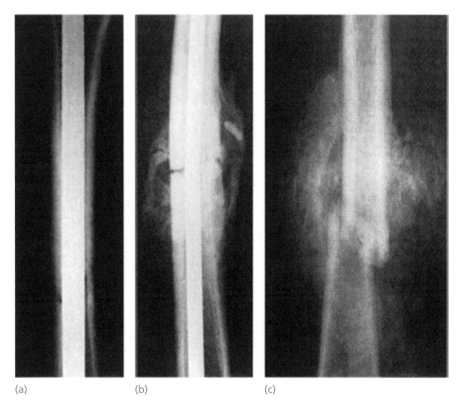

(a) (b) (c)

Figure 23.4 Callus and movement Three different cases of femoral shaft fractures. **(a)** and **(b)** are both 6 weeks post fixation: **(a)** the Kuntscher nail fitted tightly, preventing movement, and there is no callus; **(b)** the nail fitted loosely, permitting some movement, so there is callus. **(c)** This patient had cerebral irritation and thrashed around wildly; at 3 weeks, callus is excessive.

A spiral fracture in the upper limb takes 6–8 weeks to unite; in the lower limb it needs twice as long. Add 25% if the fracture is not spiral or if it involves the femur. Children's fractures unite more quickly.

Union

Union is complete repair; the ensheathing callus is calcified. Clinically, the fracture site is painless on palpation and weight-bearing. *X-rays* show bridging callus. The fracture line is completely or almost obliterated and crossed by bone trabeculae. Repair is complete and further protection is unnecessary.

Delayed union

In delayed union, the fracture healing is not taking place at the expected rate and time, but healing is still possible with appropriate measures. Clinically, the fractured limb has local swelling and movement or partial weight-bearing is painful.

Non-union

This is a bone that has failed to unite. Unless there is bone loss, non-union is usually defined as fracture that has not healed 9 months post operation and there is no visible progress of healing during the last 3 months. Typical causes are:

- mechanical instability
- impaired vascularity
- infection.

A painless pseudoarthrosis may form and non-unions may be *hypertrophic* or *atrophic* (**23.5**).

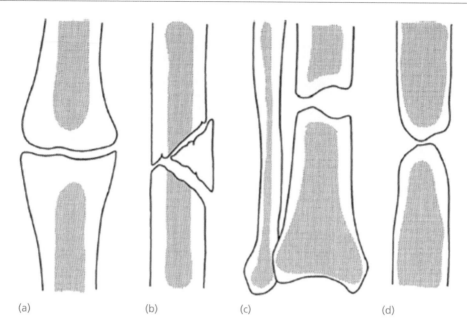

(a)   (b)   (c)   (d)

Figure 23.5 Non-unions Aseptic non-unions are generally divided into hypertrophic and atrophic types. Hypertrophic non-unions often have florid streams of callus around the fracture gap – the result of insufficient stability. They are sometimes given colourful names, such as elephant's foot (a). In contrast, atrophic non-unions usually arise from an impaired repair process; they are classified according to the X-ray appearance as necrotic (b); gap (c); atrophic (d).

CLINICAL FEATURES OF FRACTURES

HISTORY

There is usually a history of injury, then inability to use the limb, but beware that the fracture may be remote from the point of impact. Note the patient's age and mechanism. If a fracture occurs with trivial trauma, suspect a pathological lesion. Pain, bruising and swelling are common but not discriminatory. *Deformity* is more suggestive of a fracture or dislocation.

Always enquire about symptoms elsewhere:

- increasing pain
- numbness or loss of movement
- skin pallor or cyanosis
- associated features such as blood in the urine, abdominal pain, difficulty with breathing or transient loss of consciousness.

Multiply injured patients should be managed as described in Chapter 22. Do not forget the

ABCs: look for, and if necessary attend to, **A**irway obstruction (with **C**ervical spine immobilization), **B**reathing problems, **C**irculatory problems.

LOCAL SIGNS

Injured tissues must be handled gently – deliberately eliciting crepitus or abnormal movement is unnecessarily painful when *X-ray* will provide the required information. Nevertheless, a systematic approach is always helpful.

PHYSICAL EXAMINATION

1 Examine the most obviously injured part.
2 Test for artery and nerve damage.
3 Look for associated injuries in the region.
4 Look for associated injuries in distant parts.

Look

Swelling, bruising and deformity may be obvious. Check whether the skin is intact. If the skin is breached and communicates with the fracture, the injury is '*open*'.

Feel

Palpate for localized tenderness at the site of any potential fracture or dislocation-associated injuries. For example, isolated fractures of the proximal fibula are unusual, so check for an ankle injury. Vascular and nerve abnormalities should be tested for, both before and after treatment.

Move

Crepitus and abnormal movement may be present. It is more important to ask if the patient can move the joints distal to the injury.

IMAGING

- *X-ray* examination is mandatory (**23.6**). Remember the '*rule of twos*'.

X-RAY EXAMINATION: RULE OF TWOS

Two views A fracture or a dislocation may be missed in one plane. At least two orthogonal views (anteroposterior and lateral), and sometimes more, must be taken.

Two joints In the forearm or leg, one bone may be fractured and angulated. Angulation, however, is impossible unless the other bone is also broken, or a joint dislocated. The joints above and below the fracture must both be included.

Two limbs In children, the appearance of immature epiphyses may confuse the diagnosis of a fracture; X-rays of the uninjured limb can be used for comparison.

Two injuries Severe force often causes injuries at more than one level. Thus,

---

with fractures of the calcaneum or femur, it is important also to check the pelvis and spine.

Two occasions Some fractures are notoriously difficult to detect soon after injury, but another X-ray examination a week or two later may show the lesion (e.g. scaphoid and stress fractures).

- *Computed tomography (CT)* may be helpful in lesions of the spine or for complex joint fractures; indeed, these cross-sectional images are essential for accurate visualization of fractures in 'difficult' sites such as the calcaneum or acetabulum.
- *Magnetic resonance imaging (MRI)* may be the only way of showing whether a fractured vertebra is threatening to compress the spinal cord.
- *Radioisotope scanning* may be helpful in diagnosing a suspected stress fracture or other undisplaced fractures.
- *Ultrasound* can be used in children to diagnose fracture.

DESCRIPTION

Patient characteristics and comorbidities, secondary injuries and last but not least the fracture pattern and displacement are important features that will help the surgeon begin to formulate a management plan. The AO/OTA classification offers an easy-to-use and globally accepted system for all bones.

Pattern of the fracture

- *Transverse fractures* are slow to unite because the area of contact is small but may be stable under compression if opposed.
- *Spiral fractures* unite more rapidly but are not stable under compression.
- *Comminuted fractures* are often slow to unite because they are:
  - associated with more severe soft-tissue damage
  - likely to be unstable.

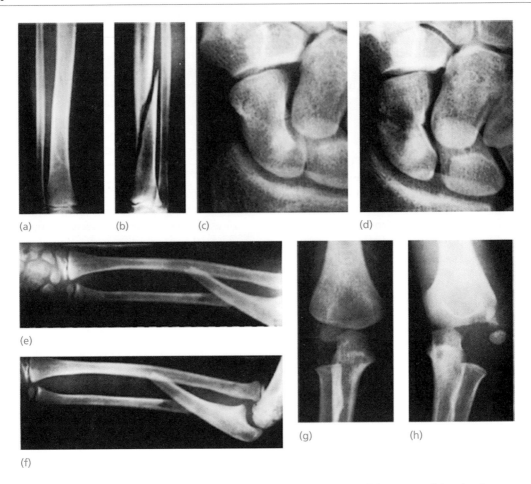

(a)   (b)   (c)   (d)

(e)

(g)   (h)

(f)

Figure 23.6 X-ray examination must be 'adequate' (a,b) Two views of the same tibia: the fracture may be 'invisible' in one view and perfectly plain in a view at right angles to that. **(c,d)** More than one occasion: a fractured scaphoid may not be obvious on the day of injury, but clearly seen 2 weeks later. **(e,f)** Two joints: the first X-ray **(e)** did not include the elbow; this was, in fact, a Monteggia fracture-the head of the radius is dislocated; **(f)** shows the dislocated radiohumeral joint. **(g,h)** Two limbs: sometimes the abnormality can be appreciated only by comparison with the normal side; in this case there is a fracture of the lateral condyle on the left side **(h)**.

Displacement

Displacement occurs partly due to the force of injury, partly gravity and partly the pull of attached muscles. For each fracture, four components must be assessed.

'Anterior angulation' could mean that the apex of the angle points anteriorly or that the distal fragment is tilted anteriorly: in this chapter, it is always the latter meaning that is intended ('anterior tilt of the distal fragment' is probably clearer).

FOUR COMPONENTS OF DISPLACEMENT
Translation (shift) – backwards, forwards, sideways
Angulation (tilt) – in any direction
Rotation (twist) – in any direction along the longitudinal bone axis
Length – impaction or distraction

SECONDARY INJURIES

 Certain fractures are likely to cause secondary injuries and these should always be assumed to have occurred until proved otherwise.

Thoracic injuries Fractured ribs or sternum may be associated with injury to the lungs or heart.

Spinal cord injury Neurological examination is essential in spinal fractures to:

* establish what has been damaged
* obtain baseline for later comparison.

Pelvic and abdominal injuries Fractures of the pelvis may be associated with visceral injury. If a urethral or bladder injury is suspected, diagnostic urethrograms or cystograms may be necessary.

Pectoral girdle injuries Fractures and dislocations around the pectoral girdle may damage the brachial plexus or large vessels at the base of the neck.

TREATMENT OF CLOSED FRACTURES

 Treat the whole patient, not only the fracture (see Chapter 22).

Displaced fractures are *manipulated* to reduce them then *splinted* to maintain position until they unite. Joint *movement* and function must be preserved. Fracture healing is promoted by physiological loading of the bone, so muscle activity and early *weight-bearing* are encouraged. These objectives are covered by:

* reduce
* hold
* exercise.

The risks and benefits of the different available methods to hold the fracture (non-operative vs operative) and the speed with which the patient can commence mobilization and weight-bearing need to be carefully considered.

The fact that the fracture is closed is no cause for complacency. The most important factor in determining the tendency for a fracture to unite is the state of the surrounding soft tissues and blood supply. Tscherne has devised a helpful classification. Good skeletal stability aids soft-tissue recovery.

TSCHERNE CLASSIFICATION OF CLOSED FRACTURES

Grade 0 Simple fracture with little or no soft-tissue injury
Grade 1 Fracture with superficial abrasion or bruising
Grade 2 More severe fracture with deep soft-tissue contusion and swelling
Grade 3 Severe injury with marked soft-tissue damage and threatened compartment syndrome

REDUCTION

After initial resuscitation, fractures should be attended to as soon as possible. Increasing swelling in the hours following fracture makes reduction increasingly difficult. Reduction is not required:

* when there is little or no displacement
* when displacement does not matter initially (e.g. clavicle fractures)
* when it is unlikely to succeed (e.g. vertebral compression fractures).

Aim for *adequate apposition* and *normal alignment* of the bone fragments. Increased contact surface area will decrease time to union but, for non-articular surfaces, it does not need to be anatomical. Certain deformities are less well tolerated (e.g. rotation or angular deformity out of the plane of motion of the joints above and below).

SECTION 3 TRAUMA

CLOSED REDUCTION

Under appropriate anaesthesia and muscle relaxation when required, closed reduction can be achieved in three stages (**23.7**).

STAGES IN CLOSED REDUCTION

1 The distal part of the limb is pulled in the line of the bone.
2 As the fragments disengage, they are repositioned (by reversing the original direction of force if this can be deduced).
3 Alignment is adjusted in each plane.

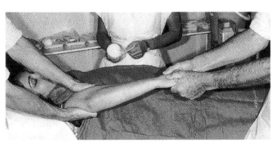
(a)

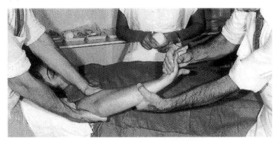
(b)

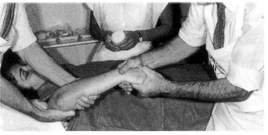
(c)

Figure 23.7 Closed reduction (a) Traction in the line of the bone; **(b)** disimpaction; **(c)** pressing fragment into reduced position.

INDICATIONS FOR CLOSED REDUCTION

All minimally displaced fractures
Most fractures in children
Fractures that are not unstable after reduction or can be stabilized in some form of splint or cast

---

Fractures requiring fixation can also be reduced using closed methods prior to stabilization. Traction, which reduces fracture fragments through *ligamentotaxis* (ligament pull), can usually be applied by using a fracture table or bone distractor.

OPEN REDUCTION

Operative reduction is sometimes indicated. As a rule, however, open reduction is merely the first step to fracture fixation.

INDICATIONS FOR OPEN REDUCTION

When closed reduction fails (e.g. difficulty controlling fragments or soft-tissue interposition)
When articular fragments need accurate positioning
For traction (avulsion) fractures in which the fragments are held apart

---

HOLDING REDUCTION

The word 'immobilization' has been deliberately avoided because the objective is seldom complete immobility; usually it is the prevention of displacement.

There are several available methods of holding reduction:

- continuous traction
- cast splintage
- functional bracing
- internal fixation
- external fixation.

Do not overlook closed methods: they are often very successful and lower risk than the alternatives. The muscles surrounding a fracture, if they are intact, act as a fluid compartment; traction or compression creates a hydraulic effect that is capable of splinting the fracture. Remember, too, that the objective is to splint the fracture, not the entire limb. Even unstable fractures may achieve equivalent functional outcomes to operatively treated fractures in the correct patients (e.g. unstable ankle fractures in patients over 60 years of age).

CONTINUOUS TRACTION

Traction is applied to the limb distal to the fracture, exerting a continuous pull in the long axis of the bone, with a counterforce. It can also be used as a temporizing measure (e.g. acetabular fractures with femoral head subluxation or dislocation).

Traction cannot *hold* a fracture still; it can pull a long bone straight and hold it out to length but maintaining accurate reduction can be difficult.

Meanwhile, the patient can *move* the joints and exercise the muscles.

Types of traction

A number of traction methods are available (**23.8**).

Russell traction A padded sling is placed behind the knee and skin traction to the lower leg. Traction cords and pulleys are used as illustrated (**23.8d**).

Traction by gravity This method is used in upper limb injuries. Thus, with a collar and cuff, the weight of the arm provides continuous traction to the humerus. This may be augmented with a humeral splint.

Skin traction Skin traction will sustain a pull of no more than 4–5 kg. Holland strapping or one-way-stretch Elastoplast is stuck to the shaved skin and held on with a bandage. The malleoli are protected by Gamgee tissue, and cords or tapes are used for traction.

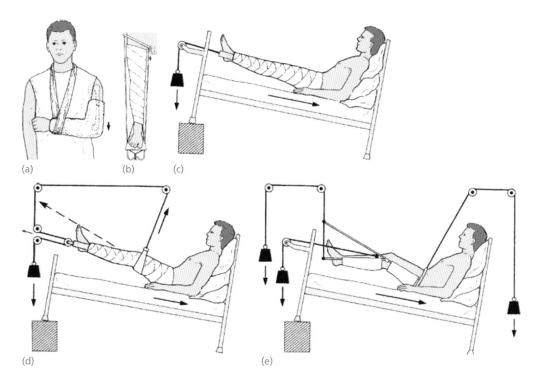

Figure 23.8 Methods of traction (a) Traction by gravity. **(b–d)** Skin traction: **(b)** fixed; **(c)** balanced; **(d)** Russell. **(e)** Skeletal traction with a splint and a knee-flexion piece.

Skeletal traction   A stiff wire or pin is inserted – usually behind the tibial tubercle for hip, thigh and knee injuries, or through the calcaneum for tibial fractures – and cords tied to them for applying traction. The fracture is reduced and held by fixed traction, balanced traction or a combination.

Complications

Circulatory embarrassment   Traction tapes and bandages may constrict the circulation; for this reason 'gallows traction' should never be used for children over 12 kg in weight.

Nerve injury   In older people, leg traction may predispose to peroneal nerve injury and cause a foot drop.

Pin-site infection   Pin sites must be kept clean and should be checked daily.

Cast splintage

Plaster is safe, as long as the practitioner is alert to the danger of a tight cast and the need to prevent pressure sores. Joints encased in plaster cannot move and are liable to stiffen. Adhesions and contractures can form during periods of immobility. Newer substitutes have some advantages over plaster – they are impervious to water, and also lighter – but as long as they are used as full casts, the basic drawback is the same.

Technique

The fracture is reduced, stockinette threaded over the limb and the bony prominences padded. Plaster is then applied. While it is setting, it is moulded away from bony prominences; with shaft fractures, three-point pressure can be applied to keep the intact periosteal hinge under tension and thereby maintain reduction.

   If the fracture is recent, further swelling is likely; the plaster and stockinette may therefore need to be split from top to bottom, exposing the skin. Check *X-rays* are essential and the plaster can be wedged if further correction of angulation is necessary.

   Rotation is only controlled if the joints above and below are included. In the lower limb, the knee is held slightly flexed, the ankle at a right angle and the tarsus and forefoot neutral. In the upper limb, the position of the splinted joints varies with the fracture. Splintage must not be discontinued (though a functional brace may be substituted) until the fracture is consolidated; if plaster changes are needed, check X-rays are essential.

Complications

Tight cast   The cast may be put on too tightly, or it may become tight if the limb swells. The patient complains of diffuse pain. The only safe course is to split the cast and ease it open:

* throughout its length
* through all the padding down to skin.

Pressure sores   Even a well-fitting cast may press upon the skin over a bony prominence. There is localized pain in sensate patients, and the cast should be windowed and the area inspected.

Skin abrasion or laceration   This is really a complication of removing plasters. Complaints of nipping or pinching during plaster removal should never be ignored.

Loose cast   If it is loose, the cast should be replaced as it is no longer holding the fracture.

Functional bracing

Functional bracing is one way of preventing joint stiffness while still permitting fracture splintage and loading. Segments of a cast are applied only over the shafts of the bones, leaving the joints free; the cast segments are connected by metal or plastic hinges that allow movement of the joint in one plane. They are typically applied only when the fracture is beginning to unite.

Technique

Considerable skill is needed to apply an effective brace. A hinged cast or splint is applied, which holds the fracture snugly but permits joint movement; functional activity is encouraged. Unlike internal fixation, functional bracing holds the fracture through compression of the soft tissues.

INTERNAL FIXATION

Bone fragments may be fixed with:

- screws
- plates held by screws
- an intramedullary rod or nail (with or without interlocking screws)
- circumferential bands
- a combination of methods.

Properly applied, internal fixation holds a fracture securely so that movement can begin immediately. The greatest danger is infection, which can be a devastating complication.

Indications

> **MOST IMPORTANT INDICATIONS FOR INTERNAL FIXATION**
>
> Fractures that cannot be reduced except by operation
>
> Fractures that are inherently unstable and prone to redisplace after reduction plus those liable to be pulled apart by muscle action
>
> Pathological fractures in which bone disease may inhibit healing
>
> Multiple fractures where early fixation reduces the risk of general complications
>
> Fractures in patients who present nursing difficulties (e.g. paraplegics, those with multiple injuries and the very elderly)

Types of internal fixation

The type of internal fixation used must be appropriate to the situation (**23.9**).

Interfragmentary lag screws   Screws that are partially threaded exert a compression or 'lag' effect when inserted across two fragments. A similar effect is achieved by overdrilling the 'near' cortex. This technique is useful for reducing single fragments onto the main shaft of a tubular bone or fitting together fragments of a metaphyseal fracture.

Cerclage and tension-band wires   These are loops of wire passed around two bone fragments, tightened to compress the fragments. Care needs to be taken not to entrap nerves or vessels.

Plates and screws   These are useful for articular, metaphyseal and diaphyseal fractures.

- *Neutralization (protection).* Plates resist torque and shortening when used to bridge a fracture and supplement the effect of interfragmentary lag screws.
- *Compression.* Plates achieve absolute stability through compression of suitable fractures to promote primary bone healing.
- *Buttressing.* The plate resists axial load by applying force against the axis of deformity.
- *Tension-band.* Using a plate in this manner on the tensile surface of the bone allows compression to be applied to the biomechanically more advantageous side of the fracture.
- *Bridging.* The plate bridges simple or multifragmentary fractures to restore correct length, axis and rotation with minimal soft-tissue stripping.

Intramedullary nails   These are suitable for long bones. A nail (or long rod) is inserted into the medullary canal to splint the fracture; rotational forces are resisted with *interlocking bolts* proximal and distal to the fracture. Nails are used with or without prior reaming of the medullary canal; reamed nails achieve an interference fit in addition to the added stability from interlocking screws.

Complications

Infection   Iatrogenic infection is now the most common cause of chronic osteomyelitis, which can necessitate multiple revision surgeries and delay healing. The operation and quality of the patient's tissues (i.e. tissue handling) can influence the risk of infection.

Non-union   If the bones have been fixed rigidly with a gap between the ends, the fracture may fail to unite. Other causes of non-union are stripping of the soft tissues and damage to the blood supply.

Implant failure   Metal is subject to fatigue and can fail unless some bone union of the fracture has occurred.

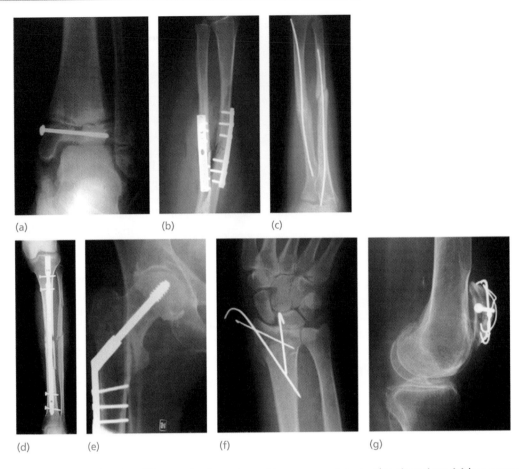

(a)   (b)   (c)

(d)   (e)   (f)   (g)

Figure 23.9 Internal fixation The method used must be appropriate to the situation: **(a)** lag screws – interfragmentary compression; **(b)** plate and screws – here at the forearm diaphysis; **(c)** flexible intramedullary nails – for long bones in children, particularly forearm bones and femur; **(d)** interlocking nail and screws – ideal for long bone shaft fractures in adults; **(e)** dynamic compression screw and plate – ideal for the proximal and distal ends of the femur; **(f)** simple K-wires – for fractures around the elbow and wrist; **(g)** tension-band wiring – for olecranon fractures or fractures of the patella.

 Recurrence of or increasing pain at the fracture site is a danger signal and must be investigated promptly.

Refracture   It is important not to remove metal implants too soon if removal is required, or the bone may refracture. A year is the minimum and 18–24 months safer; several weeks after removal the bone is still weak, and care or protection is needed.

EXTERNAL FIXATION

A fracture may be held by transfixing screws or wires that pass through the bone above and below the fracture and are attached to an external frame.

Indications

MOST IMPORTANT INDICATIONS FOR EXTERNAL FIXATION

Fractures associated with severe soft-tissue damage or contamination

Fractures around joints that are potentially suitable for internal fixation but the soft tissues are too swollen to allow safe surgery; can be combined with percutaneous fixation

> Patients with severe multiple injuries where external fixation can be a temporizing measure
>
> Bone lengthening or bone transport procedures
>
> Infected fractures, for which internal fixation might not be suitable

Technique

The bone is transfixed above and below the fracture with Schanz screws or tensioned wires and these are then connected to each other by rigid frames or bars (**23.10**).

The fractured bone can be thought of as broken into segments – a simple fracture has two segments whereas a two-level (segmental) fracture has three, and so on. Each segment should be held securely, ideally with the half-pins or tensioned wires straddling the length of that segment.

The wires and half-pins must be inserted with care. Knowledge of 'safe corridors' is essential so as to avoid injuring nerves or vessels; in addition, the entry sites should be irrigated during drilling to prevent thermal injury to the bone The fracture is then reduced by traction and connecting the various groups of pins by rods.

Complications

Damage to soft-tissue structures Transfixing pins or wires may damage nerves or blood vessels or they may tether ligaments and inhibit joint movement.

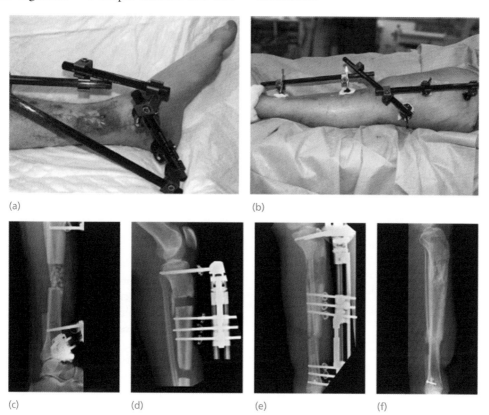

(a)   (b)

(c)   (d)   (e)   (f)

Figure 23.10 **External fixation of fractures** External fixation is widely used for 'damage control' (a,b) temporary stabilization of fractures in order to allow the patient's general condition or the state of soft tissues to improve prior to definitive surgery or (c–f) reconstruction of limbs using distraction osteogenesis. (c) A bone defect after surgical resection with gentamicin beads used to fill the space temporarily. (d) Bone transport from a more proximal osteotomy. (e) 'Docking' of the transported segment and (f) final union and restoration of structural integrity.

Overdistraction This may inhibit bone union.

Pin-track infection Meticulous pin-site care will reduce this.

RESTORATION OF FUNCTION

The objectives are to:

- reduce oedema
- preserve joint movement
- restore muscle power
- guide the patient back to normal activity.

OEDEMA

Swelling is almost inevitable after a fracture and may cause skin stretching and blisters. Persistent oedema can lead to joint stiffness. Elevation and exercise help reduce it. The essence of soft-tissue care may be summed up like this: elevate and exercise; never dangle, never force.

Elevation

An injured limb usually needs to be elevated to the same level as the heart or above to reduce swelling. The patient is allowed and encouraged to exercise the limb actively, but not to let it dangle. When the plaster is finally removed, a similar routine of activity, punctuated by elevation, is practised until circulatory control is fully restored.

Injuries of the upper limb also need elevation. A sling must not be a permanent passive arm-holder; the limb must be elevated intermittently or, if needed, continuously.

Active exercise

Active movement helps to pump away oedema fluid, stimulates the circulation, prevents soft-tissue adhesion and promotes fracture healing. Even in plaster, static muscle contraction can still be performed. Remember that the unaffected joints need exercising too; it is too easy to neglect a stiffening shoulder while caring for an injured wrist or hand.

Assisted movement

Forced movements should never be permitted, but gentle assistance during active exercises may help to retain function or regain movement after fractures involving the articular surfaces.

Functional activity

As the patient's mobility improves, an increasing amount of directed activity is included. Experience is the best teacher and the patient is encouraged to use the injured limb as much as possible. Rehabilitation units may be useful, particularly for severely injured patients.

OPEN FRACTURES

INITIAL MANAGEMENT

Patients with open fractures may have multiple injuries; a rapid general assessment is the first step and any life-threatening conditions must be addressed (see Chapter 22).

When the treatment of the patient allows the fracture to be dealt with, the wound is first carefully inspected; any gross contamination is removed, the wound is photographed to record the injury and the area is then covered with a saline-soaked dressing under an impervious seal to prevent desiccation. This is left undisturbed until the patient is in the operating theatre. The patient is given antibiotics, usually co-amoxiclav or cefuroxime, but clindamycin if the patient is allergic to penicillin. Tetanus prophylaxis is administered: toxoid for those previously immunized, human antiserum if not. The limb is then splinted until surgery is undertaken.

The limb circulation and distal neurological status will need to be checked repeatedly, particularly after any fracture reduction manoeuvres.

 Compartment syndrome is not prevented by an existing open fracture; vigilance for this complication is essential.

CLASSIFYING THE INJURY

Treatment is determined by the type of fracture and soft-tissue injury, and the degree of contamination. *Gustilo's classification* can be carried out at the time of debridement.

- *Type I.* The wound is usually a small, clean puncture through which a bone spike has protruded. There is little soft-tissue damage with no crushing and the fracture is not comminuted.
- *Type II.* The wound is more than 1 cm long, but there is no skin flap. There is not much soft-tissue damage and no more than moderate crushing or comminution.
- *Type III.* There is a large laceration, extensive damage to skin and underlying soft tissue and, in the most severe examples, vascular compromise. The injury is caused by high energy and contamination can be significant.
  - *Type III A.* The fractured bone can be adequately covered by soft tissue.
  - *Type III B.* There is extensive periosteal stripping and soft-tissue cover is not possible without use of local or distant flaps.
  - *Type III C.* There is an arterial injury which needs to be repaired.

The incidence of wound infection correlates directly with the extent of soft-tissue damage, rising from less than 2% in type I to more than 20% in type III fractures.

PRINCIPLES OF TREATMENT

All open fractures, no matter how trivial they may seem, must be assumed to be contaminated; it is important to try to prevent them from becoming infected.

THE FOUR ESSENTIALS OF OPEN FRACTURE TREATMENT

Antibiotic prophylaxis (**Table 23.1**)
Urgent wound and fracture debridement
Early definitive wound cover
Stabilization of the fracture

Debridement

The operation aims to render the wound free from foreign material and of dead tissue, leaving a clean surgical field and tissues with a good blood supply throughout. Bone ends must be fully delivered and the entire zone of injury assessed and debrided. Even full-thickness skin flaps in the zone of injury can necrose if inappropriately retained. Appropriately skilled surgeons in soft-tissue reconstruction as well as bone fixation should make treatment decisions together wherever possible.

Tourniquet use should be kept to a minimum to avoid further insult and allow accurate assessment of vascularity. It may be sited but not inflated during the debridement unless absolutely necessary.

Wound excision The wound margins are excised, back to healthy, viable tissue.

Wound extension Thorough cleansing necessitates adequate exposure. If extensions are needed, they should not jeopardize the creation of skin flaps for wound cover if this should be needed. The lines of fasciotomy incisions are safe (**23.11**).

Delivery of the fracture Examination of the fracture surfaces cannot be adequately performed without extracting the bone from within the wound. The simplest (and gentlest) method is to bend the limb in the manner in which it was forced at the moment of injury; the fracture surfaces will be exposed through the wound without any additional damage to the soft tissues (**23.12**).

Removal of devitalized tissue Dead muscle is purplish, mushy, does not contract when stimulated and does not bleed when cut. All doubtfully viable tissue should be removed. The fracture ends can be curetted or nibbled away until seen to bleed.

Wound cleansing All foreign material and tissue debris is removed by excision or through lavage with copious quantities of saline. A common mistake is to inject fluid through a small aperture using a syringe – this only serves to push contaminants further in; up to 12 L of

Table 23.1 Antibiotics for open fractures[1]

	Type I	Type II	Type IIIA	Type IIIB/IIIC
As soon as possible (within 3 hours of injury)	Co-amoxiclav[2]	Co-amoxiclav[2]	Co-amoxiclav[2]	Co-amoxiclav[2]
At debridement	Co-amoxiclav[2] and gentamicin	Co-amoxiclav[2] and gentamicin	Co-amoxiclav[2] and gentamicin	Co-amoxiclav[2] and gentamicin
At definitive fracture cover	Wound cover is usually possible at debridement Delayed closure unnecessary	Wound cover is usually possible at debridement If delayed, gentamicin and vancomycin (or teicoplanin) at the time of cover	Wound cover is usually possible at debridement If delayed, gentamicin and vancomycin (or teicoplanin) at the time of cover	Gentamicin and vancomycin (or teicoplanin)
Continued prophylaxis	Only co-amoxiclav[2] continued after surgery	Only co-amoxiclav[2] continued between procedures and after final surgery	Only co-amoxiclav[2] continued between procedures and after final surgery	Only co-amoxiclav[2] continued between procedures and after final surgery
Maximum period	24 hours	72 hours	72 hours	72 hours

[1] Based on the Standards for the Management of Open Fractures of the Lower Limb, BOA/BAPRAS, 2009.
[2] Or cefuroxime (clindamycin for those with penicillin allergy).

saline may be needed to irrigate and clean an open fracture of a long bone. Adding antibiotics or antiseptics to the solution has no added benefit.

Nerves and tendons As a general rule, it is best to leave cut nerves and tendons alone, though if the wound is absolutely clean and no dissection is required – and provided the necessary expertise is available – they can be repaired.

Wound closure

A small, uncontaminated wound in a type I or II fracture may be sutured (after debridement), provided this can be done without tension. In more severe injuries, immediate fracture stabilization and wound cover using split-skin grafts, local or distant flaps are ideal, provided that both orthopaedic and plastic surgeons are satisfied with a clean, viable wound achieved after debridement. In the absence of this combined approach at the time of debridement, the fracture is temporarily stabilized and the wound left open and dressed with an impervious dressing. Vacuum dressings are popular and have theoretical benefits but do not alter patient outcomes.

Return to surgery for a 'second look' should have definitive fracture fixation and wound coverage as objectives. It should be done within 48–72 hours, and not later than 5 days. Open fractures do not fare well if left exposed for long periods, and multiple returns to theatre for repeated debridement can be self-defeating.

Stabilizing the fracture

Stabilizing the fracture also aids soft-tissue recovery. If there is no obvious contamination and definitive wound cover can be achieved at the time of debridement, open fractures of all types can be treated as for a closed injury. This ideal scenario of judicious soft-tissue and bone debridement, wound cleansing, immediate stabilization and cover is only possible if surgeons with orthopaedic and plastic surgical expertise are present at the time of initial surgery.

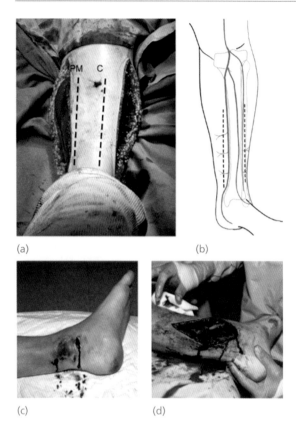

(a)   (b)

(c)   (d)

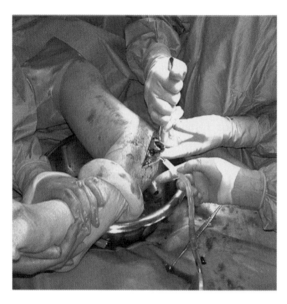

Figure 23.12 **Delivering the fracture** Debridement is only possible if the fracture is adequately seen; for this, the fracture ends have to be delivered from within.

Figure 23.11 **Wound extensions for access in open fractures of the tibia** Wound incisions (extensions) for adequate access to an open tibial fracture are made along standard fasciotomy incisions: 1 cm behind the posteromedial border of the tibia and 2–3 cm lateral to the crest of the tibia as shown in this example of a two-incision fasciotomy. The dotted lines mark out the crest (C) and posteromedial corner (PM) of the tibia (a). These incisions avoid injury to the perforating branches supplying areas of skin that can be used as flaps to cover the exposed fracture (b). (c,d) This clinical example shows how local skin necrosis around an open fracture is excised and the wound extended proximally along a fasciotomy incision.

If wound cover is delayed, external fixation or even internal fixation (that will subsequently be removed at the time of definitive fixation) can be used as a temporary measure.

If external fixation is used, it can be exchanged for internal fixation at the time of definitive wound cover as long as:

- the delay to wound cover is less than 7 days
- wound contamination is not visible
- internal fixation can control the fracture as well as the external fixator.

Aftercare

In the ward, the limb is elevated and its circulation carefully watched. Wound cultures are seldom helpful as osteomyelitis, if it were to ensue, is often caused by hospital-derived organisms; this emphasizes the need for meticulous debridement and early appropriate wound closure or coverage.

SEQUELS TO OPEN FRACTURES

Skin

If split-thickness skin grafts are used inappropriately (e.g. to cover tendons or bone), particularly where flap cover is more suited, there can be areas of contracture or friable skin that breaks down intermittently.

Bone

Infection involves the zone of injury and any implants. Identifying the causal organism without tissue samples is difficult but, at best guess, it is likely to be *Staphylococcus aureus* (including methicillin-resistant varieties) or *Pseudomonas*. Suppression by appropriate antibiotics, as long as the fixation remains stable, may allow the fracture to proceed to union, but further surgery is likely to be needed later, when the antibiotics are stopped.

In late presentation, the implants and all avascular pieces of bone should be removed; robust soft-tissue cover (ideally a flap) is needed. An external fixator can be used to bridge the fracture. If the resulting defect is too large for bone grafting at a later stage, the patient should be referred to a centre with the necessary experience and facilities for bone transport/limb reconstruction.

Joints

When an infected fracture communicates with a joint, the principles of treatment are the same as with bone infection, namely debridement and drainage, drugs and splintage.

GUNSHOT INJURIES

Missile wounds are looked upon as a special type of open injury. Tissue damage is produced by:

- direct injury in the immediate path of the missile
- contusion of muscles around the missile track
- bruising and congestion of soft tissues at a greater distance from the primary track.

With high-velocity missiles there is marked cavitation and tissue destruction over a wide area. Bone splinters act as secondary missiles. With low-velocity missiles (e.g. civilian handguns) cavitation is much less. With all gunshot injuries debris is sucked into the wound, which is therefore contaminated.

Emergency treatment

As always, the arrest of bleeding and general resuscitation take priority. Each wound should be covered with a sterile dressing and the area examined for artery or nerve damage. Antibiotics should be given immediately, following the recommendations for open fractures.

Definitive treatment

LOW-VELOCITY WOUNDS

Low-velocity wounds with relatively clean entry and exit wounds can be treated as Gustilo type I injuries, by superficial debridement, splintage of the limb and antibiotic cover; the fracture is then treated in the same way as similar open fractures. If the injury involves soft tissues only, with minimal bone splinters, the wound may be safely treated without surgery but with local wound care and antibiotics.

HIGH-VELOCITY WOUNDS

High-velocity injuries demand thorough debridement and, if necessary, splitting of fascial compartments to prevent ischaemia. The fracture is stabilized and the wound is treated as for a Gustilo type III fracture. Comminuted fractures are best managed by external fixation. The method of wound closure will depend on the state of tissues after several days; in some cases, delayed primary suture is possible but, as with other open injuries, close collaboration between plastic and orthopaedic surgeons is needed.

CLOSE-RANGE WOUNDS

Although the missiles may be technically low-velocity, close-range shotgun injuries are treated as high-velocity wounds because the mass of shot transfers large quantities of energy to the tissues.

COMPLICATIONS OF FRACTURES

The general complications of fractures (blood loss, shock, fat embolism, cardiorespiratory failure, etc.) are dealt with in Chapter 22.

Local complications can be divided into *early* (arising during the first few weeks following injury) and *late* (Table 23.2).

Table 23.2 Local complications of fractures

Early		Late
Urgent	Less urgent	
Visceral injury	Fracture blisters	Delayed union
Vascular injury	Plaster	Non-union
Nerve injury	Pressure sores	Malunion
Compartment syndrome	Heterotopic ossification	Avascular necrosis
Haemarthrosis	Ligament injury	Growth disturbance
Infection	Tendon lesions	Bed sores
Gas gangrene	Nerve compression	Muscle contracture
	Joint stiffness	Joint instability
	Complex regional pain syndrome (algodystrophy)	Osteoarthritis

EARLY COMPLICATIONS

VISCERAL INJURY

Fractures around the trunk are often complicated by injuries to underlying viscera (e.g. lung, bladder or urethra). These injuries require early recognition and emergency treatment.

VASCULAR INJURY

Arteries may be cut, torn, compressed or contused, either by the initial injury or subsequently by swelling, bone fragments, reduction manoeuvres or surgery. Even if its outward appearance is normal, the intima may be detached and the vessel blocked by thrombus. The effects vary from transient diminution of blood flow to profound ischaemia, tissue death and peripheral gangrene (**23.13**).

Clinical features

The patient may complain of paraesthesia or numbness in the toes or the fingers. The injured limb is cold and pale, or slightly cyanosed, and the pulse is weak or absent. *X-rays* will probably

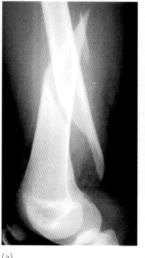 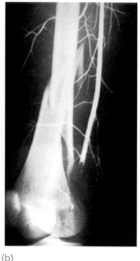 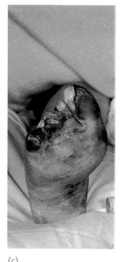

(a)　　　　　　　　　　(b)　　　　　　　　　　(c)

Figure 23.13 **Vascular injury** This patient was brought into hospital with a fractured femur and early signs of vascular insufficiency. **(a)** The plain X-ray looked as if the proximal bone fragment might have speared the popliteal artery. **(b)** The angiogram confirmed these fears. **(c)** Despite vein grafting, the patient developed peripheral gangrene.

Table 23.3 Common vascular injuries

Injury	Vessel
First rib fracture	Subclavian
Shoulder dislocation	Axillary
Humeral supracondylar fracture	Brachial
Elbow dislocation	Brachial
Pelvic fracture	Presacral and internal iliac
Femoral supracondylar fracture	Femoral
Knee dislocation	Popliteal
Proximal tibial	Popliteal or its branches

Table 23.4 Common nerve injuries

Injury	Nerve
Shoulder dislocation	Axillary
Humeral shaft fracture	Radial
Humeral supracondylar fracture	Radial or median
Elbow medial condyle	Ulnar
Monteggia fracture-dislocation	Posterior interosseous
Hip dislocation	Sciatic
Knee dislocation	Peroneal

show one of the 'high-risk' fractures listed in Table 23.3. If a vascular injury is suspected, an angiogram or duplex should be performed immediately; if it is positive, emergency treatment must be started without further delay.

Treatment

All bandages and splints should be removed. The fracture is re-X-rayed and, if the position of the bones suggests that the artery is being compressed or kinked, prompt reduction is necessary. If there is no improvement, the vessels must be explored by operation – preferably with the benefit of preoperative or perioperative angiography. A cut vessel can be sutured, or a segment may be replaced by a vein graft; if it is thrombosed, endarterectomy may restore the blood flow. If vessel repair is undertaken, stable fixation is a must and where it is practicable, the fracture should be fixed internally.

NERVE INJURY

Nerve injury is particularly common with fractures of the humeral shaft or injuries around the elbow or the knee. The telltale signs should be looked for *and documented* during the initial examination and again after reduction of the fracture.

Common nerve injuries are listed in Table 23.4.

INDICATIONS FOR EARLY EXPLORATION

Nerve injury associated with open fracture
Nerve injury with fractures that need internal fixation
Presence of a concomitant vascular injury
Nerve damage diagnosed after manipulation of the fracture

Closed nerve injuries

In closed injuries, the nerve is seldom severed, and spontaneous recovery should be awaited – it occurs in 90% of cases within 4 months. If recovery has not occurred within the expected time, and if nerve conduction studies and electromyography (EMG) fail to show evidence of recovery, the nerve should be explored.

Open nerve injuries

With open fractures, the nerve injury is more likely to be complete. In these cases, the nerve should be explored at the time of debridement and repaired at debridement or wound closure.

Acute nerve compression

Nerve compression sometimes occurs with fractures or dislocations around the wrist. Complaints of numbness or paraesthesia in the distribution of the median or ulnar nerves should be taken seriously; if there is no improvement within 48 hours of fracture reduction or splitting of bandages around the splint, the nerve should be explored and decompressed.

COMPARTMENT SYNDROME

Bleeding, oedema or inflammation (infection) may increase the pressure within one of the osseofascial compartments; there is reduced capillary flow leading to muscle ischaemia, further oedema, greater pressure and yet more profound ischaemia. Nerve is capable of regeneration but muscle, once infarcted, can never recover and is replaced by inelastic fibrous tissue (*Volkmann's ischaemic contracture*). A similar cascade of events may be caused by swelling of a limb inside a tight plaster cast.

Clinical features

High-risk injuries are fractures of the elbow, forearm bones, proximal third of the tibia, and also multiple fractures of the hand or foot, crush injuries and circumferential burns. Other precipitating factors are operation (usually for internal fixation) or infection.

The classic features of ischaemia are the five Ps. The earliest of these 'classic' features is severe pain and this may be the only feature.

CLASSIC FEATURES OF ISCHAEMIA: THE FIVE PS
Pain
Paraesthesia
Pallor
Paralysis
Pulselessness

Ischaemic muscle is highly sensitive to stretch. If the limb is unduly painful, swollen or tense, the muscles in the affected compartments should be tested by stretching them.

Confirmation of the diagnosis can be made by measuring the intracompartmental pressures. In high-risk injuries or unconscious patients, continuous compartment pressure monitoring may be justified. A split catheter is introduced into the compartment and the pressure is measured close to the level of the fracture. A differential pressure (ΔP) – the difference between diastolic pressure and compartment pressure – of less than 30 mmHg (4.00 kilopascals) is an indication for immediate compartment decompression. A normal reading can never be taken to exclude a compartment syndrome, though, and clinical suspicion should take precedence.

Treatment

The threatened compartment (or compartments) must be promptly decompressed. Casts, bandages and dressings must be completely removed and the limb should be nursed flat (elevating the limb causes a further decrease in end capillary pressure and aggravates the muscle ischaemia). Compartment syndrome is a clinical diagnosis and, if the surgeon believes there is a compartment syndrome present, fasciotomy is justified even if a predetermined pressure threshold has not been reached. If the clinical signs are 'soft', the limb should be examined at 30-minute intervals and, if there is no improvement within 2 hours of splitting the dressings down to the skin, fasciotomy should be performed as a matter of urgency.

 Muscle will be dead after 4–6 hours of total ischaemia – there is no time to lose in performing fasciotomy.

In the case of the leg, 'fasciotomy' means opening all four compartments through medial and lateral incisions (**23.14**). The wounds should

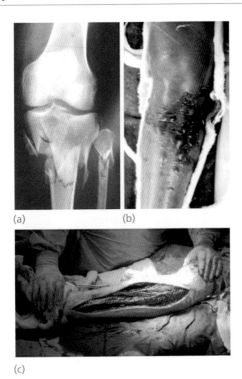

(a)   (b)

(c)

Figure 23.14 Compartment syndrome (a) X-ray showing a complex proximal tibial fracture. All tibial fractures should be monitored for signs of compartment syndrome. Severe pain is the most important clinical feature. Regular clinical evaluation is important. **(b)** Swelling, blistering and skin necrosis associated with late, severe compartment syndrome that progressed quickly, unchecked underneath a complete plaster cast. **(c)** four compartment fasciotomies required in the context of lower limb compartment syndrome.

be left open, negative pressure wound therapy can be applied, and inspected 2 days later:

- *if there is muscle necrosis*, debridement can be carried out
- *if the tissues are healthy*, the wounds can be sutured (without tension) or skin-grafted.

HAEMARTHROSIS

Fractures involving a joint may cause acute haemarthrosis. The joint is swollen and tense and the patient resists any attempt at moving it. Blood can be aspirated using aseptic technique if symptoms require.

INFECTION

Open fractures may become infected; closed fractures hardly ever do unless they are opened by operation. Post-traumatic wound infection is now the most common cause of chronic osteitis. The management of early and late infection is summarized above.

GAS GANGRENE

This terrifying condition is caused by clostridial infection (especially *Clostridium welchii*). These are anaerobic organisms that can survive and multiply only in tissues with low oxygen tension; the prime site for infection, therefore, is a dirty wound with dead muscle that has been closed without adequate debridement. Toxins produced by the organisms destroy the cell wall and rapidly lead to spreading tissue necrosis.

Clinical features

Symptoms usually appear within 24 hours. There is intense pain and swelling around the wound, and a brownish discharge may be seen; gas formation is usually not very marked. There is little or no pyrexia but the pulse rate is increased and a characteristic smell becomes evident. Rapidly the patient exhibits signs of systemic sepsis and may lapse into coma and death.

 It is essential to distinguish gas gangrene, which is characterized by myonecrosis, from anaerobic cellulitis, in which superficial gas formation is abundant but toxaemia usually slight. Failure to recognize the difference may lead to unnecessary amputation for the non-lethal cellulitis.

Prevention

Deep, penetrating wounds in muscular tissue are dangerous; they should be explored, all dead tissue should be completely excised and, if there is the slightest doubt about tissue viability, repetitive debridement should be performed. There is no effective antitoxin against *Clostridium perfringens* (*C. welchii*).

Treatment

The key to life-saving treatment is early diagnosis. Fluid replacement and intravenous antibiotics are started immediately. Hyperbaric oxygen has been used as a means of limiting the spread of gangrene. However, the mainstay of treatment is prompt decompression and aggressive debridement up to amputation.

FRACTURE BLISTERS

These may be clear fluid-filled vesicles or blood-stained. They are due to elevation of the epidermal layer of skin from the dermis. They should not be punctured and incisions through blisters are generally avoided or only undertaken when limb swelling has decreased.

PLASTER AND PRESSURE SORES

These should be prevented by padding the bony points and by moulding plasters so that pressure is distributed to the soft tissues around the bony points. They are accompanied by localized burning pain. A window must immediately be cut in the plaster, or warning pain quickly abates and skin necrosis proceeds unnoticed.

Even traction on a Thomas splint requires skill in nursing care; careless selection of ring size, excessive fixed (as opposed to balanced) traction, and neglect can lead to pressure sores around the groin and iliac crest.

LATE COMPLICATIONS

DELAYED UNION

If the time before union is unduly prolonged, the term 'delayed union' is used.

Causes

BIOLOGICAL

Inadequate blood supply Fractures cause tearing of both the periosteum and interruption of the intramedullary blood supply. If not accurately reduced or there is excessive motion, the fracture edges will become necrotic and dependent on the formation of an ensheathing callus mass to bridge the break. If the zone of necrosis is extensive, as might occur in highly comminuted fractures, union may be hampered.

Severe soft tissue damage Severe damage to the soft tissues affects fracture healing by:

- reducing muscle splintage
- damaging the local blood supply
- diminishing or eliminating the osteogenic input from muscle mesenchymal stem cells.

Periosteal stripping Overenthusiastic stripping of periosteum during internal fixation is an avoidable cause of delayed union.

BIOCHEMICAL

Imperfect splintage Excessive traction or movement will delay callus ossification. In the forearm and leg, a single-bone fracture may be held apart by an intact bone.

Over-rigid fixation Completely rigid fixation delays rather than promotes fracture union. Union by primary bone healing is slow, but provided stability is maintained throughout, it does eventually occur.

Infection Both biology and stability are hampered by active infection: not only is there bone lysis, necrosis and pus formation, but implants loosen.

PATIENT-RELATED

In a less than ideal world, there are patients who are:

- immense
- immoderate
- immovable
- impossible!

These factors must be accommodated in an appropriate fashion.

Clinical features

Fracture tenderness persists. On *X-ray*, the fracture line remains visible and there is very little or incomplete callus formation or periosteal reaction. However, the bone ends are not sclerosed or atrophic. The appearances suggest that, although the fracture has not united, it may eventually.

Treatment

CONSERVATIVE TREATMENT

The two important principles are:

* to eliminate or optimize possible causes
* to promote healing by providing the most appropriate environment.

Immobilization should be sufficient to prevent shear at the fracture site, but fracture loading is an important stimulus to union and can be enhanced by:

* muscular exercises
* full or at least partial weight-bearing.

The watchword is patience; however, at a certain point prolonged immobilization outweighs the advantages of non-operative treatment.

OPERATIVE TREATMENT

If union is delayed for more than 6 months and there is no sign of callus formation, internal fixation and bone grafting may be indicated. Care should be taken to damage the biological environment as little as possible.

NON-UNION

Delayed union may progress to 'non-union' – it becomes apparent that the fracture will never unite without intervention. Movement can be elicited at the fracture site and typically pain diminishes.

Imaging

The fracture is clearly visible on *X-ray*. There may be exuberant callus that is failing to bridge, or atrophy.

* In *hypertrophic non-union* osteogenesis is still active but not quite capable of bridging the gap.
* In *atrophic non-union*, osteogenesis seems to have ceased.

Causes

Four questions must be addressed to identify the cause of non-union (**23.15**).

QUESTIONS TO HELP IDENTIFY THE CAUSE OF NON-UNION	
Contact	Was there sufficient contact between the bone fragments?
Alignment	Was the fracture adequately aligned to reduce shear?
Stability	Was the fracture held with sufficient stability?
Stimulation	Was the fracture sufficiently 'stimulated'?

There may also be biological and patient-related reasons for non-union:

* poor soft tissues
* infection
* drug abuse, anti-inflammatory or cytotoxic immunosuppressant medication
* non-compliance.

Treatment

CONSERVATIVE TREATMENT

Non-union is occasionally symptomless or minimally symptomatic, needing no treatment, a splint or functional brace. Pulsed electromagnetic fields and low-frequency, pulsed ultrasound may also be used in an attempt to stimulate bone union.

OPERATIVE TREATMENT

With hypertrophic non-union and in the absence of deformity, rigid fixation may lead to union. With atrophic non-union, fixation alone is not enough. Fibrous tissue in the fracture gap as well as the hard, sclerotic bone ends are excised and the fracture grafted. In severe resorption, bone lengthening or transport may be required.

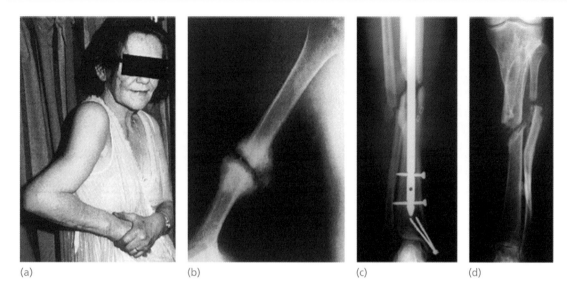

(a) (b) (c) (d)

Figure 23.15 Non-union (a) This patient has an obvious pseudarthrosis of the humerus. The X-ray **(b)** shows a typical hypertrophic non-union. **(c,d)** Examples of atrophic non-union.

MALUNION

When the fragments join with unacceptable angulation, rotation or shortening, the fracture is defined as 'malunited'. Causes are:

- failure to reduce a fracture adequately
- failure to hold reduction
- gradual collapse of comminuted or osteoporotic bone.

Clinical features

Rotational deformity may be missed unless the limb is clinically compared with the contralateral side.

X-rays are essential to check the position of the fracture while it is uniting, particularly during the first 2–3 weeks. At this stage, it is sometimes difficult to decide what constitutes 'malunion'; acceptable norms differ and these are discussed under the individual fractures.

Treatment

Incipient malunion may call for treatment even before the fracture has fully united; the decision on the need for remanipulation or correction may be extremely difficult.

- *In adults*, fractures should be reduced as near to the anatomical position as possible. Angulation of more than 10–15 degrees in a long bone or a noticeable rotational deformity may need remanipulation, or by osteotomy and fixation. Deformity in the plane of motion of a nearby joint may be better tolerated.
- *In children*, angular deformities near the bone ends (and especially if the deformity is in the same plane as that of movement of the nearby joint) will usually remodel; rotational deformities will not.
- *In the lower limb*, shortening of more than 2 cm is seldom acceptable to the patient.
- *The patient's expectations* (often prompted by cosmesis) may be quite different from the surgeon's. Early discussion with the patient and a guided view of the X-rays will help in deciding the need for treatment and may prevent later misunderstanding of what degree of deformity is considered acceptable.
- Very little is known about *the long-term effects of small angular deformities* on joint function. Malalignment of more than 15 degrees in any plane may cause asymmetrical loading of joints and late development of secondary osteoarthritis; particularly in large weight-bearing joints.

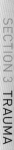

SECTION 3 TRAUMA

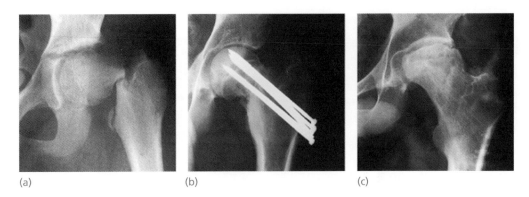

(a)   (b)   (c)

Figure 23.16 Avascular necrosis (a) Displaced fractures of the femoral neck are at considerable risk of developing avascular necrosis. Despite internal fixation within a few hours of the injury **(b)**, the head-fragment developed avascular necrosis. **(c)** X-ray after removal of the fixation screws.

AVASCULAR NECROSIS

Certain regions are notorious for their propensity to develop ischaemia and bone necrosis after injury (**23.16**) (see also Chapter 6). The clinical and radiological effects may not be seen until 18 months or later.

REGIONS AT PARTICULAR RISK OF DEVELOPING ISCHAEMIA/NECROSIS AFTER INJURY
Femoral head Proximal scaphoid Lunate (following dislocation) Body of the talus

Clinical features

If the bone collapses, the patient may complain of pain. *X-rays* show the characteristic increase in density, due to disuse osteoporosis in the surrounding parts, and collapse of trabeculae. Where normal bone meets the necrotic segment, a zone of increased radiographic density may be produced by new bone formation.

Treatment

Treatment usually becomes necessary when joint function is threatened. In elderly people with necrosis of the femoral head, an arthroplasty is the obvious choice; in younger people, realignment osteotomy (or, in some cases, arthrodesis) may be wiser. Avascular necrosis in the scaphoid or talus may need no more than symptomatic treatment, but arthrodesis of the wrist or ankle is sometimes needed.

GROWTH DISTURBANCE

Damage to an open physis may lead to abnormal or arrested growth, particularly with fractures that split the epiphysis leading to asymmetrical growth. If the entire physis is damaged, there may be slowing or complete cessation of growth (see 'Injuries of the physis' later in this chapter).

BED SORES

Bed sores occur in elderly or paralysed patients. The skin over the sacrum and heels is especially vulnerable. Careful nursing and early activity can usually prevent sores. Treatment of established sores is difficult – it may be necessary to excise the necrotic tissue and apply skin grafts. Negative pressure wound therapy may be used for sacral bed sores.

HETEROTOPIC OSSIFICATION

This sometimes occurs after an injury, particularly dislocation of the elbow and acetabular fractures, and is accentuated in craniocerebral injury. It is thought to be due to muscle damage, but it may also occur without a local injury in unconscious or paraplegic patients.

Clinical features

Soon after the injury, the patient complains of pain with local swelling and soft-tissue tenderness. *X-rays* are normal but a bone scan may show increased activity. Over the next 2–3 weeks, the pain gradually subsides, but joint movement is limited; X-rays may show fluffy calcification in the soft tissues. By 8 weeks, the bony mass is easily palpable and clearly defined on X-rays.

Treatment

The joint should be rested in the position of function until pain subsides; gentle active movements are then begun. Months later, when the ossification is mature, it may be helpful to excise the bony mass. Indomethacin or radiotherapy should be given to help prevent recurrence.

TENDON LESIONS

Tendinitis may affect the tibialis posterior tendon following medial malleolar fractures. The risk can be reduced by accurate reduction.

Rupture of the extensor pollicis longus tendon may occur 6–12 weeks after a fracture of the lower radius. Direct repair is seldom possible so transfer of the extensor indicis proprius tendon to the distal stump of the ruptured thumb tendon may be needed.

Late rupture of the long head of biceps after a fractured neck of humerus usually requires no treatment.

NERVE COMPRESSION

Nerve compression may damage the common peroneal nerve if an elderly or emaciated patient lies with the leg in full external rotation. Radial palsy may follow the faulty use of crutches. Both are due to lack of supervision.

Bone or joint deformity may result in local nerve entrapment with typical features such as numbness or paraesthesia, loss of power and muscle wasting in the distribution of the affected nerve.

COMMON SITES OF NERVE COMPRESSION

Ulnar nerve, due to a valgus elbow following a malunited lateral condyle or supracondylar fracture
Median nerve, following injuries around the wrist
Posterior tibial nerve, following fractures around the ankle

Treatment is by early decompression; in the case of the ulnar nerve this may require anterior transposition.

MUSCLE CONTRACTURE

Following arterial injury or compartment syndrome, the patient may develop ischaemic contractures *(Volkmann's ischaemic contracture)*. Nerves sometimes recover, at least partially; thus, the patient presents with deformity and stiffness, but numbness is inconstant. The most commonly affected sites are the forearm and hand, leg and foot.

In a severe case affecting the forearm, there will be forearm and hand wasting with clawing of the fingers. If the wrist is passively flexed, the patient can extend the fingers. Detachment of the flexors at their origin and along the interosseous membrane in the forearm may improve the deformity, but function is no better if sensation and active movement are not restored. A pedicle nerve graft, using the proximal segments of the median and ulnar nerves may restore protective sensation, and tendon transfers (wrist extensors to finger and thumb flexors) will allow active grasp.

Ischaemia of the hand may follow forearm injuries or swelling. The intrinsic hand muscles fibrose and shorten, flexing the metacarpophalangeal joints, but the interphalangeal joints remain straight. The thumb is adducted across the palm (Bunnell's 'intrinsic-plus' position).

Ischaemia of the calf muscles may follow injuries or operations involving the popliteal artery or its divisions. One of the causes of late claw-toe deformity is an undiagnosed compartment syndrome.

JOINT INSTABILITY

Following injury, a joint may give way due to:

- *ligamentous laxity*
- *muscle weakness*
- *bone loss.*

Injury may lead to *recurrent dislocation*. The commonest sites are the shoulder (Bankart or Hill–Sachs lesions) and the patella (medial patellofemoral ligament).

A more subtle form of instability is seen after fractures around the wrist. Patients complaining of persistent discomfort or weakness after wrist injury should be fully investigated for *chronic carpal instability* (see Chapters 15 and 26).

JOINT STIFFNESS

Sometimes the joint itself has been injured; a haemarthrosis forms and leads to synovial adhesions. More often the stiffness is due to oedema and fibrosis of the capsule, ligaments and muscles around the joint, or adhesions of the soft tissues to each other or to the underlying bone. All are made worse by prolonged immobilization and holding joints in non-functional positions.

In a small percentage of patients with fractures of the forearm or leg, early post-traumatic swelling is accompanied by tenderness and progressive stiffness of the distal joints. These patients are at great risk of developing a *complex regional pain syndrome*. This must be recognized early and skilled physiotherapy commenced.

Treatment

The best treatment is prevention by mobilization. If a joint has to be splinted, make sure that it is held in the 'position of safe immobilization'.

Joints that are already stiff take time to mobilize, but prolonged and patient physiotherapy can work wonders. If the situation is due to intra-articular adhesions, arthroscopic-guided releases

may help. Occasionally, adherent or contracted tissues need to be released (e.g. when knee flexion is prevented by quadriceps adhesions).

COMPLEX REGIONAL PAIN SYNDROME

Complex regional pain syndrome (CRPS) is an advanced atrophic disorder which is much more common than originally believed and that it may follow relatively trivial injury.

Two types of CRPS are recognized:

- *Type 1* – a reflex sympathetic dystrophy that develops after an injurious or noxious event
- *Type 2* – causalgia that develops after a nerve injury.

The patient complains of continuous pain, often described as 'burning'. There is local swelling, redness and warmth, as well as tenderness and moderate joint stiffness. As the weeks go by, the skin becomes pale and atrophic, movements are increasingly restricted and the patient may develop fixed deformities. *X-rays* characteristically show patchy rarefaction of the bone.

Treatment

The earlier the condition is recognized and treatment begun, the better the prognosis. Elevation and active exercises are essential. In the early stage, anti-inflammatory drugs and adequate analgesia are helpful. Involvement of a pain specialist who is familiar with desensitization methods, regional anaesthesia, and use of drugs such as amitriptyline, carbamazepine and gabapentin may help. In combination with prolonged and dedicated physiotherapy, this is the mainstay of treatment.

OSTEOARTHRITIS

A fracture involving a joint may severely damage the articular cartilage and give rise to post-traumatic osteoarthritis. Irregularity of the joint surface may cause localized stress and predispose to secondary osteoarthritis years later. If there is a large step, intra-articular osteotomies may help.

Malunion of a metaphyseal fracture may radically alter the mechanics of a nearby joint and give rise to secondary osteoarthritis.

STRESS (FATIGUE) FRACTURES

A stress or fatigue fracture is one occurring in the normal bone of a healthy patient due to repetitive bending and compression stresses.

- In repeated *bending stress*, osteoclastic resorption exceeds osteoblastic formation and a zone of relative weakness develops, ultimately leading to a breach in the cortex. This process affects young adults undertaking strenuous physical routines. Athletes in training, dancers and military recruits build up muscle power quickly but bone strength only slowly; this accounts for the high incidence of stress fractures in these groups.
- *Compressive stresses* act on soft cancellous bone; with frequent repetition, an impacted fracture may result.
- *A combination of compression and shearing stresses* may account for the osteochondral fractures that characterize some of the so-called osteochondritides.
- *Spontaneous fractures* occur with even greater ease in people with osteoporosis or osteomalacia and in patients treated with drugs that affect bone remodelling in a similar way. These are often referred to as *insufficiency fractures*.

SITES AFFECTED BY STRESS FRACTURES

Shaft of humerus (adolescent cricketers)
Pars interarticularis of fifth lumbar vertebra (causing spondylolysis)
Pubic rami (inferior in children, both rami in adults)
Femoral neck (at any age)
Femoral shaft (mainly lower third)
Patella (children and young adults)
Tibial shaft (proximal third in children, middle third in athletes and military recruits, distal third in the elderly)

Distal shaft of the fibula (the 'runner's fracture')
Calcaneum (adults)
Navicular (athletes)
Metatarsals (especially the second)

Clinical features

There may be a history of unaccustomed and repetitive activity or one of a strenuous physical exercise programme. A common sequence of events is:

1 pain *after* exercise
2 pain *during* exercise
3 pain *without* exercise.

The patient is usually healthy. The affected site may be swollen or red. It is sometimes warm and usually tender; the callus may be palpable. 'Springing' the bone (attempting to bend it) is often painful.

Imaging

X-RAYS

Early on, the fracture is difficult to detect; radioscintigraphy will show increased activity. X-rays may show a small transverse cortical defect and/or localized periosteal new-bone formation, which can easily be missed or misdiagnosed (**23.17**). These appearances have, at times, been mistaken for those of an osteosarcoma, a horrifying trap for the unwary.

Compression stress fractures (especially of the femoral neck and upper tibia) may show as a hazy transverse band of sclerosis with peripheral callus (in the tibia).

Small osteoarticular fractures may occur, most commonly the dome of the medial femoral condyle at the knee or the upper surface of the talus at the ankle. Later, ischaemic necrosis of the detached fragment may render the lesion more obvious.

MRI

The earliest changes are revealed by MRI.

SECTION 3 TRAUMA

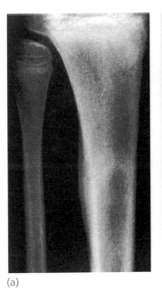
(a)

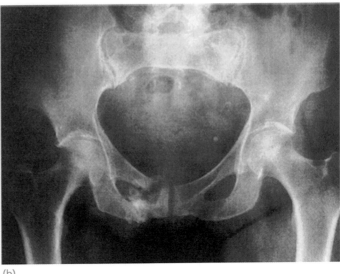
(b)

Figure 23.17 Stress fractures Stress fractures are often missed or wrongly diagnosed. **(a)** This tibial fracture was at first thought to be an osteosarcoma. **(b)** Stress fractures of the pubic rami in elderly women can be mistaken for metastases.

Diagnosis

 Many disorders, including osteomyelitis, scurvy and non-accidental injury, may be confused with stress fractures. The great danger, however, is a mistaken diagnosis of osteosarcoma; scanning shows increased uptake in both conditions and even biopsy may be misleading.

Treatment

Most stress fractures need no treatment other than support and avoidance of the painful activity until the lesion heals, which can take many months.

An important exception is stress fracture of the femoral neck. This should be suspected in all elderly people who complain of pain in the hip for which no obvious cause can be found. If the diagnosis is confirmed by bone scan, the femoral neck should be internally fixed with screws as a prophylactic measure.

PATHOLOGICAL FRACTURES

Pathological fractures occur in abnormal bone.

HISTORY

Bone that fractures spontaneously, or after trivial injury, must be regarded as abnormal until proved otherwise. Older patients should always be asked about previous illnesses or operations. A malignant tumour, no matter how long ago it occurred, may be the source of a late metastatic lesion. A history of gastrectomy, intestinal malabsorption, chronic alcoholism or prolonged drug therapy suggests a metabolic bone disorder.

Symptoms such as loss of weight, pain, a lump, cough or haematuria suggest that the fracture may be through a secondary deposit.

In younger patients, a history of several previous fractures may suggest a diagnosis of osteogenesis imperfecta.

EXAMINATION

Local signs of bone disease (sinus, old scar, swelling or deformity) should not be missed. The site of the fracture may suggest the diagnosis: patients with involutional osteoporosis develop fractures of the vertebral bodies and corticocancellous junctions of long bones; a fracture through the shaft of the bone in an elderly patient, especially in the subtrochanteric region, may be due to metastasis.

CAUSES OF PATHOLOGICAL FRACTURE

Generalized bone disease

- Osteogenesis imperfecta
- Postmenopausal osteoporosis
- Metabolic bone disease
- Myelomatosis
- Polyostotic fibrous dysplasia
- Paget's disease

Local benign conditions

- Chronic infection
- Solitary bone cyst
- Fibrous cortical defect
- Chondromyxoid fibroma
- Aneurysmal bone cyst
- Chondroma
- Monostotic fibrous dysplasia

Primary malignant tumours

- Chondrosarcoma
- Osteosarcoma
- Ewing's tumour

Metastatic tumours

- Carcinoma in breast, lung, kidney, thyroid, colon and prostate

General examination may be informative. Congenital dysplasias, fibrous dysplasia, Cushing's syndrome and Paget's disease all produce characteristic appearances. The patient may be wasted (possibly due to malignant disease). The lymph nodes or liver may be enlarged. It should be noted whether there is a mass in the abdomen or pelvis. Old scars should not be overlooked, and rectal and vaginal examinations are mandatory.

- Under the age of 20, the common causes of pathological fracture are benign bone tumours and cysts.
- Over the age of 40, the common causes are multiple myeloma, metastatic lesions and Paget's disease.

Imaging

The bone surrounding the fracture must be examined for features such as cyst formation, cortical erosion, abnormal trabeculation and periosteal thickening. The type of fracture is important too: vertebral compression fractures may be due to severe osteoporosis or osteomalacia, but they can also be caused by skeletal metastases or myeloma.

Additional investigations

- *Radionuclide imaging* may help with the diagnosis and reveal other deposits.
- *Additional X-rays* of other bones, the lungs and the urogenital tract may be necessary to exclude malignant disease.
- Investigations should always include a full blood count, erythrocyte sedimentation rate (ESR), protein electrophoresis, and tests for syphilis and metabolic bone disorders.
- *Urine examination* may reveal blood from a tumour or Bence–Jones protein in myelomatosis.

Biopsy

Some lesions are so typical that a biopsy is unnecessary (solitary cyst, fibrous cortical defect, Paget's disease). Others are more obscure, requiring a biopsy for diagnosis. The principles of management of primary bone tumours must be followed until the diagnosis is established (Chapter 9).

Treatment

The principles of fracture treatment remain the same: *reduce, hold, exercise*. However, the method is influenced by the underlying pathology (Chapter 9) and condition of the bone (23.18).

Generalized bone disease In most of these conditions (including Paget's), the bones fracture more easily but heal quite well provided that the fracture is properly immobilized. Internal fixation is therefore advisable. Patients with osteomalacia, hyperparathyroidism, renal osteodystrophy and Paget's disease will need systemic treatment.

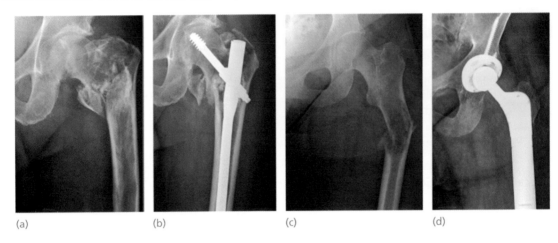

(a)   (b)   (c)   (d)

Figure 23.18 Pathological fractures–treatment (a,b) Paget's disease of the femur increases the brittleness of bone, making it more likely to fracture. Intramedullary fixation allows the entire femur to be supported. **(c,d)** A fracture through a solitary metastasis from a previously excised renal cell carcinoma can be resected in order to achieve cure. In this case, replacement of the proximal femur with an endoprosthesis is needed.

Local benign conditions Fractures through benign cyst-like lesions usually heal quite well. Treatment is therefore the same as for simple fractures in the same area, although in some cases it will be necessary to take a biopsy before immobilizing the fracture. When the bone has healed, the tumour can be dealt with by curettage or local excision.

Primary malignant tumour The fracture may need splinting but this is a prelude to definitive treatment of the tumour (see Chapter 9).

Metastatic tumours Metastasis is a frequent cause of pathological fracture in older people. Breast cancer is the commonest source and the femur the commonest site.

- *Fracture of a long-bone shaft* should be treated by internal fixation. Remember the implant will function as a load-*bearing* and not a load-*sharing* device and will need to be strong enough not to break due to fatigue failure during the lifespan of the patient.
- *Fracture near a bone end* can often be treated by excision and total joint or endoprosthetic replacement (e.g. hip). Preoperatively, imaging studies should be performed to detect other bone lesions; these may be amenable to prophylactic fixation as part of the same procedure.

- *Pathological compression fractures of the spine* cause severe pain due to spinal instability and treatment options should include operative stabilization. If there are either clinical or imaging features of actual or threatened spinal cord or cauda equina compression, the segment should also be decompressed. Postoperative irradiation is given as usual.

With all types of metastatic lesion, the primary tumour should be sought if not known, investigated and treated as well.

INJURIES OF THE PHYSIS

Over 10% of children's fractures involve injury to the physis which is a relatively weak part of the bone. The fracture most commonly runs transversely through the hypertrophic or the calcified layer of the growth plate, often veering off into the metaphysis at one of the edges to include a triangular lip of bone. This has little effect on longitudinal growth, however, if the fracture traverses the cellular 'reproductive' layers of the physis, it may result in premature ossification of the injured part and growth disturbance.

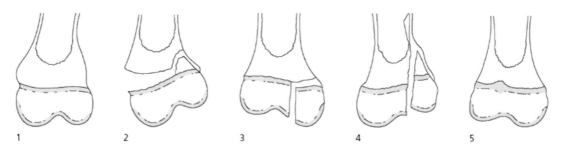

Figure 23.19 Physeal injuries *Type 1* – separation of the epiphysis–which usually occurs in infants but is also seen at puberty as a slipped femoral epiphysis. *Type 2* – fracture through the physis and metaphysic – is the commonest; it occurs in older children and seldom results in abnormal growth. *Type 3* – an intra-articular fracture of the epiphysis–needs accurate reduction to restore the joint surface. *Type 4* – splitting of the physis and epiphysis – damages the articular surface and may also cause abnormal growth; if it is displaced, it needs open reduction. *Type 5* – crushing of the physis – may look benign but ends in arrested growth.

Classification

The Salter and Harris classification is widely used and distinguishes five types of physeal injury (**23.19**).

Mechanism of injury

Physeal fractures usually result from falls or traction.

 Non-accidental injury should always be considered by the treating doctors and surgeons and investigated appropriately.

Clinical features

Deformity is usually minimal, but any injury in a child followed by pain and tenderness near the joint should arouse suspicion, and X-ray examination is essential.

Imaging

On *X-ray*, the physis itself is radiolucent and the epiphysis may be incompletely ossified making diagnosis more difficult. Telltale features are:

- widening of the physeal 'gap'
- joint incongruity
- tilting of the epiphyseal axis.

If there is the faintest suspicion of a physeal fracture but the diagnosis has not been made, a repeat X-ray after 4 or 5 days is strongly advised.

Treatment

UNDISPLACED FRACTURES

These may be treated by splinting or a cast for 2–4 weeks (depending on the site of injury and the age of the child). With undisplaced type 3 and type 4 fractures, a check X-ray after 4 days and again at about 10 days is needed in order not to miss late displacement.

DISPLACED FRACTURES

These should be reduced as soon as possible. With types 1 and 2, this can usually be done closed; the part is then splinted securely for 3–6 weeks. Type 3 and type 4 fractures demand perfect anatomical reduction which may be achieved closed and then held in a cast for 4–6 weeks. If a type 3 or 4 fracture cannot be reduced accurately closed, immediate open reduction and internal fixation with smooth K-wires is essential. The limb is then splinted for 4–6 weeks.

Complications

Type 1 and type 2 injuries These have an excellent prognosis and bone growth is not affected. Exceptions to this are injuries around the knee involving the distal femoral or proximal tibial physis; both growth plates are undulating in shape. Transverse fractures may therefore pass through the proliferative zone. Complications such as malunion or non-union may also occur if the diagnosis is missed and the fracture remains unreduced.

Type 3 and type 4 injuries   These may result in premature fusion or asymmetrical growth.

Type 5 fractures   These cause premature fusion and growth retardation. The size and position of the bony bridge across the physis can be assessed by CT or MRI and, if less than one-third the width of the physis, can be excised and replaced by a fat graft, with some prospect of preventing or diminishing the growth disturbance.

Established deformity   Whether from asymmetrical growth or from malunion of a displaced fracture (e.g. a valgus elbow due to proximal displacement of a lateral humeral condylar fracture), established deformity should be treated by corrective osteotomy.

INJURIES TO JOINTS

If the injuring force is great enough, the ligaments may tear, or the bone to which they are attached may be pulled apart. The articular cartilage may be damaged, too, if the joint surfaces are compressed or if there is a fracture into the joint (**23.20**).

Sprains, strains and ruptures

A *sprain* is any painful wrenching (twisting or pulling) movement of a joint, but the term is generally reserved for joint injuries less severe than actual complete tearing of the capsule or ligaments. *Strain* is a physical effect of stress, in this case tensile stress associated with some stretching of the ligaments; in colloquial usage, 'strained ligament' is often meant to denote an injury somewhat more severe than a 'sprain', which possibly involves tearing of some fibres. If the stretching or twisting force is severe enough, the ligament may be strained to the point of complete *rupture*.

STRAINED LIGAMENT

Only some of the fibres in the ligament are torn and the joint remains stable. The joint is painful and swollen and the tissues may be bruised. Tenderness is localized to the injured ligament and tensing the tissues on that side causes pain.

Treatment

The joint should be firmly strapped or braced to support the injured ligament but range of motion permitted. Active movements are encouraged when tolerated.

RUPTURED LIGAMENT

The joint is unstable. Sometimes the ligament holds and the bone to which it is attached is avulsed and may be amenable to reattachment.

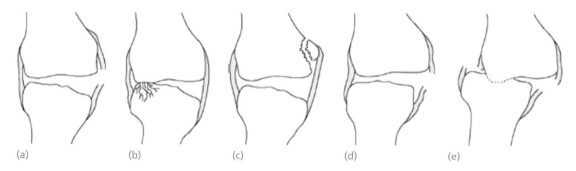

(a)   (b)   (c)   (d)   (e)

Figure 23.20 Joint injuries Severe stress may cause various types of injury. (**a**) A ligament may rupture, leaving the bone intact. If the soft tissues hold, the bone on the opposite side may be crushed (**b**), or a fragment may be pulled off by the taut ligament (**c**). Subluxation (**d**) means the articular surfaces are partially displaced; dislocation (**e**) refers to complete displacement of the joint.

SECTION 3 TRAUMA

The joints most likely to be affected are the ones that are insecure by virtue of their shape or least well protected by surrounding muscles:

- knee
- ankle
- finger joints.

Pain is severe and there may be considerable bruising; if the joint is swollen, this is probably due to a haemarthrosis and typically comes on quickly. The joint is often too painful to elicit instability in the first few days. *X-rays* may show a detached flake of bone from the origin or insertion.

Treatment

Torn ligaments heal by fibrous scarring. Direct repair may be suitable in some injuries, such as rupture of the ulnar collateral ligament of the metacarpophalangeal joint of the thumb. In others (e.g. medial collateral ligament ruptures of the knee), non-operative treatment in a brace may be suitable. Physiotherapy or exercises are commenced to maintain muscle strength and later proprioceptive exercises are added.

Avulsions may benefit from reattachment of the fragment if the piece is large enough. Non-operative treatment may result in some residual instability that impairs function, in which case surgical reconstruction should be considered.

DISLOCATION AND SUBLUXATION

Dislocation means that the joint surfaces are completely displaced and are no longer in contact; *subluxation* implies a lesser degree of displacement, such that the articular surfaces are still partly apposed.

Clinical features

Following an injury, the joint is painful and the patient tries to avoid movement. The contour of the joint is abnormal. The limb is often held in a characteristic position. *X-rays* in multiple planes will clinch the diagnosis but appropriate views must be taken; they will also show whether there is an associated bony injury affecting joint stability, i.e. a fracture-dislocation.

Apprehension test If the dislocation is reduced by the time the patient is seen, the joint can be tested by stressing it as if almost to reproduce the suspected dislocation: the patient develops a sense of impending disaster and resists further manipulation.

Recurrent dislocation If the ligaments and joint margins are damaged, repeated dislocation may occur. This is seen especially in the shoulder and patellofemoral joint.

Habitual (voluntary) dislocation Some patients acquire the knack of dislocating (or subluxing) the joint by voluntary muscle contraction. Ligamentous laxity may make this easier. It is important to recognize this because such patients are seldom helped by operation, which can lead to worsening of their symptoms, and require focused physiotherapy to train appropriate muscle patterning.

Treatment

The dislocation is reduced as soon as possible which may require sedation or general anaesthetic, and sometimes a muscle relaxant as well. The joint is then rested or immobilized until soft-tissue swelling reduces – usually after 2 weeks. Controlled movements then begin in a functional brace; progress with physiotherapy is monitored. Occasionally, surgical reconstruction for residual instability is needed.

Complications

Many of the complications of fractures are seen also after dislocations:

- vascular injury
- nerve injury
- avascular necrosis of bone
- heterotopic ossification
- joint stiffness
- secondary osteoarthritis.

The principles of diagnosis and management of these conditions are discussed in 'Complications of fractures' earlier in this chapter.

▪ Fractures of the clavicle	551	
▪ Fractures of the scapula	552	
▪ Scapulothoracic dissociation	553	
▪ Acromioclavicular joint injuries	553	
▪ Sternoclavicular dislocation	555	
▪ Dislocation of the shoulder	556	
▪ Fractures of the proximal humerus	559	
▪ Fractures of the shaft of the humerus	562	

The great bugbear of upper limb injuries is stiffness. In elderly patients especially, it is as important to preserve movement as it is to treat the fracture.

FRACTURES OF THE CLAVICLE

A fall on the shoulder or the outstretched hand may fracture the clavicle; the lateral fragment is pulled down by the weight of the arm, while the medial fragment is held up by the sternomastoid muscle.

Clinical features

The fracture is often displaced, producing a lump along the 'collar-bone'. Fractures of the outer third are easily mistaken for acromioclavicular injuries. Vascular and neurological complications are rare.

Imaging

* *X-rays* show that the fracture is usually in the middle third of the bone and the lateral fragment lies below the medial. Outer-third injuries need special views to define any fracture.

* A *computed tomography (CT) scan* is occasionally needed to define the fracture configuration to exclude a sternoclavicular dislocation or to show if a fracture has healed.

Treatment

UNDISPLACED MIDDLE-THIRD FRACTURES
Accurate closed reduction is neither possible nor essential. In most cases, all that is needed is to support the arm in a sling until the pain subsides (usually 1–3 weeks). Thereafter, active shoulder exercises should be encouraged; this is particularly important in older patients.

DISPLACED MIDDLE-THIRD FRACTURES
There is less agreement about the management of displaced middle-third fractures. Treating those with shortening of more than 2 cm by simple splintage incurs a risk of symptomatic malunion – mainly pain and lack of power during shoulder movements – and an increased incidence of non-union. There is therefore a growing trend towards internal fixation of acute clavicular fractures associated with severe displacement, fragmentation or shortening (24.1). Specific contoured locking plates are available. Another advantage is that the

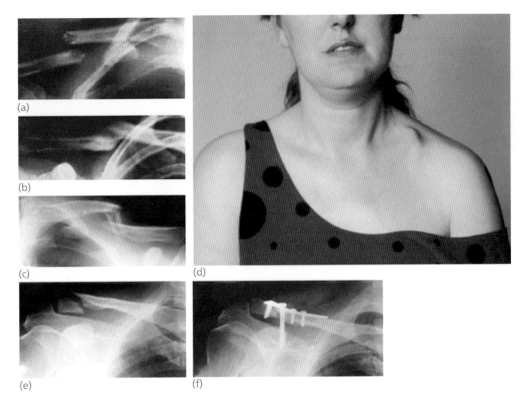

24.1 Fractured clavicle (a) The common site and displacement. Often the fracture unites in a some-what faulty position **(b)** but this seldom worries the patient. However, the severely displaced fracture shown in **(c)**, though it united well enough, left an unsightly deformity **(d)**; it would have been better treated by open reduction and internal fixation with a small plate and screws. Fractures of the outer (lateral) third with elevation of the clavicular shaft due to rupture of the coracoclavicular ligament may also require internal fixation **(e,f)**.

patient can mobilize the arm and return to work and independence more quickly.

OUTER-THIRD FRACTURES

By contrast, outer-third fractures are quite troublesome and may need open reduction and internal fixation (e24.1).

Complications

Despite deformity, damage to the lung or vessels beneath the clavicle is very rare.

Malunion This is inevitable in displaced fractures; in children, the bone is soon remodelled, but in adults the slight deformity has to be accepted unless there is a very unsightly bump with skin irritation.

Non-union This sometimes occurs in middle-third fractures and is treated by bone graft and plating.

FRACTURES OF THE SCAPULA

The *body of the scapula* is fractured by a crushing force, which usually also fractures ribs and may dislocate the sternoclavicular joint. The *neck of the scapula* may be fractured by a blow or by a fall on the shoulder.

Clinical features

Shoulder movements are painful but possible. If breathing also is painful, thoracic injury must be excluded.

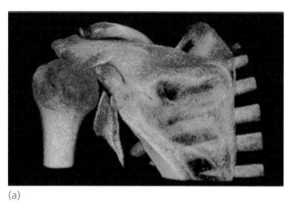
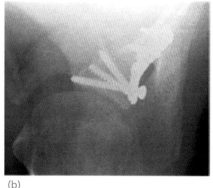

(a)   (b)

24.2 Glenoid fracture – imaging (a) Three-dimensional CT of a glenoid fracture. **(b)** X-ray after open reduction and internal fixation.

Imaging

- Scapular fractures can be difficult to define on plain *X-rays* because of the surrounding soft tissues. X-rays may show a comminuted fracture of the *body* of the scapula, or a fractured *scapular neck* with the outer fragment pulled downwards by the weight of the arm.
- *CT* is useful for demonstrating *glenoid* or *body* fractures (e24.2).

Treatment

Reduction is usually unnecessary. The patient wears a sling for comfort and from the start practises active exercises of the shoulder, elbow and fingers.

Check repeatedly for dislocation of the shoulder; a large glenoid fragment may require open reduction and internal fixation (**24.2**).

SCAPULOTHORACIC DISSOCIATION

This is a high-energy injury in which the shoulder is literally wrenched away from the torso.

> ⚠ There is a great chance of death due to the associated vascular rupture.

Treatment requires resuscitation and then reconstruction of the vascular, neurological and musculoskeletal injuries. The arm rarely recovers.

ACROMIOCLAVICULAR JOINT INJURIES

A fall on the shoulder strains or tears the acromioclavicular ligaments, and upward subluxation of the clavicle may occur; more severe injury also tears the coracoclavicular ligaments, resulting in complete dislocation of the joint (**24.3**).

Clinical features

The patient can usually point to the site of injury. If there is tenderness but no deformity (or very little deformity), it is probably a strain or a subluxation. With dislocation, the patient is in more pain and a prominent 'step' can be seen and felt (**24.4**).

X-rays

The films show either a subluxation with only slight elevation of the clavicle, or dislocation with considerable separation. A stress view, taken with the patient holding a 5 kg weight in each hand, may reveal the displacement more clearly.

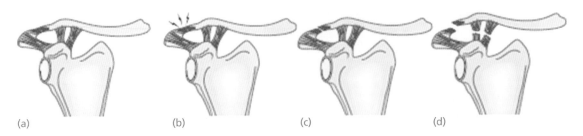

24.3 Acromioclavicular joint injuries **(a)** Normal joint. **(b)** Sprained acromioclavicular joint; no displacement. **(c)** Torn capsule and subluxation but coracoclavicular ligaments intact. **(d)** Dislocation with torn coracoclavicular ligaments.

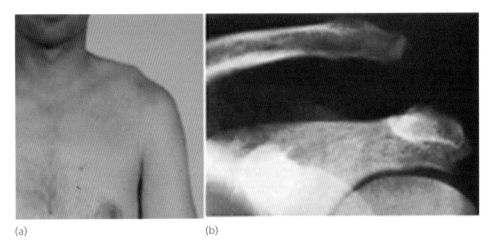

24.4 Acromioclavicular dislocation **(a)** The clinical picture is unmistakable: a definite step in the contour at the outer end of the clavicle. **(b)** X-ray showing complete separation of the acromioclavicular joint.

Treatment

SPRAINS AND SUBLUXATION

These do not usually affect function and require no special treatment; the arm is rested in a sling until pain subsides (usually no more than 1 week), and shoulder exercises are then begun.

DISLOCATION

This is poorly controlled by padding and strapping. Nevertheless, surgery is controversial and it is doubtful whether it improves the outcome except in those whose work or hobbies involve using the arm above shoulder height for long periods. One of the more reliable techniques is to reduce the dislocation by open operation, then reconstruct the ligament and support it with a graft.

Complications

Discomfort and weakness of the shoulder Long-standing, unreduced dislocation of the acromioclavicular joint, though still compatible with reasonably good function, may leave the patient with an ill-defined feeling of discomfort and weakness of the shoulder, especially when attempting strenuous overhead activities. If the symptoms warrant active treatment, reconstructive surgery can be advised, but the patient must be warned that improvement cannot be guaranteed. One approach is to excise a small segment of the lateral end of the clavicle and then to tether the 'floating' clavicle by transferring the coracoacromial ligament to the lateral end of the clavicle; the structure may be further stabilized by

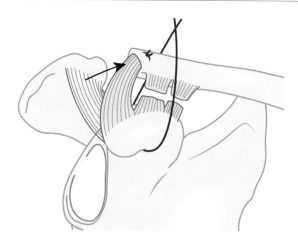

24.5 Modified Weaver Dunn operation The lateral end of the clavicle is excised; the acromial end of the coracoacromial ligament is detached and fastened to the lateral end of the clavicle. Tension on the ligament is lessened by placing a 'sling' around the clavicle and the coracoid process. (Dotted lines show former position of coracoacromial ligament.)

holding the clavicle down with a screw between the clavicle and the coracoid process (**24.5**).

Osteoarthritis A very late complication is osteoarthritis of the acromioclavicular joint; this can usually be managed conservatively, but if pain is marked, the outer end of the clavicle can be excised.

STERNOCLAVICULAR DISLOCATION

ANTERIOR DISLOCATION

This uncommon injury is caused by a fall on the shoulder. The inner end of the clavicle springs forward, producing a visible and palpable prominence. The joint can usually be reduced quite easily by direct pressure on the prominent clavicle while the shoulders are relaxed. The problem is keeping it there. Splintage is unsatisfactory and internal fixation carries unnecessary risks – great vessels and pericardium are too close for comfort! The patient should be persuaded to accept the slight residual deformity and mild discomfort during strenuous activity (**24.6**).

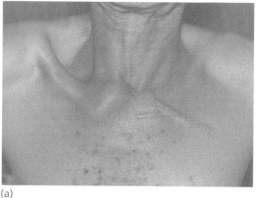

(a)

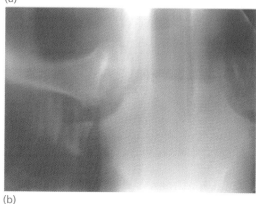

(b)

24.6 Sternoclavicular dislocation (a) The bump over the sternoclavicular joint may be obvious, though this is difficult to demonstrate on plain X-ray. (b) Tomography (or better still CT) will show the lesion.

POSTERIOR DISLOCATION

> ⚠ Posterior dislocation is very rare, but it can cause compression of the large vessels in the neck and should be reduced as a matter of urgency.

Closed reduction can sometimes be achieved by lying the patient supine with a sandbag between the shoulder blades and then pulling on the arm with the shoulder abducted and extended; the joint reduces with a snap. The shoulders are braced backwards with a figure-of-eight bandage, which is kept in place for 3 weeks. If closed reduction fails, operative reduction is called for. The displaced clavicle is pulled forward with a hook.

SECTION 3 TRAUMA

DISLOCATION OF THE SHOULDER

The glenohumeral joint is very shallow and stability is maintained largely by the glenoid labrum (which slightly deepens the socket) and the surrounding ligaments and muscles. Traumatic dislocation is common; humeral head displacement is usually anterior, less often posterior. In this chapter, acute dislocations are described. Chronic instability is described in Chapter 13.

ANTERIOR DISLOCATION

Anterior dislocation is caused either by a fall on the backward-stretching hand or by forced abduction and external rotation of the shoulder. The head of the humerus is driven forward, tearing the capsule or avulsing the glenoid labrum, and usually ends up just below the coracoid process. There may be an associated fracture of the proximal end of the humerus.

Clinical features

Pain is severe. The patient supports the arm with the opposite hand and is loath to permit any kind of examination. The lateral outline of the shoulder is flattened and a small bulge may be seen and felt just below the clavicle (e24.3). Looking from above, the usual forward bulge is altered compared with the other side.

> ⚠ The arm must always be examined for nerve and vessel injury *before* reduction is attempted.

X-rays

These show the overlapping shadows of the humeral head and glenoid fossa, with the head usually lying below and medial to the socket. A *lateral view* is essential to show whether or not the head is in the socket.

Treatment

In those with recurrent dislocations, the reduction may be achieved spontaneously by the patient or by the doctor with no sedation. Otherwise, for those with a first dislocation, prompt reduction can be achieved under sedation; if the muscle spasm and pain are overwhelming, a general anaesthetic may be required. *X-rays* prior to dislocation are mandatory to exclude a fracture-dislocation.

While the patient is waiting, they can be placed in the prone position with the arm hanging over the side of the bed – the dislocation may reduce (*Stimson's method*). Otherwise, the simplest and safest method is to pull on the arm in slight abduction and flexion while the body is steadied by an assistant who has wrapped a towel around the torso for countertraction (*Hippocratic method*).

An X-ray is taken to confirm reduction and exclude a fracture. When the patient is fully awake, active abduction is gently tested to exclude an axillary nerve injury or rotator cuff tear. The arm is then supported in a sling.

For those over 30 years of age, stiffness is more of a risk than recurrent dislocation so movements are begun after 1 week. For those under 30 years, recurrence is more of a risk and so the sling is retained for 3 weeks before mobilizing.

> ⚠ X-ray before and after reducing the shoulder.
>
> Examine the axillary and musculocutaneous nerve before and after reduction.
>
> Direct blow to the shoulder: X-ray for associated cervical spine injury.

Complications

Rotator cuff tear   The rotator cuff is often torn, particularly in older people. This is suggested by the patient's inability to initiate abduction of the arm. An ultrasound or magnetic resonance imaging (MRI) will readily confirm the diagnosis. The lesion may later require surgical repair.

Nerve injury   The axillary nerve may be injured; the patient is unable to contract the deltoid muscle and there may be a small patch of anaesthesia over the muscle. The lesion is usually a neurapraxia, which recovers spontaneously after a few weeks. This must be distinguished from a rotator cuff tear.

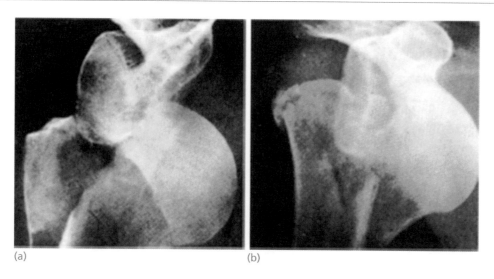

(a)   (b)

24.7 Anterior fracture-dislocation Anterior dislocation of the shoulder may be complicated by fracture of **(a)** the greater tuberosity or **(b)** the neck of the humerus – this often needs open reduction and internal fixation.

Occasionally, the posterior cord of the brachial plexus, the median nerve or the musculocutaneous nerve may be injured. This is alarming, but these injuries usually recover with time.

Vascular injury The axillary artery may be damaged before or during reduction. The limb should always be examined for signs of ischaemia.

Fracture-dislocation If there is an associated fracture of the proximal humerus, open reduction and internal fixation may be necessary (**24.7**).

Recurrent dislocation If the glenoid labrum has been damaged or detached, recurrent dislocation is likely (**24.8**).

POSTERIOR DISLOCATION

This is much rarer than an anterior dislocation but is commonly missed. It should always be suspected if the patient had suffered an epileptic fit or a severe electric shock. It is otherwise caused

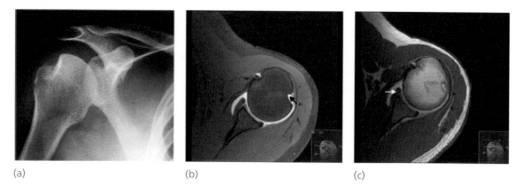

(a)   (b)   (c)

24.8 Recurrent dislocation of the shoulder **(a)** The classic X-ray sign is a depression in the posterosuperior part of the humeral head (the Hill–Sachs lesion). **(b,c)** MRI scans showing both the Hill–Sachs lesion and a Bankart lesion of the glenoid rim (arrows).

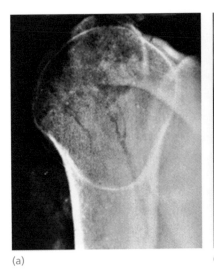
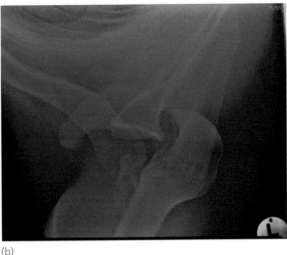

(a)   (b)

24.9 Posterior dislocation of the shoulder (a) The characteristic X-ray image. Because the head of the humerus is internally rotated, the anteroposterior X-ray shows a head-on projection giving the classic 'electric light-bulb' appearance. **(b)** Locked (unreduced) posterior dislocation.

by forced internal rotation of the abducted arm or by a direct blow on the front of the shoulder.

Clinical features

The diagnosis is frequently missed because, in the anteroposterior X-ray, the humeral head may seem to be in contact with the glenoid socket. However, clinically the condition is unmistakable because the arm is held in medial rotation and is locked in that position.

X-rays

In the *anteroposterior* view, the humeral head looks somewhat like a light bulb because it is medially rotated (24.9). A *lateral view* is essential; it shows posterior subluxation and, sometimes, indentation of the humeral head.

Treatment

The arm is pulled and rotated laterally, while the head of the humerus is pushed forwards. After reduction, the management is the same as for anterior dislocation. The management of late-presenting posterior dislocation is complicated.

INFERIOR DISLOCATION

 Inferior dislocation is rare but it demands early recognition because the consequences are potentially very serious.

Dislocation occurs with the arm in nearly full abduction/elevation. The humeral head is levered out of its socket and lies in the axilla; the arm remains fixed in abduction.

Mechanism of injury and pathology

The injury is caused by a severe hyper-abduction force. With the humerus as the lever and the acromion as the fulcrum, the humeral head

POSSIBLE SERIOUS SOFT-TISSUE INJURY

Avulsion of the capsule and surrounding tendons
Rupture of muscles
Fractures of the glenoid or proximal humerus
Damage to the brachial plexus and axillary artery

is lifted across the inferior rim of the glenoid socket; it remains in the subglenoid position, with the humeral shaft pointing upwards. Soft-tissue injury may be severe.

Clinical features

The startling picture of a patient with his arm locked in almost full abduction should make diagnosis quite easy. The head of the humerus may be felt in or below the axilla. Always examine for neurovascular damage.

X-rays

The humeral shaft is shown in the abducted position with the head sitting below the glenoid. It is important to search for associated fractures of the glenoid or proximal humerus (**24.10**).

Treatment

Inferior dislocation can usually be reduced by pulling upwards in the line of the abducted arm,

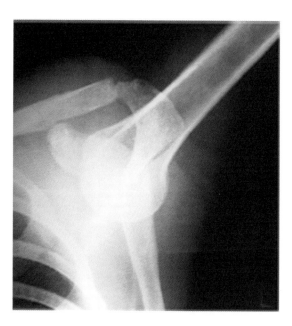

24.10 Inferior dislocation of the shoulder You can see why the condition is called *luxatio erecta*. The shaft of the humerus points upwards and the humeral head is displaced downwards.

with countertraction downwards over the top of the shoulder. If the humeral head is stuck in the soft tissues, open reduction is needed. It is important to examine again, after reduction, for evidence of neurovascular injury.

RECURRENT DISLOCATION

This is discussed in Chapter 13.

FRACTURES OF THE PROXIMAL HUMERUS

IN ADULTS

Fractures of the proximal humerus usually occur after middle age and are most common in osteoporotic individuals. The patient falls on the outstretched hand, fracturing the surgical neck; one or both tuberosities may also be fractured.

Clinical features

Pain may not be very severe because the fracture is often firmly impacted. However, the appearance of a large bruise in the upper arm is very suspicious. The patient should be examined for signs of axillary nerve or brachial plexus injury.

Imaging

X-ray examination is needed.

- *In elderly patients*, X-rays often appear to show a single, impacted fracture extending across the surgical neck; sometimes a separate fracture of the greater tuberosity is also seen. However, with good definition X-rays, several undisplaced fragments may be visible.
- *In younger patients*, the fragments are usually more clearly defined. Axillary and scapular lateral views should always be obtained, to exclude dislocation of the shoulder.

Neer's classification is used to assess fractures.

> **NEER'S CLASSIFICATION OF PROXIMAL HUMERUS FRACTURES**
>
> *One-part fracture* The fragments are undisplaced or firmly impacted (i.e. the humerus appears to be 'in one piece').
> *Two-part fracture* The neck fracture is displaced (i.e. there are only two fragments, the humeral head and the rest of the bone).
> *Three-part or four-part fracture* In addition to the neck fracture, one or both of the tuberosities is also fractured (**24.11**).

This system sounds systematic and straightforward, but it is not easy to distinguish the radiographic outlines of comminuted fractures (**24.12**).

In common with so many other complex fractures, a *CT scan* will help to diagnose the fracture configuration and plan treatment (**24.13**).

As the fracture heals, the humeral head is sometimes seen to be subluxated downwards (inferiorly); this is due to muscle atony and it usually recovers once exercises are begun.

Treatment

IMPACTED OR MINIMALLY DISPLACED FRACTURES

These need no treatment apart from a short period of rest with the arm in a sling. Active movements are begun as soon as practicable, but the sling is retained until the fracture has united (usually after 6 weeks). The elbow and hand are, of course, actively exercised from the start.

TWO-PART FRACTURES

These can usually be reduced closed; the arm is then bandaged to the chest for 3–4 weeks, after which shoulder exercises are commenced (the elbow and hand are, of course, exercised throughout). If the fragments cannot be reduced, fixation, particularly in younger patients, is considered.

THREE-PART FRACTURES

- *In young, active individuals,* these usually require open reduction and internal fixation with either a nail or a locking plate and screws (**24.14**).
- *In elderly patients with osteoporotic bone,* the results are less certain and manipulative

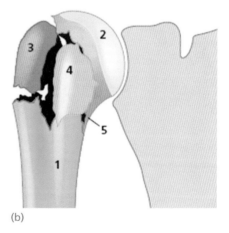

(a)   (b)

24.11 Fractures of the proximal humerus Diagram of **(a)** the normal and **(b)** a fractured proximal humerus, showing the four main fragments, two or more of which are seen in almost all proximal humeral fractures: 1, shaft of humerus; 2, head of humerus; 3, greater tuberosity; 4, lesser tuberosity. In this diagram, there is a sizeable medial calcar spike, 5, suggesting a low risk of avascular necrosis.

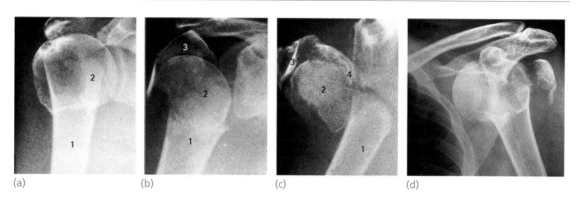

(a)   (b)   (c)   (d)

24.12 X-rays of proximal humeral fractures Classification is all very well, but X-rays are more difficult to interpret than line drawings. **(a)** Two-part fracture. **(b)** Three-part fracture involving the neck and the greater tuberosity. **(c)** Four-part fracture. (1, shaft of humerus; 2, head of humerus; 3, greater tuberosity, 4, lesser tuberosity.) **(d)** X-ray showing fracture dislocation of the shoulder.

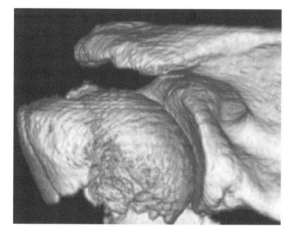

24.13 CT with 3D reconstruction Advanced imaging provides a much clearer picture of the injury, allowing better preoperative planning.

reduction followed by physiotherapy may be equally satisfactory in the long term. Alternatives for osteoporotic patients include bone sutures, intramedullary nails or locking plates.

FOUR-PART FRACTURES

Because they carry additional risks of incomplete reduction, non-union and avascular necrosis of the humeral head, these are best treated by prosthetic replacement, particularly in elderly patients.

Complications

Avascular necrosis This is a risk (10–50%) in three- and four-part fractures due to the complex but fragile blood supply to the humeral head. The risk is even higher in fracture dislocations.

Malunion This usually causes little disability, but loss of rotation may make it difficult for the patient to reach behind the neck or up the back.

Shoulder dislocation Combined fracture and dislocation of the shoulder is difficult to manage. The dislocation should be reduced (this may require an operation) and the fracture can then be tackled in the usual way.

Vascular and nerve injuries These may occur with three-part and four-part fractures and should be sought at the initial examination and after reduction or surgery.

Stiffness Shoulder stiffness is common. It can be minimized by starting exercises as early as possible.

IN CHILDREN

In children, fractures of the proximal humerus are often angulated and will remodel well following simple treatment in a sling for a few weeks. Occasionally, the fracture is through a benign (or very rarely malignant) bone lesion (**24.15**).

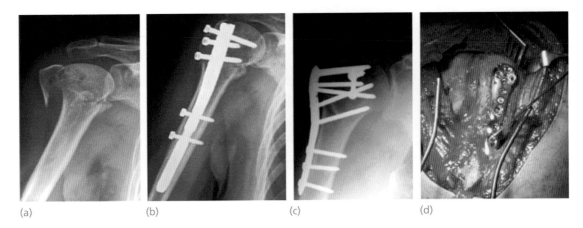

(a)   (b)   (c)   (d)

24.14 Proximal humerus fractures – treatment (a) Three-part fracture, treated by (b) locked nail fixation. (c) Four-part fracture fixed with a locked plate; the intraoperative picture (d) shows how the plate was positioned.

FRACTURES OF THE SHAFT OF THE HUMERUS

POSSIBLE CAUSES OF HUMERUS SHAFT FRACTURES

A fall on the hand may twist the humerus, causing a *spiral fracture.*

A fall on the elbow with the arm abducted may hinge the bone, causing an *oblique or transverse fracture.*

A direct blow to the arm causes either a *transverse or comminuted fracture.*

A fracture of the shaft in an elderly patient may be through a metastasis.

Clinical features

The arm is painful, bruised and swollen.

> ⚠ Active extension of the wrist and fingers should be tested *before and after treatment* because the radial nerve may be damaged.

Testing of the wrist and fingers is best done by assessing active extension of the metacarpophalangeal (MCP) joints; active extension of the wrist can be misleading because extensor carpi

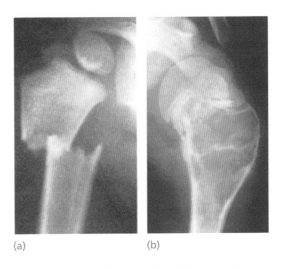

(a)   (b)

24.15 Fractures of the proximal humerus in children (a) The typical metaphyseal fracture. Reduction need not be perfect as remodelling will compensate for malunion. (b) Fracture through a benign cyst.

radialis longus is sometimes supplied by a branch arising proximal to the injury.

X-rays

The fracture is usually obvious, but don't forget to look for features suggesting a pathological lesion (e.g. fracture through a bone cyst or metastasis).

Treatment

NON-OPERATIVE TREATMENT

Fractures of the humerus require neither perfect reduction nor total immobilization; the weight of the arm with an external cast is usually enough to pull the fragments into alignment. The cast is applied from the shoulder to the wrist with the elbow flexed to 90 degrees; after 2–3 weeks, it may be replaced by a shorter cast (shoulder to elbow) or by a removable brace. Exercises of the shoulder can be started within 1 week, but abduction is avoided until the fracture has united. It takes at least 6 weeks for simple spiral fractures to heal. Other fractures may take 3 months or even longer.

OPERATIVE TREATMENT

Patients often find the hanging cast uncomfortable, tedious and frustrating; they can feel the fragments moving and that is sometimes quite distressing. The temptation is to 'do something', and the 'something' usually means an operation. It is as well to remember:

- the complication rate after internal fixation of the humerus is high
- the great majority of humeral fractures unite with non-operative treatment

- there is no good evidence that the union rate is higher with fixation (and the rate may be lower if there is distraction with nailing or periosteal stripping with plating).

There are, nevertheless, some well-defined indications for surgery.

> **INDICATIONS FOR SURGERY ON HUMERUS SHAFT FRACTURES**
>
> Severe multiple injuries
> An open fracture
> Segmental fractures
> Displaced intra-articular extension of the fracture
> A pathological fracture
> A 'floating elbow' (simultaneous unstable humeral and forearm fractures)
> Radial nerve palsy after manipulation
> Non-union
> Problems with nursing care in a dependent person

Fixation (**24.16**) can be achieved with:

- a compression plate and screws
- an interlocking intramedullary nail or semi-flexible pins
- an external fixator.

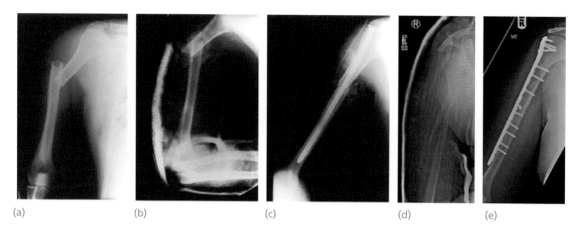

(a) (b) (c) (d) (e)

24.16 Fractured shaft of humerus – treatment (a,b) Most shaft fractures can be treated in a hanging cast or functional brace, but beware the upper third fracture which tends to angulate at the proximal border of a short cast. This fracture would have been better managed by **(c)** intramedullary nailing or open reduction and internal fixation. **(d)** Segmental fracture of the humerus. **(e)** Open reduction and internal fixation.

Complications

Nerve injury   Radial nerve palsy (wrist-drop and paralysis of the MCP extensors) may occur with oblique fractures of the middle-distal shaft. In closed injuries, the nerve is very seldom divided, so there is no hurry to operate. Passive and active movements of the wrist and hand are encouraged while recovery is awaited. However, if the nerve is normal before manipulation and fails after, exploration is indicated in case it has been snagged on the fracture.

If there is no sign of recovery by 12 weeks, the nerve should be explored. In complete lesions (*neurotmesis*), nerve grafting is undertaken but the results are not always satisfactory. If so, function can be largely restored by tendon transfers:

- pronator teres to extensor carpi radialis brevis for wrist extension
- flexor carpi radialis to extensor digitorum for MCP extension
- palmaris longus to abductor pollicis longus for thumb abduction.

Non-union   Midshaft fractures can take months to heal and occasionally fail to unite. Non-union is probably higher with surgical than with non-operative care. This is treated by bone grafting and internal fixation. Care must be taken not to injure the radial nerve.

Stiffness   Joint stiffness is common. It can be minimized by early activity, but transverse fractures (in which shoulder abduction is ill-advised) may limit shoulder movement for several weeks.

Elbow and forearm injuries

25

- Fractures of the distal humerus in children   565
- Fractures of the distal humerus in adults   574
- Fracture-dislocation of the elbow   576
- Simple dislocation of the elbow   576
- Fractured capitellum   577
- Isolated dislocation of the radial head   578
- Pulled elbow in children   578
- Fractures of the proximal end of the radius   578
- Fractures of the olecranon   580
- Fractures of the radius and ulna   582
- Fracture of a single forearm bone   585
- Monteggia fracture-dislocation of the ulna   586
- Galeazzi fracture-dislocation of the radius   587

FRACTURES OF THE DISTAL HUMERUS IN CHILDREN

The elbow is second only to the distal forearm for frequency of fractures in children. Most of these injuries are supracondylar fractures, the remainder being divided between condylar, epicondylar and proximal radial and ulnar fractures. Boys are injured more often than girls and more than one-half of the patients are under 10 years old.

The usual accident is a fall directly on the point of the elbow or onto the outstretched hand with the elbow forced into valgus or varus. Pain and swelling are often marked and examination is difficult. X-ray interpretation also has its problems: the bone ends are largely cartilaginous and therefore radiographically incompletely visualized.

Points of anatomy

 A good knowledge of the normal anatomy is essential if fracture displacements are to be recognized.

The elbow is a complex hinge. Its stability is due largely to the shape and fit of the bones that make up the joint and this is liable to be compromised by any break in the articulating structures. The surrounding soft-tissue structures also are important, especially the capsular and collateral ligaments.

With the elbow extended, the forearm is normally in slight valgus in relation to the upper arm, the average carrying angle in children being about 15 degrees. When the elbow is flexed, the forearm comes to lie directly upon the upper arm. Malunion of a supracondylar fracture will inevitably disturb this relationship.

SECTION 3 TRAUMA

Since the epiphyses are in some part cartilaginous, only the secondary ossific centres can be seen on X-ray; they should not be mistaken for fracture fragments! The average ages at which they appear are easily remembered by the mnemonic CRITOE. Epiphyseal displacements will not be detectable on X-ray before these ages, but they are inferred from radiographic indices such as *Baumann's angle* (25.1).

CRITOE: AVERAGE AGE AT WHICH SECONDARY OSSIFIC CENTRES APPEAR	
Capitellum	2 years
Radial head	4 years
Internal (medial) epicondyle	6 years
Trochlea	8 years
Olecranon	10 years
External (lateral) epicondyle	12 years

SUPRACONDYLAR FRACTURES
IN CHILDREN

These are among the commonest fractures in children. The distal fragment may be displaced and/or tilted either posteriorly or anteriorly.

- *Posterior displacement and tilt* (95% of all cases), suggests a hyperextension injury, usually due to a fall on the outstretched hand. The jagged end of the proximal fragment pokes into the soft tissues anteriorly, sometimes injuring the brachial artery or median nerve.
- *Anterior displacement* is rare.

Clinical features

Following a fall, the child is in pain and the elbow is swollen; with a posteriorly displaced fracture, the S-deformity of the elbow is usually obvious.

> ⚠ With supracondylar fractures, it is essential to feel the pulse and check the capillary return as well as to check distal nerve function. Exclude forearm ischaemia by excluding forearm pain on passive extension of the fingers.

X-rays

- *Undisplaced fractures* are easily missed; there may be no more than subtle features of a soft-tissue haematoma.

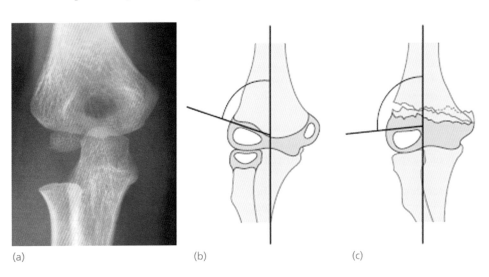

(a)   (b)   (c)

25.1 Baumann's angle Anteroposterior X-rays are sometimes difficult to make out, especially if the elbow is held flexed after reduction of the supracondylar fracture. Measurement of Baumann's angle is helpful. This is the angle subtended by the longitudinal axis of the humeral shaft and a line through the coronal axis of the capitellar physis, as shown in (a) the X-ray of a normal elbow and the accompanying diagram (b). Normally, this angle is less than 80 degrees. If the distal fragment is tilted in varus, the increased angle is readily detected (c).

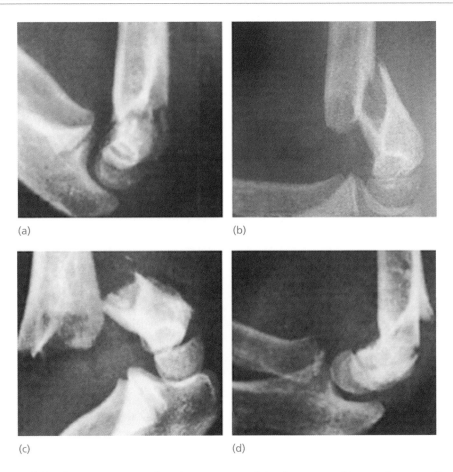

(a)   (b)

(c)   (d)

25.2 Supracondylar fractures X-rays showing supracondylar fractures of increasing severity: **(a)** undisplaced; **(b)** distal fragment posteriorly angulated but in contact; **(c)** distal fragment completely separated and displaced posteriorly; **(d)** a rarer variety with anterior angulation.

- In the common *posteriorly displaced fracture*, the distal fragment is tilted backwards and/or shifted backwards.
- In the rare *anteriorly displaced fracture*, the fragment is tilted forwards (**25.2**).

The anteroposterior (AP) X-ray is often difficult to interpret because it is taken with the elbow flexed. The degree of sideways tilt (angulation) may therefore not be appreciated. This is where Baumann's angle is most helpful; wherever possible it should be accurately measured and compared with that of the uninjured side (see **25.1**).

Treatment

If there is even a suspicion of a fracture, the elbow is gently splinted in 30 degrees of flexion to prevent movement and possible neurovascular injury during the X-ray examination.

UNDISPLACED FRACTURES

The elbow is immobilized at 90 degrees and neutral rotation in a lightweight splint or cast and the arm is supported by a sling.

 It is essential to obtain an X-ray 5–7 days later to check that there has been no displacement.

The splint is retained for 3 weeks and supervised movement is then allowed.

SECTION 3 TRAUMA

POSTERIORLY ANGULATED FRACTURES WITH INTACT POSTERIOR CORTICAL HINGE

Swelling is usually not severe and the risk of vascular injury is low. If the posterior cortices are in continuity, the fracture can be reduced under general anaesthesia by gentle traction and then flexion of the elbow with pressure on the olecranon to correct the posterior angulation. Intraoperative *X-rays* are then taken to confirm anatomical reduction. K-wire fixation is usually required due to the tendency of the fracture to redisplace. There is controversy on whether to perform lateral pinning vs cross-pinning (from the medial and lateral aspect) but there is good evidence that reduction is maintained with lateral pinning alone, minimizing the risk of ulnar nerve injury as it courses around the medial epicondyle. If medial pinning is required for improved stability, a small incision is made over the medial epicondyle (to place the wire directly on bone) and the wire is inserted at 30 degrees of elbow flexion to avoid injury to the ulnar nerve.

Following reduction and pinning, a backslab is applied and the circulation should be rechecked. The splint and K-wires are removed at 3 weeks and the elbow is gently mobilized.

POSTERIORLY DISPLACED FRACTURES

These are usually associated with *significant swelling*. Neurovascular injury or circulatory compromise can occur due to fracture displacement and swelling. The fracture should be reduced under general anaesthesia as soon as possible. Inline traction is performed and an *AP intraoperative X-ray* is taken to confirm there is no medial or lateral translation. Once corrected, the elbow is then flexed with firm pressure on the olecranon to reduce the posterior translation and the forearm is pronated. K-wire fixation is then performed as above. The K-wires should be either divergent or parallel and spread widely at the fracture site to avoid redisplacement (**25.3**). The postoperative management is the same as for simple angulated fractures but the neurovascular status should be checked repeatedly in the first 24 hours.

Open reduction   This is sometimes necessary. The fracture is exposed from the lateral side or anteriorly when there is a vascular injury. The haematoma is then evacuated, and the fracture is reduced and stabilized with K-wire fixation.

INDICATIONS FOR OPEN REDUCTION
A fracture that simply cannot be reduced closed
An open fracture
A fracture associated with vascular injury

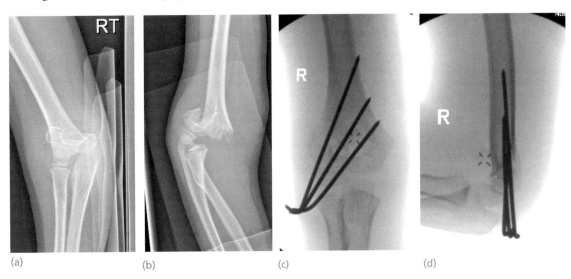

(a)   (b)   (c)   (d)

25.3 Posteriorly displaced supracondylar fracture (a–d) Fracture in a 7-year-old boy, managed by closed reduction and divergent lateral K-wire fixation.

SECTION 3 TRAUMA

Continuous traction Overhead traction with a screw through the olecranon is also described. Once the swelling subsides, a further attempt can be made at reduction.

INDICATIONS FOR CONTINUOUS TRACTION

A severely displaced fracture that cannot be reduced by manipulation

When intraoperative imaging is not available

For severe open injuries or multiple injuries of the limb

ANTERIORLY DISPLACED FRACTURES

The fracture is reduced by pulling on the forearm with the elbow semi-flexed, applying thumb pressure over the front of the distal fragment and then extending the elbow fully. These injuries are typically unstable and require K-wire stabilization. A posterior slab is then applied and retained for 3 weeks as previously described. Thereafter, the wires are removed and the child is allowed to regain elbow motion.

Complications

VASCULAR INJURY

The great danger of supracondylar elbow fractures is *injury to the brachial artery*. Severely displaced fractures can present with a white, pulseless hand (caused by forearm ischaemia). This is a surgical emergency requiring urgent operative management.

A closed reduction is performed (converted to an open reduction when unsuccessful) and the fracture is stabilized with K-wire fixation as described. If distal perfusion is restored, the patient is monitored closely for 24 hours for the possible development of *compartment syndrome* or loss of distal perfusion. However, if distal perfusion fails to return, brachial artery exploration +/− repair is indicated.

Compartment syndrome can occur after reperfusion following brachial artery injury, or due to excessive swelling of the forearm. Untreated, muscle necrosis and nerve injury develop.

- The *early cardinal signs* are increasing pain despite splintage and pain on passive extension of the fingers.
- *Late signs* are reduced capillary return and blunted sensation.

All tight dressings should be split and the arm elevated to heart level. Unless there is rapid improvement, urgent vascular intervention +/− forearm fasciotomy is indicated.

NERVE INJURY

Anterior interosseous nerve The anterior interosseous nerve (branch of the median nerve) is the most frequently injured nerve in posteriorly displaced supracondylar fractures. This is diagnosed by failure to make the 'OK sign' (touching the tip of the index finger and thumb together). The loss of function is usually temporary and recovery can be expected in 3–4 months.

If a nerve, documented as intact prior to manipulation, is then found to be compromised after manipulation, entrapment in the fracture is suspected and immediate exploration should be arranged.

Ulnar nerve This may be damaged by careless pin placement. It is safest to perform a mini-open approach on the medial side of the elbow and identify the nerve before placing the smooth K-wire. If the injury is recognized, and the pin removed, recovery will usually follow.

MALUNION

Malunion with a cubitus varus deformity or posterior translation is common. Residual posterior translation causing a flexion block can remodel in young children (see Chapter 14) but varus angulation persists (**25.4**). Cubitus varus used to be

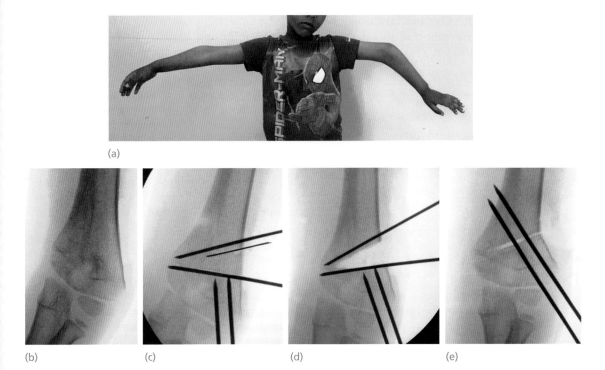

(a)

(b)   (c)   (d)   (e)

25.4 Supracondylar fractures – complications (a) Varus deformity of the left elbow following incomplete correction of the varus displacement in a supracondylar fracture, the 'gunstock deformity' becomes more obvious when the arms are raised. **(b–e)** X-ray showing the malunion and resultant surgical management with a closing wedge osteotomy (correction temporarily marked with wires prior to definitive K-wire fixation).

considered simply a cosmetic problem, but recent evidence suggests that severe cases (>20 degrees of varus) can result in problems years later:

- ulnar nerve subluxation
- snapping of the medial head of triceps
- rotatory instability of the radiocapitellar joint.

 In surgical treatment of supracondylar fractures in children, beware of leaving varus angulation of the distal fragment. Double-check the position and measure Baumann's angle.

ELBOW STIFFNESS

Full movement may take months to return and must not be hurried. Forced movement will only make matters worse and may contribute to the development of heterotopic ossification.

FRACTURES OF THE LATERAL CONDYLE IN CHILDREN

The distal humeral epiphysis begins to ossify at the age of about 2 years and fuses with the shaft at about 16 years; between these ages, the condylar or epicondylar parts of the epiphysis may be sheared off or avulsed by the sudden pull of the forearm muscles during a fall on the hand. Only two of these injuries are at all common (**25.5**):

- fracture-separation of the entire condyle on the lateral side
- separation of the epicondyle on the medial side.

Clinical features

If the child falls with the elbow stressed in varus, a large fragment, including the lateral condyle,

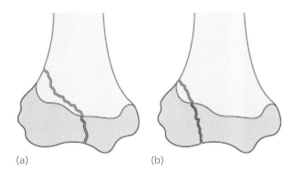

(a)   (b)

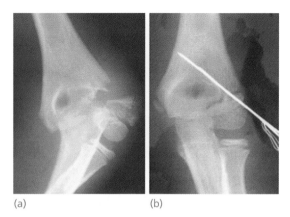

(a)   (b)

25.5 Physeal fractures of the lateral condyle
(a) The commonest is a fracture starting in the metaphysis and running along the physis of the lateral condyle into the trochlea (Salter–Harris Type II injury). **(b)** Less common is a fracture running right through the lateral condyle to reach the articular surface in the capitulo trochlear groove (Salter–Harris Type IV): although uncommon, this latter injury is important because of its potential for causing growth defects.

25.6 Fractured lateral condyle – treatment
If displacement is more than 2 mm **(a)**, open reduction and internal fixation is the treatment of choice **(b)**.

can be avulsed by the attached wrist extensors. The fracture line usually runs along the physis to enter the joint through the trochlea or (less often) through the capitulotrochlear groove.

The extent of the injury is often not appreciated because the capitellar epiphysis is largely cartilaginous and only the ossific centre in the fragment is visible on *X-ray*. If the fracture runs through the trochlea, the elbow joint can dislocate. The fragment may be grossly displaced and capsized.

with a screw or K-wires (**25.6**). Care must be taken to minimize posterior dissection on the fracture fragment as avascular necrosis can occur. The arm is immobilized in a cast. The wires are moved after 4 weeks and the cast can then be discarded.

COMPLICATIONS

Non-union and malunion   If the condyle is left displaced, *non-union* is inevitable; with growth, the elbow becomes increasingly valgus, and ulnar nerve palsy is then likely to develop. *Malunion*, likewise, can result in cubitus valgus (**25.7**). If deformity is marked, it should be corrected by supracondylar osteotomy.

 The condylar fragment is always larger than the image shown on X-ray.

Treatment

UNDISPLACED FRACTURES

An undisplaced fracture can be treated by splinting the elbow for 3–4 weeks and then starting exercises. A check *X-ray* should be obtained at 1 week and at 2 weeks due to the high incidence of late fracture displacement.

DISPLACED FRACTURES

A displaced fracture requires operative reduction via a lateral approach with the fragment fixed in position

SEPARATION OF THE MEDIAL EPICONDYLAR APOPHYSIS IN CHILDREN

If the wrist is forced into extension, the medial epicondylar apophysis is avulsed by the attached wrist flexors; if the elbow opens up on that side, the epicondylar fragment may be pulled into the joint. The inner side of the elbow is swollen and acutely tender. The *X-ray* has to be studied very carefully to detect the tiny ossific centre which marks the epicondylar fragment (**25.8**).

Treatment

Minor displacement may be disregarded; the elbow is splinted for 2–3 weeks to relieve pain, and

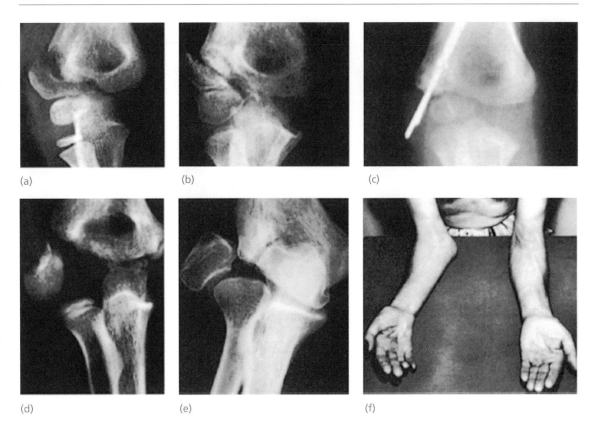

(a)   (b)   (c)

(d)   (e)   (f)

25.7 Fractured lateral condyle – complications (a,b) A large fragment of bone and cartilage is avulsed; even with reasonable reduction, union is not inevitable. **(c)** Open reduction with fixation is often wise. **(d)** Sometimes the condyle is capsized; if left unreduced, non-union is inevitable **(e)** and a valgus elbow with delayed ulnar palsy **(f)** is the likely sequel.

exercises are then encouraged. However, if the epicondyle is markedly displaced, it should be reduced and stabilized with a K-wire (or screw in an older child). If it is trapped in the joint (as can happen following an elbow dislocation that has spontaneously reduced), it must be freed. Manipulation with the elbow in valgus and the wrist hyperextended (to pull on the flexor muscles) may be successful; if this fails, the joint must be opened and the fragment retrieved before being replaced.

APOPHYSITIS

This is separate pathology. It is a painful traction injury of the medial epicondyle apophysis, and it occurs in young athletes as a result of repeated forced valgus moments of the elbow, such as when bowling a ball or throwing 'Little leaguers' elbow'. The condition usually settles with rest.

FRACTURE OF THE MEDIAL CONDYLE IN CHILDREN

This is much rarer than a lateral condyle fracture. It can be difficult to visualize on a plain *X-ray*. An *arthrogram or magnetic resonance imaging (MRI) scan* can be helpful. These are treated in the same way as lateral condyle fractures.

FRACTURE-SEPARATION OF THE ENTIRE DISTAL HUMERUS EPIPHYSIS (TRANSPHYSEAL FRACTURE) IN CHILDREN

Up to the age of 7 years, the distal humeral epiphysis is a solid cartilaginous segment with maturing centres of ossification. With severe

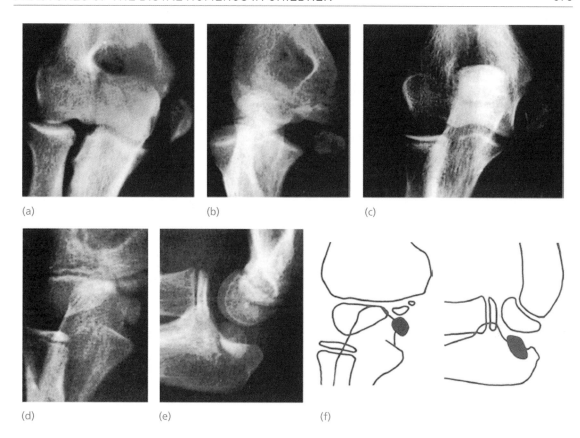

(a)   (b)   (c)

(d)   (e)   (f)

25.8 Fractured medial epicondyle (a) Avulsion of the medial epicondyle following valgus train. **(b)** Avulsion associated with dislocation of the elbow; **(c)** after reduction. Sometimes the epicondylar fragment is trapped in the joint **(d,e)**; the serious nature is then liable to be missed unless the surgeon specifically looks for the trapped fragment, which is emphasized in the tracings **(f,g)**.

injury, it may separate en bloc. This can occur with fairly severe violence, such as a birth injury or child abuse. It usually occurs in younger children, under 3 years of age.

 Be alert to the possibility of non-accidental injury as a cause of transphyseal fracture.

Clinical features

The child is distressed and the elbow is swollen. The history may be deceptively uninformative.

X-rays

In a very young child, in whom the bony outlines are still unformed, the X-ray may look normal in an undisplaced or minimally displaced injury. When displaced, there is medial displacement of the proximal radius and ulna from the distal humerus – something that can be mistaken for a dislocation (**25.9**).

Treatment

The injury is treated like a supracondylar fracture.

UNDISPLACED FRACTURES

The elbow is merely splinted in flexion for 2 weeks; any resulting deformity (which is rare) can be dealt with at a later age.

DISPLACED FRACTURES

If a fracture is obviously displaced, it should be accurately reduced and held with smooth percutaneous wires (otherwise there is a high incidence

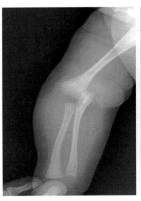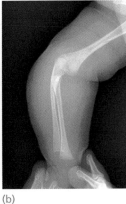

(a)   (b)

25.9 Transphyseal fracture (a,b) Fracture of the distal humerus in a 3-month-old child. Note the medial translation of the proximal radius and ulna that could be misinterpreted as a dislocation. Cubitus varus malunion is common after such injuries. It is important to investigate non-accidental injury as a cause.

of cubitus varus). An *arthrogram* is often needed due to the absence of distal humeral ossification centres in the infant or young child. The wires are removed at 3 weeks.

FRACTURES OF THE DISTAL HUMERUS IN ADULTS

There are three types of distal humeral fracture:

- extra-articular supracondylar
- intra-articular unicondylar
- bicondylar with varying degrees of comminution.

EXTRA-ARTICULAR SUPRACONDYLAR FRACTURES

Supracondylar fractures are rare in adults. When they do occur, they are usually displaced and unstable or severely comminuted (high-energy injuries).

Treatment

Closed reduction is unlikely to be stable and K-wire fixation is not strong enough to permit early mobilization. Open reduction and internal fixation are therefore the treatment of choice. The distal humerus is approached through a posterior exposure and reflection of the triceps tendon. A transverse or oblique fracture can usually be reduced and fixed with a single contoured plate and screws. Comminuted fractures may require double plates and transfixing screws.

INTRA-ARTICULAR UNICONDYLAR AND BICONDYLAR FRACTURES

Except in osteoporotic individuals, intra-articular condylar fractures should be regarded as high-energy injuries with soft-tissue damage. A severe blow on the point of the elbow drives the olecranon process upwards, splitting the condyles apart. Swelling is considerable and the bony landmarks are difficult to feel.

 The patient should be carefully examined for evidence of *vascular or nerve injury*; vascular insufficiency must be addressed as a matter of urgency.

Imaging

- On *X-ray*, the fracture extends from the lower humerus into the elbow joint; it may be difficult to tell whether one or both condyles are involved, especially with an undisplaced condylar fracture. Sometimes, the fracture extends into the metaphysis as a T-shaped or Y-shaped break, and the bone between the condyles may be comminuted.
- *Computed tomography (CT) scans* are very helpful to plan surgery.

Treatment

These are usually severe injuries associated with joint damage; prolonged immobilization will certainly result in a stiff elbow. Early movement is therefore a prime objective.

UNDISPLACED FRACTURES

These can be treated by applying a posterior slab with the elbow flexed almost 90 degrees; gentle movements are commenced after 2 weeks, but only after obtaining another X-ray at 1 week and 2 weeks to exclude late displacement.

DISPLACED FRACTURES

Open reduction and internal fixation through a posterior approach is the treatment of choice. The best exposure is obtained by performing an intra-articular olecranon osteotomy. The ulnar nerve should be identified and protected throughout. The fragments are reduced and held temporarily with K-wires.

- A *unicondylar fracture without comminution* can then be fixed with screws; if the fragment is large, a contoured plate is added to prevent redisplacement.
- *Bicondylar and comminuted fractures* will require double plate and screw fixation (25.10), and sometimes also bone grafts in the gaps.

Postoperatively, movement is encouraged but should never be forced.

The fracture heals in about 8 weeks but the elbow often does not regain full movement; in severe injuries, movement may be markedly restricted, however beautiful the postoperative X-ray.

In elderly osteoporotic patients, elbow hemi- or total replacement is often a more reliable option.

Complications

Vascular injury   Always check the circulation – repeatedly! Vigilance is required to make the diagnosis and institute treatment as early as possible.

Nerve injury   There may be damage to either the median or the ulnar nerve. It is important to examine the hand and record the findings before treatment is commenced and again after treatment. The ulnar nerve may shut down following surgery but it usually recovers in time.

Stiffness   Comminuted fractures of the elbow always result in some degree of stiffness. However, the disability may be reduced by encouraging an energetic exercise programme. Late operations to improve elbow movement are difficult but can be rewarding.

Heterotopic ossification   Severe soft-tissue damage may lead to heterotopic ossification. Forced movement should be avoided.

Treatment

UNDISPLACED FRACTURES

These can be treated by resting the arm in a sling for 4–5 days and then starting movement.

DISPLACED FRACTURES

Treatment is by operative reduction and fixation with small buried screws. If this proves too

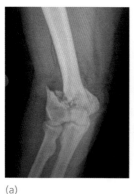 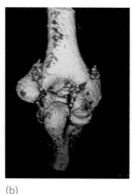 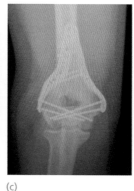 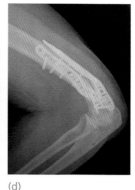

(a)   (b)   (c)   (d)

25.10 Bicondylar fractures X-rays taken (a,b) before and (c,d) after open reduction and internal fixation. An excellent reduction was obtained in this case; however, the elbow sometimes ends up with considerable loss of movement even though the general anatomy has been restored.

difficult, the fragment is best excised. Movements are commenced as soon as discomfort permits.

FRACTURE-DISLOCATION OF THE ELBOW

The combination of radial head fracture, coronoid fracture and lateral collateral ligament injury is known as the *'terrible triad'* – a fitting acknowledgement of the severe instability and poor outcome in these cases. The injury is now well understood and no longer earns the 'terrible' title, but, as with other elbow injuries, stiffness is a common problem. The treatment is usually surgical, with radial head fixation or replacement and lateral ligament repair. Coronoid fixation is required only if the fracture extends to the medial facet, and opinion varies about repair of the medial ligament.

Complications

Vascular injury

 Absence of the radial pulse is a warning that the brachial artery may be damaged. If there are other signs of ischaemia, this should be treated as an emergency.

Splints must be removed and the elbow should be straightened somewhat. If there is no improvement, an *arteriogram* is performed; the brachial artery may have to be explored.

Nerve injury The median or ulnar nerve is sometimes injured. Spontaneous recovery usually occurs after 6–8 weeks.

Stiffness Loss of 20–30 degrees of extension is not uncommon after elbow fracture dislocation. Physiotherapy may help, but forceful manipulation must be avoided.

Heterotopic ossification Heterotopic bone formation may occur in the damaged soft tissues in front of the joint. In former years, 'myositis ossificans' was a fairly common complication, usually associated with forceful reduction and overenthusiastic passive movement of the elbow. Nowadays it is rarely seen, but one should be alert for signs such as excessive pain, tenderness, and slow recovery of active movements. *X-rays* may show soft-tissue ossification as early as 4–6 weeks after injury. If the condition is suspected, exercises are stopped and the elbow is splinted in comfortable flexion until pain subsides; gentle active movements and continuous passive motion are then resumed. Anti-inflammatory drugs may help to reduce stiffness; they are also used prophylactically to reduce the risk of heterotopic bone formation.

A bone mass which markedly restricts movement and elbow function should be excised once the bone is 'mature' (i.e. has well-defined cortical margins and trabeculae). This is followed by anti-inflammatory medication, bisphosphonates or radiotherapy to prevent recurrence.

Osteoarthritis Secondary osteoarthritis (OA) is a late complication. Symptoms can usually be treated conservatively, but if pain and stiffness are intolerable, total elbow replacement can be considered.

SIMPLE DISLOCATION OF THE ELBOW

A fall on the outstretched hand may dislocate the elbow. In 90% of cases, the forearm bones are pushed backwards and dislocate posteriorly or posterolaterally. Provided there is no associated fracture, reduction will usually be stable and recurrent dislocation unlikely.

Clinical features

Deformity is usually obvious and the bony landmarks are displaced. In very severe injuries, pain and swelling are so marked that examination of the elbow is impossible; however, the hand should be examined for signs of vascular or nerve damage.

X-ray examination is essential (**25.11**):

- to confirm the presence of a dislocation
- to identify any associated fractures.

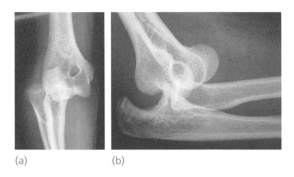

(a) (b)

25.11 Dislocation of the elbow X-rays showing (a) lateral and (b) posterior displacement.

Treatment

The patient should be fully relaxed under anaesthesia. The surgeon pulls on the forearm while the elbow is slightly flexed. With one hand, sideways displacement is corrected, then the elbow is further flexed while the olecranon process is pushed forward. Unless almost full flexion can be obtained, the olecranon is not in the trochlear groove.

After reduction, the elbow should be put through a full range of movement to see whether it is stable. Nerve function and circulation are checked again and the *X-ray* is repeated to confirm that the joint is reduced and that there are no associated fractures.

The arm is held in a light cast with the elbow flexed to just above 90 degrees and the wrist supported in a collar and cuff. After 1 week, the cast can be removed and gentle exercises begun; at 3 weeks, the collar and cuff are discarded. Elbow movements are allowed to return spontaneously and should never be forced.

Complications

These are similar to those described for 'Fracture-dislocation of the elbow', but are usually less serious or prevalent.

FRACTURED CAPITELLUM

This is an articular fracture which occurs only in adults. The patient falls on the hand, usually with the elbow straight. The anterior part of the capitellum is sheared off; there may be a tiny cartilaginous shell or a large single or comminuted fracture.

Fullness in front of the elbow is the most notable feature. The lateral side of the elbow is tender and flexion is grossly restricted.

Imaging

In the lateral *X-ray* view, the capitellum (or part of it) is seen in front of the lower humerus, and the radial head is not opposed to it. The images can be difficult to interpret and a *CT scan* is invaluable in planning treatment (**25.12**).

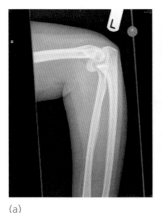

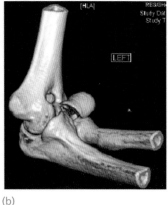

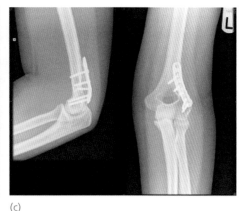

(a) (b) (c)

25.12 Fractured capitellum (a) Lateral X-ray; **(b)** 3D CT reconstruction; and **(c)** surgical fixation.

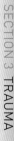

SECTION 3 TRAUMA

Treatment

Small fragments are excised. Larger fragments can be fixed with a screw from behind or with modern buried screws from in front.

ISOLATED DISLOCATION OF THE RADIAL HEAD

Isolated dislocation of the radial head is very rare; if it is seen, search carefully for an associated fracture of the ulna (the Monteggia injury), which may be difficult to detect in a child because the fracture is often incomplete. Even a minor deformity of the ulna may prevent full reduction of the radial head dislocation.

PULLED ELBOW IN CHILDREN

In young children, the elbow is sometimes injured by a sharp tug on the wrist. The child is in pain; the elbow is held in extension and he or she will not allow it to be moved. There are no *X-ray* changes. What has happened is that the radius has been pulled distally and the annular ligament has slipped up over the head of the radius. A dramatic cure is achieved by forcefully supinating and then flexing the elbow; the ligament slips back with a snap.

FRACTURES OF THE PROXIMAL END OF THE RADIUS

Fractures of the proximal end of the radius are fairly common in young adults and children. A fall on the outstretched hand with the elbow extended and the forearm pronated causes impaction of the radial head against the capitellum. In adults, this may fracture the *head of the radius*; in children, it is more likely to fracture the *neck of the radius* (possibly because the head is largely cartilaginous). In addition, the articular cartilage of the capitellum may be bruised or chipped; this cannot be seen on *X-ray* but is an important complication.

Clinical features

Following a fall on the outstretched arm, the patient complains of pain and local tenderness posterolaterally over the proximal end of the radius. A further clue is a marked increase in pain on pronation and supination of the forearm.

X-rays

- *In children*, the fracture is through the neck; the proximal fragment may be tilted forwards and outwards (**25.13, 25.14**).
- The *typical adult fracture* is a vertical split or marginal fracture through the radial head; less often there is a transverse neck fracture. Sometimes the head is crushed or comminuted (**25.15**). Impacted fractures are easily missed unless several views are obtained. The wrist also should be very carefully examined to exclude a concomitant injury of the distal radioulnar joint – the Essex-Lopresti lesion. If this is not recognized early, it can be almost impossible to treat.

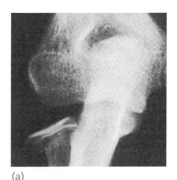

(a)

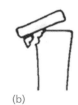

(b)

25.13 Fractured neck of radius in a child Up to 30° of tilt is acceptable. Greater degrees of angulation should be reduced; never excise the radial head in a child.

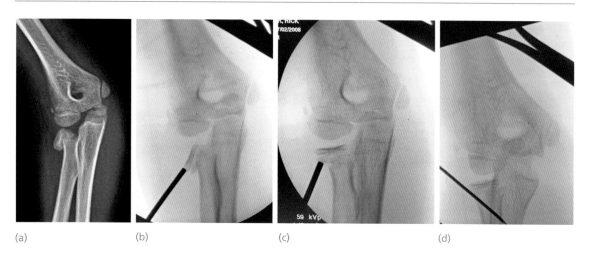

(a) (b) (c) (d)

25.14 (a–d) Restoring the radial head in a child with wire passed through the skin.

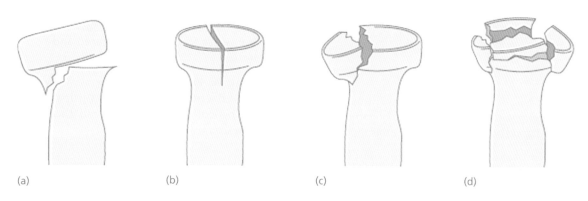

(a) (b) (c) (d)

25.15 Fractures of the radial head (a) In children the injury usually causes a fracture of the neck of the radius. **(b–d)** In adults the injury is usually a vertical split **(b)**, a marginal fragment **(c)** or a comminuted fracture of the head of the radius **(d)**.

Treatment

CHILDREN

In fractures of the radial neck, up to 30 degrees of radial head tilt and up to 3 mm of transverse displacement are acceptable. The arm is rested in a collar and cuff, and exercises are commenced after 1 week.

Displacement of more than 30 degrees should be corrected. With the patient's elbow extended, traction and varus force are applied; the surgeon then pushes the displaced radial fragment into position with his or her thumb. If this fails, open reduction is performed; there is no need for internal fixation. Following operation, the elbow is splinted in 90 degrees of flexion for 1–2 weeks and then movements are encouraged.

 The head of the radius must never be excised in children because this will interfere with the synchronous growth of the radius and ulna.

Fractures that are seen 1 week or longer after injury should be left untreated (except for light splintage).

ADULTS

Undisplaced fractures of the radial head These can be treated by supporting the elbow in a collar and cuff for 2 weeks; active flexion, extension and rotation are encouraged.

Displaced fractures These are treated by open reduction and fixation with small screws for the head and a small pre-contoured plate for the neck.

Comminuted fractures Historically, these been treated by excising the radial head. However, if there is associated medial ligament injury or olecranon fracture or disruption of the distal radioulnar joint, the risk of proximal migration of the radius is considerable and the patient may develop intractable symptoms of pain and instability in the forearm. In such cases, every effort should be made to reconstruct the radial head or, if it has to be excised, it should be replaced by a metal prosthesis.

Complications

> ⚠️ Beware excision of radial head fractures – it can lead to intractable elbow or forearm instability.

Recurrent instability of the elbow This can occur if the medial collateral ligament was injured and the radial head then excised.

Instability of the distal radioulnar joint Also known as an Essex-Lopresti lesion, this can occur if the radial head is excised with a rupture of the interosseous membrane of the forearm.

OA of the radiocapitellar joint A very rare late complication of adult injuries, this may call for excision of the radial head.

FRACTURES OF THE OLECRANON

Two types of olecranon injury are seen:

- a *comminuted fracture*, which is due to a direct blow or a fall on the elbow
- a *clean transverse fracture*, due to traction when the patient falls onto the hand while the triceps muscle is contracted (**25.16**).

Clinical features

A graze or bruise over the elbow suggests a comminuted fracture: the triceps is intact and the

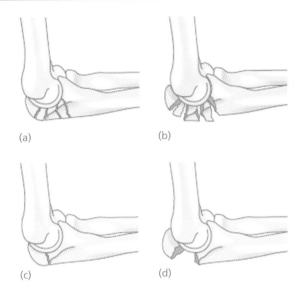

25.16 Fractured olecranon (a,b) Comminuted fractures, undisplaced and displaced. **(c,d)** Transverse fractures, undisplaced and displaced.

elbow can be extended against gravity. With a transverse fracture, there may be a palpable gap and the patient is unable to extend the elbow against resistance.

X-rays

A properly orientated lateral view is essential to show details of the fracture, as well as the associated joint damage. The position of the radial head should be checked: it may be dislocated. The ulna may also be displaced forwards.

Treatment

COMMINUTED FRACTURES

An *undisplaced comminuted fracture* with the triceps intact can occasionally be treated conservatively if the patient is old and osteoporotic; internal fixation is challenging and immobilizing the elbow will lead to stiffness. The arm is rested in a sling until the pain subsides; a further *X-ray* is obtained to ensure that there is no displacement, and the patient is then encouraged to start active movements.

Comminuted fractures in others should be treated by operation, using meticulous technique to preserve the soft-tissue attachments. Modern metal plates are specially contoured for these fractures and can 'bridge' across the fragments.

TRANSVERSE FRACTURES

Undisplaced An undisplaced transverse fracture that does not separate when the elbow is flexed can be treated by immobilizing the elbow in a cast in about 60 degrees of flexion for 1 week; then exercises are begun. The fracture must be examined carefully with repeat *X-rays* to make sure it does not distract.

Displaced In theory, these can be held by splinting the arm absolutely straight – but stiffness in that position would be disastrous. Operative treatment is therefore preferred. The fracture is reduced under vision and held by one of two methods (**25.17**):

- *tension-band wiring* – two stiff wires driven across the fracture, leaving their ends protruding proximally and distally to anchor a tight loop of wire which will pull the fragments together

- a contoured *low-profile plate* and screws.

Early mobilization should be encouraged.

Complications

Stiffness This used to be common, but secure internal fixation and early mobilization minimize the residual loss of movement.

Non-union This sometimes occurs after inadequate reduction and fixation of a transverse fracture. If elbow function is good, it can be ignored; if not, rigid internal fixation and bone grafting will be needed.

Osteoarthritis OA is a late complication, especially if the articular surface in the trochlear notch is poorly reduced. This can usually be treated with modification of activities and occasional cortisone injections. Joint replacement is considered for severe symptoms but heavy work and sport would not be permissible afterwards.

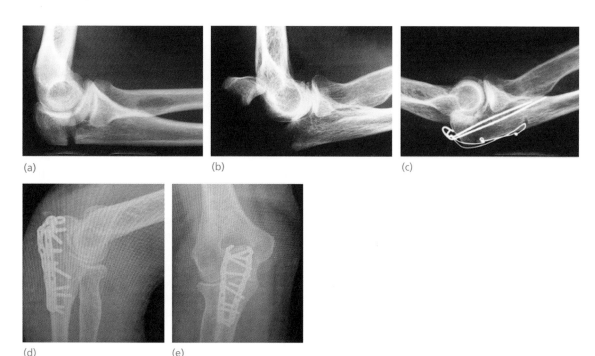

(a) (b) (c)

(d) (e)

25.17 Fractured olecranon (a) Slightly displaced transverse fracture. **(b)** Markedly displaced transverse fracture – the extensor mechanism is no longer intact. Treatment in this case was by open reduction and tension-band wiring **(c)**. **(d,e)** Unstable comminuted fracture fixed with locking plate.

FRACTURES OF THE OLECRANON IN CHILDREN

A fracture of the olecranon in a child is rare. When it does occur, it is usually due to a direct blow onto the tip of the flexed elbow or a fall on the outstretched hand. Most are undisplaced and are treated in a splint for 3–4 weeks. If displaced, they should be reduced and held with K-wires.

FRACTURES OF THE RADIUS AND ULNA

A twisting force (usually a fall on the hand) produces spiral fractures with the bones broken at different levels. A direct blow or an angulating force causes transverse fractures of one or both bones at the same level. The bone fragments are easily displaced by contraction of strong muscles attached to the radius. Bleeding and swelling in the muscle compartments of the forearm may cause circulatory impairment.

Injuries to the bones of the forearm should be considered intra-articular fractures, because the forearm is a quadrilateral joint, with the proximal distal radioulnar joint at one end and the distal radioulnar joint at the other. Disruption of any one part, the radioulnar joints or the shafts of the long bones, will usually disrupt another part of the quadrilateral ring (25.18). Malalignment is likely to affect forearm rotation especially in the skeletally mature.

Clinical features

The diagnosis is usually quite obvious, but the wrist and hand must be carefully examined for signs of nerve damage or circulatory impairment.

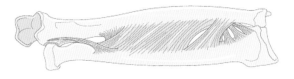

25.18 The forearm is a quadrilateral joint A break or angulation in one part will affect another part.

Repeated examination of forearm fractures is necessary in order to detect an impending compartment syndrome. Pain out of proportion to the injury is the cardinal symptom. The signs are the five Ps.

COMPARTMENT SYNDROME IN FOREARM FRACTURES IN CHILDREN: THE FIVE Ps
Pain on passive extension of the fingers (the most sensitive test – do not wait for the others!) **P**araesthesia **P**aralysis **P**allor **P**eripheral pulses absent

X-rays

In adults, the fractures are easy to see; in children, they are often incomplete and the bones may appear bent rather than broken.

Treatment

CHILDREN

In children, closed reduction is usually successful because the tough periosteum tends to guide and then control the reduction; fragments can be held in a well-moulded, full-length cast extending from the axilla to the metacarpal shafts (to control rotation). The cast is applied with the elbow at 90 degrees. If the radial fracture is proximal to pronator teres, the forearm is supinated; if it is distal to pronator teres, the forearm is held in neutral. The position is checked by *X-ray* after 1 week and, if it is satisfactory, splintage is retained until both fractures are united (usually 6–8 weeks) (25.19).

Throughout this period, hand and shoulder exercises are encouraged. If reduction is impossible or unstable, fixation with percutaneous wires or intramedullary nails is needed (25.20). The pins are inserted with great care taken to avoid the growth plates.

Childhood fractures usually remodel well. One can accept 20 degrees of angulation in the distal third of the radius, 15 degrees in the middle third and 10 degrees in the proximal third, as

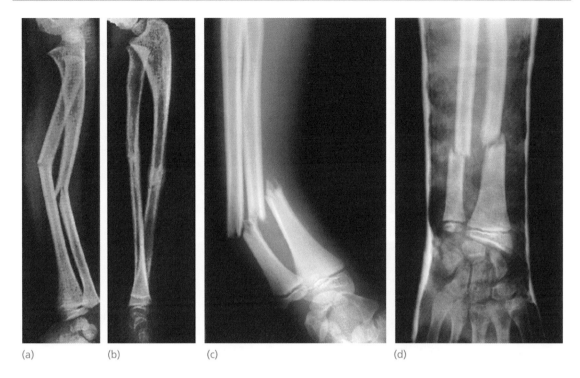

(a)   (b)   (c)   (d)

25.19 Fractured radius and ulna in children Greenstick fractures **(a)** need only correction of angulation **(b)** and plaster splintage. Complete fractures **(c)** are harder to reduce; however, provided alignment is corrected and held in plaster **(d)**, remodelling will restore the anatomy.

long as there is at least 2 years or more of growth left. One can accept 100% translation as long as there is no more than 1 cm of shortening.

ADULTS

Unless the fragments are in close apposition, reduction is difficult and redisplacement in the cast almost inevitable. Consequently, most surgeons opt for open reduction and internal fixation from the outset. The fragments are held by plates and screws (**25.21**). The deep fascia is left open to prevent a build-up of pressure in the muscle compartments, and only the skin and subcutaneous tissues are sutured.

After the operation, the arm is kept elevated until the swelling subsides, and during this period active exercises of the hand are encouraged. If the fracture is not comminuted and the patient is reliable, early range-of-movement exercises are commenced, but lifting and sports are avoided. It takes 8–12 weeks for the bones to unite.

Complications

Nerve injury Nerve injuries are rarely caused by the fracture, but they may be caused by the surgeon! Exposure of the radius in its proximal third risks damage to the posterior interosseous nerve, where it is covered by the superficial part of the supinator muscle. Surgical technique is particularly important here; the anterior Henry approach is safest to protect the nerve. Nerves are also at risk if a radius plate is ever removed.

Compartment syndrome Fractures (and operations) of the forearm bones are always associated with swelling of the soft tissues, with the attendant risk of a compartment syndrome. The threat is even greater, and the diagnosis more difficult, if the forearm is wrapped up in plaster. The byword is 'watchfulness'; if there are any signs of circulatory embarrassment, treatment must be prompt and uncompromising with a complete release (**25.22**).

SECTION 3 TRAUMA

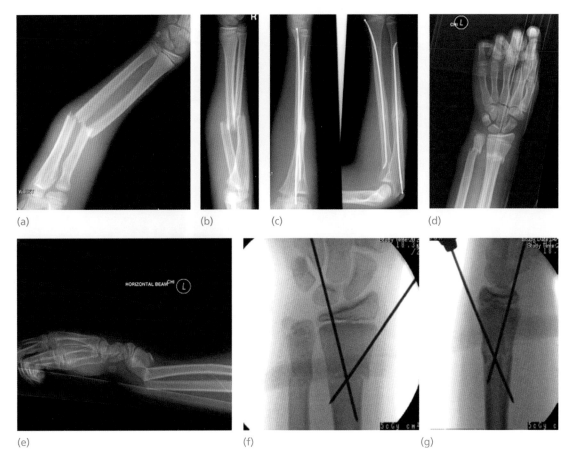

(a)　　　　　　　　(b)　　(c)　　　　　　(d)

(e)　　　　　　　　　　　　(f)　　　　　　　(g)

25.20 Forearm fractures in children A displaced forearm fracture (a,b) is fixed with flexible intramedullary nails (c). An unstable distal third diaphyseal fracture (d,e) is treated with percutaneous wires (f,g).

Delayed union and non-union Most fractures of the radius and ulna heal within 8–12 weeks. However, one of the bones may take longer than usual, and immobilization may have to be continued beyond the usual time. High-energy and open fractures are at risk of developing non-union, which will require bone grafting and internal fixation. Occasionally, cross-union occurs where the radius and ulna heal to each other (e25.1).

Malunion With closed reduction, there is always a risk of malunion, resulting in angulation or rotational deformity of the forearm, cross-union of the fragments, or shortening of one of the bones and disruption of the distal radioulnar joint. If pronation or supination is severely restricted, and there is no cross-union, mobility may be improved by a corrective osteotomy.

Complications of plate removal These are common and include:

- damage to vessels and nerves
- infection
- fractures through screw holes (see **25.21**).

 Removal of plates and screws is often regarded as a fairly innocuous procedure. Beware!

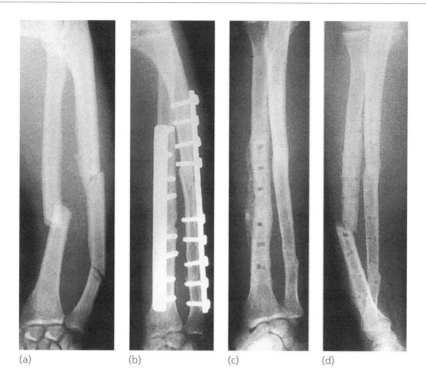

(a) (b) (c) (d)

25.21 Fractured radius and ulna in adults (a,b) Forearm fractures in adults have a strong tendency to redisplace after closed reduction and are therefore usually treated by internal fixation with sturdy plates and screws. Removal of the implants is not without risk. In this case **(c,d)**, the radius fractured through one of the screw holes.

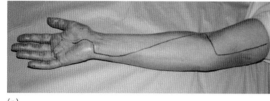

(a)

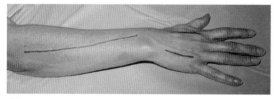

(b)

25.22 Compartment syndrome Incisions to relieve a compartment syndrome in the forearm.

FRACTURE OF A SINGLE FOREARM BONE

Fracture of either the radius or the ulna alone is uncommon. Its importance lies in the fact that deformity or shortening of one bone (while the partner bone remains intact) usually involves a concomitant disruption of either the proximal or distal radioulnar joint. This associated injury must always be looked for by obtaining a full-length *X-ray* of the forearm, including the elbow and wrist.

Clinical features

Ulnar fractures are easily missed – even on X-ray. If there is local tenderness, a further X-ray 1–2 weeks later is wise. Always examine the elbow and wrist.

X-rays

The fracture may be anywhere in the radius or ulna. The ulna is particularly prone to the so-called 'nightstick fracture' when the victim's arm is raised to protect the face and the assailant's weapon strikes the ulna. The fracture line is transverse and displacement is slight. In children, the intact bone sometimes bends without actually breaking ('*plastic deformation*').

 Always X-ray the elbow and wrist to exclude a dislocation.

Treatment

ISOLATED FRACTURE OF THE ULNA

The fracture may be undisplaced with good bone apposition, in which case a forearm cast leaving the elbow free can be sufficient. However, it takes about 8 weeks before full activity can be resumed. Angular or rotation alignment will affect forearm rotation; rigid internal fixation will therefore be preferable for many patients to allow earlier activity and reduce the risk of displacement or non-union.

ISOLATED FRACTURE OF THE RADIUS

Radius fractures are prone to rotary and angular displacement; to achieve reduction in children the forearm needs to be supinated for upper third fractures, neutral for middle third fractures and pronated for lower third fractures. The position is sometimes difficult to hold in children and just about impossible in adults; if so, internal fixation with a compression plate and screws in adults, and preferably intramedullary nails in children, is better (e25.2).

MONTEGGIA FRACTURE-DISLOCATION OF THE ULNA

The injury originally described by Monteggia was a fracture of the shaft of the ulna associated with disruption of the proximal radioulnar joint and dislocation of the radiocapitellar joint.

Nowadays, the term also includes fractures of the olecranon combined with radial head dislocation.

Clinical features

The cause is usually a fall on the hand and forced pronation of the forearm. The radial head usually dislocates forwards and the upper third of the ulna fractures and bows forwards. The forearm deformity is obvious but the radial head dislocation may be missed.

X-rays

Any apparently isolated fracture of the ulna should raise the suspicion of a proximal radial dislocation (**25.23**).

A good lateral view of the elbow will confirm the diagnosis: normally, the head of the radius points directly to the capitellum; if it is dislocated, it lies in a plane anterior to the capitellum.

Treatment

The secret of successful treatment is to restore the length of the fractured ulna; only then can the dislocated proximal radioulnar joint be fully reduced and remain stable. In adults, this means an operation. The ulnar fracture must be accurately reduced, with the bone restored to full length, and then fixed with a plate and screws. The radial head usually reduces once the ulna has been fixed. Stability must be tested through a full range of movement. If the radial head does not reduce, or it is not stable after reduction, open reduction should be performed.

If the elbow is completely stable, flexion/extension and rotation can be started very soon. If there is doubt, the arm should be immobilized in plaster with the elbow flexed for 6 weeks.

Complications

Unreduced dislocation If the diagnosis has been missed or the dislocation imperfectly reduced, the radial head remains dislocated and limits both elbow flexion and forearm rotation.

- *In children*, no treatment is advised until the end of growth, and then only if function is significantly impaired.

SECTION 3 TRAUMA

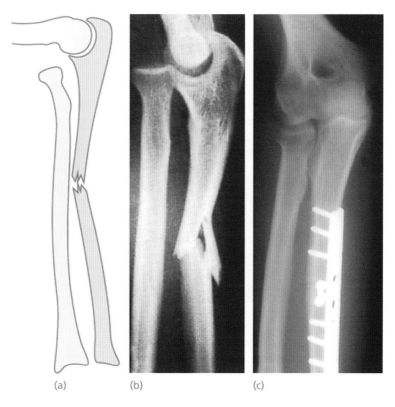

(a) (b) (c)

25.23 Monteggia fracture-dislocation of the radius and ulna (a–c) The Monteggia injury is a fracture of the ulna and dislocation of the proximal end of the radius. X-rays that include the elbow joint will show that the head of the radius no longer points to the capitellum. In a child **(a)**, closed reduction and plaster is usually satisfactory; in the adult **(b,c)**, the crucial step is to restore the ulna to its full length by reducing the fracture and holding it with internal fixation; in most cases the radial head will then reduce by itself but if it does not then open reduction is required.

• *In adults*, operative reduction or excision of the radial head may be needed.

GALEAZZI FRACTURE-DISLOCATION OF THE RADIUS

The counterpart of the Monteggia injury is a fracture of the distal third of the radius and dislocation or subluxation of the distal radioulnar joint.

Clinical features

The Galeazzi fracture is much more common than the Monteggia. Prominence or tenderness over the lower end of the ulna is the striking feature. It is important also to test for an ulnar nerve lesion, which is common.

X-rays

The displaced fracture in the lower third of the radius is obvious; check the inferior radioulnar joint for subluxation or dislocation.

Treatment

As with the Monteggia fracture, the important step is to restore the length of the fractured bone. In children, closed reduction is often successful; in adults, reduction is best achieved by open operation and compression plating of the radius (**25.24**). An *X-ray* is taken to ensure that the distal radioulnar joint is reduced and stable.

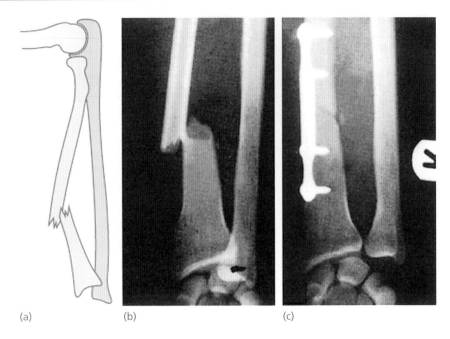

(a)   (b)   (c)

25.24 Galeazzi fracture-dislocation (a) In the Galeazzi fracture-dislocation, it is the radius that is fractured and thereby 'shortened', causing the head of the ulna to dislocate. **(b,c)** X-rays before and after reduction and plating.

- *If it is reduced and stable*, no further action is needed; the arm is rested for a few days, after which gentle active movements are encouraged.
- *If it is reduced but unstable*, the radioulnar joint should be fixed with a K-wire and the forearm splinted in an above-elbow cast for 6 weeks.
- *If there is a large ulnar styloid fragment*, it should be reduced and fixed.

Wrist injuries

26

■ Fractures of the distal radius in adults   589
■ Fractures of the distal radius in children   595
■ Injuries of the carpus   597

FRACTURES OF THE DISTAL RADIUS IN ADULTS

The distal end of the radius is subject to many different types of fracture, depending on factors such as age, transfer of energy, mechanism of injury and bone quality. Treatment options depend on whether the fracture is intra- or extra-articular and the degree of fragmentation of the joint surface and the metaphysis.

LOW-ENERGY DORSALLY DISPLACED FRACTURE (COLLES' FRACTURE)

The injury which Abraham Colles described in 1814 is a transverse fracture of the radius just above the wrist, with dorsal displacement of the distal fragment. It is the most common of all fractures in older women, the high incidence being related to the onset of postmenopausal osteoporosis. Thus, the patient is usually an older woman who gives a history of falling on her outstretched hand.

Clinical features

We can recognize the most common fracture pattern (as Colles did long before radiography was invented) by the 'dinner-fork' deformity, with prominence on the back of the wrist and a depression in front. In patients with less deformity, there may only be local tenderness and pain on wrist movements.

X-rays

The radius is fractured at the corticocancellous junction, about 2 cm from the wrist; often the ulna styloid is also fractured. Characteristically, the distal fragment is shifted and tilted both dorsally and towards the radial side. In some cases, the fracture is impacted; in others, it may be severely comminuted.

Treatment

UNDISPLACED FRACTURES

If the fracture is undisplaced, a dorsal splint is applied for 1–2 days until the swelling has resolved, then the cast is completed. The fracture is stable and the cast can usually be removed after 4 weeks to allow mobilization.

DISPLACED FRACTURES

Displaced fractures must be reduced under anaesthesia (haematoma block, Bier's block or axillary block). The hand is grasped and traction

SECTION 3 TRAUMA

is applied in the length of the bone to disimpact the fragments; the distal fragment is then pushed into place by pressing on the dorsum while manipulating the wrist into moderate flexion, ulnar deviation and pronation. The position is then checked by *X-ray* (26.1). If it is satisfactory, a dorsal plaster slab is applied, extending from just below the elbow to the metacarpal necks and two-thirds of the way round the circumference of the wrist. It is held in position by a crepe bandage. Flexion and ulnar deviation of 20 degrees in each direction is adequate (26.2).

 Extreme positions of flexion and ulnar deviation must be avoided.

The arm is kept elevated for the next day or two; shoulder and finger exercises are started as soon as possible. If the fingers become swollen, cyanosed or painful, there should be no hesitation in splitting the bandage.

It is essential to check the position again by X-ray 7 days later and again at 14 days. Later collapse is not uncommon. Often the fracture redisplaces in the cast; if so, remanipulation usually fails and surgery is considered.

The fracture usually unites in about 5 weeks and, even in the absence of radiological proof of union, the slab may then be discarded and exercises begun.

 With a *Colles' fracture*, avoid too much flexion in plaster!

COMMINUTED AND UNSTABLE LOW-ENERGY FRACTURES

If plaster immobilization alone cannot hold the fracture, then surgery is considered. Options include percutaneous K-wire fixation or a volar locking plate. The plates have a special design such that the screws lock into the plate which holds the plate–bone combination very firmly even in relatively osteoporotic and comminuted bone, allowing early functional movement.

If wires are used, the plaster and wires are removed after 5 weeks and exercises begun. Plates are designed to stay indefinitely and allow earlier movement and thus return to function. They are, however, very expensive and need technical skill to use safely and effectively. The final outcomes and complication rates for the two methods appear the same. Early mobilization and thus earlier return to function might tempt certain patients towards a plate if the device is available and affordable.

For very unstable fractures and osteoporotic bone, external fixation may be added to prevent collapse around the wires. Proximal pins are placed through the radius and distal pins through the shaft of the second metacarpal. Bone grafts may be added if the radius has markedly collapsed. However, with the advent of locking plates, external fixation is rarely used nowadays.

Outcome

As Colles himself recognized, the outcome of these fractures in an older age group with lower

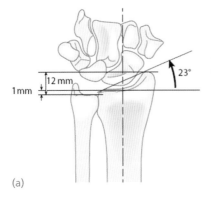

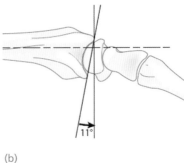

(a)   (b)

26.1 Distal radius fracture – normal angles (a,b) Make sure that the articular congruency is restored.

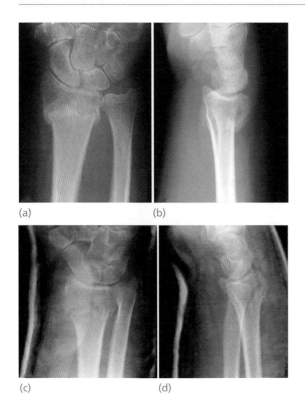

(a)   (b)

(c)   (d)

26.2 Colles' fracture (a,b) The typical Colles' fracture is both displaced and angulated towards the dorsum and towards the radial side of the wrist. **(c,d)** Note how, after successful reduction, the radial articular surface faces correctly both distally and slightly volarwards.

functional demands is usually good, regardless of the cosmetic or the radiographic appearance. Poor outcomes can usually be improved by performing a corrective osteotomy. The amount of displacement that can be accepted depends on patient factors such as:

- age
- comorbidity
- functional demands
- handedness
- quality of bone

and treatment factors such as surgical skill and implants available.

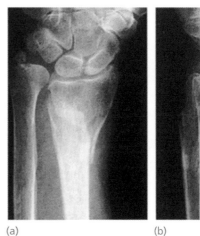

(a)   (b)

26.3 Smith's fracture (a,b) Here, in contrast to Colles' fracture, the displacement of the lower radial fragment is forwards – not backwards.

VOLAR DISPLACED FRACTURE (SMITH'S FRACTURE AND BARTON'S FRACTURE)

Smith (a Dubliner, like Colles) described a similar fracture about 20 years later. However, in *Smith's fracture*, the distal fragment is displaced and tilted anteriorly (which is why it is sometimes called a 'reversed Colles' fracture') (**26.3**). It is caused by a fall on the back of the hand.

Barton's fracture is an oblique fracture which runs from the volar surface of the distal end of the radius into the wrist joints. The fragment is often displaced anteriorly, carrying the carpus with it as a fracture-dislocation (**26.4**). The significance of recognizing this fracture is that it can be expected to be unstable.

Treatment

The fracture may be easily reduced, but it is just as easily redisplaced. Internal fixation, using a small anterior buttress plate, is recommended.

 Volar displaced fractures are very unstable and usually need surgery.

SECTION 3 TRAUMA

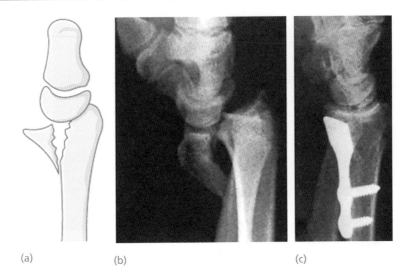

(a)   (b)   (c)

26.4 Fracture-subluxation (Barton's fracture) (a,b) The true Barton's fracture is a split of the volar edge of the distal radius with anterior (volar) subluxation of the wrist. This has been reduced and held **(c)** with a small anterior plate.

FRACTURE OF THE RADIAL STYLOID PROCESS

This injury is caused by forced radial deviation of the wrist, usually the result of a fall. The fracture line is transverse or oblique, just proximal to the radial styloid process. The fragment is often undisplaced but the injury is commonly associated with a carpal ligament injury and this should be looked for. The energy transfer which breaks the radial styloid can rupture the scapholunate ligament or fracture the scaphoid. These associated injuries must always be carefully excluded.

Treatment

If the styloid fragment is displaced, it should be reduced and held with screws or K-wires (**26.5**). Associated ligamentous injuries should be addressed.

COMMINUTED INTRA-ARTICULAR FRACTURE IN YOUNGER ADULTS

In the young adult, a comminuted intra-articular fracture is a high-energy injury. A poor outcome will result unless intra-articular congruity, fracture alignment and length are restored and movements started as soon as possible.

Treatment

The simplest option is a manipulation and cast immobilization but only if a perfect reduction is achieved. If the fracture is extremely comminuted, open reduction can disrupt the soft-tissue envelope; percutaneous wires may be the most suitable option (**26.6**). In fractures where the anatomy is not restored and there are identifiable fragments (computed tomography (CT) scanning can help to decide), open reduction and volar plate fixation may be necessary. Sometimes, special implants or a separate dorsal approach is required as well (**26.7**).

 High-energy distal radius fractures are very different from low-energy osteopaenic 'Colles' fractures.

COMPLICATIONS OF DISTAL RADIUS FRACTURES (LOW-ENERGY AND HIGH-ENERGY)

There are a number of possible complications with distal radius fracture (**26.8**).

Circulatory impairment Circulation in the fingers must be checked; the bandage holding the slab may need to be split or loosened.

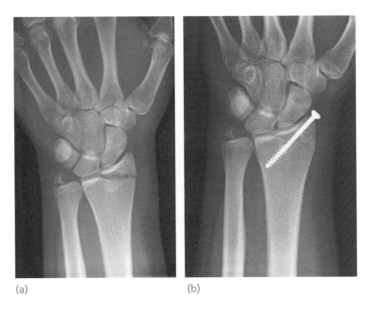

26.5 Fractured radial styloid (a) X-ray; **(b)** fixation with cannulated percutaneous screw.

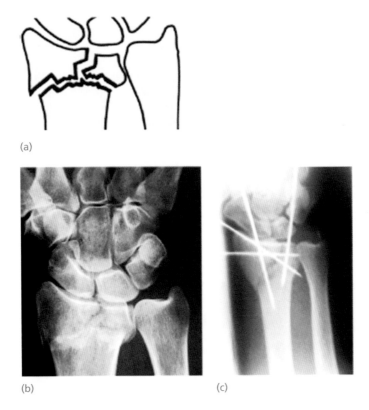

26.6 Comminuted fracture of the distal radius The 'die-punch fragment' of the lunate fossa of the distal radius **(a,b)** must be perfectly reduced and fixed; here, this has been achieved by closed reduction and percutaneous K-wire fixation **(c)**. The wires can be used as 'joy sticks' to manipulate the fragment back before fixation.

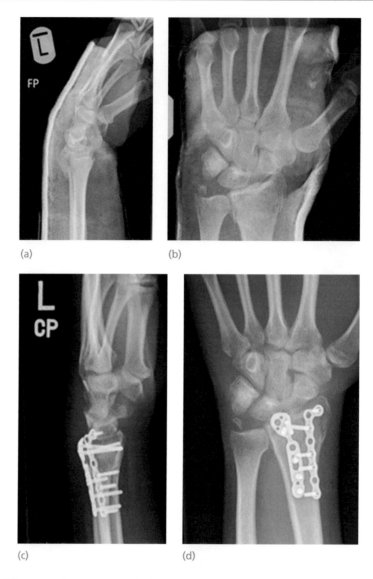

26.7 Comminuted fractures in younger adults (a) dorsal subluxation and **(b)** intra-articular comminution fixed with **(c,d)** dorsal plates.

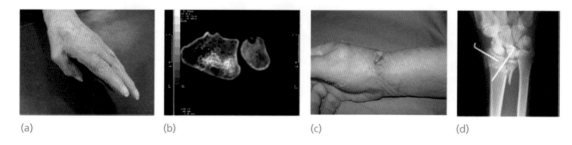

26.8 Distal radius fracture complications (a) Rupture of extensor pollicis longus; **(b)** malunion – CT scan showing incongruity of the DRUJ; **(c)** infected K-wire; **(d)** failed fixation as the wires have cut through the osteoporotic bone.

Nerve injury The median nerve may be compressed by swelling in the carpal tunnel. If the symptoms are mild, they may resolve with release of the dressings and elevation of the arm. If symptoms are severe or persistent, the transverse carpal ligament should be divided.

Malunion This is common, either because reduction was not complete or because displacement within the plaster was overlooked. In most cases, treatment is not necessary. However, if disability is marked, the radial deformity can be corrected by osteotomy.

Associated radioulnar and carpal injuries Compression fractures in osteoporotic bone may result in shortening of the radius relative to the ulna (positive ulnar variance) and displacement of the distal radioulnar joint (DRUJ), which can be painful.

Ligament strains around the wrist are more common than generally recognized and may be a source of pain and weakness long after the fracture has healed.

Tendon rupture Rupture of the extensor pollicis longus tendon occasionally occurs several weeks after the fracture. The frayed fibres cannot easily be sutured; a tendon transfer, using one of the extensor tendons of the index finger, will restore lost function.

Joint stiffness Stiffness of the shoulder, elbow and fingers can be avoided by encouraging active movement.

Complex regional pain syndrome This troublesome condition (formerly called Sudeck's atrophy or reflex sympathetic dystrophy) may appear after any wrist fracture. Early signs are swelling and tenderness of the finger joints – a warning not to neglect the daily exercises. The hand becomes waxy, stiff and painful. It is hypersensitive to temperature ('vasomotor instability'); the forearm hair may overgrow.

Secondary osteoarthritis Injuries around the wrist joint may eventually lead to secondary osteoarthritis (OA) but this is very unusual. If pain and weakness interfere significantly with function, partial arthrodesis, total arthrodesis or even joint replacement of the wrist may be needed.

FRACTURES OF THE DISTAL RADIUS IN CHILDREN

The distal radius and ulna are among the commonest sites of childhood fractures. The break may occur through the distal radial physis or in the metaphysis of one or both bones. Metaphyseal fractures are often incomplete or greenstick.

The usual injury is a fall on the outstretched hand with the wrist in extension; the distal fragment is usually forced posteriorly. Lesser force may do no more than buckle one metaphyseal cortex (a type of compression fracture, or *torus fracture*) or buckle one cortex and break the other (*greenstick fracture*).

Clinical features

The wrist is painful, and often quite swollen; sometimes there is an obvious 'dinner-fork deformity'.

X-rays

Physeal (i.e. growth plate) fractures are almost invariably Salter–Harris Type I or II, with the epiphysis shifted and tilted backwards and radially (**26.9**). *Metaphyseal* (i.e. distal shaft) fractures may appear as either torus or greenstick fractures. If only the radius is fractured, the ulna may be bent though not fractured.

Treatment

PHYSEAL FRACTURES

These are reduced, under anaesthesia, by pressure on the distal fragment. The arm is immobilized in a full-length cast with the wrist slightly flexed and ulnar deviated, and the elbow at 90 degrees. The cast is retained for 4 weeks. These fractures do not interfere with growth. Even if reduction is not absolutely perfect, further growth and modelling will obliterate any deformity within a year or two.

BUCKLE FRACTURES

These require no more than 3–4 weeks in a splint or plaster.

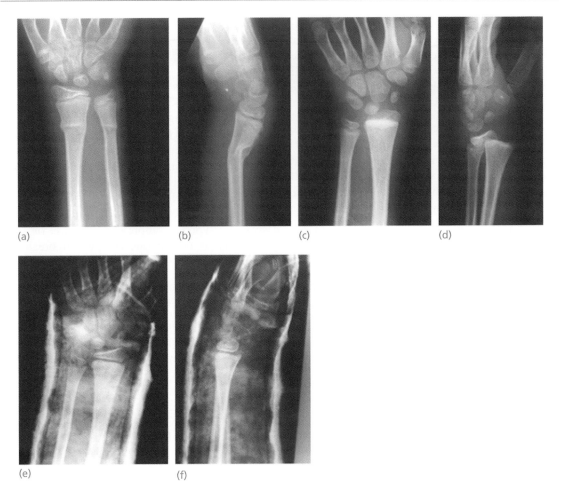

(a)   (b)   (c)   (d)

(e)   (f)

26.9 Distal forearm fractures in children **(a,b)** In older children, the fracture is usually slightly more proximal than a true Colles' fracture, and often merely a greenstick or buckling injury. **(c,d)** In young children, physeal fractures are usually Salter–Harris Type I or II. In this case, accurate reduction has been achieved **(e,f)**.

GREENSTICK FRACTURES

These fractures are usually easy to reduce – but apt to redisplace in the cast! Some degree of angulation can be accepted:

- *in children under the age of 10 years*, up to 30 degrees
- *in children over 10 years*, up to 15 degrees.

If the deformity is greater, the fracture is reduced by thumb pressure and the arm is immobilized in a full-length cast with the wrist and forearm in neutral and the elbow flexed 90 degrees. The cast is changed and the fracture re-X-rayed at 1 week; if it has redisplaced,

a further gentle manipulation can be carried out and held with a K-wire. The cast is finally discarded after 6 weeks.

COMPLETE FRACTURES

Complete fractures can be embarrassingly difficult to reduce – especially if the ulna is intact. The fracture is manipulated in much the same way as a Colles' fracture; the reduction is checked by *X-ray* and a full-length cast is applied with the wrist neutral and the forearm supinated. After 1 week, a check X-ray is obtained; the cast is kept on for 6 weeks. If the fracture slips, especially if the ulna is intact, it should be stabilized with a percutaneous K-wire.

Wiring should be considered in all cases where the fracture fragment is displaced 100% or more as the risk of redisplacement is very high.

Complications

Forearm swelling and a threatened compartment syndrome   These are prevented by:

- avoiding overforceful or repeated manipulations
- splitting the plaster
- elevating the arm for the first 24–48 hours
- encouraging exercises.

Malunion   As a late sequel, malunion is uncommon in children under 10 years of age. Deformity of as much as 30 degrees will straighten out with further growth and remodelling over the next 1–2 years. This should be carefully explained to the worried parents.

Radioulnar discrepancy   Premature fusion of the radial epiphysis may result in bone length disparity and subluxation of the radioulnar joint. If this is troublesome, the radius can be lengthened and, if the child is near to skeletal maturity, the ulnar physis can be fused surgically.

INJURIES OF THE CARPUS

Injuries of the wrist comprise soft-tissue strains and fractures or dislocations of individual carpal bones. However, they should never be regarded as isolated injuries: the entire carpus suffers, and sometimes, long after the fracture has healed, the patient still complains of pain and weakness in the wrist.

COMMONEST CARPAL INJURIES

Simple self-limiting sprains of the joint capsule and interosseous ligaments
More serious unstable tears of the joint capsule and interosseous ligaments
Fracture of a carpal bone (usually the scaphoid)
Injury of the triangular fibrocartilage complex (TFCC) and distal radioulnar joint
Dislocations of the lunate or the bones around it

Clinical assessment

Following a fall, the patient complains of pain in the wrist, perhaps accompanied by swelling. Tenderness can often be localized to a particular spot, providing a clue to the diagnosis. Movements are likely to be restricted and painful.

Imaging

Fractures are often quite obvious, but sometimes multiple views – and examination on multiple occasions – are needed to detect an undisplaced crack. Follow the 'three golden rules'.

THREE GOLDEN RULES

1 Accept only high-quality images.
2 If the initial X-rays are 'normal', treat the clinical diagnosis and immobilize the wrist. Bear in mind that 10–15% of scaphoid fractures are not visible on initial X-rays.
3 Early MRI reduces uncertainty and streamlines care.

If *MRI* is not available, repeated *X-rays* are needed 2 weeks later (as shifting of the bones and resorption at the fracture line can make the fracture more apparent). If there is still doubt after a further 2 weeks, X-ray again.

Initially, four standard views are obtained:

- posteroanterior (PA) with wrist in ulnar deviation
- lateral
- semi-pronated oblique
- semi-supinated oblique.

An anteroposterior (AP) view with the fist clenched can be added if there is a suspicion of a scapholunate injury.

Study the shape of the carpus and the relationship of the bones to each other. Familiarity with the normal anatomy is essential. Unusual gaps (e.g. between the scaphoid and the lunate) suggest disruption of ligaments; more subtle changes appear in the alignment of the bones. In the lateral X-ray, the axes of the radius, lunate, capitate and third metacarpal are co-linear, and the scaphoid projects at an angle of about 45 degrees

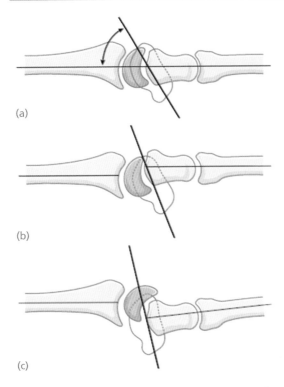

(a)

(b)

(c)

26.10 Carpal instability – X-ray patterns (a) Normal lateral view. The radius, capitate and middle metacarpal lie in a straight line and the scaphoid axis is angled at 45° to the line of the radius. **(b)** Dorsal intercalated segmental instability (DISI). The lunate is tilted dorsally and the scaphoid is tilted somewhat volarwards; the axes of the capitate and metacarpals now lie behind (dorsal to) that of the radius. **(c)** Volar intercalated segmental instability (VISI). The lunate and scaphoid are tilted somewhat volarwards and the capitate and metacarpals lie anterior (volar) to the radius.

to this line. With traumatic instability, the linked carpal segments collapse (like the buckled carriages of a derailed train). Two patterns of carpal instability are recognized (**26.10, 26.11**).

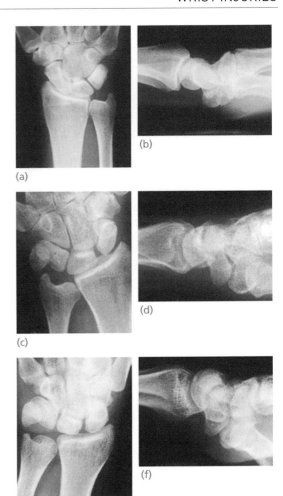

(a)

(b)

(c)

(d)

(e)

(f)

26.11 Carpal injuries (a,b) Normal appearances in AP and lateral X-rays. **(c,d)** Following a 'sprained wrist' this patient developed persistent pain and weakness. X-rays showed **(c)** scapholunate dissociation and **(d)** dorsal rotation of the lunate (the typical DISI pattern). **(e,f)** This patient, too, had a sprained wrist. The AP and lateral X-rays show foreshortening of the scaphoid and volar rotation of the lunate (VISI).

THE TWO PATTERNS OF CARPAL INSTABILITY
Dorsal intercalated segmental instability (DISI) The lunate is torn from the scaphoid and tilts backwards.
Volar intercalated segment instability (VISI) The lunate is torn from the triquetrum and tilts forwards.

Principles of management

A diagnosis of 'wrist sprain' should not be accepted until a more serious injury has been excluded with certainty. Even with apparently trivial injuries, ligaments are sometimes torn and the patient may later develop carpal instability.

If the initial *X-rays* seem to be normal but the clinical signs suggest a carpal injury, a splint or plaster should be applied and the X-ray examination repeated 2 weeks later; a fracture or dislocation may then be more obvious. A *magnetic resonance imaging (MRI) scan* is very helpful to settle uncertainty and allow either earlier definitive treatment or reassurance that there is not a serious injury after all.

MRI arthrogram and *wrist arthroscopy* are the most sensitive methods to detect ruptures of the scapholunate and lunotriquetral ligament or TFCC.

FRACTURE OF THE SCAPHOID

Scaphoid fractures account for almost 75% of all carpal fractures but are rare in children and in the elderly. The usual mechanism is forced hyperextension of the wrist.

Fractures occur in three anatomical locations:

* distal tubercle
* waist
* proximal pole.

Some fractures, especially distal oblique and waist fractures, are unstable, which predisposes to *non-union* or *malunion*.

The blood supply of the scaphoid arises from the dorsal distal pole. This means that the proximal pole has a poor blood supply and is less likely to heal than the distal pole and may actually crumble away (*avascular necrosis*).

Clinical features

There may be slight fullness in the anatomical snuffbox; precisely localized tenderness in the same place is an important diagnostic sign. However, examination must also include:

* pressure backwards over the scaphoid tubercle
* palpation over the proximal pole
* telescoping of the thumb base.

If any of these are positive, the suspicion for a scaphoid fracture should be high.

Imaging

X-RAYS

X-rays should include AP, lateral and two oblique views; even then, the fracture may not be seen in the first few days after the injury. Two weeks later, the break is usually much clearer, due to bone resorption at the fracture site and slight displacement of fragments. The crack is usually transverse through the narrowest part of the bone (the waist), but it may be more proximal or more distal. Always look for signs of associated carpal displacement (**26.12**).

CT

A CT scan is more sensitive for diagnosing a scaphoid fracture; it is particularly useful in confirming the alignment of the bone fragments if surgery is planned, or to confirm whether the fracture has united or not.

MRI

This is the definitive way to confirm or exclude a diagnosis of scaphoid fracture if the technique is available.

Treatment

If the X-ray looks normal but the clinical features are suggestive of a fracture, the patient must not be discharged. The diagnosis has to be confirmed one way or another. The usual advice is to return for a second X-ray 2 weeks later. Meanwhile, the wrist is immobilized in a cast extending from the upper forearm to just short of the metacarpophalangeal joints of the fingers, but incorporating the proximal phalanx of the thumb; the wrist is held dorsiflexed and the thumb forwards in the 'glass-holding' position (the so-called scaphoid plaster) (**26.13a**). An alternative is to arrange an *MRI scan* (or, if not available, a *CT scan*) which will definitely detect the fracture even if it was not visible on the X-ray.

If a fracture is confirmed, treatment will depend on the type of fracture and the degree of displacement (**26.13b–i**).

 Take at least four X-rays of possible *scaphoid fractures*. Even then, X-rays might be normal initially. If any doubt, put in plaster and either re-X-ray in 2 weeks or get an MRI scan.

SECTION 3 TRAUMA

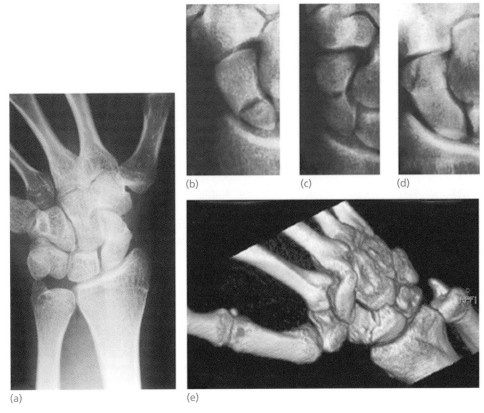

(b)   (c)   (d)

(a)   (e)

26.12 Fractures of the scaphoid – diagnosis (a) The initial AP view often fails to show the fracture. The fracture may be **(b)** through the proximal pole, **(c)** the waist, or **(d)** the scaphoid tubercle. **(e)** A CT scan is useful for showing the fracture configuration.

FRACTURE OF THE SCAPHOID TUBERCLE

These are treated in a cast for 4–6 weeks. There are usually no complications but occasionally there is a non-union needing excision of a small fragment or grafting of a larger fragment.

UNDISPLACED FRACTURES OF THE WAIST

These can be treated in two ways: plaster or percutaneous fixation.

Plaster Around 90% of waist fractures should heal in plaster (a neutral forearm cast from the upper forearm to just short of the metacarpophalangeal joints of the fingers; the thumb is not incorporated) for 6–8 weeks. The plaster is then removed and the wrist examined clinically and radiologically. If there is no tenderness and the *X-ray* shows full healing, the wrist is left free; a *CT scan* is the most reliable means of confirming union if in doubt.

If the scaphoid is tender, or the fracture is still visible on X-ray, the cast is reapplied for a further 4 weeks. At that stage, one of two pictures may emerge:

- the wrist is painless and the fracture has healed – the cast can be discarded
- the X-ray shows signs of delayed healing (bone resorption and cavitation around the fracture). Union can be hastened by bone grafting and internal fixation.

Percutaneous fixation This should be considered for those patients who do not want to endure prolonged plaster immobilization and who want to get back to work or sport earlier (but they must still avoid impact or heavy load on the wrist until the fracture is healed). A screw is passed through a small incision in the front of the scaphoid tubercle. Special cannulated screws and technical perfection are essential.

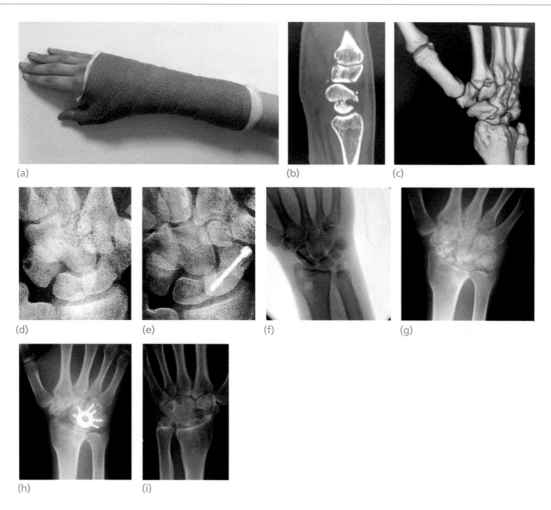

26.13 Fractures of the scaphoid – treatment (a) Scaphoid plaster – the thumb is optional. (b,c) CT scan showing collapse, which needs a graft from the front to wedge it open. (d) Delayed union, treated successfully by (e) bone grafting and screw fixation. (f) Waist fracture treated with distal radius graft. (g) Non-union with avascular necrosis and secondary OA can be treated by (h) scaphoid excision and four-corner fusion or (i) proximal row carpectomy.

DISPLACED FRACTURES

These can also be treated in plaster, but the outcome is less predictable: it may not heal or may heal in a poor position. It is better to reduce the fracture (closed if possible, otherwise open) and to fix it with a compression screw. This should increase the likelihood of union and reduce the time of immobilization.

PROXIMAL POLE FRACTURES

These may heal in plaster, and probably will if left long enough. However, the risk of non-union and the disadvantages of prolonged immobilization are such that early surgical fixation (through a small dorsal incision) should be considered.

Complications

Non-union By 2–3 months, it may be obvious that the fracture will not unite. If so, screw fixation with bone grafting should be considered. The aim is to reduce the pain from the non-union and to reduce the chance of secondary OA. Bone graft on a vascular pedicle can be taken from the back of the distal radius. Once a fracture of the waist fails to heal, it starts to collapse into a 'hump back' deformity. A wedge of bone taken from the iliac crest can be carved into shape and placed into the non-union to restore the proper shape and encourage healing.

Avascular necrosis The proximal fragment may die, because of the precarious blood supply. It appears dense on X-ray. Although revascularization and union are theoretically possible in some cases, this is unpredictable. Surgery should be considered. For small proximal pole fragments, the bone can be stabilized by a very small screw; if there is space, a bone graft from the distal radius is inserted. There may be a greater chance of healing if the graft is attached to an arterial pedicle. Free microvascular grafts have been suggested.

Osteoarthritis Non-union or avascular necrosis may lead to secondary OA of the wrist. Salvage procedures include proximal row carpectomy, partial wrist fusion and radiocarpal fusion (**26.13g–i**).

FRACTURES OF THE OTHER CARPAL BONES

Fractures of other carpal bones (**26.14**) are all rare; they can easily be overlooked. Careful examination, and meticulous inspection of *X-rays*, especially after a significant fall or blow, is mandatory. If in any doubt, *CT* or *MRI* is invaluable.

Undisplaced fractures are usually treated by splinting until healed. Displaced fractures will need open reduction and internal fixation.

ULNAR-SIDED WRIST INJURIES

TYPES OF ULNAR-SIDED WRIST INJURY
The *ulnar styloid* is broken off in about half of distal radius fractures. It almost never needs treatment.   The *DRUJ* can be dislocated, in isolation or with a displaced distal radius fracture.   The *TFCC* can be perforated or torn from its attachment.   With sudden supination (e.g. playing tennis or golf), the *extensor carpi ulnaris* (ECU) can be pulled out of its sheath.

Clinical features

The patient complains of pain and often clunking. The ulnar corner must be examined very thoroughly. There is tenderness over the injured site (e.g. the DRUJ, the ulna fovea – the dent at the front of the base of the ulna styloid – or the ECU sheath) and pain on rotation of the forearm. The distal ulna may be unstable; the *piano-key sign* is elicited by holding the patient's forearm pronated and pushing sharply forwards on the head of the ulna. Remember, though, that the ulna is the fixed point and it is the radius that is unstable. The ECU may be seen and felt to clunk out of its groove on rotation.

Investigation

X-ray examination may show a fracture or signs of incongruity of the distal radioulnar joint. *MRI* and *arthroscopy* help to confirm the diagnosis.

Treatment

An acute dislocation of the DRUJ usually resolves if the arm is held in supination for 6 weeks; occasionally, a K-wire is needed to maintain the reduction. If the dislocation is irreducible, this may be due to trapped soft tissue, which will have to be removed. Chronic instability may require reconstructive surgery.

An unstable TFCC tear should be reattached. A displaced fracture at the base of the ulnar styloid, if painful and associated with instability of the radioulnar joint, should be fixed with a small screw. An acute ECU sheath tear can be treated with either repair or an above-elbow cast in pronation for 6 weeks.

SCAPHOLUNATE LIGAMENT RUPTURE

A fall on the outstretched hand, rather than breaking a bone, may tear the all-important scapholunate ligament. There is pain and swelling with tenderness over the dorsum just distal to Lister's tubercle. Pushing backwards on the scaphoid tubercle is very painful and, if performed while moving the wrist radialwards and ulnarwards, it can elicit a clunk (*Watson's test*).

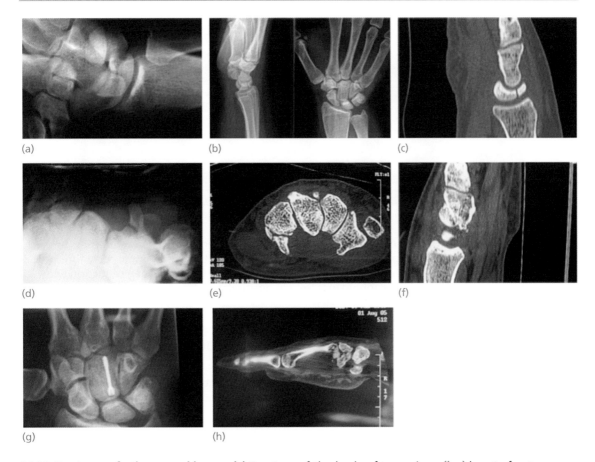

26.14 Fractures of other carpal bones **(a)** Fracture of the body of trapezium; **(b,c)** lunate fractures; **(d)** hook of hamate fracture; **(e)** hook of hamate CT; **(f)** capitate fracture fixed with a screw **(g)**; **(h)** fracture of body of hamate.

What is thought to be a sprain giving rise to persistent tenderness over the dorsum of the wrist may be shown by X-ray or arthrography to be a much more significant injury due to disruption of the ligament between scaphoid and lunate. The pathognomonic features are foreshortening of the scaphoid (**26.15**), dorsal tilt of the lunate (DISI, see **26.10**) and the appearance of a large gap between scaphoid and lunate.

Treatment

If the patient is seen early (i.e. less than 4 weeks after injury), the scapholunate ligament should be repaired directly with interosseous sutures, and protected by K-wires for 6 weeks and a cast

for 8–12 weeks. If the diagnosis presents later, a complicated reconstruction is considered but the results are unpredictable.

LUNATE AND PERILUNATE INJURIES

A fall with the hand forced into dorsiflexion may tear the tough ligaments that normally bind the carpal bones. The lunate usually remains attached to the radius, and the rest of the carpus is displaced backwards (*perilunate dislocation*). Usually, the hand immediately snaps forwards again but, as it does so, the lunate may be levered out of position to be displaced anteriorly (*lunate dislocation*). Sometimes the scaphoid remains attached to the radius and the force of

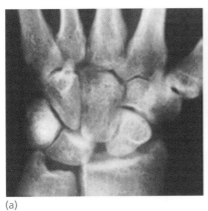
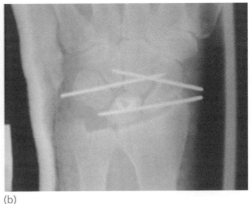

(a)   (b)

26.15 Scapholunate dissociation After a fall, this patient complained of pain and tenderness in the anatomical snuffbox. X-ray **(a)** shows that the scaphoid is intact but the image is markedly foreshortened and there is a wide gap between the scaphoid and the lunate. **(b)** After open reduction and repair of the dorsal ligaments, the scaphoid was held in position with K-wires.

the perilunar dislocation causes it to fracture through the waist (*trans-scaphoid perilunate dislocation*). Rarely, the lunotriquetral ligament is torn in isolation, causing a VISI deformity (see **26.10**).

Clinical features

The wrist is painful and swollen and is held immobile. If the carpal tunnel is compressed, there may be paraesthesia or blunting of sensation in the territory of the median nerve, and weakness of palmar abduction of the thumb.

X-rays

Most dislocations are *perilunate*. In the *AP view*, the carpus is diminished in height and the bone shadows overlap abnormally. One or more of the carpal bones may be fractured (usually the scaphoid). *Lunate* dislocation can be recognized by the abnormal shape of the lunate AP X-ray image – triangular instead of quadrilateral.

In the *lateral view*, it is easy to distinguish a lunate from a perilunate dislocation (**26.16**). The dislocated lunate is tilted forwards and is displaced in front of the radius, while the capitate and metacarpal bones are in line with the radius. With a perilunate dislocation, the lunate is not displaced forwards.

Treatment

CLOSED REDUCTION

Pulling on the hand with the wrist in extension and applying thumb pressure to the displaced bones may succeed. A plaster slab is applied, holding the wrist neutral. Percutaneous K-wires may be needed to hold the reduction.

OPEN REDUCTION

If closed reduction fails, open reduction is imperative. The carpus is exposed by an anterior approach, which has the advantage of decompressing the carpal tunnel. While an assistant pulls on the hand, the lunate is levered into place and kept there by a K-wire which is inserted through the lunate into the capitate. If the scaphoid is fractured, this too can be reduced and fixed with a screw or K-wires. Torn ligaments should be repaired through palmar and dorsal (**26.17**). At the end of the procedure, the wrist is splinted. Fingers, elbow and shoulder are exercised throughout this period. The splint and K-wires are removed at 8 weeks.

Complications

Avascular necrosis of the lunate   This may follow disruption of its blood supply. The X-ray shows progressive increase in bone density. Treatment is required only if symptoms demand it. If the wrist is stiff and painful, removal of the lunate and the adjacent bones may be considered.

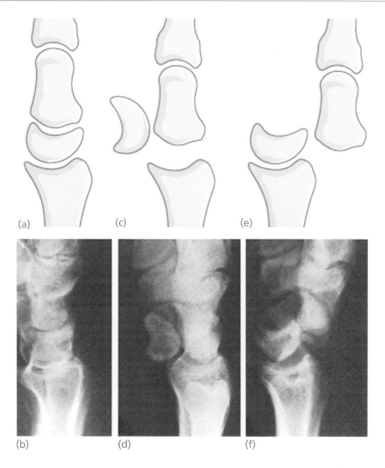

26.16 Lunate and perilunate dislocations **(a,b)** Lateral X-ray of normal wrist; **(c,d)** lunate dislocation; **(e,f)** perilunate dislocation.

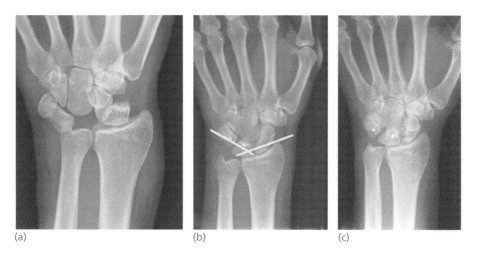

26.17 Perilunate dislocation **(a)** Lunate still in its original position while the rest of the carpus is dislocated around it. **(b)** The dislocation has been reduced and held with K-wires. **(c)** The lunotriquetral ligament is reattached with ligament anchors.

Hand injuries

27

■ Principles of treatment   607
■ Carpometacarpal injuries   608
■ Fracture of the metacarpals   609
■ Skier's thumb (torn ulnar collateral ligament
  of the metacarpophalangeal joint)   611

■ Fractured phalanges   612
■ Finger joint injuries   614
■ Closed tendon injuries   616
■ Open injuries of the hand   617
■ Burns   623

Hand injuries – the commonest of all injuries – are important out of all proportion to their apparent severity, because of the need for perfect function. Local oedema and stiffness of the joints – common accompaniments of all injuries – are more threatening in the hand than anywhere else. Fractures may heal and joints re-stabilize, and yet the patient may still be left with a useless hand because of insufficient attention to splintage, the prevention of swelling, the preservation of movement and rehabilitation.

 In all hand injuries, the danger of *stiffness* is ever present, and a stiff finger can be worse than no finger. The principles of soft-tissue care should never be neglected:

- elevate
- keep splintage to a minimum
- move
- exercise.

PRINCIPLES OF TREATMENT

Assessment

The history should include:

- details of the accident
- the patient's age
- occupation
- leisure activities
- 'handedness'.

Superficial injuries and severe fractures are obvious, but deeper injuries are often poorly disclosed. Thorough assessment is important in the *initial examination*.

INITIAL EXAMINATION

Circulation
Soft–tissue cover
Bones
Joints
Nerves
Tendons

Treatment

Closed injuries and small wounds can often be treated under regional block anaesthesia. Large wounds and multiple fractures are better dealt with under general anaesthesia.

Definitive treatment is dictated by the nature of the injury, but common to all injuries are four important requirements.

FOUR BASIC REQUIREMENTS OF TREATMENT

Safe splintage
Prevention of swelling
Dedicated rehabilitation
Adequate soft-tissue cover

SPLINTAGE

Splintage must be kept to a minimum. If only one finger is injured, it alone should be splinted – either by strapping it to its neighbour so that both move as one ('buddy-strapping'), or by fashioning a splint that does not impede movement in the uninjured fingers. If the whole hand is splinted or bandaged, this must always be in the *'position of safe immobilization'* – with the knuckle joints flexed at least 70 degrees, the finger joints straight and the thumb abducted (**27.1**). That way, the ligaments are at full stretch, so if they do become adherent it is still possible to regain movement with physiotherapy.

PREVENTION OF SWELLING

This means keeping the hand elevated and performing early and repeated active exercises.

PHYSIOTHERAPY AND REHABILITATION

These are best undertaken by a dedicated and experienced hand therapist.

SKIN COVER

Treatment of the skin takes precedence over treatment of the fracture.

TREATMENT OF SKIN DAMAGE

Thorough wound washout followed by
    suture
Skin grafting
Local flaps
Pedicled flaps or (occasionally) free flaps

CARPOMETACARPAL INJURIES

DISLOCATION OF THE CARPOMETACARPAL JOINTS

Dislocation of the finger carpometacarpal (CMC) joints is caused by forceful dorsiflexion of the wrist combined with a longitudinal impact. Thus, it is seen typically in boxers and in motorcyclists. There may be an associated intra-articular fracture at the base of the metacarpals.

The thumb CMC may dislocate, often leaving a small triangular fragment of bone left attached to the carpus ('Bennett's fracture').

The *X-rays* must be carefully inspected. If there is any doubt about the nature of the injury, a *computed tomography (CT) scan* will usually help.

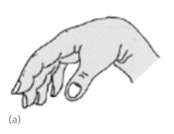
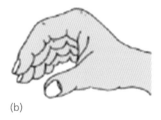
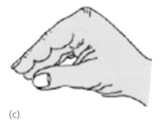

(a)   (b)   (c)

27.1 Splintage of the hand – Three positions of the hand: (a) the position of relaxation; **(b)** the position of function (ready for action); and **(c)** the position of safe immobilization, with the ligaments taut.

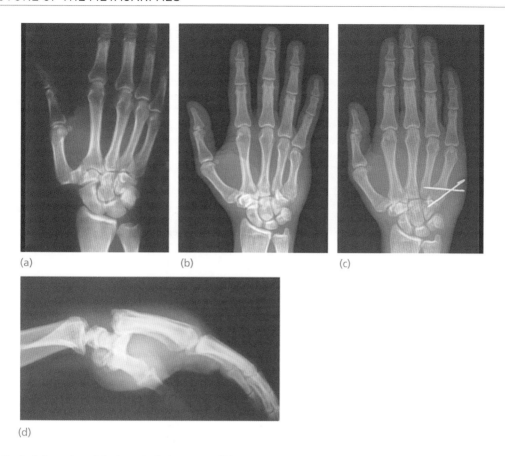

(a)   (b)   (c)

(d)

27.2 CMC dislocation **(a)** Thumb dislocation. **(b)** Dislocation of the fourth and fifth CMC joints treated by closed reduction and Kirschner wires **(c)**. Complete CMC dislocation **(d)**.

Treatment

The dislocation is reduced by traction, manipulation and thumb pressure. A protective slab is worn for 6 weeks, during which time the fingers are kept moving. The reduction is usually unstable, and so percutaneous wires should be used and removed after 5–6 weeks (**27.2**). With a larger fragment, a screw can be used (**27.3**).

Complications

If the CMC joint is seriously damaged or subluxated, osteoarthritis may ensue. Treatment is usually conservative, but if pain becomes intolerable, an operation may be needed – either arthrodesis of the joint or excision of the trapezium.

FRACTURE OF THE METACARPALS

The metacarpal bones are vulnerable to blows and falls upon the hand, or the force of a boxer's punch. The bones may fracture at their base, in the shaft or through the neck.

Clinical features

If the fragments are displaced, there may be a bump on the back of the hand, or one of the knuckles may be flattened. The metacarpal head can be prominent in the palm, a particular problem with grip if the index finger is involved. There is considerable swelling and local tenderness.

SECTION 3 TRAUMA

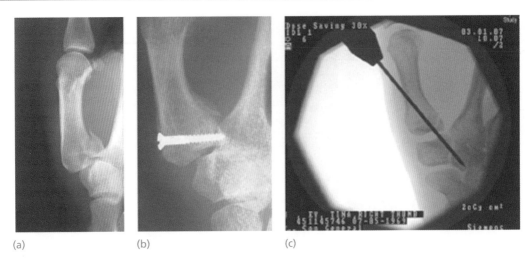

(a)   (b)   (c)

27.3 Bennett's fracture-subluxation (a) This fracture at the base of the thumb metacarpal with extension into the CMC joint is inherently unstable. It is therefore best treated by reduction and internal fixation with a small screw **(b)** or a percutaneous K-wire **(c)**.

X-rays

Fractures of the base of the metacarpal are usually impacted. Fractures of the shaft are either transverse or oblique; there may be shortening or angulation of the fragments. Fractures of the metacarpal neck may result in forward tilting of the distal fragment.

Treatment

UNDISPLACED FRACTURES

Fractures that are undisplaced (or only slightly displaced) require only a firm crepe bandage (for comfort), which is worn for 2–3 weeks. This should not be allowed to interfere with active movements of the fingers, which must be practised assiduously.

DISPLACED FRACTURES OF THE SHAFT

Most can be left alone. In the midshaft, angular deformity is usually not marked; even if it is, it does not interfere much with function. No plaster is needed and early movement is encouraged. Rotational deformity is unusual as the intermetacarpal ligaments tend to maintain alignment.

Marked angulation or any rotation would be an indication for open reduction and internal fixation with small plates and screws. Careful attention should be given to correcting rotation, otherwise the finger will go awry during flexion. A useful guide is to remember that in flexion every finger should point towards the thenar crease (compare with the other side). After operation, movements are started as soon as possible (**27.4**).

DISPLACED FRACTURES OF THE NECK

With fractures of the metacarpal neck, angulation of up to 70 degrees in the fifth metacarpals and 20 degrees in the second and third can be accepted. If the displacement is too great, fixation with percutaneous intramedullary wires passed from the base is usually preferred.

FRACTURES OF THE HEAD

In a closed injury with displaced fragments, tiny buried screws are needed to hold the fragments in place. Occasionally the joint is so badly damaged that primary replacement is considered (Silastic, pyrocarbon or polythene–metal).

Head fractures are associated with a punching injury. If an opponent's tooth has punctured the skin over the metacarpal head – a 'fight-bite' – then the joint will surely become infected.

Immediate exploration and thorough washout of the wound, however small, is essential to avoid destruction of the joint (**27.5**).

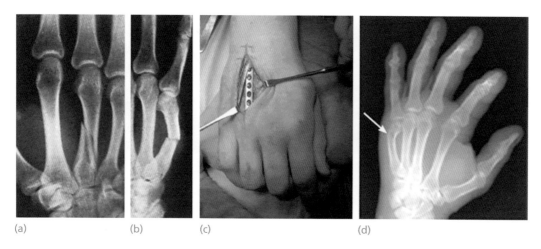

(a)   (b)   (c)   (d)

27.4 Metacarpal fractures (a) A spiral fracture of a single metacarpal is usually held adequately by neighbouring bones and muscles. **(b)** A displaced transverse fracture will often require internal fixation with rigid wires or a small plate **(c)**. Fractures of the metacarpal neck **(d)** can usually be managed by early mobilization.

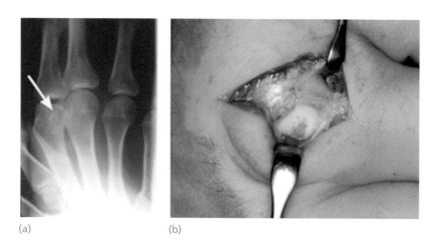

(a)   (b)

27.5 A 'fight-bite' The underlying metacarpal head was damaged by the attacker's tooth.

> ⚠ A *fight bite* from an opponent's tooth over the knuckle must be thoroughly washed out immediately.

Complications

Malunion Angulation may result in a visible bump or a flattened knuckle, but function is usually good.

Stiffness Metacarpal fractures invariably unite and, even if angulation persists, malunion is less disabling than stiffness of the hand. Early movement and the avoidance of swelling are essential.

SKIER'S THUMB (TORN ULNAR COLLATERAL LIGAMENT OF THE METACARPOPHALANGEAL JOINT)

In former years, gamekeepers who twisted the necks of little animals ran the risk of tearing the ulnar collateral ligament of the thumb (MCP) joint. The injury came to be known as *gamekeeper's*

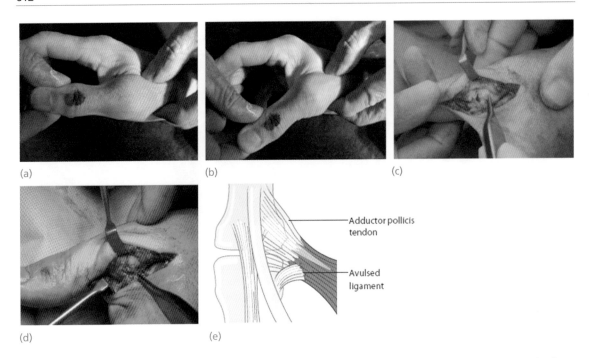

27.6 Skier's thumb (a,b) The ulnar collateral ligament has ruptured. Urgent repair is indicated **(c,d)**. **(e)** A Stener lesion – when the ligament is trapped proximal to adductor pollicis.

thumb. Nowadays, it is seen in skiers who fall onto the extended thumb, forcing it into hyperabduction and is known as *skier's thumb.* A small flake of bone may be pulled off at the same time.

Clinical features

The ulnar side of the joint is swollen and very tender, yet the condition is often under-diagnosed as a simple 'sprain'. Before testing the ligament, an *X-ray* must be obtained to exclude any fracture. The thumb is stressed in abduction and, if there is laxity (compared with the normal side), a ligament injury is diagnosed; local anaesthetic into the joint can help (**27.6**). The ligament can become jammed proximally under the adductor pollicis tendon (the so-called Stener lesion) and requires operative repair. An *ultrasound scan* can be helpful in clarifying the degree of injury.

Treatment

PARTIAL TEARS

These can be treated by immobilization of the thumb in a cast or splint for 4 weeks. This is followed by increasing movement and pinching and gripping exercises.

COMPLETE TEARS

Complete tears need operative repair. Care should be taken during the exposure not to injure the superficial radial nerve branches. Postoperatively, the joint is immobilized in a removable thumb splint (leaving the interphalangeal joint free) for 6 weeks. Gentle flexion–extension movements out of the splint are allowed early to prevent stiffness, but no pinch against the repair is permissible for 6 weeks.

FRACTURED PHALANGES

The fingers are usually injured by direct violence, and there may be considerable swelling or open wounds. Injudicious treatment may result in a stiff finger which, in some cases, can be worse than no finger.

Treatment

Open wounds should always be treated first. Skin must be preserved and carefully sutured, and wound healing must not be jeopardized by the treatment of the fractures.

UNDISPLACED FRACTURES

These need the minimum of splintage. The type of splint depends on the fracture and the direction of potential instability. This may necessitate strapping the finger to its uninjured neighbour ('buddy-strapping') or a splint on the digit alone. Early movement, without compromising stability, is encouraged.

DISPLACED FRACTURE OF THE PROXIMAL OR MIDDLE PHALANX SHAFT

The bone should be straightened under local anaesthesia, carefully avoiding malrotation; the injured finger is then splinted, leaving the other fingers free. The splint can be discarded after 3 weeks.

- *Basal fractures* with extension are manipulated and held with a dorsal blocking splint with the MCP joint at 90 degrees.
- *Angulated basal fractures* are manipulated with a pencil between the digits as a lever and then held with neighbour strapping which pulls the injured finger to the next one.
- *Spiral fractures* are held with 'derotation taping' to the next digit, using tension in the tape to unwind the fracture.
- *Transverse fractures* may be held in a gutter splint or neighbour splint.

If reduction cannot be held in this way, fixation with K-wires, a small plate or screws is indicated, depending on the type of fracture (27.7). Surgery is challenging and invites stiffness. Meticulous attention to surgical technique and postoperative rehabilitation is needed.

PILON FRACTURES OF THE MIDDLE PHALANX

These are quite common injuries and can be very troublesome. The head of the proximal phalanx impacts into the base of the middle phalanx,

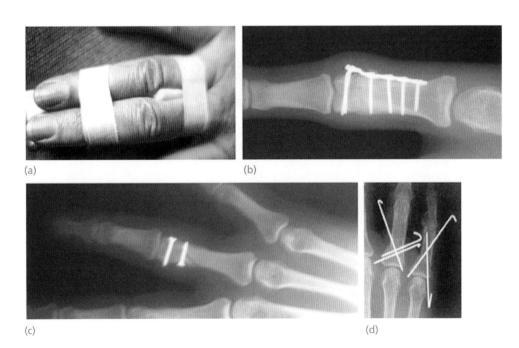

(a)   (b)

(c)   (d)

27.7 Phalangeal fractures Depending on the 'personality' of the fracture, the equipment available and the experience of the surgeon, these injuries can be treated by neighbour strapping (a), plate fixation (b), percutaneous screw fixation (c) or percutaneous wire fixation (d).

causing the latter to splay open in several pieces. These injuries are best treated with dynamic distraction using a spring-loaded external fixator which rotates around the head of the proximal phalanx and disimpacts the distal fragment. The results can be surprisingly good (see **27.9d–h**).

CONDYLAR FRACTURES

The convex distal joint surface of the phalanges can be fractured, usually by an angulation force. One or both condyles may be fractured. If the fragment is not displaced, it is best to disregard the fracture, strap the finger to its neighbour and concentrate on regaining movement. An *X-ray* should be taken after a week to ensure there is no displacement.

If the fracture is displaced, there is a risk of permanent angular deformity and loss of movement at the joint. The fracture should be anatomically reduced, either closed or by open operation and

fixed with small K-wires or mini-screws. The finger is splinted for a few days and then supervised movements are commenced.

FRACTURES OF THE DISTAL PHALANX

Distal phalangeal fractures are usually due to crushing injuries or a blow from a hammer. The soft-tissue damage must be treated (**27.8**); the fracture can be ignored.

FINGER JOINT INJURIES

SPRAINS

Partial or complete tears of the ligaments are common and usually due to forced angulation at the joint. Milder injuries require no treatment; with more severe strains, the finger should be splinted for 1–2 weeks. However, the patient

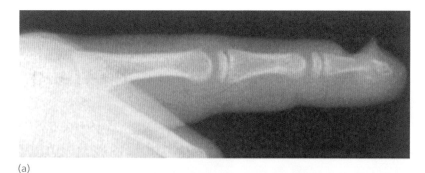

(a)

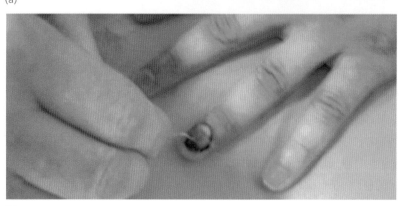

(b)

27.8 Distal phalangeal injury (a) A fracture of the tuft, caused by a hammer blow, is treated by a protective dressing. The subungual haematoma should be evacuated using a red-hot paper clip tip **(b)** or a small drill.

should be warned that the joint may remain slightly swollen, stiff and painful for several months.

METACARPOPHALANGEAL JOINT DISLOCATION

This is rare. A hyperextension force may dislocate the phalanx backwards, and the volar capsule may be torn. If the metacarpal head has been forced like a button through the hole, closed reduction may be impossible. Sometimes one or other collateral ligaments are avulsed, pulling off a triangular fragment of bone.

For a dislocation, closed reduction is attempted by pulling on the thumb and levering the phalanx forwards. If this fails, the joint is exposed from the dorsum and, while strong traction is applied, the metacarpal head is levered into place. The joint is then strapped in the flexed position for 1 week before mobilizing.

A collateral ligament avulsion is usually treated by strapping the finger to its neighbour for 3–4 weeks. A markedly displaced or unstable fracture can be fixed with a small screw or bone suture.

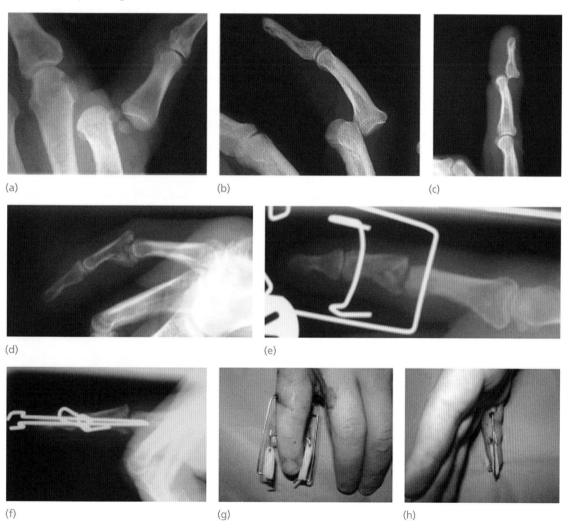

(a)   (b)   (c)
(d)   (e)
(f)   (g)   (h)

27.9 Finger dislocation (a) MCP dislocation in the thumb occasionally buttonholes and needs open reduction; **(b,c)** interphalangeal dislocations are easily reduced (and easily missed if not X-rayed). A comminuted pilon fracture **(d)** is best treated by dynamic external fixation **(e–h)**.

INTERPHALANGEAL JOINT DISLOCATION

Dislocation at the proximal joint is common and is easily reduced by pulling on the finger.

- *If there is no associated fracture*, minimal splintage is needed. However, the patient should be warned that swelling and slight loss of movement may persist for months.
- *If there is a fracture*, the joint may be unstable, requiring surgery under local anaesthesia with wires or even a spring-loaded external fixator (**27.9a,b**).

CLOSED TENDON INJURIES

MALLET FINGER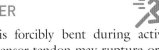

If the fingertip is forcibly bent during active extension, the extensor tendon may rupture or a flake of bone may be avulsed from the base of the distal phalanx. This sometimes occurs when the finger is stubbed when making a bed or catching a ball.

A pure soft-tissue injury can be treated by splinting the distal joint continuously in extension for 8 weeks and then at night only for another 4 weeks (**27.10**). If there is a large flake of bone, a shorter term of splintage will usually suffice. Operative fixation is rarely needed; it is unlikely to improve outcome in any but the most markedly displaced fractures. The risk of stiffness and wound problems is rather high.

FLEXOR TENDON AVULSION

Avulsion of the flexor tendon from the base of the distal phalanx is a rare injury, but it should not be missed. It usually affects the left ring finger; it is sometimes known as a 'rugby jersey finger', reflecting the fact that it is often caused when the finger is caught in an opponent's shirt. The patient cannot actively flex the tip of the finger.

X-rays sometimes show a fragment of avulsed bone either at the tip or further down the finger (**27.11**).

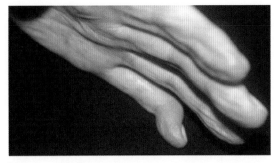
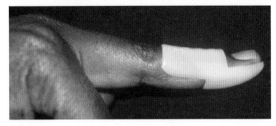
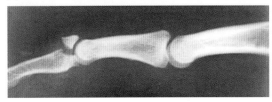
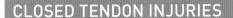

27.10 'Mallet finger' (a,b) The typical deformity in the little finger. This is best treated with a splint for 6 weeks. (c) Sometimes a small fragment is avulsed from the base of the distal phalanx; this also can be treated with a splint – surgery may make the outcome worse.

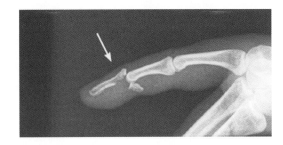

27.11 Flexor tendon avulsion Avulsion at the distal interphalangeal joint.

 Treatment of flexor tendon avulsion is urgent and requires operative reattachment of the tendon.

SECTION 3 TRAUMA

OPEN INJURIES OF THE HAND

Open injuries range from clean cuts to ragged lacerations, crushing, injection of foreign material, pulp defects and amputations. Knowing the mechanism of injury helps considerably in assessing the type and degree of damage.

Clinical assessment

Examination must be gentle and painstaking. It may have to be repeated in the operating theatre when the patient is anaesthetized.

 With *hand laceration*, even a tiny cut may be associated with life-changing tendon or nerve damage.

- *Skin damage* is important, but remember that even a tiny, clean cut may conceal nerve or tendon injury.
- The *circulation* to the hand and fingers must be assessed.

- *Sensation* and *motor activity* are tested in the territory of each nerve.
- *Tendons* are examined with similar care. Note the posture of the hand and fingers; comparison with the opposite hand may show that the normal postural tension in one or other finger is absent, suggesting a tendon injury.
- If the patient will allow it, active wrist and finger movements are then assessed.
  - *Flexor digitorum profundus* (*FDP*) is tested by holding the proximal finger joint straight and instructing the patient to bend the distal joint.
  - *Flexor digitorum superficialis* (*FDS*) is tested by asking the patient to flex one finger at a time while the examiner holds the other fingers in full extension; this immobilizes all the deep flexors because they have a common muscle belly, so any active flexion of the injured finger must be performed by the superficial flexor (**27.12**).
- *X-rays* are obligatory: they may show fractures or foreign bodies.

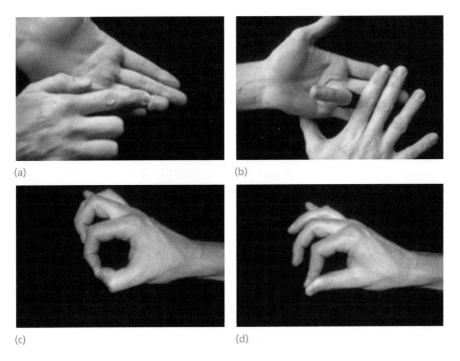

(a)   (b)

(c)   (d)

27.12 Testing the flexor tendons Testing for (a) FDP lesser fingers, (b) FDS lesser fingers, (c) FDP index, (d) FDS index.

Severe lacerations and fractures can produce a daunting picture. Yet even a 'mangled hand' deserves painstaking examination to see what is salvageable.

Treatment

PREOPERATIVE CARE

The patient will need painkillers. All wounds should be thoroughly rinsed with sterile saline. For clean wounds, antibiotics should be omitted to avoid the plague of antibiotic resistance that the unfettered use of antibiotics will bring. Prophylaxis against tetanus may also be needed. The wound is covered with a sterile dressing and the hand is lightly splinted.

 Thoroughly wash every wound, under local anaesthetic if needed. *Avoid antibiotics* unless really needed for contaminated wounds or bites.

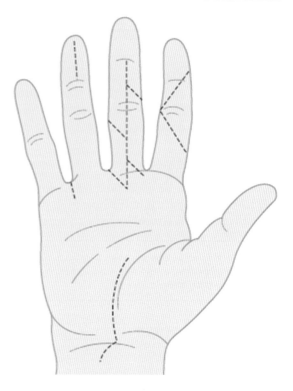

27.13 Hand incisions 'Permissible' incisions in hand surgery. Incisions must not cross a skin crease or an interdigital web or else scarring may cause contracture and deformity.

WOUND EXPLORATION

Under general or regional anaesthesia, the wound is cleaned and explored. A pneumatic tourniquet is essential unless there is a crush injury and muscle viability is in doubt. Skin is too precious to waste, and only obviously dead skin should be excised. For adequate exposure, the wound may need enlarging.

 Incisions must never cross a skin crease or an interdigital web because healing will result in a soft-tissue contracture across the crease (27.13).

Through the enlarged wound, loose debris is picked out, dead tissues are excised and the wound is thoroughly irrigated with isotonic crystalloid solution. A more thorough assessment of the extent of the injury is then undertaken.

TISSUE REPAIR

Fractures These are reduced and held with K-wires or plates or an external fixator depending on the configuration (**27.14**). Bone defects can be treated with bone graft or may be simply bridged with a metal device for later expert attention. The *joint capsule and ligaments* are repaired with fine sutures.

Arteries and veins Repair (or grafting) may be needed if the hand or finger is ischaemic.

Severed nerves These are sutured under high magnification with very thin sutures. If the repair cannot be achieved without tension, a nerve graft (e.g. from the posterior interosseous nerve at the wrist or sural nerve at the ankle). More recently, dissolvable nerve guides have been used to bridge the gap in digital nerves, allowing biological regeneration across the gap.

Extensor tendon repair This is not easy and the results not as reliable as some have suggested. Repair and postoperative management should be meticulous.

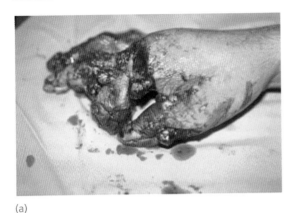

(a)

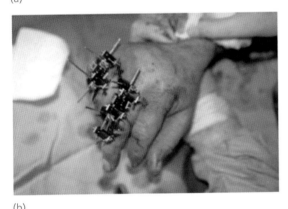

(b)

27.14 Open injuries (a) A mangled hand; (b) open fractures treated with external fixation.

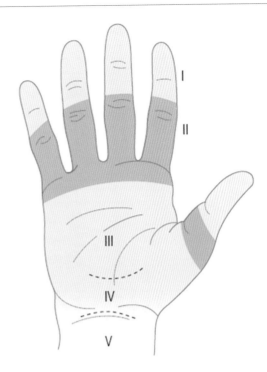

27.15 The zones of injury (I) Distal to the insertion of FDS. (II) Between the opening of the flexor sheath (the distal palmar crease) and the insertion of flexor superficialis. (III) Between the end of the carpal tunnel and the beginning of the flexor sheath. (IV) Within the carpal tunnel. (V) Proximal to the carpal tunnel.

Flexor tendon repair This is more challenging, particularly in the region between the distal palmar crease and the flexor crease of the proximal interphalangeal joint (Zone II), where both the superficial and deep tendons run together in a common sheath (27.15). This area has been called — rather portentously – 'no man's land'. Primary repair with at least four threads across the cut and fastidious postoperative supervision gives the best outcome, but calls for a high level of expertise and specialized physiotherapy (27.16). If the necessary facilities are not available, the wound should be washed out and loosely closed, and the patient transferred to a special centre. A delay of several days, with a clean wound, is unlikely to affect the outcome. Tendon grafting, sometimes with a temporary silicone 'spacer', may be needed.

Superficialis tendon Division of the *superficialis tendon alone* should also be repaired. Even though the loss of superficialis action does not altogether prevent finger flexion, it noticeably weakens the hand and may lead to a swan-neck deformity of the finger.

Cuts above the wrist, in the palm or distal to the superficialis insertion These have a better outcome than injuries in 'no man's land'.

 Amputation of a finger as a primary procedure should be avoided unless the damage involves many tissues and is clearly irreparable.

CLOSURE

The tourniquet is deflated and bipolar diathermy is used to stop bleeding; haematoma formation leads to poor healing and tendon adhesions.

SECTION 3 TRAUMA

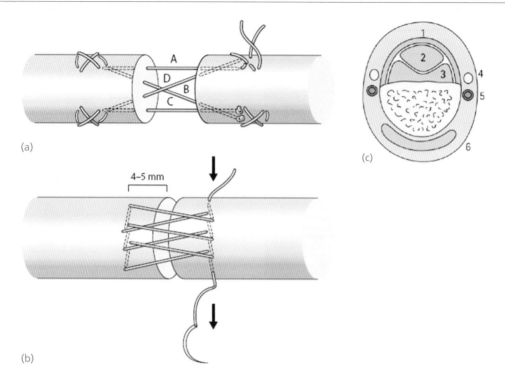

(a)

(c)

4–5 mm

(b)

27.16 Flexor tendon repair A core 4-strand suture **(a)** is supplemented by circumferential sutures **(b)**. **(c)** The relationship of the important structures in 'no man's land': 1, the tendon sheath; 2, FDP; 3, FDS; 4, digital nerve; 5, artery; 6, extensor tendon.

Unless the wound is contaminated, the skin is closed – either by direct suture without tension or, if there is skin loss, by skin grafting (skin grafts are conveniently taken from the inner aspect of the upper arm). If tendon or bare bone is exposed, this must be covered by a rotation skin flap or a pedicled flap. If the wound is very large, a free flap with a microvascular attachment may be needed. If a severely mutilated finger has to be sacrificed, its skin can be used as a rotation flap or a source of graft to cover an adjacent area of loss.

DRESSING AND SPLINTAGE

The wound is covered with a single layer of paraffin gauze and ample wool roll. A light plaster slab holds the wrist and hand in the position of safe immobilization (wrist extended, MCP joints flexed to 70 degrees, interphalangeal joints straight, thumb abducted, 27.17). This is the position in which the MCP and interphalangeal ligaments are fully stretched and fibrosis is therefore least likely to cause contractures.

> ⚠ It is important to splint in the position of safe immobilization. Failure to appreciate the importance of the hand position in plaster is the commonest cause of *persistent stiffness* after injury.

The rule is slightly modified in two circumstances:

- *after primary flexor tendon repair*, the wrist is held in about 20 degrees of flexion to take tension off the repair
- *after extensor tendon repair*, the MCP joints are flexed to only about 30 degrees so that there is less tension on the repair.

Postoperative management

The hand is kept elevated in a roller towel or high sling, which can be removed several times a day to exercise the elbow and shoulder. As soon as possible, the sling is discarded but dependency of the limb must be avoided.

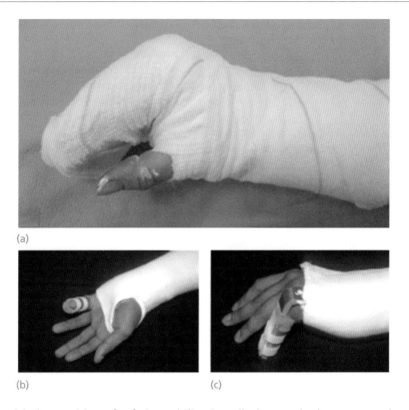

(a)

(b)   (c)

27.17 Splintage (a) The 'position of safe immobilization'. **(b,c)** For a single metacarpal or phalangeal injury immobilize only the affected ray.

Rehabilitation

Movements of the hand must be commenced within a few days at most. Splintage should allow as many joints as possible to be exercised, consistent with protecting the repair. Extensor tendon injuries are splinted for about 4 weeks. Various protocols are followed for flexor tendon injuries, including passive, active or elastic-band-assisted flexion. Early movement promotes tendon healing and excursion. In all cases, the risk of rupture is balanced against the need for early mobilization. Close supervision and attention to detail are essential.

Once the tissues have healed, the hand is increasingly used for more and more complex tasks, especially those that resemble the patient's normal work activities. The importance of an experienced hand therapist cannot be overestimated.

Delayed tendon repair

Primary suture may have been contraindicated by wound contamination, undue delay between injury and repair, massive skin loss or inadequate operating facilities. In these circumstances, secondary repair or tendon grafting may be necessary.

INJURY OF THE PROFUNDUS TENDON WITH AN INTACT SUPERFICIALIS

Unless the patient's work or hobby demands active flexion of the fingertip, fusion or tenodesis of the distal interphalangeal joint is the most reliable option.

INJURY OF BOTH THE SUPERFICIALIS AND PROFUNDUS TENDONS

If both tendons have been divided and have retracted, a tendon graft is needed. Full passive joint movement is a prerequisite.

- *If the pulley system is in good condition and there are no adhesions,* the tendons are excised from the flexor sheath and replaced with a tendon graft (palmaris longus, plantaris or a toe extensor). Rehabilitation is the same as for a primary repair.

- *If the pulleys are damaged*, the skin cover poor, the passive range of movement limited or the sheath scarred, a two-stage procedure is preferred.

1 The tendons are excised and the pulleys reconstructed with extensor retinaculum or excised tendon. A Silastic rod is sutured to the distal stump of the profundus tendon and is left free in the palm or distal forearm. Rehabilitation is planned to maintain a good passive range of movement. A smooth gliding surface forms around the rod.

2 No less than 3 months later, the rod is removed through two smaller incisions and a tendon graft (palmaris longus, plantaris or a lesser toe extensor) is sutured to the proximal and distal stumps of FDP at exactly the right tension.

Rehabilitation is as for a primary repair.

PULP AND FINGERTIP INJURIES

In full-thickness wounds without bone exposure, the best results come with simple non-adherent dressings. These are changed every few days until the wound has re-epithelialized. This might take a few weeks but the alternatives of skin grafts or skin flaps invite cold intolerance and poor sensory recovery. If bone is exposed and length of the digit is important for the individual patient, an advancement flap or neurovascular island flap should be considered. If not, primary cover can be achieved by shortening the bone and tailoring the skin flaps ('terminalization').

In young children, the fingertips recover extraordinarily well from injury and they should almost always be treated with dressings rather than grafts or terminalization.

Thumb length should never be sacrificed lightly. Sophisticated techniques such as a free microsurgical toe transfer or metacarpal lengthening may be suitable when the injury leaves the thumb too short for proper function.

NAIL-BED INJURIES

These are often seen in association with fractures of the terminal phalanx. If appearance is important, meticulous repair and split-thickness grafting under magnification will give the best cosmetic result.

THE SEVERELY MUTILATED HAND

This should be dealt with by a team with special skills in hand surgery. In exceptional cases, a new finger or thumb can be constructed by neurovascular microsurgical transfer of a toe, or a lost thumb can be replaced by rotating a surviving finger (pollicization) to restore oppositional movement (**27.18**).

REPLANTATION

With modern microsurgical techniques and appropriate skill, amputated digits or hands can be replanted. An amputated part should be wrapped in sterile saline gauze and placed in a plastic bag, which is itself placed in watery ice. The 'cold ischaemic time' for a *finger*, which contains so little muscle, is about 30 hours, but the 'warm time' less than 6 hours. For a *hand or forearm*, the cold ischaemic time is only about 12 hours and the warm time much less.

After resuscitation and attention to other potentially life-threatening injuries, the patient and the amputated part should be transferred to a centre where the appropriate surgical skills and facilities are available.

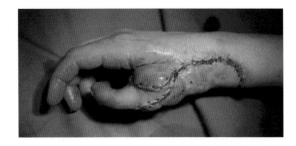

27.18 Late reconstruction The second toe has been transferred to replace the thumb, which was severed in an accident.

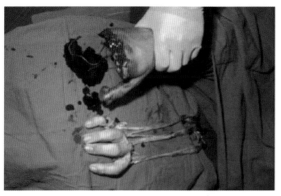
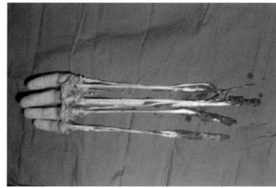

(a)   (b)

27.19 Avulsion This is not replantable.

Indications and relative contraindications

The decision to replant depends on the patient's age, their social and professional requirements, the condition of the part (whether clean-cut, mangled, crushed or avulsed), and the warm and cold ischaemic time. Furthermore, and perhaps most importantly, it depends on whether the replanted part is likely to give better function than an amputation.

- *The thumb* should be replanted whenever possible. Even if it functions only as a perfused 'post' with protective sensation, it will give useful service.
- *Multiple digits* also should be replanted, and in a child even a single digit.
- *Proximal amputations* (through the palm, wrist or forearm) likewise merit an attempt at replantation.

Other parts do less well.

- *Single digits* do badly if replanted. There is a high complication rate, including stiffness, non–union, poor sensation, and cold intolerance; a replanted single finger is likely to be excluded from use.

- Severely *crushed, mangled or avulsed* parts may not be replantable (**27.19**).
- Parts with a *long ischaemic time* may not survive.

 General medical disorders or other injuries may engender unacceptable risks from the prolonged anaesthesia needed for replantation.

BURNS

In general, these should be managed in a specialized burns unit because of the devastating loss of function that can follow burns to the hand.

- *Superficial burns* are covered with a moist dressing and the hand is elevated. Early movement is encouraged.
- *Partial-thickness burns* are dressed in an antimicrobial cream and splinted in the position of safety.
- *Full-thickness burns* do not heal and require skin grafting.
- *Constricting burns* may need urgent release to preserve the circulation (escharotomy).

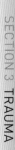

SECTION 3 TRAUMA

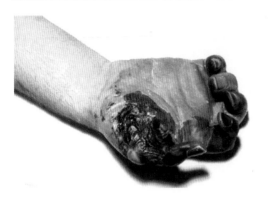

27.20 Frostbite

- *Electric burns* can cause very widespread damage that may only become apparent a few days later.
- *Chemical burns* require copious irrigation; particular neutralizing agents are suitable for certain chemical burns.
- *Frostbite* needs special attention, with slow rewarming and management of blisters and tissue loss. Amputation is often required, once the area of dead and viable tissue has been demarcated (**27.20**).

Spine and thorax injuries

28

■ Stable and unstable injuries   625
■ Mechanism of injury   626
■ Principles of diagnosis and management   626
■ Cervical spine injuries   630

■ Thoracolumbar injuries   636
■ Neural injuries   640
■ Fractures of the thoracic cage   641

STABLE AND UNSTABLE INJURIES

STABILITY DEFINED

A stable injury is one in which the vertebral components will not be displaced by normal physiological loads.
An unstable injury is one in which there is a significant risk of displacement and damage to the neural tissues.

The current preferred classification system is the AO/ASIF (Arbeitsgemeinschaft für Osteosynthesefragen/Association for the Study of Internal Fixation) system which reverts back to the original two-column theory (from the three-column theory of Denis):

- *anterior column* consisting of vertebral body and disc
- *posterior column* consisting of pedicles, laminae, facets and posterior ligamentous complex (PLC).

AO/ASIF CLASSIFICATION OF SPINAL INJURIES

Type A injuries Anterior column compression fractures which tend to be stable
Type B injuries Involve anterior and posterior columns with distraction; these are unstable
Type C injuries Double-column injuries with rotation or sheer; these are unstable

Fortunately, only 10% of spinal fractures are unstable and less than 5% are associated with cord damage.

Primary pathophysiological changes Injury may be limited to the vertebral column and soft-tissue components, varying from strains to fracture-dislocations. The spinal cord and/or nerve roots may be injured, either by the initial trauma or by ongoing structural instability of a vertebral segment.

Secondary pathophysiological changes Following a spinal injury, biochemical changes may lead to more gradual cellular disruption and extension of the initial neurological damage.

SECTION 3 TRAUMA

MECHANISM OF INJURY

Traction (avulsion) injury Resisted muscle effort may avulse transverse processes; in the cervical spine, the seventh spinous process can be avulsed ('clay-shoveller's fracture').

Direct injury Penetrating injuries from knives or projectiles rarely cause vertebral column instability but do commonly result in direct neurological injury.

Indirect injury This occurs most commonly in a fall from a height when the spinal column collapses in its vertical axis, or else during violent free movements of the neck or trunk (**28.1**). A variety of forces may be applied to the spine (often simultaneously):

- axial compression
- flexion
- lateral compression
- flexion-rotation
- shear
- flexion-distraction
- extension.

Healing

- *Bony injuries* tend to heal but the patient may be left with kyphosis or loss of height.
- *Ligamentous injuries* seldom heal to a stable state and will potentially lead to progressive kyphosis, chronic pain and further neurological sequelae.

PRINCIPLES OF DIAGNOSIS AND MANAGEMENT

Assessment and resuscitation according to a recognized protocol, such as the ATLS® protocol, precedes the assessment of the spinal injury. Adequate oxygenation and perfusion help minimize secondary spinal cord injury. Spinal precautions need to be followed until the patient has been resuscitated and other life-threatening injuries have been managed. Immobilization continues until spinal injury has been excluded by both clinical and radiological assessment.

Temporary immobilization with a semi-rigid collar and sandbags may be used when transferring a spinal injury patient into a computed

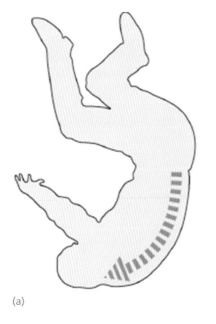
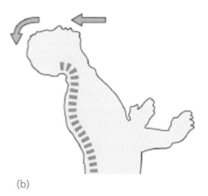

(a)   (b)

28.1 Mechanism of injury The spine is usually injured in one of two ways: **(a)** a fall onto the head or the back of the neck; or **(b)** a blow on the forehead that forces the neck into hyperextension.

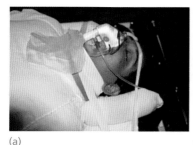
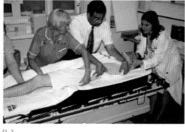
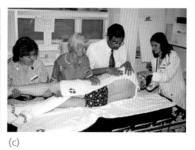

(a)   (b)   (c)

28.2 Spinal injuries – early management (a) Quadruple immobilization: the patient is on a backboard, the head is supported by sandbags and held with tape across the forehead, and a semi-rigid collar has been applied. **(b,c)** The log-rolling technique for exposure and examination of the back.

tomography (CT) or magnetic resonance imaging (MRI) scanner (**28.2**). *Log-rolling* (i.e. turned over 'in one piece') with spinal precautions is mandatory to avoid further injury, and the patient should be transferred to a pressure care mattress as soon as possible to avoid bedsores.

HISTORY

A high index of suspicion is essential since symptoms and signs may be minimal. The history is important and, with any high-energy injury such as high-speed traffic accidents or falls from heights, the emphasis should be on excluding a vertebral column injury.

 Unconscious and polytraumatized patients need to be considered as having an unstable spinal injury until proven otherwise.

Any history of trauma with neck/back pain or neurological symptoms needs careful examination and investigation to exclude spinal injury.

EXAMINATION

Physical examination

 Look, feel but *do not move!*

LOOK, FEEL BUT DO NOT MOVE!

- *The head and face* are thoroughly inspected for bruises or grazes which could indicate indirect trauma to the cervical spine. Note the attitude of the head; torticollis may allude to an underlying axial cervical spine injury.
- *The neck* is inspected for deformity, bruising or penetrating injury.
- *The patient is log-rolled* to avoid movement of the vertebral column.
- *The spine* is inspected from occiput to coccyx for deformity, penetrating injury, haematoma or bruising. The spinous processes are palpated for tenderness, haematoma, gap or a step which may indicate instability.
- *A digital rectal examination* completes the log-roll, and anal tone, sensation and voluntary 'pinch' are documented.

SHOCK

- *Hypovolaemic shock* is suggested by tachycardia, peripheral shutdown and, in later stages, hypotension.
- *Neurogenic shock* occurs due to loss of the sympathetic pathways in the spinal cord. The peripheral vessels dilate, causing hypotension with warm well-perfused limbs, but the heart, with no sympathetic innervation, remains bradycardic and there is paralysis.
- *Spinal shock* is physiological dysfunction following structural injury rarely lasts for more than 48 hours. The neurological level cannot be determined until this resolves. Below the level of the injury, the muscles are flaccid, the reflexes are absent and sensation is lost. While

the primitive reflexes (anal 'wink' and the bulbocavernosus reflex) are absent, there is spinal shock and the neurological level cannot be accurately determined.

Neurological examination

A full neurological examination, testing each dermatome, myotome and reflex, should be carried out in every case; this may have to be repeated several times during the first few days. This should include testing for *sacral sparing*, which suggests a partial lesion and the potential for further recovery. The unconscious patient is difficult to examine; a spinal injury must be assumed until proven otherwise.

FEATURES SUGGESTIVE OF A SPINAL CORD LESION

History of a fall or rapid deceleration
Head injury
Diaphragmatic breathing
Flaccid anal sphincter
Hypotension with bradycardia
Pain response above, but not below, the clavicle
Priapism (an important finding since it occurs almost immediately with 'complete' cord injuries and settles in a few hours)

For tests for nerve root function, see **Table 28.1**.

The neurological examination should be recorded on the ASIA scoring system (https://asia-spinalinjury.org/international-standards-neurological-classification-sci-isncsci-worksheet/), which is the standard neurological classification of spinal cord injury.

IMAGING

X-RAY

X-ray examination is mandatory for all accident victims complaining of pain or stiffness in the neck or back, all patients with head injuries or severe facial injuries (cervical spine), patients with rib fractures or severe seat-belt bruising (thoracic spine), and those with severe pelvic or abdominal

Table 28.1 Tests for nerve root motor function

Nerve root	Test	Tendon reflex
C5	Elbow flexion	Biceps
C6	Wrist extension	Brachioradialis
C7	Wrist flexion	Triceps
	Finger extension	
C8	Finger flexion	
T1	Finger abduction	
L1,2	Thigh abduction	
L3,4	Knee extension	Quadriceps
L5, S1	Knee flexion	Tendo Achillis
L5	Great toe extension	
S1	Great toe flexion	

injuries (thoracolumbar spine). Accident victims who are unconscious should have spine X-rays as part of the routine workup.

Movement should be kept to a minimum. In the cervical spine, anteroposterior (AP) and lateral views (with coverage from C1 to T1) and open-mouth views are needed.

CT

'Difficult' areas, such as the lower cervical and upper thoracic segments, which are often obscured by shoulder and rib images, may require CT. CT is also ideal for showing structural damage to individual vertebrae and displacement of bone fragments into the vertebral canal (**28.3**).

MRI

For displaying the intervertebral discs, ligamentum flavum and neural structures, MRI is the method of choice. MRI may also help with decisions about spinal stability by demonstrating disruption to the PLC.

TREATMENT

OBJECTIVES OF TREATMENT

To preserve neurological function
To minimize a perceived threat of neurological compression

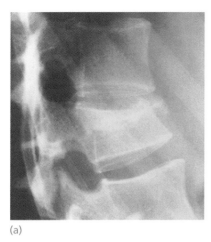
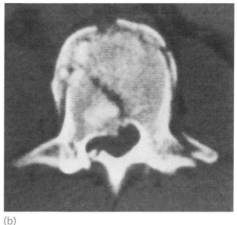

(a)   (b)

28.3 X-ray diagnosis (a) This X-ray showed the fracture, but it needed a CT scan **(b)** to reveal the large fragment encroaching on the spinal canal.

To restore alignment of the spine
To stabilize the spine
To rehabilitate the patient

INDICATIONS FOR URGENT SURGICAL STABILIZATION

An unstable fracture with progressive neurological deficit
An unstable fracture in a polytraumatized patient (relative indication)

Patients with no neurological injury

If the spinal injury is stable, these may be managed with bed rest until pain and muscle spasm subside. For pain control, bracing may be used.

If the spinal injury is unstable, it should be held secure until the tissues heal and the spine becomes stable. In the cervical spine, this should be done as soon as possible by traction in bed through tongs or a halo device attached to the skull. Unstable thoracolumbar injuries are more often treated by internal fixation.

Patients with neurological injury

Once out of spinal shock, the full extent of the neurological injury is assessed. Spinal injury patients need a multidisciplinary team to manage their multisystem physiological impairment and malfunction, including the spinal injury; early transfer to a spinal injury centre should be done when available. High-dependency care is required during the acute injury phase.

- *Stable injuries* are usually due to penetrating injuries which very rarely cause instability.
- Conservative treatment can be used for *unstable injuries* where surgical skills and resources are not available, but surgical stabilization leads to shorter hospitalization, earlier rehabilitation and improved outcomes. *Complete* spinal cord injuries do not benefit from decompression but it is required in *incomplete* lesions.

Methods of treatment

CERVICAL SPINE

Collars *Soft collars* are limited to minor sprains. *Semi-rigid collars* are used in the acute setting but do not provide enough stability for unstable injury patterns. *Four-poster braces* apply pressure to the mandible, occiput, sternum and thoracic spine but can be uncomfortable and cause pressure sores.

Tongs Pins are inserted into the outer table of the skull, tongs mounted and traction applied to reduce the injury and maintain reduction (**28.4**).

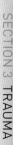

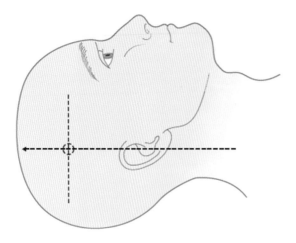

28.4 Cone's calliper pin location The intersection of a vertical line through the external auditory meatus and a horizontal line 1 cm above the ear pinna marks the location for the pin insertion.

Halo ring A ring attached to the skull by at least four pins can be used for initial traction and reduction and then attached to a plaster vest or a fitted body orthosis. Complications such as pin loosening, pin-site infection and (in elderly patients) respiratory distress should be checked for.

Operative fixation This is necessary in some cases. Various procedures are available, depending on the level and pattern of injury.

- *Odontoid fractures* can be fixed with lag screws.
- *Burst fractures* can be decompressed through an anterior approach.
- Facet dislocations can be reduced through a posterior approach.

The spine can be stabilized anteriorly with plates, posteriorly with wires between the spinous processes or small plates between the lateral masses.

THORACOLUMBAR SPINE

Beds and mattresses These are designed to avoid pressure sores and facilitate turning the patient.

Bracing This prevents flexion by three-point fixation. It is suitable for some burst fractures, seat-belt injuries and compression fractures.

Operative decompression and stabilization The aim of surgery is to reduce the fracture, hold the reduction and decompress the neural elements. The surgical approach can be either anterior or posterior.

- *The anterior approach* is suitable to address anterior neural compression or to augment posterior fixation. The vertebral body is removed for canal decompression and reconstructed with bone graft or a cage.
- *The posterior approach* is most commonly used for most fracture patterns. Some fractures can be reduced indirectly from posterior by distraction with instrumentation such as pedicle screw systems. Supplementary bone graft is used to achieve fusion.

CERVICAL SPINE INJURIES

Clinical features

The patient usually gives a history of a fall from a height, diving into a pool or a vehicle accident. In an unconscious patient, an unstable cervical spine injury needs to be excluded.

An abnormal position of the neck is suggestive, and careful palpation may elicit tenderness. Postpone movement where possible until after X-ray. Pain or paraesthesia in the limbs is significant, and the patient should be examined for evidence of spinal cord or nerve root damage.

Imaging

Plain *X-rays* must be adequate and examined methodically.

- *On the AP view*, the lateral outlines should be intact, and the spinous processes and tracheal shadow in the midline. An open-mouth view is necessary to show C1 and C2 and check for odontoid and lateral mass fractures.
- *The lateral view* must include seven cervical vertebrae and the upper half of T1 to visualize the cervicothoracic junction. Follow the four curves running down the front of the vertebral bodies, the back of the bodies, the bases of and along the tips of the spinous processes

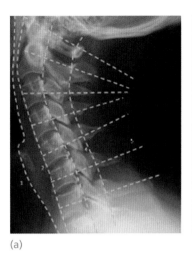
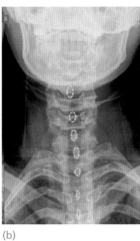
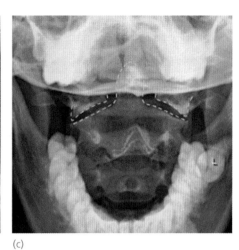

(a)   (b)   (c)

28.5 Cervical spine (a) Lateral view, the radiological lines are: 1, soft-tissue line; 2, anterior vertebral body line; 3, posterior vertebral body line; 4, spinolaminar line. 5, The lines of convergence are drawn down the spinous processes and should converge posteriorly. **(b)** AP view confirms alignment of the spinous processes. **(c)** Open-mouth view should show a centrally placed dens with congruous and symmetrical C1/C2 lateral mass joints.

(**28.5**). The prevertebral soft-tissue shadow should be less than 5 mm in width above the trachea and less than one vertebral body's width below that level; any increase suggests a prevertebral haematoma.

- *Children's X-rays* can be particularly difficult to interpret.
  - An increased atlantoaxial interval (up to 5 mm) may be due to normal ligamentous laxity.
  - Unfused growth plates in the odontoid process or spinous processes can be mistaken for undisplaced fractures.
  - Even a normal-looking spine does not exclude the possibility of a cord injury (spinal cord injury without obvious radiographic abnormality, SCIWORA).

UPPER CERVICAL SPINE

Occipital condyle fracture

This is usually a high-energy injury and not isolated. *CT* is required to visualize it. Impacted and undisplaced fractures can be treated by brace immobilization for 8–12 weeks. Displaced fractures are best managed by using a halo vest or by operative fixation.

Occipitocervical dislocation

This is also usually a high-energy injury and not isolated. Associated arterial and pharyngeal disruption is often fatal. On the lateral view *X-ray*, the tip of the odontoid should be no more than 5 mm in vertical alignment and 1 mm in horizontal alignment from the basion. *CT scans* are more reliable where the distance between the dens and the clivus should be less than 12 mm. It is usually unstable and requires immediate reduction without traction and fitting of a halo vest. Stabilization is by means of an occipitocervical instrumented fusion posteriorly if severe, or a 6- to 8-week period in the halo vest.

C1 RING FRACTURE

Axial loading may cause a 'burst' fracture of the ring of the atlas (*Jefferson's fracture*). There is usually no neurological damage. On the open-mouth view *X-ray*, the lateral masses are spread away from the odontoid peg and *CT* helps define the fracture.

Hyperextension can fracture either the anterior or posterior arch. These injuries are usually stable and are managed with a semi-rigid collar until union occurs. If the C1 lateral masses have a combined overhang on C2 of more than 7 mm on the open-mouth view, the injury is likely to be unstable and require surgical intervention. Fractures of the atlas are associated with injury elsewhere in the cervical spine in up to 50% of cases.

C2 traumatic spondylolisthesis

These fractures are typically caused by hyperextension (Forsyth mechanism) causing anterior translation at C2. This results in a pars fracture, which may extend into the posterior body and cause a C2/3-disc disruption (**28.6**). Neurological injury is unusual. Stability is determined by the C2/3-disc status and facet integrity. Undisplaced fractures are assessed with supervised flexion/extension views; if there is less than 3.5 mm of C2/3 subluxation, they can be treated in a semi-rigid orthosis for 6–12 weeks until union. If there is more displacement but no kyphotic angulation, reduction with inline traction may be needed, followed by a semi-rigid collar and infrequently surgery. Rarely there is associated C2/3 facet dislocation which will require open reduction and stabilization.

These injuries are frequently incorrectly called a '*hangman's fracture*'. Judicial hanging caused the fracture and death by spinal cord injury due to a distractive force.

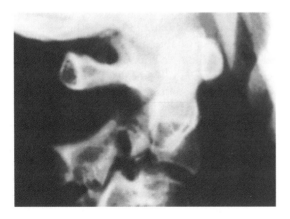

28.6 Traumatic spondylolisthesis Fracture of the pars interarticularis of C2.

C2 odontoid process fracture

Odontoid fractures are uncommon. They usually occur due to flexion due to high-energy injuries or, less commonly, in elderly patients as a result of low-energy trauma with forced hyperextension. There is seldom neurological injury due to the large canal size at this level. They are usually visible on plain *X-ray* and are classified according to Anderson and D'Alonzo (**28.7**).

ANDERSON/D'ALONZO CLASSIFICATION OF ODONTOID PROCESS FRACTURES
Type I Avulsion fracture of the tip of the odontoid process due to traction by the alar ligaments *Type II* Fracture at the junction of the odontoid process and the body of the axis. This is the most common (and potentially the most dangerous) type *Type III* Fracture through the body of the axis

- *Type I fractures* are stable and can be treated in a rigid collar until discomfort subsides.
- *Type II fractures* are often unstable and prone to non-union. Undisplaced fractures can be treated in a halo vest. Displaced fractures need to be reduced by traction and held either by anterior screw fixation or posterior C1/2 fusion. If these cannot be performed, immobilization can be applied by using a halo vest with repeated X-ray monitoring.
- *Type III fractures*, if undisplaced, are treated in a halo vest for 8–12 weeks. If displaced, the fracture must be reduced by traction and either flexion or extension before immobilization in a halo vest for 8–12 weeks. A collar may be used in elderly patients with poor bone but there is a higher risk of non-union.

LOWER CERVICAL SPINE

Fractures from C3 to C7 tend to produce characteristic patterns according to the mechanism. The Subaxial Cervical Spine Injury Classification (SLIC) scoring system (Vaccaro) guides

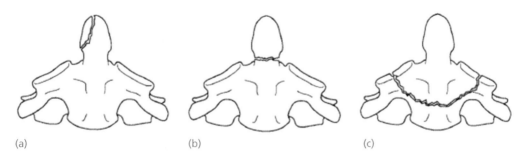

28.7 Odontoid fractures (a) *Type I* – fracture through the tip of the odontoid process. **(b)** *Type II* – fracture at the junction of the odontoid process and the body. **(c)** *Type III* – fracture through the body of the axis. Neurological symptoms occur in a significant number of cases.

management and incorporates three main characteristics (**Table 28.2**).

CHARACTERISTICS USED IN SLIC SYSTEM

Morphology of the injury – based on the available imaging, consists of compression, distraction and translation/rotation of the vertebral bodies
Discoligamentous complex (DLC) – considers the integrity of the disc, anterior and posterior ligamentous structures, defined as disrupted, intact and indeterminate; DLC is considered directly proportional to stability
Neurological status of the patient – linked with the severity of the injury

---

The more traditional mechanistic descriptions remain in common use.

Flexion injuries

These include distractive flexion and compressive flexion injuries. Depending on the instantaneous axis of rotation during the injury, there is a spectrum from posterior ligament disruption ranging to anterior column compression.

Wedge compression fractures

These are caused by a compressive flexion force. Clinical examination and flexion X-rays are required to determine if the posterior elements are intact, and the injury stable.

Table 28.2 The SLIC scale

Characteristic	Points
Morphology	
No abnormality	0
Compression	1
Burst	+1 = 2
Distraction	3
Disrupted	4
Discoligamentous complex	
Intact	0
Indeterminate	1
Disrupted	2
Neurological status	
Intact	0
Root injury	1
Complete cord injury	2
Incomplete cord injury	3
Continuous cord compression in setting of neurological deficit	+1

 If there appears to be posterior displacement of a vertebral body fragment, this suggests a *burst fracture*, which is potentially unstable, and CT or MRI should be performed.

BURST OR 'TEARDROP' FRACTURES

These occur due to axial compression while flexed, such as when diving into a pool. In-line force tends to create a burst; if the neck is more flexed, it is more likely to see the teardrop fragment from the anteroinferior edge of the fractured vertebra created by shearing force (**28.8**). In both types, posterior displacement of a body fragment can injure the cord. Disruption of the anterior column makes these highly unstable, requiring immobilization. *CT* shows the fracture pattern and retropulsion while *MRI* confirms the disc and PLC.

- *Conservative treatment* has a limited role due to the injury being highly unstable with high chance of kyphosis and spinal cord compression. These patients are often quadriplegic and prolonged traction carries significant morbidity.

- *Surgical management* is preferred. The aim is to stabilize the injury. Decompression is attempted but of secondary importance as cord injury is often already established. After initial stabilization in traction, anterior corpectomy with bone grafting and plate fixation is performed. Posterior stabilization may be added if required.

Posterior ligament injury, dislocations and fracture dislocations

These injuries are caused by distractive flexion mechanisms. Structures fail sequentially from posterior to anterior with progressive instability and increasing risk of neurological injury.

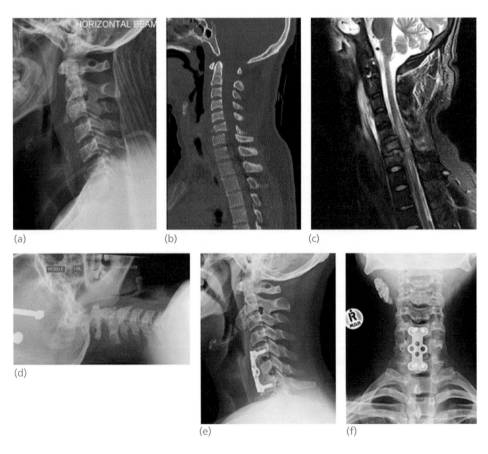

28.8 Teardrop fracture (a) An innocuous-looking fracture at C6 with large prevertebral swelling heralds the 'teardrop' fracture; note the mild retrolisthesis; **(b)** CT details the interspinous widening and retrolisthesis of C6; **(c)** MRI reveals the posterior interspinous ligament disruption and spinal cord injury. **(d)** Cervical traction helps maintain alignment until surgery. **(e,f)** Surgical stabilization with corpectomy and anterior cervical plating.

POSTERIOR LIGAMENT INJURY

If there is midline tenderness over the spine or a palpable gap, this should be suspected. Lateral *X-rays* may reveal a gap but it may be hidden if the neck is extended. Flexion views will reveal it but should not be forced if there is pain. If they cannot be done, protect in a semi-rigid collar and try again at 10 days. More than 11 degrees of angulation or more than 3.5 mm anterior translation on the flexion view is considered unstable and may require fixation if conservative treatment fails.

DISLOCATIONS

Bilateral facet joint dislocations There is complete disruption of the PLC and spinal instability, often with cord damage. Lateral *X-rays* show anterior vertebral translation more than half a body width and spinous processes aligned on AP views (no rotation).

Unilateral facet joint dislocations These are distractive flexion-rotation injuries and cord injury is less common. On a lateral *X-ray*, the vertebra displaces less than one-half a body width and rotation of the facets is seen cephalad to the injury. On an AP X-ray, the alignment of the spinous processes is distorted.

 Dislocations must be reduced urgently.

Closed cervical reduction can be performed if the patient is awake and cooperative, there are X-ray facilities and traction equipment is available. Traction of 5 kg is applied and increased in steps up to 30 kg as required. Repeat neurological assessment after each addition and abandon if the neurology deteriorates. Initial reduction is easier in 20 degrees of flexion. Once reduced, they should be stabilized on the next available operating list with anterior, posterior or combined approaches. Anterior approaches are required if the disc needs to be addressed. Stabilization is achieved with lateral mass screws for posterior approaches. Facet fracture may prevent reduction and can be seen on CT.

Hyperextension injury (distraction or combined compression and extension)

Strains via this mechanism are common but more severe injuries rare. With compressive extension, the posterior elements are compressed; if the disc and vertebral body are intact, they tend to be stable. With distraction, anterior structures fail in sequence. They are more common in a stiff spine where pinching of the cord may cause an acute central cord syndrome. If stable, they are treated in a semi-rigid collar for 6–8 weeks.

Injuries at more than one level

Care should be taken to continue to thoroughly assess the rest of the spine even when an injury is spotted. The high energies involved can typically create injuries at more than one level.

Avulsion of C7 spinous process (clay shoveller's fracture)

This occurs with severe contraction of the attached muscles. It is a stable injury and can be rehabilitated as pain allows.

Acute post-traumatic cervical disc herniation

Disc herniation may cause severe pain radiating to one or both limbs and neurology. Rarely, it may cause sudden paresis requiring urgent decompression. The lesion is shown on *MRI*. Milder cases can be managed conservatively initially. Failed treatment requires anterior discectomy and interbody fusion.

SPRAINED NECK (WHIPLASH INJURY)

Soft-tissue sprains (or wrenching injuries) of the neck are now very common after car accidents. The incidence is much lower in countries with legal systems that do not award compensation for them. It usually follows a rear-end collision in which the occupant's body is thrown forwards and the head jerked backwards with hyperextension. Women are affected more often than men. There is disagreement about the exact pathology and there is no correlation between the amount of damage to the vehicle and the severity of complaints.

Pain and stiffness of the neck usually appear during the next 12–48 hours, occasionally later. Some complain of more ill-defined symptoms such as headache and paraesthesiae in the arms. There is muscular tenderness and restricted movements. *X-ray* examination may show reduced cervical lordosis, a sign of muscle spasm. The presence of true neurological signs should prompt an *MRI*.

Simple pain-relieving measures, including analgesic medication, may be needed during the first few weeks. However, the emphasis should be on graded exercises for return of neck movement.

The long-term prognosis is variable and a small group of patients appear never to be free of symptoms.

> ### NEGATIVE PROGNOSTIC INDICATORS IN WHIPLASH INJURY
>
> Increasing age
> Severity of symptoms at the outset
> Prolonged duration of symptoms
> Presence of pre-existing intervertebral disc degeneration

THORACOLUMBAR INJURIES

Most injuries of the thoracolumbar spine occur in the transitional area (T11–L2) between the relatively rigid thoracic spine and the more mobile lumbar spine. The upper thoracic vertebrae are protected by the rib cage and fractures in this region tend to be stable. However, the spinal canal in that area is relatively narrow, so cord damage is not uncommon; when it does occur, it is usually complete.

The spinal cord ends at L1 and below that level it is the lower nerve roots that are at risk.

Pathogenesis

Pathogenic mechanisms fall into three main groups.

> ### PATHOGENIC MECHANISMS IN THORACOLUMBAR INJURIES
>
> *Low-energy insufficiency fractures* – mild compressive stress in osteoporotic bone
> *Minor fractures of the vertebral processes* – compressive, tensile or torsional strains
> *High-energy fractures or fracture-dislocations* – motor vehicle collisions, falls or diving from heights, sporting events, horse-riding and collapsed buildings

It is mainly in the high-energy group that one encounters neurological complications, but lesser fractures also sometimes cause nerve damage. The common mechanisms of injury are:

- compression
- rotation/translation
- distraction.

COMPRESSION

Compression leads to failure of the vertebral body under axial loading. The mildest cases show wedging of the body (**28.9**). As the energy increases, there can be retropulsion into the canal and interpedicular widening. Lateral compression may cause a scoliotic deformity. When there is more than 50% loss of height, the posterior tension-band is likely to have failed, leading to instability.

ROTATION/TRANSLATION

Shear or rotational forces tend to create unstable injuries. There is commonly neurology and they are identified by pedicle or spinous process malalignment.

DISTRACTION

This is a 'Chance fracture' or seat-belt injury, caused by flexion with a distraction moment. Posterior disruption can be bony, ligamentous or both. Around 50% have associated intra-abdominal injuries They are usually unstable and require stabilization.

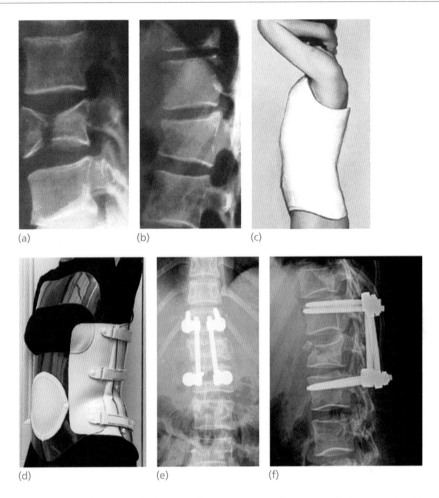

(a)   (b)   (c)

(d)   (e)   (f)

28.9 Wedge-compression fractures (a) Central compression fracture of the vertebral body and **(b)** anterior wedge compression fracture with less than 20% loss of vertebral body height. If the fracture is stable without injury to the PLC, it can be managed conservatively with 8–12 weeks in **(c)** a plaster 'jacket' or **(d)** a lightweight removable orthosis. **(e,f)** Unstable compression fractures may need posterior internal fixation if there is disruption of the PLC.

Examination

Patients complaining of back pain following an injury or showing signs of bruising and tenderness over the spine, as well as those suffering head or neck injuries, chest injuries and pelvic fractures, should undergo a careful examination of the spine and a full neurological examination, including rectal examination.

Imaging

- *X-rays* should be carefully examined for loss of vertebral height or splaying of the vertebral body. Widening of the distance between the pedicles or an increased distance between successive spinous processes suggests posterior column damage. The lateral view is examined for vertebral alignment and structural integrity. Look particularly for evidence of fragment retropulsion towards the spinal canal.
- *Helical CT scans* show better osseous detail, provide additional views and don't require potentially damaging manoeuvres to get the correct views.
- *MRI* may also be needed to evaluate neurological or other soft-tissue injuries.

Treatment

Treatment depends on:

- the type of anatomical disruption
- whether the injury is stable or unstable
- whether there is neurological involvement
- the presence or absence of concomitant injuries.

Fractures of the transverse processes

The transverse processes can be avulsed with sudden muscular activity. This typically requires only symptomatic treatment. If the fracture is at L5, this may herald a vertical shear injury of the pelvis.

Fractures of the pars interarticularis

These are typically stress fractures and should be suspected if there is a sudden onset of back pain during the course of strenuous activity (*traumatic spondylolysis*). It is best seen in oblique *X-rays*, but a thin fracture line is easily missed; a week or two later, an *isotope bone scan* may show a 'hot' spot. *CT scan* will demonstrate the fracture and also differentiate between an acute and a chronic fracture. Bilateral fractures occasionally lead to spondylolisthesis.

Rest for several months will usually allow an acute fracture to heal. Chronic fractures with sclerosis that are 'cold' on bone scanning are unlikely to heal with rest alone.

Flexion-compression injury

This is by far the most common vertebral fracture and is due to severe spinal flexion (or minimal trauma in osteoporosis).The posterior ligaments usually remain intact. Pain may be quite severe but the fracture is usually stable and neurological injury is extremely rare.

- *Patients with minimal wedging (<20%)* and a stable fracture pattern are kept in bed for 1–2 weeks until pain subsides and are then mobilized; no support is needed.

- *Those with moderate wedging* (loss of 20–40% of anterior vertebral height) and no disruption of the posterior ligament complex can be allowed up after 1 week, wearing a thoracolumbar brace or a body cast applied with the back in extension. At 3 months, flexion-extension *X-rays* are obtained with the patient out of the orthosis; if there is no instability, the brace is discarded. If the deformity increases or neurological signs develop, stabilization is indicated.
- *In those with wedging >40%*, where it is likely that the posterior ligaments are disrupted, *or with neurological signs*, posterior instrumented fixation is indicated.

Axial compression or burst injury

Severe axial compression may 'explode' the vertebral body, causing failure of the anterior column and comminution of the posterior part of the body with potential retropulsion. If the PLC is intact, which is usually the case, the injury is stable.

AP *X-rays* may show spreading of the vertebral body (**28.10**). Posterior displacement of bone into the spinal canal (retropulsion) can be appreciated at the posterosuperior border of the vertebral body where the normal concavity of the posterior body wall becomes convex. *CT scan* clearly defines the injury.

If there is minimal anterior wedging and the fracture is stable with normal neurology, bed rest is advised until the acute symptoms settle (less than a week) and then mobilized in a thoracolumbar brace or body cast, worn for 12 weeks. If the neurology is normal, even if CT demonstrates significant retropulsion, non-operative treatment is still appropriate.

In unstable fractures with PLC disruption, most fractures require posterior pedicle screw fixation. Canal compromise of more than 50% is an indicator of instability. In cases with very severe vertebral body comminution, fixation may need to be augmented with anterior column reconstruction. Canal decompression can be indirect or direct.

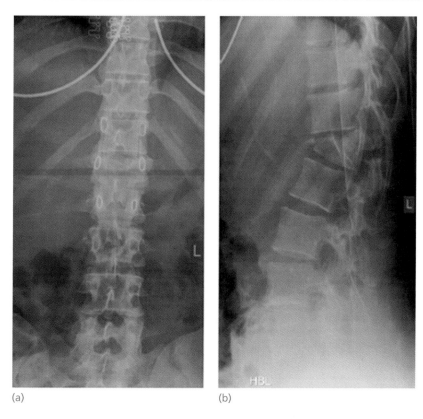

(a)   (b)

28.10 Lumbar burst fracture An 18-year-old female fell from a trampoline sustaining L1 burst fracture, ASIA D. **(a)** AP X-ray showing pedicle widening and interspinous gap; **(b)** lateral X-ray showing kyphosis at L1 with mild retrolisthesis.

- *Indirect decompression* is achieved with pedicle screw fixation and posterior distraction.
- If the posterior wall fragment flips 180 degrees ('reversed cortical sign'), the PLC is disrupted and indirect reduction is not possible. In this case, *direct decompression* would be required if indicated via the anterior approach.

JACK-KNIFE INJURY (CHANCE FRACTURE)

Combined flexion and posterior distraction (seen typically in severe seat-belt injuries) may cause the mid-lumbar spine to jack-knife around an axis anterior to the vertebral column. There is little crushing of the vertebral body; the tear passes transversely through the bones or the ligament structures, or both. Because the posterior elements fail, it is unstable in flexion but neurological damage is uncommon. Around 50% have associated intra-abdominal injuries.

Bony injury usually heals quite rapidly with 3 months in a body cast or well-fitting brace. Posterior stabilization may allow more rapid rehabilitation. Ligamentous Chance injuries require stabilization.

FRACTURE-DISLOCATION

Segmental displacement may occur with various combinations of flexion, compression, rotation and shear. The spine is grossly unstable and there is often neurological damage to the lower cord or cauda equina.

X-rays may show fractures through the vertebral body, pedicles, articular processes and

SECTION 3 TRAUMA

laminae; there may be varying degrees of sub-luxation or even bilateral facet dislocation. *CT* helps demonstrate the degree of spinal canal occlusion.

There is little place for conservative man-agement. For those with neurological deficits, surgical stabilization allows easier nursing care, lower morbidity, decreased hospitalization and earlier rehabilitation. Fixation often requires two vertebral levels instrumented above and below the injury due to the degree of instability. Neurological outcome is mostly dictated by the initial neural injury.

NEURAL INJURIES

The spinal cord, nerve roots or both may be damaged. Cervical lesions may cause quadriple-gia, thoracolumbar lesions paraplegia and the damage may be partial or complete.

- *Neurapraxia* causes motor paralysis (flaccid), burning paraesthesia, sensory loss and visceral paralysis below the level of the cord lesion. The lesion may initially appear complete but recovery begins within minutes or hours and soon becomes full.
- *Cord transection* causes motor paralysis, sen-sory loss and visceral paralysis below the level of the cord lesion. Initially, the motor paraly-sis is flaccid. The cord below the level of the lesion then recovers from this initial period and exhibits reflex activity. Within 48 hours, the bulbocavernosus reflex returns. With 4 weeks, tendon reflexes return. Tone and reflexes increase and there is clonus.
- *Root transection* causes motor paralysis, sen-sory loss and visceral paralysis in the root distribution. Unlike cord transection, recov-ery may occur and residual motor paralysis remains permanently flaccid.

ANATOMICAL LEVELS

- *Cervical spine.* Cord transection cephalad to C3 is usually fatal due to loss of phrenic nerve

(C3-5). Below the C5 vertebra, the upper limbs are partially spared.
- *Between T1 and T10.* The first lumbar cord segment in adults arises at the level of T10, therefore cord transection at this level spares the thoracic cord but will cause paralysis of lower limbs and viscera.
- *Below T10.* The conus medullaris sits between T10 and L1 with the L2–S4 roots arising from it then forming the cauda equina.
- *Lumbar roots* innervate:
  - sensation to the groin and lower limb apart from the portion supplied by the sacral segment
  - motor power to the muscles controlling the hip and knee
  - the cremasteric reflexes and knee jerks – cord transection with root escape carries a much better prognosis than cord and root transection.

INCOMPLETE CORD INJURY SYNDROMES

Persistence of any sensation distal to the injury (e.g. perianal pinprick) suggests an incomplete lesion.

Central cord syndrome This is the common-est. Initial flaccid weakness is followed by lower motor neuron paralysis of the upper limbs with upper motor neuron (spastic) paralysis of the lower limbs, and intact perianal sensation (sacral sparing). Bladder control may be variable.

Anterior cord syndrome There is complete paralysis and anaesthesia but deep pressure and position sense are retained in the lower limbs (dorsal column sparing).

Posterior cord syndrome This causes loss of deep pressure and proprioception.

Brown-Séquard syndrome Caused by cord hemi-section, this syndrome is usually due to penetrating injuries. Motor power is lost on the side of the injury and pain and temperature sen-sation on the opposite side.

MANAGEMENT OF TRAUMATIC PARAPLEGIA AND QUADRIPLEGIA

Skin Pressure sores can develop rapidly so 2-hourly log-rolling, pressure care and pressure-reducing mattresses are required.

Bladder training This is begun as soon as possible. Partial recovery may lead to an autonomic bladder or an expressible bladder. If high volume residuals are a problem, urological investigation and intervention may be required.

Bowel training Enemas, aperients and abdominal exercises are needed.

Paralysed muscles The development of flexion contractures can be prevented by moving the muscles through a full range of passive motion twice a day. Splinting may be needed later. Calipers are used to keep the knees straight and the feet plantigrade. Tenotomies may be needed to address flexion contractures. Heterotopic ossification is common and excision may be needed once the bone is mature.

TENDON TRANSFERS

Tendon transfers may be used to compensate for lost function. In cervical injuries, attempts are made to restore a pinch grip (normally powered by C8 or T1).

- If C5–6 *deltoid and biceps only are working*, a posterior-deltoid to triceps transfer using interposition tendon grafts will replace the lost C7 function of elbow extension.
- If C6 *brachioradialis is working*, it can be transferred to become a wrist extensor. Using the *Moberg procedure*, a primitive thumb pinch can be recreated with thumb interphalangeal joint fusion and tenodesis of the basal joint of the thumb with flexor pollicis longus. Active wrist extension then creates passive flexion of the basal joint of the thumb.
- If C7 *extensor carpi radialis longus and brevis* are available, one of them can be transferred into the flexor pollicis longus to provide active thumb flexion (normally C8).

FRACTURES OF THE THORACIC CAGE

FRACTURES OF THE STERNUM

The sternum may be fractured by a direct blow or indirectly during spine flexion.

There is severe pain over the sternum. Fractures can be difficult to see on *X-ray*. If the mechanism was anything other than a direct blow, the spine should be imaged.

Most are minimally displaced and are treated with pain control and breathing exercises; severe displacement requires fixation.

RIB FRACTURES

Rib fractures are almost always due to direct injury but can occur on coughing in osteoporotic patients.

There is sharp localized pain, worse on deep breathing or coughing. Fractures can be difficult to see on *X-ray*. Flail segments should be checked for. If this or multiple rib fractures are compromising respiratory function, rib fixation should be considered.

In most cases, treatment is needed only for pain. Breathing exercises are encouraged.

 Even a benign-looking rib fracture can occasionally penetrate the pleura and lead to increasing compromise due to a slowly developing tension pneumothorax. The patient should be advised to return for review if they are struggling with breathing.

COMPLEX THORACIC INJURIES

 Complex fractures of the thorax include secondary injuries to mediastinal structures. These conditions require emergency treatment. They are dealt with in Chapter 22.

SECTION 3 TRAUMA

Pelvic injuries

29

- Initial assessment 643
- Isolated fractures 644
- Fractures of the pelvic ring 645
- Fractures of the acetabulum 649
- Injuries of the sacrum and coccyx 652

Pelvic injuries may result in fractures of the pelvic ring, acetabular fractures or both.

 Fractures of the pelvis are relatively rare (less than 5% of skeletal injuries) but are particularly serious due to associated blood loss and injuries to viscera that can be fatal.

The pelvis is stabilized by ligaments (**29.1**). The overall mortality in pelvic trauma is 9%, although this is significantly increased (up to 50%) if the patient is haemodynamically unstable at presentation.

INITIAL ASSESSMENT

CLINICAL ASSESSMENT

A fracture of the pelvis should be suspected in any multiply injured patient. Pelvic binders are applied as soon as possible to such patients on scene. If pelvic binders are not available, a sheet can be wrapped round the pelvis and tightened with a windlass mechanism using a bar or stick. The feet can also be internally rotated and tied

together. These interventions help reduce the pelvic volume in anterior instability and reduce haemorrhage. The patient may be severely shocked due to blood loss and visceral damage. Resuscitation should be started even before the examination is complete (the Advanced Trauma Life Support – ATLS – approach is described in Chapter 22). In settings with trauma networks, these patients are typically taken directly to level 1 (major) trauma centres.

Local bruising or abrasions may be obvious; ecchymoses often extend into the thigh and perineum, and there may be gross swelling of the labia or scrotum.

 Bleeding from the urethra or genitalia suggests serious visceral damage. *Abdominal tenderness and guarding* suggest intraperitoneal bleeding, possibly due to rupture of the spleen or liver.

Repeated assessment of an unstable pelvis will lead to disruption of any clot formed; this may worsen haemorrhage. The pelvis is palpated and gently compressed to determine if there is tenderness consistent with a fracture, but the pelvis

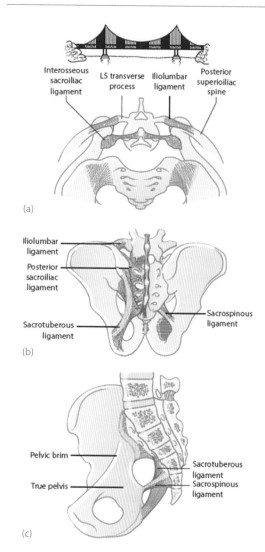

29.1 Posterior ligamentous stabilizers of the pelvis (a) Superior view; the anterior sacro-iliac ligament and the iliolumbar ligament. **(b)** Posterior view; the posterior sacroiliac ligament, sacrotuberous ligament and sacrospinous ligament. **(c)** Lateral view; the sacrotuberous ligament and sacrospinous ligament.

is not 'sprung' or vigorously tested for stability to avoid provoking further bleeding.

During *rectal examination* (which is mandatory), the coccyx and sacrum can be felt; more importantly, the position of the prostate can be gauged: if it is abnormally high, it suggests a urethral injury. A ruptured bladder should be suspected in patients who do not void or in whom a bladder is not palpable after adequate intravenous fluid replacement. Bladder rupture may be intra-peritoneal or extraperitoneal.

> ⚠ Intraperitoneal bladder rupture may be associated with massive haemorrhage.

Neurological examination is essential. If the patient is unconscious, it must be noted that this needs to be performed later. There may be damage to the lumbosacral plexus (e.g. a foot drop due to damage to the L5 nerve root).

IMAGING

During the primary survey, an anteroposterior (AP) view *X-ray* of the pelvis is obtained (**29.2**). This is carefully assessed for any signs of fracture or diastasis. Inlet and outlet views allow visualization of the pelvic ring and Judet views, visualization of the acetabulum. These may be required later but, in the trauma setting, the next imaging performed is usually a *computed tomography (CT) scan* which allows fine assessment of osseous detail and relationships. If contrast is administered, it also allows assessment of the urinary tract. If the pelvic binder is still *in situ* when the CT is performed, it is very important to perform an AP X-ray of the pelvis after the binder is removed (**29.3**).

TYPES OF FRACTURE

Pelvic ring fractures and acetabular fractures are usually the result of a high-energy injury. However, isolated pelvic fractures can occur.

ISOLATED FRACTURES

AVULSION FRACTURES

A piece of bone is pulled off by violent muscle contraction; this is usually seen in sports participants and athletes. The most common are the anterior inferior iliac spine (rectus femoris) and

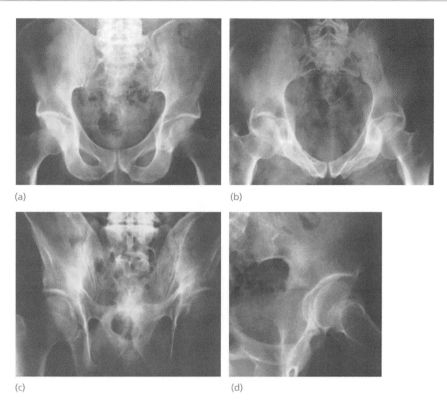

(a)

(b)

(c)

(d)

29.2 Pelvic X-rays (a) AP; **(b)** inlet view; **(c)** outlet view; and **(d)** right and left oblique views, similar to this view of the left half of the pelvis.

the ischial tuberosity (hamstring). Other sites include the anterior superior iliac spine (sartorius) and the pubis (adductor longus). Most can be treated as muscle injuries. Occasionally, reduction and fixation are required to facilitate high-demand activities (e.g. large piece of ischium avulsed and retracted).

DIRECT FRACTURES

A direct blow to the pelvis, usually after a fall from a height, may fracture the ischium or the iliac blade. Bed rest until pain subsides is usually all that is needed.

STRESS FRACTURES

Fractures of the pubic rami are fairly common in severely osteoporotic patients. Posterior insufficiency fractures also occur, although less frequently and are harder to diagnose. *Magnetic resonance imaging (MRI)* of the pelvis can be useful to confirm the diagnosis. These fractures usually unite and patients can weight-bear as tolerated.

FRACTURES OF THE PELVIC RING

Pelvic ring fractures are usually due to a high-energy injury. Think of the pelvic ring as a 'polo mint'. It is impossible to break a polo mint in one place. If you see an injury anteriorly in the ring, look posteriorly for the disruption of the sacroiliac joint or sacral fracture. In order to understand the fracture, and therefore to make decisions about its treatment, the two commonly used classifications are:

- *Young and Burgess* (pelvic ring injury classified by mechanism)
- *Tile* (assesses stability and guides need for fixation).

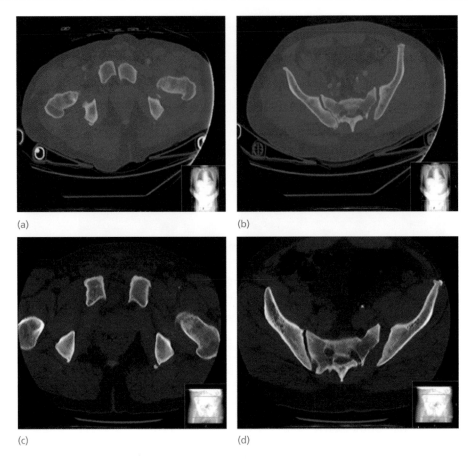

(a)　　(b)

(c)　　(d)

29.3 Pelvic ring fracture (a) The pubic symphysis and **(b)** the sacroiliac joints with the binder applied. There is a pubic symphysis injury which can be seen with the step across the symphysis, with a left sacroiliac joint injury which can be appreciated with the subtle widening of the left side compared to the right. When the binder is removed, the significant widening of **(c)** the pubic symphysis and **(d)** the left sacroiliac joint can be seen.

Young and Burgess classification

ANTEROPOSTERIOR COMPRESSION

Anteroposterior compression (APC) injuries are usually seen in mechanisms such as motor-cyclists straddling the petrol tank at impact or horse riders who have been fallen on by the horse. Initially, the pubic symphysis is disrupted; as the force of energy increases, the sacroiliac joints posteriorly are disrupted – the so-called 'open-book' injury (**29.4**). The sacroiliac ligaments may be torn; there may be a fracture of the posterior part of the ilium or a vertical sacral fracture. This fracture pattern increases the pelvic volume and is associated with the largest amount of blood loss. The displacement of the pubic symphysis can only be assessed with the pelvic binder off.

YOUNG AND BURGESS CLASSIFICATION: APC	
APC I	Less than 2.5 cm of widening at the pubic symphysis
APC II	Symphysis widening of more than 2.5 cm with anterior widening of a sacroiliac joint; the posterior ligaments are intact
APC III	Widening of the symphysis of more than 2.5 cm with dislocation of a sacroiliac joint

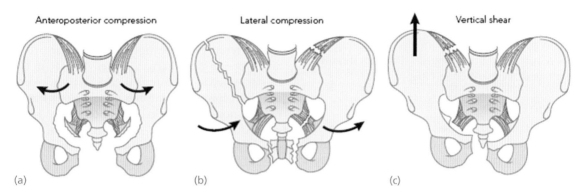

29.4 Fractures of the pelvic ring (a) APC with lateral rotation causes disruption of the anterior part of the ring – the 'open-book' injury. **(b)** Lateral compression causes the ring to buckle and break, fracturing the pubic rami on one or both sides; posteriorly, the iliac blade may break or the sacrum is crushed. **(c)** Vertical shear injury, causing disruption of both the sacroiliac and symphyseal regions on one side.

LATERAL COMPRESSION

Side-to-side compression of the pelvis causes the ring to buckle and break. This is usually due to a side-on impact.

YOUNG AND BURGESS CLASSIFCATION: LATERAL COMPRESSION
LC I   Rami fracture and ipsilateral anterior sacral alar fracture
LC II Rami fracture and ipsilateral posterior ilium fracture dislocation
LC III Ipsilateral lateral compression and contralateral APC pattern injury (windswept pelvis)

VERTICAL SHEAR

Vertical shear injuries are usually seen after a fall from height, landing on one leg leading to one hemipelvis being driven up, disrupting all posterior structures. These are usually severe, unstable injuries with gross tearing of the soft tissues and retroperitoneal haemorrhage.

COMBINATION INJURIES

In severe pelvic injuries, there may be a combination of the above (e.g. when an individual is ejected from a car or motorcycle).

Tile classification

The Tile classification aids in assessing stability and therefore whether stabilization is required. A simplified version is shown here.

TILE CLASSIFCATION
A (stable)
• *A1* – fracture not involving pelvic ring (e.g. avulsion or iliac wing fracture)
• *A2* – iliac wing fracture or anterior rami fractures
• *A3* – transverse sacral fracture
B (partially stable)
• *B1* – unilateral anterior disruption of posterior structures (SIJ widening or sacral fracture)
• *B2* – unilateral SIJ joint fracture/subluxation (anterior ring rotation)
• *B3* – bilateral SIJ/sacral fracture/subluxation
C (unstable)
• *C1* – complete unilateral posterior disruption
• *C2* – complete unilateral posterior disruption with contralateral partial disruption
• *C3* – complete bilateral posterior disruption

Treatment of pelvic ring fractures

Many pelvic ring injuries involve high energy and there may be multiple injuries. Patients should be managed as described in Chapter 22.

PELVIC BINDERS

Pelvic binders are now widespread and are a very effective means of providing initial stability, reducing the pelvic volume and haemorrhage. Correct placement is critical. The binder should be applied at the level of the greater trochanters and adequately tightened. If the binder needs to remain in place beyond 24 hours, it should be released and the pressure areas checked. If they are satisfactory, it can be reapplied if necessary.

MANAGEMENT OF THE PATIENT *IN EXTREMIS*

Massive blood loss caused by a pelvic fracture is, fortunately, rare. The first steps are as outlined as above, to apply a pelvic binder as soon as possible to reduce the pelvic volume and to resuscitate the patients according to ATLS protocols. If a binder is *in situ*, and there is persistent haemodynamic instability despite resuscitation with blood products, immediate haemorrhage control is required. Other causes and sites of haemorrhage must first be excluded (chest, abdomen, external bleeding). A trauma *CT* is preferred but, if not immediately available, an AP *X-ray* of the pelvis should be performed. It is very unlikely that bleeding in the pelvis is solely responsible for haemodynamic instability if there is a stable fracture pattern.

There are two options available according to local resources and protocols.

Immediate transfer to the operating theatre for pre-peritoneal packing Stabilization needs to be achieved. This can be done with an external fixator, in-fix or by replacing the pelvic binder if there is no other option. The pelvis is opened via the Stoppa approach; the rectus abdominis is divided in the midline and at least six large abdominal packs are inserted, three either side of the midline: one posteriorly, one in the mid-pelvis, and another anteriorly. External fixators should be sited to allow access for this approach but also for a trauma laparotomy.

Angiography and embolization Targeted embolization is preferred. This method controls arterial bleeding only (internal iliac artery and superior gluteal artery). Haemorrhage in the unstable pelvic fracture is predominantly bleeding from low-pressure veins. The venous bleeding will not be controlled by embolization. There can be high morbidity following embolization due to muscle necrosis. Unselected embolization should be used only as a last resort.

CONSERVATIVE MANAGEMENT

In stable fractures, non-operative management is generally preferred. Early mobilization with walking aids should occur to reduce the risk of complications. Patients may partially or fully weight-bear as tolerated through the affected side.

OPERATIVE MANAGEMENT

The principle is to turn an unstable ring injury into a stable one. The procedure is best performed on a radiolucent table. Reduction of a hemipelvis involves a combination of traction and rotation to correct the deformity and can be performed closed or open. Anterior instability can be addressed with an in-fix or with open reduction and plate fixation of the symphysis. Percutaneous iliosacral screws are passed to stabilize sacral fractures and sacroiliac joint injuries following reduction (**29.5**). Sometimes, in the case of a displaced

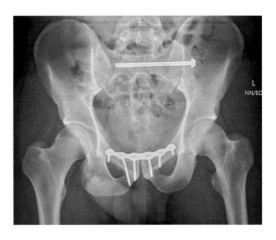

29.5 Postoperative pelvic fracture fixation
Symphysis pubis plating with a left iliosacral screw.

sacral fracture, open reduction and internal fixation is performed via a posterior approach.

Treatment of urogenital injuries

These are the commonest associated injuries. Involvement of a urologist is important to manage these injuries correctly. If a soft, silicone 16F catheter (in adults) cannot be passed by a single, gentle attempt, a suprapubic catheter is required. If the catheter is passed and drains blood-stained urine, a retrograde cystogram via the catheter is mandated. If only blood is drained or the catheter will not pass, a retrograde urethrogram should be performed. Posterior urethral tears are diagnosed by retrograde urethrography and are usually treated conservatively with catheterization for a few weeks. If there is a urine leak from the bladder or urethra, the pelvic fracture should be treated as open with antibiotics for 72 hours and debridement and fixation as soon as the patient is stable. Bladder rupture may be intraperitoneal or extraperitoneal.

 Intraperitoneal rupture of the bladder requires emergency laparotomy and direct repair.

Extraperitoneal bladder rupture may be treated conservatively unless the pelvic fracture is unstable, in which case it should be repaired at the time of fixation.

Complications

Urethral stricture   This may arise as a result of scarring from a healed tear. Rarely extrinsic pressure from fracture healing can cause urethral narrowing.

Impotence   Damage to vascular and nervous structures supplying the genitalia is as high as 30% in pelvic fractures particularly in symphyseal disruption. Early referral to a sexual dysfunction/andrological clinic should be made.

Venous thromboembolism (VTE)   Prophylaxis is essential in all patients: they should receive thromboembolus deterrent (TED) stockings,

mechanical compression and pharmacological prophylaxis prior to surgery (unless there is major bleeding). The risk is especially high following pelvic surgery. Postoperative patients should receive extended duration prophylaxis. Low-molecular-weight heparin for 6 weeks or warfarin for 3 months is commonly used.

Nerve injury   This can arise as a result of the initial injury, or as a result of surgery. It is essential to use the correct views during screw placement (inlet, outlet and lateral views). For S1 iliosacral screws, the L5 nerve root is at risk as it runs anteriorly to the sacral ala, the sacral canal posteriorly and the S1 foramen inferiorly. Always check and record nerve function preoperatively and postoperatively.

Infection   This is rare but serious. The risk is increased in open fractures, bowel and bladder injury. In these cases, definitive fixation using external fixation is sometimes the best way to manage the patient to minimize this risk.

Non-union   Sometimes seen following conservative management, this usually results in a pubic rami non-union and may not always be symptomatic. Sacral non-union does occur following operative fixation, but this risk is minimized by an accurate reduction.

FRACTURES OF THE ACETABULUM

Fractures of the acetabulum occur when the head of the femur is driven into the acetabulum, usually by a direct blow on the side or by a blow on the front of the knee, usually in a dashboard injury when the femur also may be fractured.

Patterns of fracture

It is the position of the leg (i.e. rotation and abduction/adduction) that determines the fracture pattern. The *Letournel classification* (**29.6**), although complex, allows accurate description of the fracture pattern and guides the surgical approach if operative treatment is indicated.

Elementary fractures

Posterior wall   Posterior column   Anterior wall   Anterior column   Transverse

Associated fractures

Posterior column plus   Transverse plus   T-shaped   Anterior column plus   Both-column
posterior wall   posterior wall   fracture   posterior hemitransverse   fracture

29.6 The Letournel classification of acetabular fractures

Fractures are divided into five 'elements', and five 'associated fractures'.

ELEMENTARY FRACTURES

Four *elementary fractures* correspond to four lines:

- posterior wall
- posterior column
- anterior wall
- anterior column.

The fifth elementary fracture is the transverse fracture, which is a complete fracture through the innominate bone.

Posterior wall fracture   This is the commonest type and usually occurs with the leg flexed and the knee hitting the dashboard in a motor vehicle accident. This mechanism is also associated with posterior cruciate ligament ruptures. On impact, the femoral head is thrust against the posterior wall of the acetabulum, commonly

dislocating the hip. Emergent reduction of the femoral head should be performed; if the hip remains subluxed, traction can be applied. *CT scans* are performed to look for bone fragments in the joint and marginal impaction. They are then examined under anaesthetic to determine stability and fixed via a Kocher-Langenbeck approach if unstable, marginal impaction or fragments in the joint need addressing.

Posterior column fracture   This fracture occurs when the femoral head is impacted medially. The fracture line runs from the obturator foramen through the posterior part of the dome into the sciatic notch. It is usually associated with medial migration of the femoral head. Fixation is performed via a Kocher-Langenbeck approach with care to mobilize and protect the superior gluteal neurovascular bundle.

Anterior wall fracture   The rarest fracture pattern, this occurs with the leg in external rotation and is easily mistaken for a high superior pubic ramus fracture. Here, the fracture produces a trapezoid fragment with anterior subluxation of the femoral head. If the hip is unstable or the femoral head subluxed, fixation is performed via the Stoppa or the ilioinguinal approach.

Anterior column fracture This injury occurs with the leg in external rotation. *X-rays* show disruption of the iliopectineal line with an existing fracture line through the ischiopubic ramus. Operative fixation is via the Stoppa or ilioinguinal approach. If a closed reduction is achievable, percutaneous anterior column screw fixation can be performed.

Transverse fracture This fracture occurs with the leg in abduction and internal rotation. It separates the iliac portion above from the pubic and ischial portions below; the femoral head usually follows the ischiopubic segment. Transverse fractures are associated with sacroiliac joint injuries. The position of the fracture determines the approach for fixation:

- *transtectal* (ilioinguinal or iliofemoral approach)
- *juxtatectal*
- *infratectal* (Kocher-Langenbeck approach).

ASSOCIATED FRACTURES

The five *associated fractures* are combinations of the elementary fractures. The articular surface is more severely disrupted, and the fractures usually need operative reduction and internal fixation.

T-shaped fracture In addition to the pattern described for the transverse fracture, there is a vertical fracture line typically exiting through the obturator foramen.

Transverse plus posterior wall fracture This is a transverse fracture with an additional posterior wall fracture due to dislocation of the femoral head. There may be an associated sacroiliac joint injury and there is a high incidence of sciatic nerve injury (up to 70%). Immediate management is reduction of the femoral head. Operative fixation is via the Kocher-Langenbeck approach.

Posterior column plus posterior wall fracture This is a posterior column fracture with an associated posterior wall fracture. The femoral head is dislocated and the level of the fracture is through the sciatic notch. There may be an associated sciatic nerve injury. Fixation is via the Kocher-Langenbeck approach.

Anterior column plus posterior hemitransverse fracture This is a fracture of the anterior column with an additional posterior column fracture at the posterior half of a transverse fracture. It is mostly seen in elderly patients. If fixation is required, it is performed via the Stoppa or the ilioinguinal approach.

Associated both-column fracture All articular segments are separate from the ilium – a 'floating acetabulum'. This is the most severe form of injury. Generally, the ilioinguinal approach is preferred but multiple approaches may be required.

Treatment

The treatment goals are the same as for any periarticular fracture.

TREATMENT GOALS
To restore joint congruency To provide fracture stability to allow mobilization To prevent osteoarthritis

Undisplaced fractures are usually stable and can be managed non-operatively. Patients are mobilized with ipsilateral partial weight-bearing for 6 weeks. Severe pain indicates a lack of stability. Repeat *X-rays* should be performed to look for displacement, and operative fixation needs to be considered.

If the hip is dislocated, reduction is urgent, followed by the application of skeletal traction with a distal femoral transfixion pin until definitive surgery. Fractures with more than 2 mm of displacement of the articular surface should be anatomically reduced and stabilized. Patients with >3 mm of displacement have been shown to have a poor outcome, and patients with <1 mm displacement have been shown to have less progression to osteoarthritis. Articular surface impaction is a poor prognostic factor, particularly if this is not anatomically reduced and supported.

Complications

Nerve injury With posterior fractures involving a hip dislocation, the sciatic nerve may be injured. The nerve is usually not severed, but recovery is seldom complete.

Hip abductor dysfunction This may occur following the Kocher-Langenbeck approach if there has been significant stretching of the superior gluteal nerve, or there may have been nerve damage at the time of injury.

Avascular necrosis As in all severe injuries of the hip, femoral head necrosis may occur. The changes take months or even years to develop. If this progresses to fragmentation and collapse of the femoral head, arthroplasty may be indicated.

Heterotopic bone formation This is common following the Kocher-Langenbeck approach. Any devitalized muscle should be excised, and patients are placed on prophylactic measures such as non-steroidal anti-inflammatory drugs to avoid this.

Osteoarthritis This is related to the severity of the injury, the quality of reduction and the age of the patient. Patients with imperfect reductions have a higher risk of the development of arthritis, as do patients over the age of 50 years.

INJURIES OF THE SACRUM AND COCCYX

A blow from behind, or a fall onto the 'tail' may fracture the sacrum or coccyx, or sprain the joint between them. Women are affected more commonly than men.

Bruising is considerable and tenderness is elicited when the sacrum or coccyx is palpated from behind or per rectum. Sensation may be lost over the distribution of sacral nerves.

X-rays

FINDINGS ON X-RAY

Transverse fracture of the sacrum, in rare cases with the lower fragment pushed forwards

Fractured coccyx, sometimes with the lower fragment angulated forwards

Normal appearance if the injury was merely a sprained sacrococcygeal joint

Treatment

If the fracture is displaced, reduction is worth attempting. The lower fragment may be pushed backwards by a finger in the rectum. The reduction is stable, which is fortunate. The patient is allowed to resume normal activity but is advised to use a rubber ring cushion. Occasionally, sacral fractures are associated with urinary problems, necessitating sacral laminectomy.

Persistent pain, especially on sitting, is common. If the pain is not relieved by the use of a cushion or by the injection of local anaesthetic, excision of the coccyx may be considered.

Hip and femur injuries

30

- Dislocation of the hip 653
- Femoral head fractures 656
- Hip fractures 657
- Femoral shaft fractures 665
- Supracondylar and condylar fractures of the femur 670
- Fracture-separation of the distal femoral epiphysis 673

DISLOCATION OF THE HIP

Hip dislocations are high-energy injuries, occurring in conjunction with femoral fractures or polytrauma in 40–75% of cases. The Thompson and Epstein classification helps define and plan treatment.

THOMPSON AND EPSTEIN CLASSIFICATION OF HIP DISLOCATIONS

Type I	Dislocation with no more than minor chip fractures
Type II	Dislocation with single, large fragment of posterior acetabular wall
Type III	Dislocation with comminuted fragments of posterior acetabular wall
Type IV	Dislocation with fracture through acetabular floor
Type V	Dislocation with fracture through acetabular floor and femoral head

POSTERIOR DISLOCATION

This is the commonest type (~80%). They usually occur with an axial force applied to the knee (e.g. a dashboard injury in a road traffic accident). As the femur is flexed, the femoral head is forced posteriorly, dislocating and fracturing the posterior wall (30.1).

Clinical features

In an isolated posterior hip dislocation, the leg is shortened and lies adducted, internally rotated and slightly flexed. In the presence of an ipsilateral femoral fracture, the position may not be typical.

Maintain a high index of suspicion and screen at-risk cases. Examine the knee for bruising anteriorly and ligamentous injuries, and determine the neurovascular status of the limb, particularly the sciatic nerve.

Imaging

- In the anteroposterior (AP) X-ray film, the femoral head is high-riding and appears smaller than the contralateral head. Associated head and wall fractures may be seen.
- Articular impaction and presence of bone in the joint are best seen on computed tomography (CT), but do not delay hip reduction to perform CT – this can be done after.

SECTION 3 TRAUMA

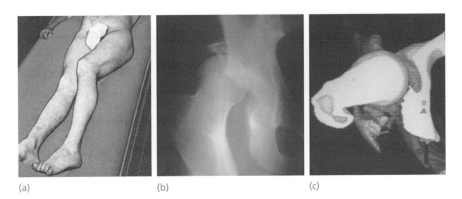

(a)   (b)   (c)

30.1 Posterior dislocation of the hip (a) Posture of a posterior dislocation: the left hip slightly flexed and internally rotated. **(b)** X-ray showing a dislocated hip with associated posterior wall fracture. **(c)** CT image revealing the full extent of the injury.

Treatment

 Check for an ipsilateral femoral neck fracture; if this is present, it needs to be fixed urgently prior to reduction to prevent displacement and blood supply disruption.

Reduction of the dislocation should occur as soon as possible as rates of osteonecrosis of the head increase as time spent dislocated increases. Reduction can be performed closed under sedation in the Emergency Department or may take place under general anaesthesia (usually not required in a posterior dislocation). Open reduction is rarely required. The pelvis is held against the bed by an assistant with pressure over the anterior superior iliac spines and initial traction is in line with the femur (adducted and internally rotated) with the knee flexed to 90 degrees. Maintaining traction, the hip is gradually flexed. Further internal rotation and adduction may be required to clear the acetabular rim. Additional pressure can be applied to the femoral head with a medial and anterior force. The hip usually reduces with a clunk.

X-rays are essential to confirm reduction and to exclude a fracture. Once closed reduction has been performed, CT is performed to look for impaction and bone fragments in the joint.

After reduction, the hip is usually stable. Stability is assessed under fluoroscopic screening.

The hip is flexed to 90 degrees and a posteriorly directed force applied, looking for subluxation.

Surgery may be required if there is:

- subluxation
- articular impaction
- presence of incarcerated fragments.

If there is persistent subluxation and surgery will not be immediate, skeletal traction should be applied with a distal femoral traction pin.

In an isolated hip dislocation with concentric hip reduction, the patient can weight-bear as tolerated, protected with the aid of crutches. Thompson and Epstein Type II and above usually require operation.

- Fixing the posterior wall fragment stabilizes *Type II injuries.*
- *Type III injuries* may require removal of fragments from the joint and, if required, the comminuted wall can be stabilized with spring plates or similar.
- *Type IV and V injuries* are reduced and then reassessed to determine if fixation is required.

Persistent displacement or instability requires surgery (**30.2**). Femoral head fracture treatment is described in 'Femoral Head Fractures' later in this chapter.

Complications

SCIATIC NERVE INJURY

The sciatic nerve is damaged in 10–20% of posterior dislocations. Nerve function must be tested

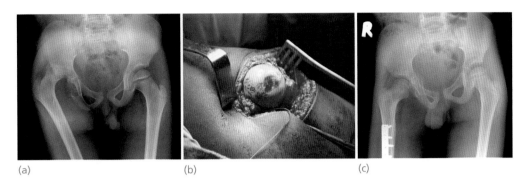

(a) (b) (c)

30.2 Posterior dislocation – late presentation A neglected traumatic posterior hip dislocation in a 10-year-old boy who presented 11 months after the initial injury with a 4 cm leg length discrepancy and severe limp. **(a)** Successful open reduction performed through a posterior hip approach **(b)**, note the chondral thinning on the posterior aspect of the head. A 1.5 cm femoral shortening osteotomy was needed to avoid excessive tension of the reduction. He resumed normal activities 6 months postoperatively **(c)**.

and documented before reduction of the hip is attempted. If, after reduction, a new onset sciatic nerve lesion occurs, the nerve should be explored. If a foot drop occurs, the ankle is splinted in a neutral position to prevent equinus deformity and to aid mobilization.

AVASCULAR NECROSIS

Avascular necrosis (AVN) is reported to occur in up to 20% of traumatic posterior dislocations. If reduction is delayed by more than 12 hours, it rises to 40%. X-ray features can appear within 6 weeks but may take up to 2 years. If there is a necrotic segment, operative treatment should be considered (see Chapter 6). In older patients, a total hip replacement is preferred.

OSTEOARTHRITIS

Secondary osteoarthritis (OA) is common due to:

* cartilage damage at the time of the dislocation
* the presence of retained fragments in the joint
* osteonecrosis.

The options are discussed in Chapter 5.

ANTERIOR DISLOCATION

These account for 10–20% of hip dislocations and are more commonly associated with femoral head fractures. There are two types.

TYPES OF ANTERIOR HIP DISLOCATION	
Type I	Pubic (superior) injuries
Type II	Obturator (inferior) injuries

The leg lies externally rotated, abducted and slightly flexed. Shortening is typically prevented by rectus femoris. Seen from the side, the anterior bulge of the dislocated head may be seen in the superior type and in the inferior type, the head can be palpated in the groin.

X-rays

In the AP view, the dislocation is usually obvious but, occasionally, the head is almost directly in front of the acetabulum and just appears larger. The lateral film shows the anterior dislocation.

Treatment

Anteriorly dislocated hips are more difficult to reduce than posteriorly dislocated hips. Reduction is still urgent but more likely to require general anaesthesia or open reduction. The affected leg is held in external rotation, abduction and flexion, before longitudinal traction is applied. The leg is gently internally and externally rotated until the hip reduces – for superior dislocations, pressure anteriorly over the palpable femoral head may

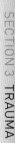

assist. Reduction usually occurs with a clunk. The subsequent treatment and risks are as for posterior dislocations.

CENTRAL DISLOCATION

A fall on the side, or a blow over the greater trochanter, may force the femoral head medially through the floor of the acetabulum. Although this is called 'central dislocation', it is really a complex fracture of the acetabulum. The condition is dealt with in Chapter 29.

FEMORAL HEAD FRACTURES

Femoral head fractures are always seen in conjunction with dislocation. Infrequently, the head may have spontaneously reduced. The classic classification is by Pipkin, describing femoral head fractures associated with posterior dislocations (30.3).

Treatment

The hip dislocation is treated as previously described. Treatment of the femoral head fracture is guided by its Pipkin classification.

TREATMENT OF FEMORAL HEAD FRACTURES	
Type I	Excise the fragment if small or fix it if large, usually with counter-sunk screws.
Type II	Treat with open reduction and internal fixation.
Type III	Stabilize the femoral neck fracture first, before any attempt to reduce and fix the dislocated femoral head.
Type IV	Fix the femoral head fracture if large enough.

Complications

Complications following a femoral head fracture include:

- OA in approximately 50%
- osteonecrosis in approximately 20%
- sciatic nerve palsy
- fracture malreduction
- non-union
- heterotopic ossification.

Pipkin classification of femoral head fractures			
Type I	Type II	Type III	Type IV
The fracture line is inferior to the fovea	The fracture fragment includes the fovea	As with types I and II but with an associated femoral neck fracture	Any pattern of femoral head fracture and an acetabular fracture (coincides with Thompson and Epstein's type V)

30.3 Pipkin classification of femoral head fractures

HIP FRACTURES

Hip fractures are defined as those that occur anywhere between the articular margin of the femoral head and 5 cm below the lesser trochanter. They are subdivided as follows:

- *intracapsular fractures* – blood supply to the head is typically damaged
- *extracapsular fractures* – blood supply is rarely damaged. These are further subdivided into:
  - *trochanteric* (including reverse oblique)
  - *subtrochanteric*.

INTRACAPSULAR HIP FRACTURES

Hip fractures typically occur in elderly patients due to falls from standing height and are secondary to osteoporosis. The hip may also fracture leading to a fall. Approximately 6–10% of patients will die within 1 month, rising to 24–33% within 12 months despite optimized management pathways.

Four per cent of elderly patients sustain another fracture at the same time (e.g. distal radius or proximal humerus). Treating, rehabilitating and caring for this group of patients has a huge health economic impact.

Younger patients suffer from femoral neck fractures secondary to high-energy injuries or underlying conditions which affect bone health and the risk of falls (e.g. alcoholism).

The Garden classification is commonly used and describes displacement (**30.4**).

GARDEN CLASSIFICATION OF FEMORAL NECK FRACTURES	
Stage I	An incomplete impacted fracture, typically valgus
Stage II	A complete but undisplaced fracture
Stage III	A complete fracture with moderate displacement
Stage IV	A severely displaced fracture

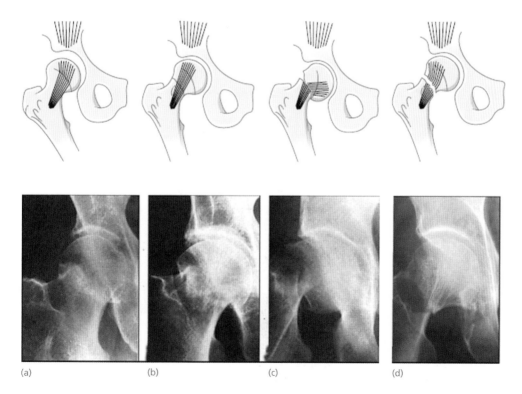

(a)   (b)   (c)   (d)

30.4 Garden classification of femoral neck fractures (a) Stage I; (b) Stage II, (c) Stage III; (d) Stage IV.

SECTION 3 TRAUMA

Extracapsular Hip Fractures

TROCHANTERIC FRACTURES

The AO/OTA (Arbeitsgemeinschaft für Osteosynthesefragen/Orthopaedic Trauma Association) system, although more complex than other systems, is a useful classification for understanding the injury and its relative stability and for planning treatment (**30.5**).

Sliding hip screw devices allow adequate stabilization of the majority of fractures, with multiple randomized trials failing to demonstrate an advantage to the use of the more expensive intramedullary devices. The exceptions are the

Type: Femur, proximal end segment, **trochanteric region fracture** 31A

Group: Femur, proximal end segment, trochanteric region, **simple pertrochanteric fracture** 31A1

Subgroups:

Isolated single trochanter fracture
31A1.1*

Two-part fracture
31A1.2

Lateral wall intact (>20.5 mm) fracture
31A1.3

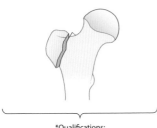
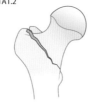
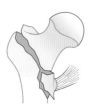

*Qualifications:
n **Greater trochanter**
o Lesser trochanter

Group: Femur, proximal end segment, trochanteric region, **multifragmentary pertrochanteric, lateral wall incompetent (≤ 20.5 mm) fracture** 31A2

Subgroups:

With 1 intermediate fragment
31A2.2

With 2 or more intermediate fragments
31A2.3

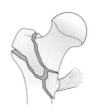
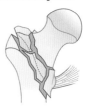

For more information about calculating the lateral wall thickness, please refer to the Appendix.

Group: Femur, proximal end segment, trochanteric region, **intertrochanteric (reverse obliquity) fracture** 31A3

Subgroups:
Simple oblique fracture
31A3.1

Simple transverse fracture
31A3.2

Wedge or multifragmentary fracture
31A3.3

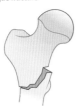
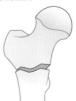
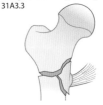

30.5 AO/OTA classification of trochanteric region fractures 31A1.1: Isolated single trochanter fracture. **31A1.2:** Two-part fracture. **31A1.3:** Lateral wall intact. **31A2.2:** Lateral wall incompetent with one intermediate fragment. **31A2.3:** Lateral wall incompetent with two or more intermediate fragments. **31A3.1:** Simple reverse oblique fracture. **31A3.2:** Simple transverse fracture. **31A3.3:** Wedge or multifragmentary fracture.

inherently unstable fractures where the biome-chanics of a sliding hip screw are not suitable to address the instability (e.g. reverse oblique and subtrochanteric fractures).

SUBTROCHANTERIC FRACTURES

These occur between the lower border of the lesser trochanter and 5 cm distal to this. If more distal, they are considered to be femoral shaft fractures. They are rare in young adults due to the thickness and strength of the posteromedial calcar femorale. In conditions with reduced bone density or weak bone (e.g. osteoporosis, metastatic deposits, as a complication of bisphosphonate use), the risk of fracture increases (**30.6**).

Clinical features

There is usually a history of a fall, followed by pain in the hip. If an elderly patient falls and can-not mobilize due to hip pain, a hip fracture needs to be excluded.

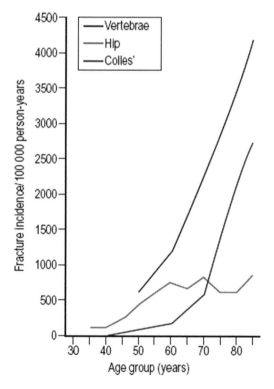

30.6 Osteoporotic fractures The incidence of osteoporotic fractures rises sharply from the menopause onwards in women.

- *In intracapsular or trochanteric fractures*, if the fracture is displaced, the limb is short and externally rotated.
- *In subtrochanteric fractures*, the leg may lie in neutral with shortening and thigh swelling.
- *Impacted intracapsular fractures* may be sta-ble enough to walk on.

In young patients, typically with high-energy injuries, up to 10% of femoral shaft fractures have an ipsilateral hip fracture, so this should be checked for.

Imaging

AP and lateral *X-rays* of the hip allow diagnosis of the fracture in the majority. If pathological lesions are suspected, views of the whole femur must be obtained. In patients with hip pain following a fall who cannot weight-bear with no fracture on plain X-rays, *magnetic resonance imaging (MRI)* (or *CT* if not available) should be performed to exclude an occult fracture (**30.7**). In settings where these are not available, a period of trial weight-bearing followed by repeat X-ray is an option.

Subtrochanteric fractures, may be transverse, oblique or spiral, and are frequently commi-nuted. The upper fragment is flexed and appears deceptively short; the shaft is adducted and dis-placed proximally. Look for three warning signs.

THREE WARNING SIGNS OF SUBTROCHANTERIC FRACTURE
Long fracture line extending proximally towards the greater trochanter and piriform fossa *Large, displaced fragment* which includes the lesser trochanter *Lytic lesions* in the femur

Treatment

Immediate treatment consists of pain relief:

- analgesia
- fascia iliaca or femoral nerve block
- skin traction or Thomas splint for subtrochanteric.

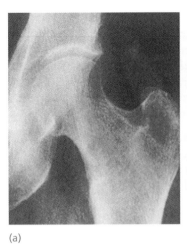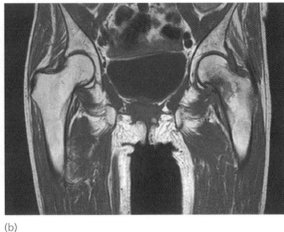

(a)   (b)

30.7 Occult femoral neck fracture (a) An elderly woman tripped on the pavement and complained of pain in the left hip. The plain X-ray showed no abnormality. (b) MRI showing occult femoral neck fracture.

Comorbidities that are amenable to rapid stabilization (e.g. cardiac ischaemia and tachycardias) are optimized. Investigations such as echocardiography are rarely justified unless they will directly and immediately influence management which, in the majority of cases, they will not.

> ⚠️ *Delay to surgery increases mortality,* so any delay needs to be justified and documented. There is good evidence of a substantial increase in the risk of mortality if the patient waits more than 24–36 hours for surgery.

Non-operative treatment is limited to those patients who would not survive the surgical intervention and, in these cases, pain relief should be attempted by regional blockade. Even in high-risk patients, surgical treatment of a hip fracture is an effective part of pain relief and palliation and allows effective nursing care.

INTRACAPSULAR HIP FRACTURES

- *In the young*, make every effort to preserve the native hip.
- *In the elderly*, high risks of re-operation (46%), non-union (30%) and osteonecrosis (14%) mean that arthroplasty should be preferred in all but the truly undisplaced and stable fracture, which is very rare.

Internal fixation Anatomical reduction is required. Percutaneous cannulated screw fixation is a straightforward technique under fluoroscopic guidance. At least three parallel screws should be used, with one buttressing the medial calcar and one the posterior cortex. The entry point should not be below the lesser trochanter to avoid a stress riser and risk of fracture. Alternatively, a sliding hip screw can be used. In elderly patients, restricting weight-bearing often means condemning the patient to bed rest and the attendant complications as they are not able to partially weight-bear. The aim should therefore be immediate full weight-bearing in all cases and constructs chosen to allow that. In young patients who have had reduction of a displaced hip fracture, particularly with posterior neck comminution, a period of 6 weeks' protected weight-bearing may be justified.

Arthroplasty For all other patients, hemiarthroplasty or total hip replacement is preferred. Independently mobile patients (using maximum one stick) who are cognitively normal and fit enough for surgery are considered to benefit from total hip replacement, as are patients with higher risk of acetabular erosion (e.g. rheumatoid arthritis, metastatic disease, Paget's disease). Hemiarthroplasty is preferred for patients not meeting these criteria. There is no good evidence of benefit for bipolar over unipolar hemiarthroplasty.

Cemented fixation is preferred and should be the default. The risk of the rare event of bone cement implantation syndrome must be minimized.

> ## MINIMIZING RISK OF BONE CEMENT IMPLANTATION SYNDROME
>
> Provide adequate fluid resuscitation
> Ensure lavage and drying of the femur prior to cementation
> Vent and avoid excessive pressurization during cementation

EXTRACAPSULAR HIP FRACTURES

Trochanteric hip fractures These are almost always treated with early internal fixation. Accurate reduction is essential to reduce the risk of failure and allow immediate full weight-bearing. This is achieved on a traction table and checked in two planes with fluoroscopy. Sliding hip screws are preferred for all but the most unstable fractures (e.g. reverse oblique and subtrochanteric), as described above. Positioning of

the screw is important to prevent cut-out. The guide wire and screw should enter above the inferior border of the lesser trochanter, pass up the middle of the femoral neck and end within the centre of the femoral head. A 'tip–apex' distance on the AP and lateral X-ray is described to identify a 'sweet-spot' for positioning this sliding screw (**30.8**): if the tip is within 25 mm of the apex when the measurement on both views is combined, there is a lower risk of the screw cutting out. If intramedullary devices are used, long devices are generally preferred as they remove the risk of fracture at the tip of a short stem, although current generation devices may have reduced this risk.

Subtrochanteric fractures These can be difficult to treat. They are associated with greater blood loss. The proximal part is abducted and externally rotated by the gluteal muscles and flexed by the psoas, making reduction more difficult. Although unnecessary soft-tissue stripping should be avoided, open reduction is preferred to a malreduced and badly fixed fracture. Your implant will not reduce the fracture for you; this needs to

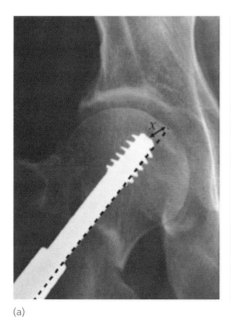
(a)

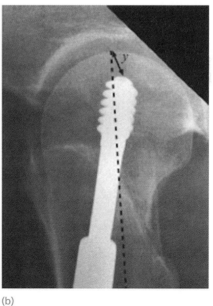
(b)

30.8 Tip–apex distance This is a measure that predicts the risk of screw cut-out from the femoral head. **(a,b)** It is the sum of the measured distances (after adjustment for magnification on the X-ray) from the tip of the screw to the apex of the femoral head – on both the AP (x) and lateral views (y). The risk of cut-out is low if the sum is less than 25 mm.

be achieved before reaming and insertion. There may be subtle fracture line extensions up to the entry point of an intramedullary nail that need to be recognized and accounted for to avoid displacement during preparation and device insertion.

Complications

GENERAL

There is a high incidence of general complications in these elderly and often frail patients. Thromboembolism, pneumonia and bed sores are constant dangers, not to mention the disorders that might have been present before the fracture. Among the survivors over 80 years of age, about half fail to resume independent walking.

OSTEONECROSIS

Osteonecrosis of the femoral head occurs in about 30% of patients with displaced intracapsular fractures and 10% of those with undisplaced fractures. X-ray changes may not become apparent for 18 months. Whether the fracture unites or not, collapse of the femoral head, if it does occur, will cause pain and progressive loss of function.

Treatment   In patients over 45 years of age, treatment is by total joint replacement. In younger patients, realignment osteotomy may be suitable for small superomedial necrotic segments. Core decompression does not have a role in traumatic osteonecrosis and arthrodesis is often mentioned but infrequently performed with unpredictable functional outcome. Even in the young population, joint replacement is often the best treatment option to address ongoing intrusive symptoms.

NON-UNION

The risk of non-union of intracapsular fractures is 30% and is particularly high in those that are severely displaced. There are many possible causes.

> **POSSIBLE CAUSES OF INTRACAPSULAR FRACTURE NON-UNION**
>
> Poor blood supply
> Imperfect reduction
> Inadequate fixation
> Tardy healing, which is characteristic of
>   intra-articular fractures

The patient complains of pain, shortening of the limb and difficulty with walking. The X-ray shows the sorry outcome.

Treatment   This depends on the age of the patient. In young patients with a relatively vertical intracapsular fracture, subtrochanteric osteotomy changes the loading to more perpendicular with the fracture line. This creates compression and may lead to healing. If the fracture line is already perpendicular to the axial load, refixation to achieve further compression and grafting may be justified. If the head shows signs of osteonecrosis, joint replacement should be preferred. In older patients, joint replacement is generally first-line treatment. For extracapsular fractures, non-union is rare. Refixation and grafting is an option but, in older patients, replacement with an endoprosthesis where necessary should be considered. In the case of failed fixation, similar strategies should be followed.

OSTEOARTHRITIS

Subarticular bone necrosis or femoral head collapse may lead, after several years, to secondary OA. If the symptoms warrant it, the joint should be replaced.

ISOLATED TROCHANTERIC FRACTURES

LESSER TROCHANTER

In adolescents, the lesser trochanter apophysis may be avulsed by psoas, usually during hurdling. Treatment is rest, followed by return to activity when comfortable. In the elderly, separation of the lesser trochanter should arouse suspicions of metastatic malignant disease and be considered pathological until proven otherwise.

GREATER TROCHANTER

In the elderly, part of the *greater trochanter* can be fractured by a direct blow after a fall. Fractures exiting below the vastus ridge benefit from the digastric effect of the abductors and vasti. Check for subtle intertrochanteric or intracapsular fractures. If not present, and displacement is less than 1 cm, treatment is non-operative and functional recovery is usually good.

Active abduction should be avoided and the patient mobilized with protected weight-bearing for 6–8 weeks.

Occasionally, the greater trochanter is fractured and the fragment widely separated in a young individual. It can be fixed back in position with cancellous screws, tension-band wiring or a trochanteric plate. Removal of metal work is often required in these patients due to soft-tissue irritation.

HIP FRACTURES IN CHILDREN

These comparatively rare injuries are usually due to high-velocity trauma (e.g. falling from a height or a car accident). The possibility of non-accidental injury should always be considered.

In infants, the area between the capital epiphysis and greater trochanter is incompletely ossified and unusually vulnerable to trauma. Fractures through the middle and basal parts of the femoral neck are the most common. Between the ages of 4 and 8 years, the ligamentum teres contributes very little to the blood supply of the epiphysis; hence its susceptibility to post-traumatic ischaemia and AVN.

Clinical features

Diagnosis can be difficult, especially in infants where the epiphysis is not easily defined on *X-ray*. *Ultrasonography, MRI and arthrography* may help. In older children, the diagnosis is usually obvious on plain X-ray examination.

It is important to establish whether the fracture is displaced or undisplaced; the former carries a much higher risk of complications.

Treatment

 Hip fractures in children should be treated as a matter of urgency, and certainly within 24 hours.

Initially, the hip is supported or splinted while investigations are carried out. Early aspiration of intracapsular haematoma is advocated by some to reduce the risk of epiphyseal ischaemia, but this is controversial, particularly in adults.

UNDISPLACED FRACTURES

These may be treated by immobilization in a plaster spica for 6–8 weeks. However, fracture position is not always maintained and there is a considerable risk of late displacement and malunion or non-union.

DISPLACED TROCHANTERIC FRACTURES

These also can be treated non-operatively with closed reduction, traction and spica immobilization. Careful follow-up is essential; if position is lost, operative fixation will be needed.

FRACTURES THROUGH THE PHYSIS OR FEMORAL NECK

Treatment for these is by closed reduction (one gentle manipulation) and then internal fixation with smooth pins or cannulated screws. If this fails, open reduction is performed (**30.9**). In small children, operative fixation is supplemented by a spica cast for 6–12 weeks.

Complications

AVASCULAR NECROSIS OF THE FEMORAL HEAD

AVN is the most common (and feared) complication. It occurs in about 30% of cases. There are several particular risk factors.

RISK FACTORS FOR AVN OF THE FEMORAL HEAD
Age >10 years High-energy injury Fracture through the proximal femoral neck Displacement

The child complains of pain and loss of movement; X-ray changes usually appear within 3 months of injury.

Treatment This is problematic; most patients end up with pain and restriction of movement, sometimes calling for reconstructive surgery.

SECTION 3 TRAUMA

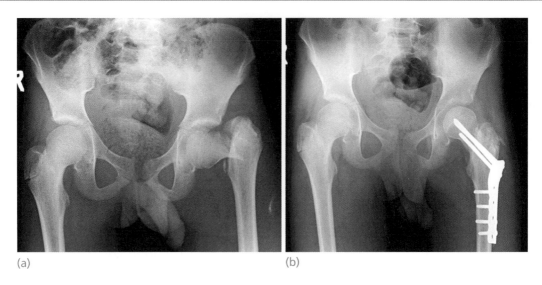

(a)   (b)

30.9 Hip fracture in child Displaced vertical basicervical fracture in a 14-year-old male (a). Anatomical reduction was achieved through an anterior open reduction and a lateral approach was used for plate fixation (b).

Arthrodesis may be considered as a late salvage procedure.

COXA VARA

Femoral neck deformity may result from malunion, AVN or premature physeal closure. If the deformity is mild, remodelling may occur. If the neck–shaft angle is less than 110 degrees, subtrochanteric valgus osteotomy will probably be needed (**30.10**).

DIMINISHED GROWTH

Physeal damage may result in retarded femoral growth. Limb length equalization may be needed.

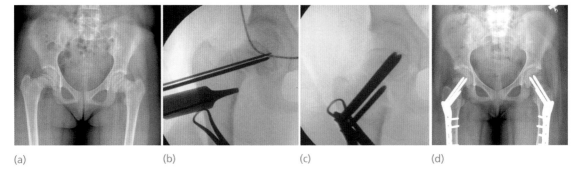

(a)   (b)   (c)   (d)

30.10 Coxa vara Bilateral pathological transcervical femoral neck fractures with resultant coxa vara in a 14-year-old female (a). The underlying cause was HIV infection. Intraoperative images demonstrate a valgus osteotomy (b,c) to correct the neck–shaft angle to improve the mechanical forces across the hip, thus enabling healing of the fractures (d).

FEMORAL SHAFT FRACTURES

The femoral shaft is surrounded by large muscles, an advantage in that open fractures are relatively rare and the healing potential is very good but a disadvantage in that fractures are often severely displaced by muscle pull, making reduction difficult.

Clinical features

This is essentially a fracture of young adults and usually results from a high-energy injury. Diaphyseal fractures in elderly patients should be considered 'pathological' until proved otherwise.

 In children, the possibility of *non-accidental injury* must be kept in mind.

- *In proximal shaft fractures*, the proximal fragment is flexed, abducted and externally rotated because of gluteus medius and iliopsoas; the distal fragment is frequently adducted.
- *In mid-shaft fractures*, the proximal fragment is flexed and externally rotated but abduction is less marked.
- *In lower-third fractures*, the proximal fragment is adducted and the knee is flexed by gastrocnemius, tilting the distal fragment.

Bleeding can be severe with up to 1 L of blood typically lost with a femoral shaft fracture.

X-rays

Adequate AP and lateral X-rays of the whole femur should be obtained. The fracture pattern should be noted; it will form a guide to treatment.

 The hip and knee joint must be included as well and an ipsilateral hip fracture excluded (**30.11**).

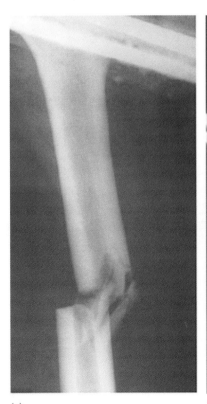
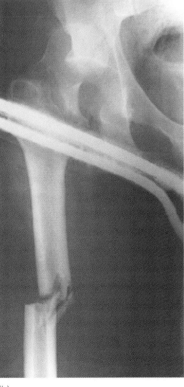

(a)   (b)

30.11 Femoral shaft fractures (a) Note that the upper fragment is adducted, suggesting that the hip may also be affected. **(b)** Always X-ray the pelvis; in this case, the hip was dislocated.

Treatment

INITIAL TREATMENT

 Traction should be applied as soon as possible at the scene of injury and before transport.

A Thomas splint or derivation thereof is critical to reduce blood loss, ease transfer and reduce pain. Its introduction led to one of the largest observed decreases in mortality in military casualties. Femoral shaft fractures often occur in polytraumatized patients, who need to be managed appropriately (see Chapter 22).

NON-OPERATIVE MANAGEMENT

Conservative treatment is rarely considered in contemporary practice due to the problems of prolonged immobility (10–14 weeks). Proximal fractures are also difficult to control and all require regular X-rays, adjustment and physiotherapy to prevent joint stiffness. Time in bed can be reduced by changing to a spica or functional bracing around the 6- to 8-week mark. Traction may be indicated, however (30.12). Methods are described in Chapter 23.

MAIN INDICATIONS FOR USE OF TRACTION

Fractures in children
Contraindications to anaesthesia
Lack of suitable skill or facilities for
    internal fixation

OPEN REDUCTION AND PLATING

Fixation with plates and screws was popular at one time but went out of favour because of the high complication rate, including implant failure. Less invasive techniques avoid the problems of widespread soft-tissue damage and stripping. There are, however, a number of circumstances in which open reduction and plating are indicated (30.13).

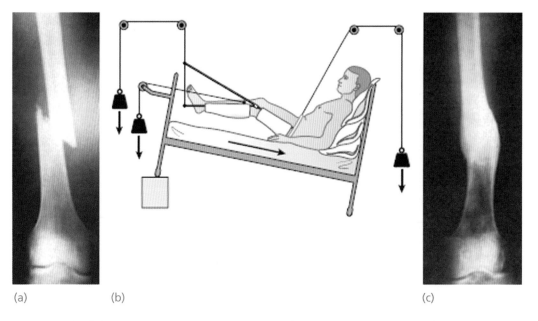

(a)   (b)   (c)

30.12 Femoral shaft fracture – conservative treatment (a) Fracture of the femur. (b) Balanced skeletal traction. (c) The fracture has healed in excellent alignment but required prolonged time in bed on traction.

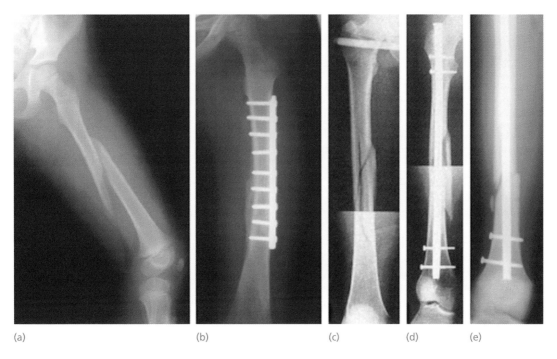

(a) (b) (c) (d) (e)

30.13 Femoral shaft fractures – internal fixation (a) Unstable shaft fractures in children and adolescents, especially those with multiple injuries, can be securely fixed **(b)** with a plate and screws. In adults, shaft fractures are usually stabilized with a locked intramedullary nail **(c,d)**; this treatment is suitable even for distal third fractures **(e)**.

MAIN INDICATIONS FOR OPEN REDUCTION AND PLATING

In the presence of well-fixed joint replacement implants

Periarticular fractures

As a treatment option when there are both shaft and femoral neck fractures

Femoral shaft fracture with an associated vascular injury

Femoral shaft fractures in children with open physes

INTRAMEDULLARY NAILING

Intramedullary nailing is the method of choice for most femoral shaft fractures. Proximal and distal locking allows control of rotation and ensures stability. An appropriate size nail for the patient should be selected. If the isthmus is tight and would require excessive reaming, consider alternatives. Reamed nails have lower failure rates than unreamed. Nails can be inserted antegrade (trochanteric or piriform fossa entry according to nail design) or retrograde. Generally, the nail should be inserted from the same side of the isthmus as the fracture for optimal control. Retrograde nails can be particularly useful for certain patients/fractures. The construct should be inserted to allow weight-bearing as soon as possible.

MAIN INDICATIONS FOR USE OF RETROGRADE NAILS

Obese patients

Bilateral fractures

When there is an ipsilateral tibial shaft fracture in association with an antegrade tibial nail through a single incision

When there is an ipsilateral hip fracture that can be addressed with cannulated screws or a sliding hip screw before insertion of the nail

EXTERNAL FIXATION

> ### MAIN INDICATIONS FOR EXTERNAL FIXATION
>
> The treatment of severe open injuries (very rare)
> Temporary stabilization in multiple injuries (damage control orthopaedics)
> Dealing with severe bone loss by bone transport (see Chapter 12)
> An option for femoral fractures in adolescents

Treatment of complex injuries

OPEN FRACTURES

Open fractures are rare in femoral shaft fractures and the good coverage with muscle means the majority can be managed with thorough debridement, stabilization and primary closure, but the general principles of open fracture management should be adhered to (see Chapter 23). In addition, it is recommended that, where available, joint decision-making occurs between specialists with orthopaedic and soft-tissue reconstruction expertise.

VASCULAR INJURY

Vascular injury must always be checked for and regular neurovascular observations performed. Do not accept 'arterial spasm' as a cause of absent pulses. The level of fractures will indicate the likely level of vascular injury, which should be assessed by *CT, angiography or arteriogram* when suspected. Warm ischaemia times beyond 4–6 hours are associated with higher rates of unsalvageable limbs and amputation. Prompt diagnosis and re-establishing perfusion is a priority. Fracture stabilization is secondary, so perfusion may need to be restored with temporary shunts before fixation and then definitive vascular bypass or repair.

ASSOCIATED KNEE INJURIES

These are easily missed but frequently associated, particularly with mechanisms such as dashboard injuries to the knee. Once the femur has been stabilized, careful assessment of knee stability should be performed with further imaging as indicated.

COMBINED NECK AND SHAFT FRACTURES

These have been addressed earlier in this chapter. The high incidence of ipsilateral injuries should be remembered and such injuries screened for both before and at the end of intervention. The femoral neck fracture takes priority for stabilization.

PATHOLOGICAL FRACTURES

These should be managed to achieve immediate weight-bearing with a construct that will outlive the patient. Solitary bone lesions need to be biopsied and a diagnosis made before treatment (see Chapter 9). Metastatic lesions in the femur are typically treated with intramedullary fixation or endoprosthetic replacement. Mirels's score is used to determine the risk of fracture through lesions and hence the need for prophylactic fixation (see Chapter 9).

PERIPROSTHETIC FRACTURES

These fractures are relatively unusual but the incidence is rising. They are classified by site, loosening of implants and bone stock with the Vancouver system.

> ### VANCOUVER CLASSIFICATION OF PERIPROSTHETIC FRACTURES
>
> *Type A*   Trochanteric region (A_G and A_L)
> *Type B*   Diaphyseal up to two cortical diameters below tip of stem
>
> - B1 Stable stem, adequate bone stock; amenable to fixation
> - B2 Loose stem, adequate bone stock; best treated with revision to bypass (30.14)
> - B3 Loose stem, inadequate bone stock; endoprosthesis or long distal fix stem with scaffold reconstruction
>
> *Type C*   Well distal to tip of stem; treat as separate fracture, avoid stress risers

Complications

GENERAL

Complications such as blood loss, shock, fat embolism and acute respiratory distress are

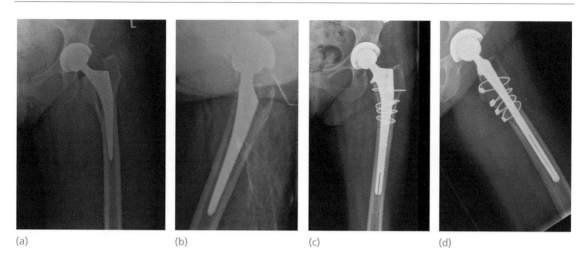

(a)   (b)   (c)   (d)

30.14 Periprosthetic femoral fracture Vancouver B2 periprosthetic fracture of the femur following a fall within a few months of primary hip replacement **(a,b)**. Stem is loose (widened metaphysis and subsidence) so revision total hip replacement is required. A stem to bypass the fracture was inserted for stable primary fixation with cabling back of the large posteromedial fragment **(c,d)**.

common in high-energy injuries such as this. These conditions are dealt with in Chapter 22. Vascular and open injuries are addressed under 'Vascular Injury' earlier in this chapter.

THROMBOEMBOLISM

Prolonged periods of immobility predispose to thrombosis. Movement and exercise are important in preventing this, supplemented by foot compression devices or prophylactic doses of anticoagulants. Formal anticoagulant treatment is required if there is thigh vein or pelvic vein thrombosis and the risks of thrombosis outweigh the risks of bleeding.

INFECTION

In open injuries, and following internal fixation, there is always a risk of infection. Prophylactic antibiotics, and careful attention to the principles of fracture surgery, should keep the incidence below 2%. Infections may be amenable to suppression until union occurs but sometimes radical debridement and alternative stabilization is required.

DELAYED UNION AND NON-UNION

If union is delayed beyond 6 months, intervention may be required (see Chapter 23). Host, local and fracture factors are addressed. Dynamization of the nail (removal of locking bolts) may be

enough, but exchange nailing to a larger nail with or without bone grafting may be required.

MALUNION

Fractures treated by traction and bracing often develop some deformity; no more than 15 degrees of angulation should be accepted. When using intramedullary nails, malrotation is the most common deformity and care should be taken to ensure a symmetrical rotational profile to the uninjured side before locking. When there are bilateral fractures, assessment is more difficult and an attitude of the distal femur, knee and foot within the expected normal range for that patient should be aimed for. If malrotation occurs, it should be addressed early before the femur unites.

JOINT STIFFNESS

The knee is often affected after a femoral shaft fracture. The joint may be injured at the same time, or it stiffens due to soft-tissue adhesions during treatment; hence the importance of early mobilization and physiotherapy.

FEMORAL FRACTURES IN CHILDREN

INFANTS <6 MONTHS OF AGE

Infants need no more than 1–2 weeks in balanced traction followed by a spica for another

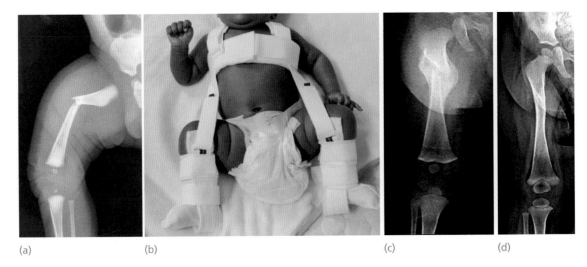

(a)   (b)   (c)   (d)

30.15 Femoral fracture in infant A proximal femoral shaft fracture in a 2-month-old child (a). This can be reliably treated in a Pavlik harness (b). Rapid union (c) and remodelling (d) are expected.

3–4 weeks. An alternative for infants under 6 months of age is a Pavlik harness. Rapid union and remodelling are expected in this age group (30.15).

 Non-accidental injury should be considered as a possible cause for children who are not yet walking.

CHILDREN 6 MONTHS–5 YEARS OF AGE

Reliable union can be achieved with skin traction or using a hip spica. X-rays will often show shortening of 1–2 cm. There is predictable overgrowth following these injuries that compensates for moderate shortening.

CHILDREN 5–11 YEARS OF AGE

These are ideally managed with flexible intramedullary nailing. They are typically retrograde with a medial and lateral entry point just proximal to the distal femoral physis.

CHILDREN >12 YEARS OF AGE (AND >50 KG)

These are usually managed with either submuscular plating or rigid intramedullary nailing with a trochanteric entry point. Traction is still an option for these children but this requires a prolonged stay in hospital.

SUPRACONDYLAR AND CONDYLAR FRACTURES OF THE FEMUR

Supracondylar fractures of the femur are seen in young adults with high-energy trauma or elderly, osteoporotic individuals. The fracture line is just above the condyles and is described by the AO classification (30.16).

AO CLASSIFICATION OF SUPRACONDYLAR FRACTURES	
Type A	No articular splits, truly 'supracondylar'
Type B	Shear fracture of one condyle
Type C	Supracondylar and intercondylar fracture lines

The pull of the gastrocnemius flexes the knee, tilting the distal fragment with potential pressure on or injury to the popliteal artery.

Hoffa fractures are a rare but interesting variant with a fracture in the coronal plane, usually unicondylar and affecting the lateral condyle although medial and bicondylar injuries do occur.

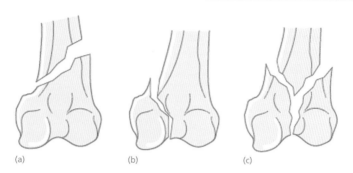

30.16 AO classification of supracondylar fractures **(a)** Type A fractures do not involve the joint surface; **(b)** type B fractures involve the joint surface (one condyle) but leave the supracondylar region intact; **(c)** type C fractures have supracondylar and condylar components.

Clinical features

The knee is swollen and deformed; movement is very painful. Always assess the distal neurovascular status.

Imaging

* AP and lateral *X-rays* of the whole femur should be obtained as a minimum. Assess the following:
  – whether it is an isolated supracondylar fracture or whether it extends into the joint
  – the plane of the fracture
  – the size of the distal segment
  – whether the bone is osteoporotic.
* *CT* is often used to delineate the fracture fully.

Treatment

NON-OPERATIVE MANAGEMENT

Non-operative treatment may be suitable if the patient is a poor candidate for surgery, usually bedbound and the fracture is only slightly displaced and extra-articular, or reduces easily with

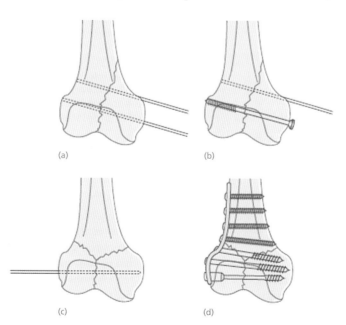

30.17 Femoral condyle fractures – treatment **(a)** A single condylar fracture can be reduced open and held with K-wires preparatory to **(b)** inserting compression screws. **(c)** T- or Y-shaped fractures are best fixed with a dynamic condylar screw and plate **(d)**.

knee flexion. Skeletal traction through the proximal tibia may be suitable with transition to a cast brace or range of motion brace as soon as pain settles and fracture stability has improved.

OPERATIVE MANAGEMENT

This is the treatment of choice: the fracture(s) can be reduced and stably fixed, allowing immediate weight-bearing and range of motion. Periods of restriction should be avoided wherever possible.

There is a range of options for fixation (**30.17**).

OPTIONS FOR FIXATION OF SUPRACONDYLAR FRACTURES

Lag screws (type B and Hoffa)
Retrograde intramedullary nails
  (type A or type C where intercondylar split stabilized or fixed before insertion)
Plates (type A, B or C depending on pattern and bone quality)

In highly comminuted fractures or elderly patients, distal femoral replacement should be considered as an option to allow immediate mobilization (**30.18**).

Complications

JOINT STIFFNESS

Knee stiffness is almost inevitable. A long period of rehabilitation is necessary but full movement is rarely regained. For marked stiffness, arthroscopic division of adhesions in the joint or even a quadricepsplasty may be needed. Unless great care is exercised during mobilization, the ultimate range of movement at the knee may be less than that at the fracture!

MALUNION

Internal fixation of these fractures is difficult and malunion – usually varus and recurvatum – is not uncommon. Corrective osteotomy may

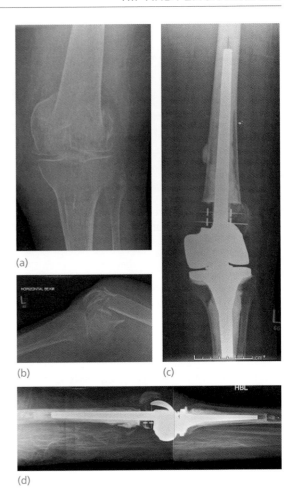

(a)   (b)   (c)   (d)

30.18 Supracondylar fracture of the femur (a,b) Highly comminuted distal femoral supracondylar fracture in a 92-year-old woman. **(c,d)** Postoperative images of a distal femoral endoprosthetic replacement.

be needed for patients who are still physically active.

NON-UNION

Although adequate exposure to allow accurate reduction of the joint surface is needed, metaphyseal stripping should be minimized as it reduces the risk of non-union. If non-union does occur, autogenous bone grafts and a revision of internal fixation will be needed, particularly if there are signs that the fixation is working loose or has failed.

OSTEOARTHRITIS

Supracondylar fractures often extend into the joint surface; anatomical restoration by accurate reduction is necessary to reduce the risk of this late complication.

FRACTURE-SEPARATION OF THE DISTAL FEMORAL EPIPHYSIS

Before skeletal maturity, the lower femoral epiphysis may be displaced – either to one side (usually laterally) or forwards by hyperextension. It is rare but important because of its potential for causing abnormal growth and deformity of the knee. It is usually a Salter–Harris type 2 lesion (30.19).

Nearly 70% of the femur's length is derived from the distal physis, so an early arrest can present a major problem.

The fracture can usually be reduced closed but close follow-up is required to ensure that the position maintained. If a type 2 lesion displaces, it can be stabilized with lag screws or K-wires across the metaphyseal spike. Occasionally, open reduction is required. Salter–Harris types 3 and 4 should be accurately reduced and fixed. Damage to the physis is not uncommon and residual deformity may require corrective osteotomy at the end of the growth period. Small areas of tethering across the growth plate can sometimes be successfully removed and normal growth restored. Shortening, if it is marked, can be treated by femoral lengthening.

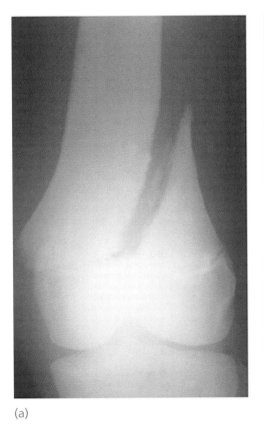

(a)

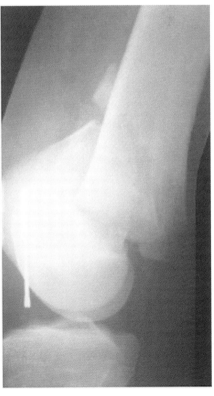

(b)

30.19 Fracture-separation of the epiphysis

Knee and leg injuries

31

▪ Acute knee ligament injuries	675
▪ Knee dislocation and multiligament injuries	678
▪ Meniscal injuries	680
▪ Osteochondral injuries	680
▪ Osteochondritis dissecans	680
▪ Patellofemoral and extensor mechanism injuries	680
▪ Tibial plateau fractures	685
▪ Knee injuries in children	688
▪ Tibia and fibula shaft fractures	690

The knee is an inherently unstable joint, relying on the strong capsule, intra- and extra-articular ligaments, muscles around the joint and cartilaginous structures for stability (31.1). The tibia is subcutaneous over a large surface area and is the most common long bone to sustain an open fracture.

ACUTE KNEE LIGAMENT INJURIES

Most ligament injuries occur while the knee is flexed as stabilizing structures are relaxed, permitting rotation. Injuries of the knee ligaments are common, particularly in sporting pursuits but also in road accidents, where they may be associated with fractures or dislocations. They range from a simple sprain to complete rupture. It is important to recognize that these injuries are seldom 'unidirectional'; they often involve more than one structure and it is therefore useful to refer to them in functional terms (e.g. anteromedial instability) as well as anatomical terms (e.g. torn medial collateral ligament (MCL) and anterior cruciate ligament (ACL)).

The cruciate ligaments provide anteroposterior (AP), rotary stability and also help resist excessive varus/valgus. Both cruciates have a double-bundle structure with each bundle taut and providing stability in different positions. Anterior displacement of the tibia in 90 degrees flexion is resisted by the anteromedial bundle of the ACL and posterior displacement by the anterolateral bundle of the posterior cruciate ligament (PCL). At 30 degrees of flexion, the MCL is the primary stabilizer to valgus stress, the semimembranosus tendon and its expansions, the posteromedial part of the capsule (posterior oblique ligament) and cruciates also contribute. The iliotibial band and lateral collateral ligament (LCL) are the primary stabilizers to varus stress between full extension and 30 degrees flexion, beyond this, the posterolateral structures (popliteus tendon and popliteofibular ligament) contribute more.

Clinical features

The patient gives a history of a twisting or wrenching injury and may have heard a 'pop'. The knee is painful and swollen – a hallmark of

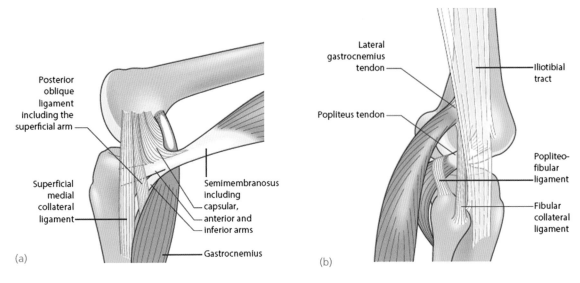

31.1 Extracapsular restraints to valgus and varus stresses on the knee (a) Restraints on valgus stresses: the deep and superficial parts of the MCL, semimembranosus and the posterior oblique ligament. **(b)** Extracapsular restraints on varus stresses: lateral collateral ligament, popliteus tendon, popliteofibular ligament and the capsule.

a ligament rupture is almost immediate onset of swelling. In MCL and LCL injuries, there is tenderness over the torn ligament and stressing the ligament is painful.

Ligament stability is assessed if pain allows (see Chapter 20). Partial tears are stable but painful on stressing. Complete tears are unstable but sometimes surprisingly painless on stressing.

Sideways tilting (varus/valgus) is examined, both in extension and at 30 degrees of flexion. Movement is compared with the normal side. If there is only instability in slight flexion, there may be an isolated collateral ligament tear; if it is unstable in full extension, there is almost certainly a more severe injury with a capsular and cruciate ligament injury.

AP stability is assessed first by placing the knees at 90 degrees with the feet resting on the couch and looking from the side for posterior sag of the proximal tibia, indicating PCL instability. *Anterior and posterior drawer* are checked while fixing the foot in place; a positive sign is a good indicator of ACL or PCL instability respectively, although a negative test does not exclude one. The *Lachman test* is a reliable way of showing up ACL instability; AP glide is tested with the knee flexed 15–20 degrees.

Imaging

- Plain *X-rays* may show that the ligament has avulsed a small piece of bone – the MCL usually from the femur (*Pellegrini-Stieda lesion*), the LCL from the fibula, the ACL from the tibial spine and the PCL from the back of the upper tibia. Another sign is an avulsion fracture off the edge of the lateral tibial condyle (the so-called 'Segond fracture'), indicating an ACL injury. Stress X-rays of the knee may provide visual evidence of instability (**31.2**).
- *Computed tomography* (*CT*) may be used to look for subtle fractures.
- Ligament injuries are usually investigated with a *magnetic resonance imaging* (*MRI*) scan; it is a good test for identifying ligament injuries and to highlight other associated features such as bone bruising.

ANTERIOR CRUCIATE LIGAMENT INJURY

The classic history is of an axial-loading twisting injury on a slightly flexed knee that typically occurs when suddenly changing direction or landing and twisting from a jump.

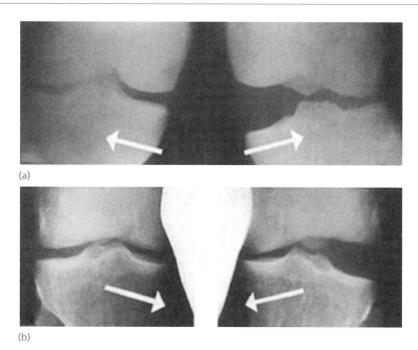

(a)

(b)

31.2 Ligament injuries Stress X-rays of two different patients showing **(a)** complete tear of the medial ligament of the left knee and **(b)** complete tear of the lateral ligament.

RISK FACTORS FOR ACL INJURY
Joint hypermobility Genetic predisposition Elevated BMI Increased tibial slope

It is very rare for the ACL to heal satisfactorily on its own, but some patients achieve a functionally stable knee with conservative treatment, helped by rehabilitation.

Treatment

Quadriceps rehabilitation and conscious knee control can minimize sagittal instability but the risk of future pivot instability, commonly leading to chondral or meniscal instability, remains. *ACL reconstruction* is commonly performed for persistent symptomatic instability aiming to stabilize the knee, reduce the risk of secondary damage and early-onset osteoarthritis (OA). Intra-articular anatomical reconstruction with four-strand autologous hamstring tendons

(semitendinosus+gracilis) or patella tendon are the most popular options. Grafts can be fixed with screws, staples and suspensory devices through tunnels drilled at the footprint of the native ACL. Stepwise structured quadriceps rehabilitation programmes are required after surgery. Return to pivoting sports is not advised for 9–12 months and recovery of normal knee function, when it is achieved, can take up to 18 months.

POSTERIOR CRUCIATE LIGAMENT INJURY

The PCL has a higher load to failure than the ACL and PCL injuries are less common. Injury is typically caused by a direct anterior blow.

Treatment

The majority of isolated PCL ruptures can be managed with quadriceps rehabilitation alone. Reconstruction is generally reserved for failed conservative management.

SECTION 3 TRAUMA

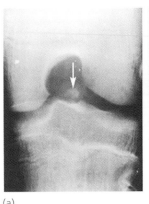
(a)
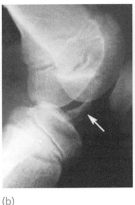
(b)
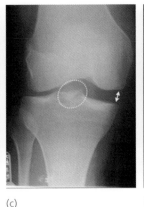
(c)
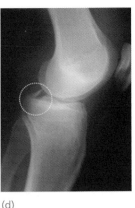
(d)

31.3 Bony avulsion fractures (a,b) AP and lateral X-rays showing a large, displaced avulsion fracture of the tibial spine consistent with a bone ACL injury. This young man injured his knee while playing football. **(c,d)** AP and lateral X-rays showing a bony avulsion of the PCL.

BONY ACL/PCL AVULSIONS

A tibial spine fracture is a traction avulsion injury of the insertion of the ACL. It typically occurs in adolescents and X-ray makes the fragment appear smaller than it is due to cartilage coverage. It may be undisplaced, have a posterior hinge or be displaced. PCL bony avulsions are from the central posterior portion of the tibia (**31.3**).

Treatment

Undisplaced avulsions are managed in a brace or cast. Displaced avulsions are best reduced and fixed with screws, anchors or wires either arthroscopically or open.

MEDIAL COLLATERAL LIGAMENT INJURY

Isolated MCL tears are caused by a pure valgus force but are relatively rare. More often, other structures such as the ACL and medial meniscus are injured at the same time.

- *Partial tears* can be managed conservatively: a brace may be needed for pain relief and to prevent further injury.
- *Complete tears* also have good healing potential with appropriate bracing; range of motion is limited from 10 degrees to full flexion, preventing full extension protects the healing ligament.

LATERAL COLLATERAL LIGAMENT INJURY

Isolated LCL tears are caused by a pure varus force and are rare. Posterolateral corner (PLC) injury needs to be excluded on examination. Isolated injuries can be managed in a brace. Bony avulsions are usually seen in PLC injuries, which may benefit from repair/reconstruction.

COMPLICATIONS

Adhesions Range of motion exercises and muscle strengthening around the knee are important parts of management in all cases to prevent stiffness, secondary to adhesions, and to improve stability.

Instability The knee may continue to give way, predisposing to secondary damage and OA.

KNEE DISLOCATION AND MULTILIGAMENT INJURIES

Traumatic knee dislocation is rare but serious (**31.4**); at least two out of four major knee ligaments will be disrupted. Although around half are high-energy injuries, approximately 40% occur in sports and 10% from falls from standing height.

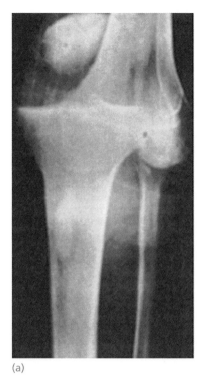

(a)

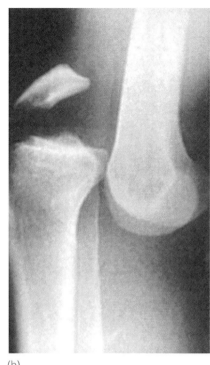

(b)

31.4 Knee dislocation X-rays showing an anterior dislocation of the knee.

The knee may have been reduced by the time it is seen so a high index of suspicion is required.

Clinical features

The injured patient should be assessed and managed according to Advanced Trauma Life Support (ATLS) principles. There is severe bruising and swelling due to joint capsule rupture. Peripheral pulses need to carefully repeatedly examined and documented as the popliteal artery may be ruptured, or more commonly, have an injury such as an intimal tear.

 The popliteal artery may be damaged and *compartment syndrome* is also a risk.

Any suspicion of vascular injury should be formally assessed with ankle brachial pressure indices (ABPI) and an index of <0.9 should prompt vascular imaging. Peroneal nerve injury occurs in 20% and should be carefully assessed.

Treatment

Dislocated knees at presentation should be reduced as soon as possible. Reduction is achieved with in-line traction avoiding hyperextension and stabilized in plaster, brace or with external fixation. Acute ischaemia is a surgical emergency and requires in-theatre angiography, vascular surgical involvement and revascularization. Traditionally, these were managed non-operatively due to the risk of stiffness, but more recent evidence favours surgical repair with 2–3 weeks. There is a wide variety of techniques described but the components contributing to the instability should be determined and repaired or reconstructed as anatomically and isometrically as possible.

Complications

Arterial damage This occurs in 8–14% of cases.

 Delay in diagnosing and revascularizing can lead to amputation.

SECTION 3 TRAUMA

Common peroneal nerve injury Injury to the common peroneal nerve results in weak or absent ankle dorsiflexion. Recovery can occur in around 20% of cases if the nerve is not completely disrupted. If there is no recovery, a transfer of tibialis posterior tendon through the interosseous membrane to the lateral cuneiform may help restore ankle dorsiflexion.

Joint instability Mild residual instability despite repair is common. Quadriceps rehabilitation can compensate for mild instability and the functional disability is rarely severe.

Stiffness Stiffness due to immobilization and scarring is common and may be more troublesome than instability. Even with early reconstruction, normal knee function is elusive.

MENISCAL INJURIES

Meniscal injuries are common both in isolation and in conjunction with ligament injuries. The menisci have an important role in load distribution, stability and congruence. Menisci are relatively poorly vascularized structures that receive their blood supply from their periphery, therefore the majority of tears have poor healing potential. They are discussed in detail in Chapter 20.

OSTEOCHONDRAL INJURIES

Patients often give a history of a patella dislocation or a blow to the front of the knee. There is an effusion and aspiration shows blood-stained fluid mixed with fat globules. Standard *X-rays* rarely reveal the osteochondral fragment unless large or the defect from which it arose and *MRI* is required to delineate.

Treatment

Small fragments can be excised if symptomatic. Large fragments, particularly from weight-bearing areas, can be fixed back with countersunk headless screws if presenting early.

- *For relatively small symptomatic lesions (<2 cm²)*, microfracture is the preferred treatment.

- *For lesions >2 cm²*, the preferred technique is more controversial. Options include:
  - microfracture
  - microfracture plus collagen scaffold
  - cartilage transplantation
  - autologous cultured chondrocytes
  - resurfacing implants.

OSTEOCHONDRITIS DISSECANS

Adolescents and young adults with intermittent knee pain are sometimes found to have developed a small segment of osteochondral necrosis, usually on the lateral aspect of the medial femoral condyle. This is probably traumatic, caused by repetitive contact with the overlying patella or an adjacent ridge on the tibial plateau. The condition is described in Chapter 20.

PATELLOFEMORAL AND EXTENSOR MECHANISM INJURIES

EXTENSOR MECHANISM INJURIES

POSSIBLE SITES OF DISRUPTION

Quadriceps tendon
Quadriceps tendon insertion to the patella
Through the patella and retinacular expansions
Origin of patellar tendon from the patella
Patellar tendon
Insertion of the patellar tendon to the tibial tubercle

In all but direct blows to the patella, the mechanism of injury is sudden resisted extension of the knee or sudden passive flexion of the knee while the quadriceps is contracting (e.g. stumbling on a stair or kicking a fixed or heavy object). The lesion tends to occur at higher levels with increasing age.

QUADRICEPS TENDON RUPTURE

The patient is usually elderly, may have a history of diabetes or rheumatoid disease, or may have been treated with corticosteroids or antibiotics such as ciprofloxacin. Occasionally, acute rupture is seen in young athletes. There is bruising and tenderness and sometimes a palpable gap or low riding patella. Assess active knee extension:

- impossible = complete rupture
- weak = partial rupture.

Diagnosis can be confirmed by *ultrasound or MRI*.

Treatment

PARTIAL TEARS

Treatment is non-operative with an extension brace or plaster cylinder followed by rehabilitation focusing on restoring knee flexion and quadriceps strength.

COMPLETE TEARS

Early operation is needed as the tendon will retract. Direct repair can be reinforced by proximal turndown techniques. Avulsions are reattached to a trough created at the site with augmentation with pull-through sutures through patellar bone tunnels. Postoperatively, the knee is braced in extension with progressively increased range of motion to prevent stiffness.

Ruptures diagnosed late are difficult to repair due to retraction. Turndown techniques may help, or augmentation with autologous hamstring tendons or synthetic meshes.

The results of acute repairs are good, with most patients regaining full power, a good range of movement and little or no extensor lag. Late repairs are less predictable.

PATELLA TENDON RUPTURE

This is an uncommon injury and usually seen in young athletes at the proximal or distal attachment of the ligament. There may be a previous history of 'tendinitis' and local injection of corticosteroid.

There is a history of sudden pain on forced extension, followed by bruising, swelling and tenderness at the site.

X-rays may show a high-riding patella and a tell-tale flake of bone at the proximal or distal attachment of the ligament. *Ultrasound or MRI* help distinguish partial and complete tears.

Treatment

ACUTE PARTIAL TEARS

These are treated in an extension brace or plaster cylinder with progressively increased flexion over 6 weeks to prevent stiffness.

ACUTE COMPLETE TEARS

These require operative repair or reattachment. The repair can be protected by inserting a temporary pull-out wire or protective figure-of-eight strong suture. Progressively increased flexion over 6 weeks is allowed to prevent stiffness.

Early repair of acute ruptures gives excellent results.

CHRONIC COMPLETE TEARS

Chronic complete tears are difficult to manage because of proximal retraction. A two-stage operation may be needed:

1. to release the contracted tissues and apply traction directly to the patella
2. at a later stage, to repair the patellar tendon and augment it with autologous hamstrings.

Late repairs are less successful and the patient may be left with a permanent extension lag.

PATELLA FRACTURES

The patella is a sesamoid bone in continuity with the quadriceps tendon and the patellar tendon with additional insertions from the vastus medialis and lateralis. The extensor 'strap' is completed by the medial and lateral extensor retinacula, which bypass the patella, inserting into the proximal tibia. The patella holds the entire extensor 'strap' away from the centre of rotation of the knee, thereby lengthening the anterior lever arm and increasing quadriceps efficiency.

> The key to managing patellar fractures is assessment of the entire extensor mechanism.

If the extensor retinacula are intact, active knee extension is still possible, even if the patella itself is fractured.

Mechanism of injury

- *Direct injury* is usually the result of a fall onto the knee or a blow against the dashboard of a car causing either an undisplaced crack or a comminuted ('stellate') fracture without severe damage to the extensor expansions.
- *Indirect injury* may be caused by the patient catching the foot against a solid obstacle and, to avoid falling, contracting the quadriceps muscle forcefully. This is a transverse fracture with a gap between the fragments and typically disrupts the extensor expansions.

Clinical features

The knee is painful and swollen; sometimes the gap can be felt. It is helpful to establish whether the patient can actively extend the knee (not just maintain a straight leg), as this will influence the choice of treatment.

X-rays

AP and lateral views are required to look for displacement and articular congruity. Patella fractures can be undisplaced or displaced and are classified as transverse, longitudinal, polar or comminuted (stellate). Displacement that creates an articular step or, in the case of a transverse fracture, a gap of more than 3 mm wide is significant.

 It is important not to confuse a fracture with a *congenital bipartite patella* (smooth line extending obliquely across the superolateral angle of the bone, often bilateral).

Treatment

UNDISPLACED OR MINIMALLY DISPLACED FRACTURES

The extensor mechanism is generally intact and treatment is protective. A knee brace locked in extension or plaster cylinder is worn for 3–4 weeks with quadriceps exercises then protected flexion in a brace permitted for 2–3 weeks.

LONGITUDINAL FRACTURES

These are inherently more stable and protected incremental increase in range of motion is permitted from 2 weeks.

DISPLACED TRANSVERSE FRACTURES

The extensor mechanism is disrupted requiring fixation. Through a longitudinal incision, the fracture is exposed and the patella repaired by the tension-band principle (**31.5**). The tears in the extensor expansions are then repaired. A backslab or hinged brace is worn until control of active knee extension is regained; this is removed every day to permit active knee-flexion exercises.

COMMINUTED (STELLATE) FRACTURES

The extensor expansions are typically intact and the patient may be able to straight leg raise; however, the articular surface is disrupted therefore reduction and fixation is generally advocated. The principle is to reduce and hold as much of the articular surface as possible. A combination of K-wires, mini fragment screws, cerclage wires or sutures is most commonly employed. Rehabilitation is the same as for transverse fractures but may need to proceed more slowly.

OUTCOME

Patients usually regain good function but, in severe injuries, there is a significant incidence of late patellofemoral OA.

DISLOCATION OF THE PATELLA

Due to femoral neck offset, the knee is in slight valgus, creating a tendency for the patella to pull laterally during quadriceps contraction. This is prevented by:

- the intercondylar groove or trochlea, which has a high lateral 'embankment'
- extensor muscle contraction, which pulls it firmly into the groove
- extensor retinacula and patellofemoral ligaments.

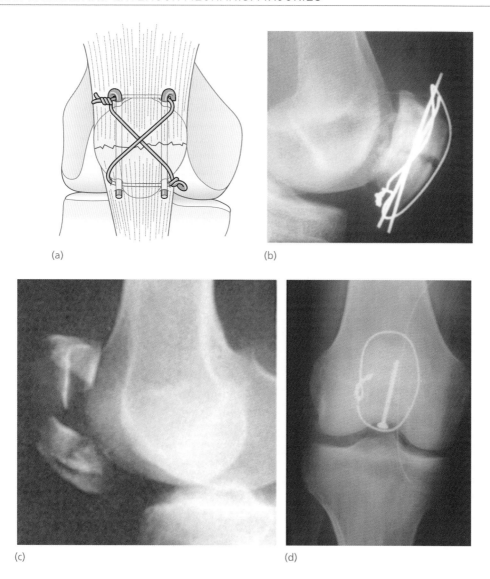

(a)

(b)

(c)

(d)

31.5 Fractured patella (a,b) Straightforward transverse fractures can be treated by tension-band wiring: the fragments are transfixed with K-wires and tightened by looping a malleable wire (1–1.25 mm) in a figure-of-eight configuration around the protruding ends of the K-wires. **(c)** For displaced comminuted fractures **(d)**, cerclage and fixation with small fragment screws preserve as many fragments as possible.

The most important static check rein on the medial side is the medial patellofemoral ligament, extending from the superomedial border of the patella towards the medial femoral condyle deep to vastus medialis.

In a normal knee, patella dislocation requires considerable force. However, dislocation occurs more easily in some people.

CONDITIONS PREDISPOSING TO PATELLA DISLOCATION

Shallow groove (trochlea dysplasia)
High patella (patella alta)
Ligaments abnormally lax (hypermobility)

Mechanism of injury

Patella dislocation may be traumatic or atraumatic. The patella dislocates laterally and the medial patellofemoral ligament and retinacular fibres may be torn.

- *Atraumatic dislocations* occur in patients with predisposing factors.
- *Traumatic dislocations* are usually due to indirect force: sudden, severe contraction of the quadriceps muscle while the knee is stretched in valgus and external rotation. Typically, this occurs in field sports when a runner dodges to one side.

First-time dislocations are most common among female adolescents. Of these, 17% will go on to become recurrent, with younger patients at greater risk.

Clinical features

In a first-time dislocation, the patient may experience a tearing sensation and a feeling that the knee has gone 'out of joint'. The patella often reduces spontaneously on knee extension. If it remains dislocated, the displaced patella sits on the lateral side of the knee and is not easily noticed but the uncovered medial femoral condyle is unduly prominent and may be mistaken for the patella (**31.6**). Patients generally resist movement of the knee. With recurrent dislocation, the features are much less marked, though still unpleasant.

After reduction, the knee looks normal, but the *apprehension test* is positive.

Imaging

- AP, lateral and tangential (skyline) *X-rays* are required for complete assessment. In unreduced dislocations, the patella is laterally displace and tilted or rotated. In 5% of cases, there is an associated osteochondral fracture. Patella alta and trochlear dysplasia (shallow trochlea; crossing sign) can be seen on lateral views.
- *MRI* is the investigation of choice when considering intervention. It allows quantification of dysplasia, contact area, patella height and morphology and soft tissue restraints.

Treatment

The patella is easily reduced with extension and medial force. The most unstable position for the patella is full extension so avoid immobilization in this position. It is safer to weight-bear and flex the knee as soon as tolerated.

NON-OPERATIVE TREATMENT

First-time dislocations are managed non-operatively. The focus is on reducing swelling, improving range of motion and confidence, with physiotherapy directed towards closed-chain exercises and vastus medialis oblique (VMO) strengthening.

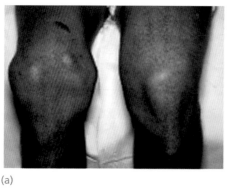
(a)

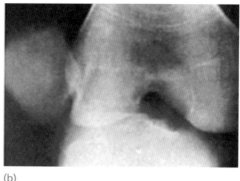
(b)

31.6 Dislocation of the patella (a) The right patella has dislocated laterally, giving a broad, flattened appearance to the knee. **(b)** X-ray showing the patella displaced to the lateral side.

OPERATIVE TREATMENT

Surgery is considered when non-operative management fails in recurrent cases with functional impairment and aims to address underlying predisposing factors. With minimal or moderate trochlear dysplasia, this may involve medial patellofemoral ligament reconstruction+/−tibial tubercle osteotomy if there is patella alta. For patients with severe dysplasia, this may involve trochleoplasty.

TIBIAL PLATEAU FRACTURES

Mechanism of injury

Fractures of the tibial plateau are caused by a varus or valgus force combined with axial loads, usually a fall from height. The classically described 'bumper fracture' with a car striking a pedestrian on the side of the knee is relatively unusual. One or both tibial condyles are crushed or split by the opposing femoral condyle, which usually remains intact.

Clinical features

The joint is swollen and may be deformed with the doughy feel of a haemarthrosis. The knee should be examined for signs of neurovascular injury: traction injury of the peroneal or tibial nerves is not uncommon. Severe fractures may also be associated with major vascular injury or represent a knee dislocation that has reduced.

Imaging

AP and lateral view *X-rays* are required but the extent of comminution or depression is only fully appreciated on *CT* scan (**31.7**). CT is very useful for surgical planning, particularly for the presence of a posterior condylar component which may require a separate posteromedial or posterolateral exposure for fixation.

The most commonly used classification is that of Schatzker (**Table 31.1**) (**31.8**).

Treatment

TYPE 1 FRACTURES

Undisplaced type 1 fractures These can be treated conservatively; a hinged cast-brace or ROM brace is fitted to allow early mobilization. Weight-bearing is restricted initially.

Displaced fractures These must be reduced and fixed.

- *Reduction* may require removal of incarcerated fragments or cartilage.
- *Fixation* can be achieved with lag screws in good bone or buttress plate in poorer bone.

TYPE 2 FRACTURES

If the knee is stable and depression less than 5 mm, or in a low-demand patient or osteoporotic fracture, non-operative treatment focused on regaining mobility and function early rather than anatomical restitution is appropriate. For others, open reduction with elevation of the plateau and internal fixation is required. Joint

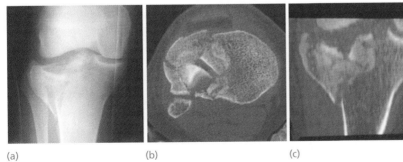
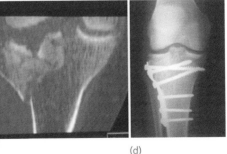

(a)   (b)   (c)   (d)

31.7 Tibial plateau fractures (a) X-rays provide information about the position of the main fracture lines and areas of articular surface depression. **(b,c)** CT reconstructions reveal the extent and direction of displacements. **(d)** Postoperative X-ray showing perfect fixation with a buttress plate and screws.

Table 31.1 Schatzker classification of tibial plateau fractures

Classification	Description
Type 1	A vertical split of the lateral condyle. May be virtually undisplaced, or the condylar fragment may be pushed inferiorly and tilted The damaged lateral meniscus may be trapped in the crevice Usually occurs in younger people
Type 2	A vertical split of the lateral condyle combined with central depression The lateral fragment, which may just be the rim or a larger portion of the lateral condyle, is displaced laterally with widening of the joint If not reduced, may lead to a valgus deformity
Type 3	Depression of the articular surface with an intact condylar rim If depression is not too severe, the joint is usually stable and may tolerate early movement
Type 4	Fracture of the medial tibial condyle Two types: • a depressed, crush fracture of osteoporotic bone • a high-energy fracture resulting with a condylar split running obliquely from the intercondylar eminence to the medial cortex May be associated LCL rupture and a traction injury of the peroneal nerve – the severity of these injuries should not be underestimated
Type 5	Fracture of both condyles Both condyles are split but there is a column of the metaphysis in between that remains in continuity with the tibial shaft
Type 6	Combined condylar and subcondylar fractures A high-energy injury that may result in severe comminution Unlike type 5 fractures, the tibial shaft is effectively disconnected from the tibial condyles

surface inspection via submeniscal arthrotomy or arthroscopically is recommended. Screws can be placed in parallel just beneath the subchondral bone ('raft' screws) to support the articular surface (**31.9**). Bone graft may also help. The wedge of lateral condyle is then fixed with a buttress plate. Periarticular locking plates are popular but not always necessary. Early knee movement is encouraged to minimize joint stiffness.

TYPE 3 FRACTURES

The principles of treatment and fixation are similar to type 2 fractures. The intact lateral rim means the knee is usually stable, but the depressed fragments may need to be elevated through a metaphyseal window checking the reduction by *X-ray* or *arthroscopy*.

TYPE 4 FRACTURES

 Do not underestimate the severity and complexity of type 4 injuries.

Osteoporotic crush fractures of the medial plateau are difficult to reduce but treatment is similar to types 2 and 3. Medial condylar splits generally occur in younger patients in high-energy injuries. The fracture itself is often more complex than it appears; there may be a second, coronal plane posterior split requiring a posteromedial approach. Once the fracture is fixed with methods as described above, integrity of the lateral ligament is assessed and addressed as necessary.

TYPE 5 AND 6 FRACTURES

 Compartment syndrome must be checked for and treated urgently when it occurs.

The soft tissues often take time to settle down to permit safe surgery. Excessive soft-tissue stripping needs to be avoided. The three-column concept (medial, lateral and posterior) is useful for planning treatment. Most fractures can be

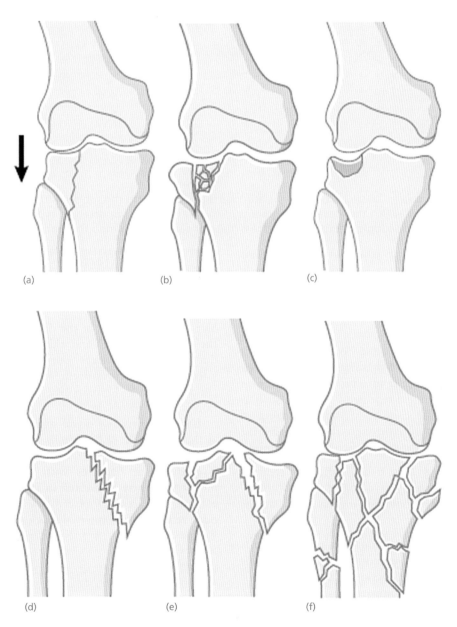

31.8 Tibial plateau fractures (a) *Type 1:* split of the lateral condyle. **(b)** *Type 2:* a split of the lateral condyle with central depression. **(c)** *Type 3:* depression of the lateral condyle with an intact rim. **(d)** *Type 4:* medial condyle fracture. **(e)** *Type 5:* bicondylar fracture with intact central portion of metaphysis still connected to the tibial shaft. **(f)** *Type 6:* combined bicondylar and metaphyseal/subcondylar fractures.

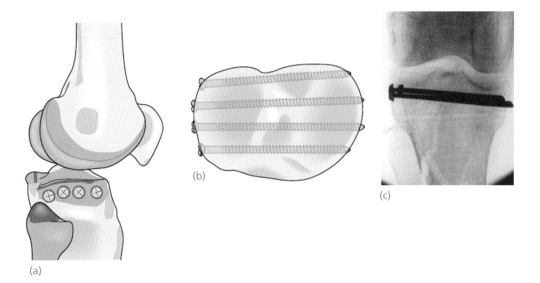

(b)

(c)

(a)

31.9 Raft screws (a–c) These cortical screws are inserted just beneath the subchondral surface and form a 'raft' above which the elevated fragments of the plateau are supported. In type 2, 5 or 6 injuries, they need to be supplemented by a buttress plate or can be performed through holes in a plate.

addressed through a combination of anterior and posteromedial approaches or percutaneously and/or the use of a fine-wire frame (**31.10**).

Complications

Compartment syndrome   With severe condylar fractures, there is a significant risk of developing a compartment syndrome. The leg and foot should be examined repeatedly for signs such as disproportionate pain on passive stretching of muscles which run through the compartment and distal neurological or vascular compromise.

Joint stiffness   The risk of stiffness is reduced by ensuring stability, avoiding prolonged immobilization and encouraging movement as early as possible.

Deformity   Some residual valgus or varus deformity is quite common but this can be compatible with good function, although constant overloading of one compartment may predispose to OA in later life.

Osteoarthritis   If, at the end of treatment, there is marked depression of the plateau, or deformity of the knee or ligamentous instability, secondary OA is likely to develop. Subsequently, this may require reconstructive/arthroplasty surgery.

KNEE INJURIES IN CHILDREN

PATELLAR SLEEVE FRACTURES

Sleeve fractures occur at the distal pole between the cartilage 'sleeve' and the ossifying patella due to forced quadriceps contraction on a flexed knee. These fractures occur most commonly in children aged 8–12 years when patella ossification is nearly complete.

Lateral *X-rays* may reveal small flecks of bone at the distal pole of the patella and patellar alta. *CT/MRI* may show this more clearly.

Undisplaced fractures with intact extensor mechanisms may be treated in long-leg casts or extension braces. Displaced fractures require open reduction and internal fixation.

PROXIMAL TIBIAL EPIPHYSEAL INJURIES

These injuries are uncommon due to the insertion of knee ligaments being distal to the tibial epiphysis. They are usually caused by a severe hyperextension and valgus strain and create a Salter–Harris type 2 fracture. Distal pulses should be checked as there is a risk of popliteal artery damage.

SECTION 3 TRAUMA

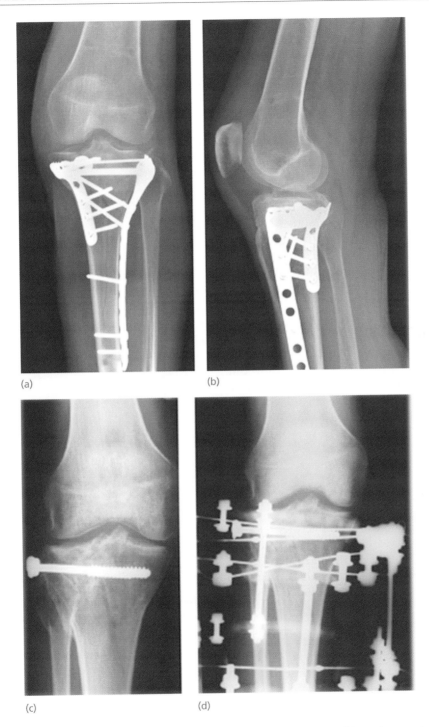

(a)　　　(b)

(c)　　　(d)

31.10 Complex tibial plateau fractures – internal fixation (a,b) Lateral locking plate and a posteromedial buttress plate to address all three (anterolateral, anteromedial and posterior) columns. (c,d) Percutaneous fixation of main fracture fragments with screws followed by stabilization of construct with fine-wire frame.

Imaging

Salter–Harris type 1 and 2 fractures may be undisplaced and difficult to see on *X-ray*. *CT* or *MRI* will demonstrate the injury. In displaced fractures, the fracture is categorized by the direction of displacement (hyperextension or flexion, varus or valgus types).

Treatment

Closed reduction is performed under anaesthesia. The fragment is reduced by gentle traction and manipulation. Fixation using smooth K-wires or screws may be needed if the fracture is unstable. The rare Salter–Harris type 3 or 4 fractures also may need open reduction and fixation.

Complications

Deformity   Subsequent angular deformity may require later operative correction.

Growth arrest   Complete growth arrest can occur and there is higher risk in more severe injuries. If the predicted leg length discrepancy is greater than 2.5 cm, tibial lengthening (or epiphysiodesis of the opposite limb) may be needed.

PROXIMAL TIBIAL METAPHYSEAL FRACTURES

This rare injury (Cozen's fracture) occurs between 4 and 8 years of age. There is a fracture of the medial cortex with valgus angulation. Most fractures can be managed non-operatively with reduction and immobilization in a varus moulded cast. The position must be carefully monitored during healing.

Rare complications include progressive valgus deformity after bony healing and possible tibial overgrowth resulting in leg lengthening.

TIBIA AND FIBULA SHAFT FRACTURES

Due to its subcutaneous position, the tibia is more commonly fractured, and more often sustains an open fracture (23.5% in one large study), than any other long bone.

Mechanism of injury

Twisting causes a spiral fracture of both bones at different levels. Angulatory forces produce transverse or short oblique fractures, usually at the same level.

- *Indirect injury* usually causes a low-energy, spiral or long oblique fracture, which may pierce the skin from within.
- *Direct injury* is usually high-energy, and crushes or splits the skin over the fracture.

Clinical features

The limb should be carefully examined.

> **WHAT TO LOOK FOR IN THE EXAMINATION OF TIBIA/FIBULA SHAFT FRACTURES**
>
> Bruising
> Severe swelling
> Crushing or tenting of the skin (**Table 31.2**)
> An open wound (**Table 31.3**)
> Degree of contamination
> Pain on passive stretch
> Weak or absent pulses
> Diminution or loss of sensation
> Inability to move the toes

 Always be on the alert for signs of an impending *compartment syndrome*.

Table 31.2 Tscherne classification of skin lesions in closed fractures

Grade	Skin lesion
IC1	No skin lesion
IC2	No skin laceration but contusion
IC3	Circumscribed degloving
IC4	Extensive, closed degloving
IC5	Necrosis from contusion

Table 31.3 Gustilo classification of open fractures

Grade	Wound	Soft-tissue injury	Bone injury
I	<1 cm long	Minimal	Simple low-energy fractures
II	>1 cm long	Moderate, some muscle damage	Moderate comminution
IIIA	Usually >1 cm long	Severe deep contusion + compartment syndrome	High-energy fracture patterns; comminuted but soft-tissue cover possible
IIIB	Usually >10 cm long	Severe loss of soft-tissue cover	Requires soft-tissue reconstruction for cover
IIIC	Usually >10 cm long	As IIIB, with need for vascular repair	Requires soft-tissue reconstruction for cover

Imaging

The entire length of the tibia and fibula, as well as the knee and ankle joints, must be seen. *CT angiography* is often used in the assessment of open fractures for the planning of soft-tissue reconstruction.

Management

> **MAIN OBJECTIVES OF MANAGEMENT OF TIBIA/FIBULA SHAFT FRACTURES**
>
> Limit soft-tissue damage and preserve (or restore) skin cover
> Prevent, or recognize and treat, a compartment syndrome
> Reduce and stabilize the fracture
> Start early weight-bearing (loading promotes healing)
> Start joint movements as soon as possible

With high-energy fractures, the most important consideration is the viability of the damaged soft tissues; often this will dictate or at least guide the optimal treatment. Further insult to the soft tissues is avoided where possible. They are more likely to require surgical stabilization (e.g. with intramedullary nailing).

NON-OPERATIVE TREATMENT

This may be suitable for some low-energy fractures. If the fracture is *undisplaced or minimally displaced*, a full-length cast from upper thigh to metatarsal necks is applied with the knee slightly flexed and the ankle at 90 degrees.

 Translation of fibular shaft fractures is unimportant. Alignment must be near-perfect and rotation absolutely perfect.

Minor degrees of angulation can be corrected by making a transverse cut in the plaster and wedging it. Regular checks of position are carried out by *X-ray*.

A change to a below-the-knee cast is possible around 4–6 weeks, when the fracture becomes 'sticky'. An alternative is a 'Sarmiento' cast, which allows knee flexion but confers some additional stability. The cast is retained (or renewed if it becomes loose) until the fracture unites, which is around 8 weeks in children but seldom less than 12 weeks in adults.

INTRAMEDULLARY NAILING

This is the method of choice for *diaphyseal fractures*. Modern nail designs allow for fractures closer to the joints to be treated. Care should be taken to identify and address any intra-articular extensions. Reamed locked intramedullary nailing achieves union in over 95% of cases (**31.11**). Locking allows immediate weight-bearing and range of motion exercises.

PLATE FIXATION

Plating can be used for *metaphyseal fractures* deemed unsuitable for nailing and complex periarticular fractures. Extensive incisions further insult the soft tissues and are avoided wherever possible with minimal access submuscular techniques preferred. It is also sometimes used for *unstable tibial shaft fractures in children* as it avoids the potential damage to the growth plate from nailing.

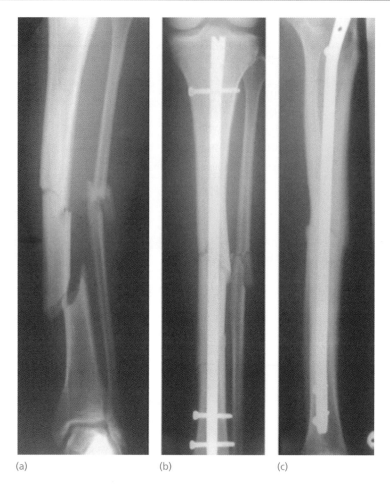

(a)   (b)   (c)

31.11 Fractured tibia and fibula – internal fixation Closed intramedullary nailing for unstable tibial fractures. **(a)** Position on admission to hospital. **(b,c)** AP and lateral views after intramedullary nailing. Active movements and weight-bearing can be commenced soon after operation.

EXTERNAL FIXATION

External fixation is a less frequently used alternative; it may avoid exposure of the fracture site and allow further adjustments. It has a particular role in *long, segmental, multifragmentary fractures* (31.12). Monolateral fixators are most commonly used as a temporizing method. It is more commonly used in children. Disadvantages include the need to span joints for sufficient stability. Circular external fixators confer greater stability and often negate the need to span joints.

Treatment of open fractures

Expert assessment and management of the soft tissues is key with degloving and the zone of injury often extending far beyond the visible wound. Two-stage surgery is commonly used to allow adequate debridement, temporary stabilization, followed by definitive bone fixation and soft-tissue reconstruction. The aim is to minimize the risk of infection while restoring function as soon as feasible. Guidelines such as the British Orthopaedic Association (BOA) Standards for Trauma (BOAST 4) provide a useful template for treatment. Primary closure may be feasible but requires expert assessment of the soft tissues to avoid high complication rates.

A suitable regimen for the treatment of open tibial fractures comprises:

SECTION 3 TRAUMA

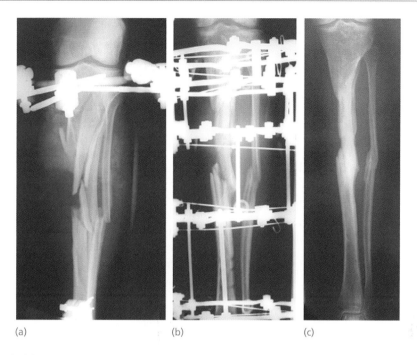

(a)　　　　　　　　(b)　　　　　　　　(c)

31.12 Fixation (a,b) Severely comminuted fractures treated by external fixation. This offers the benefit of multilevel stability and can be carried out with little additional damage to the soft tissues around the injury. **(c)** X-ray 6 months later showing fracture union in satisfactory alignment.

REGIMEN FOR THE TREATMENT OF OPEN TIBIAL FRACTURES

1 *Antibiotics*   These are started immediately (first- or second-generation cephalosporin or co-amoxiclav in most cases) and continued until definitive soft tissue cover or for a *maximum* of 72 hours, whichever is sooner.

2 *Document*   Wound photography is useful to avoid repeated exposure.

3 *Debridement*   Complete and adequate debridement involves excising and extending the wound and delivery of the bone ends. Dead, avascular or highly contaminated material is removed. Negative-pressure wound therapy is often used between stages to reduce oedema and encourage blood flow and granulation tissue formation.

4 *Lavage*   Thorough high-volume, low-pressure lavage is performed.

5 *Stabilization*   Temporary stabilization between stages can be achieved with plaster, external fixator or there is growing evidence for the use of temporary internal fixation if there is appropriate orthopaedic and soft-tissue reconstruction expertise to facilitate. Definitive fixation is most commonly performed with intramedullary nailing.

6 *Soft-tissue cover*   Definitive soft-tissue cover should be carefully planned and may require the full repertoire of soft-tissue reconstructive techniques including free flaps.

7 *Rehabilitation*   This is a critical component of achieving a successful outcome and commences as soon as the soft-tissue management allows. Orthopaedic reconstruction should aim to permit full weight-bearing and range of motion as soon as possible. A period of protected weight-bearing may be required in very unstable patterns but should be the exception.

Complications

VASCULAR INJURY

Fractures of the proximal half of the tibia may damage the popliteal artery requiring a high-index of suspicion and potential need for angiograms, exploration and repair.

COMPARTMENT SYNDROME

Tibial fractures – both open and closed – and intramedullary nailing are the commonest causes of compartment syndrome in the leg.

- *Early warning symptoms* are increasing pain and pain on passive stretch of affected muscle compartments.
- *Late signs* are numbness and absent pulses, which are worrying.

The diagnosis can be confirmed by measuring the compartment pressures in the leg and may be the only means of assessment in patients with reduced consciousness or those who are intubated. However, strong clinical suspicion must override any numerical figure obtained by the pressure monitoring.

 Once the diagnosis is made, decompression by two-incision, four-compartment open fasciotomy should be carried out with the minimum delay (**31.13**).

INFECTION

Open fractures are always at risk; even a small perforation should be treated with respect, and debridement carried out before the wound is closed.

With established infection, skeletal fixation should not be abandoned if the construct is stable; infection control and fracture union are more

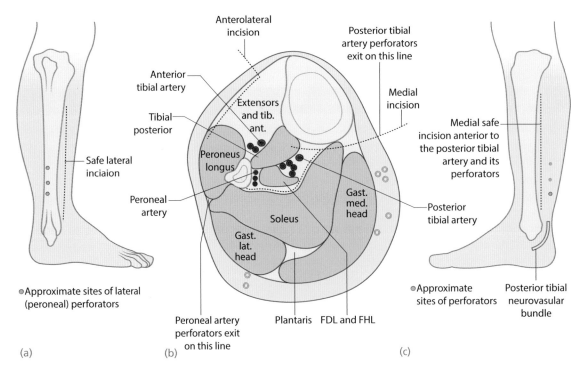

31.13 Fasciotomies for compartment decompression (a) The first incision is usually anterolateral, giving access to the anterior and lateral compartments. The superficial and deep posterior compartments also must be opened; their position is shown in **(b)**, a cross-section of the leg. This requires a second incision **(b,c)** which is made a finger's breadth behind the posteromedial border of the tibia; care must be taken not to damage the deep perforators of the posterior tibial artery. Note that the two incisions should be placed at least 7 cm apart so as to ensure a sufficient width of skin bridge without risk of necrosis.

likely if fixation is secure. However, if there is a loose implant, it should be removed and alternative stabilization achieved. Intractable infections also are unlikely to subside unless the implant is removed as part of treatment.

MALUNION

Slight shortening (up to 1.5 cm) is usually of little consequence, but angulation should be prevented at all stages. The normal ankle compensates more readily for a valgus deformity than for a varus one; however, anything more than 7 degrees in either plane is unacceptable. Malunion nearer the ends of the tibia is more likely to lead to early OA. Deformity, if marked, should be corrected by tibial osteotomy.

DELAYED UNION AND NON-UNION

High-energy fractures and fractures associated with bone loss or deep infection are slow to unite and liable to non-union. If there is a failure of union to progress on *X-ray* by 6 months, secondary intervention should be considered. Bone grafting may solve some 'slow' unions; in others, a different mode of fixation may be needed.

JOINT STIFFNESS

Prolonged cast immobilization is liable to cause stiffness of the ankle and foot, which may persist for 12 months or longer in spite of active exercises. This can be avoided by changing to a functional brace as soon as it is safe to do so, usually by 4–6 weeks.

COMPLEX REGIONAL PAIN SYNDROME

This is not uncommon in fractures of the distal third of the tibia. Exercises should be encouraged throughout the period of treatment. The management of the established condition is discussed in Chapter 26.

Ankle and foot injuries

32

Injuries of the ankle	**697**	■ Fractures of the calcaneum	710
■ Ankle ligament injuries	697	■ Midtarsal injuries	712
■ Malleolar fractures of the ankle	700	■ Tarsometatarsal injuries	713
■ Pilon fractures	703	■ Metatarsal fractures	714
■ Ankle fractures in children	705	■ Metatarsophalangeal joint injuries	715
Injuries of the foot	**707**	■ Fractured toes	715
■ Fracture of the talus	707	■ Fractured sesamoids	715

INJURIES OF THE ANKLE

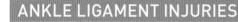

ANKLE LIGAMENT INJURIES

ACUTE LIGAMENT INJURIES

A sudden twist of the ankle momentarily tenses the structures around the joint. This may amount to no more than a painful wrenching of the soft tissues – a *sprained ankle*. If more severe force is applied, the ligaments may be strained to the point of rupture. If the tear is *partial*, healing is likely to restore full function to the joint; however, with *complete tears*, joint instability may persist.

More than 75% of ankle ligament injuries involve the lateral ligament complex, particularly the anterior talofibular ligament (ATFL) and calcaneofibular ligament (CFL) (**32.1**). Medial ligament injuries are usually seen in association with a fracture or joint injury.

Clinical features

A history of a twisting injury followed by pain, bruising and swelling is typical but could be anything from a sprain to a displaced fracture. In an ATFL sprain, tenderness is maximal just distal and slightly anterior to the lateral malleolus. The slightest attempt at passive inversion of the ankle is extremely painful. Stability assessment in the acute phase is not possible.

> ⚠ *It is essential to examine the entire leg and foot:* undisplaced fractures of the ankle, the more proximal fibula, tarsal bones and the peroneal tendon sheath are easily missed.

Imaging

* The need for *X-ray* is guided by the Ottawa ankle rules for when to X-ray. Anteroposterior, lateral and 'mortise' (15–20 degrees internally rotated) views of the ankle should be obtained. Weight-bearing views are useful in helping determine stability.

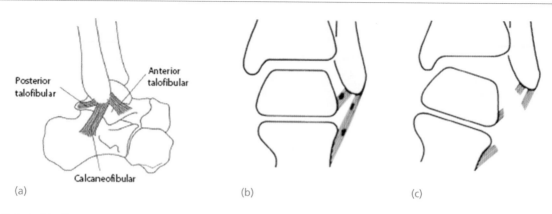

Posterior talofibular
Anterior talofibular
Calcaneofibular

(a) (b) (c)

32.1 Ankle ligament injuries (a) Schematic diagram showing the mortise-and-tenon articulation and main ligaments of the ankle. (b) The three components of the lateral collateral ligament. (c) The commonest injury is a partial tear of one or other component of the lateral ligament.

> **OTTAWA ANKLE RULES: WHEN TO X-RAY**
>
> Pain around the malleolus
> Inability to take weight on the ankle immediately after the injury
> Inability to take four steps in the Emergency Department
> Bone tenderness at the posterior edge or tip of either of the malleoli or the base of the fifth metatarsal bone

- *Computed tomography (CT)* and *magnetic resonance imaging (MRI)* may be needed to fully characterize an injury or in those who have persistent pain, swelling, instability and impaired function over 6 weeks or longer.

Treatment

NON-OPERATIVE TREATMENT

Initial treatment consists of protection, rest, ice, compression, elevation and rehabilitation (PRICER), which is continued for 1–3 weeks depending on the severity and response. Cold compresses should be applied for about 20 minutes every 2 hours, and after any activity that exacerbates the symptoms. An advice leaflet for patients is useful.

The use of oral or topical non-steroidal anti-inflammatory drugs (NSAIDs) during the acute phase can be helpful.

Functional treatment – i.e. protected mobilization without jeopardizing stability – provides earlier recovery of all grades of injury than either rigid immobilization or early operative treatment.

OPERATIVE TREATMENT

If the ankle does not start to improve within 1–2 weeks, further review is advised. Persistent problems after 12 weeks, despite physiotherapy, may include symptoms suggestive of cartilage damage or impinging scar tissue.

> **PROBLEMS SUGGESTIVE OF CARTILAGE DAMAGE OR SCAR TISSUE**
>
> Ankle pain and stiffness
> Instability
> Intermittent swelling

Arthroscopic repair or ligament substitution is now effective in many cases, allowing a return to full function and sports.

Deltoid ligament injuries

Disruption of the deltoid ligament is usually associated with a fracture of the distal fibula or tearing of the distal tibiofibular ligaments, allowing the talus to evert and externally rotate. Medial joint space is seen on *X-ray* and talar tilting may be apparent. If there is a medial injury but no lateral disruption, check for fracture or dislocation of the proximal fibula (*Maisonneuve injury*).

TREATMENT

- *If the medial joint space is reduced*, the ligament will heal. This often requires accurate reduction and fixation of fibular fractures or diastasis.
- *If it will not reduce*, it should be explored to remove any incarcerated tissue.

RECURRENT ANKLE INSTABILITY

Recurrent sprains and instability are potentially associated with cartilage damage, and warrant careful investigation by *MRI*, *arthroscopy* and examination under anaesthesia.

Lateral ligament instability

Lateral ligament laxity can be detected through talar tilt and anterior drawer tests.

TESTS FOR LATERAL LIGAMENT LAXITY

Positive talar tilt test, i.e. on stress *X-rays*, 5 degrees more than the normal side in the symptomatic ankle is considered abnormal

Positive anterior drawer test, i.e. 5 mm more than the normal side

---

TREATMENT

Initially, modified footwear (raised outer side of the heel), peroneal strengthening and a light brace are tried. If, despite these measures, problems persist, operative intervention may be required.

- *If there is functional but not demonstrable frank instability*, arthroscopic debridement of scar tissue and physiotherapy may suffice
- *If there is demonstrable instability*, an operation to stabilize the ankle by either repair or tightening of the ligaments or alternatively to construct a check rein against the unstable movement may be required (**32.2**).

PERONEAL TENDON DISLOCATION

Acute dislocation may be mistaken for lateral ligament injury. Look for an oblique fracture of the lateral malleolus (rim fracture) or a small flake off the lateral border (retinacular avulsion). Treatment in a weight-bearing cast or boot for 6 weeks will help some.

In *recurrent dislocation*, the peroneal tendons flick forward over the fibula during dorsiflexion and eversion. Repair of the retinaculum to the fibula helps in symptomatic individuals. Associated peroneal tears should be addressed at the same time.

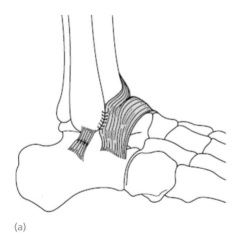

(a)

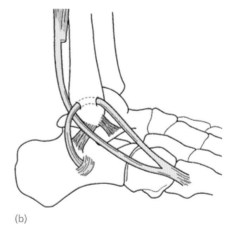

(b)

32.2 Recurrent lateral instability – operative treatment (a) The lax ATFL and CFL can be reinforced by a double-breasting technique (the Boström–Karlsson operation). (b) Another way of augmenting the lateral ligament is to reroute part of the peroneus brevis tendon so that is acts as a check rein (tenodesis) (the Chrisman operation).

MALLEOLAR FRACTURES OF THE ANKLE

Fractures of the malleoli and associated ankle fracture dislocations are common. Most are low-energy fractures and caused by a twisting, inversion injury. The ligamentous component can be just as serious as the fracture.

Mechanism of injury

The precise fracture pattern is determined by:

- the position of the foot
- the direction of force at the moment of injury.

The foot may be either pronated or supinated and the force upon the talus is towards adduction, abduction or external rotation, or a combination of these.

There is no completely satisfactory classification system.

- The *Lauge–Hansen system* groups fractures by the likely position of the foot and the direction of force at the moment of fracture and guides reduction but is relatively complex.
- The *Danis–Weber classification* focuses on the fibular fracture (Table 32.1) (32.3).

X-rays

Anteroposterior, lateral and 'mortise' views are required. The level of the fibular fracture is often best seen in the lateral view; diastasis may not be appreciated without a mortise or weight-bearing view. Further X-rays may be needed to exclude a proximal fibular fracture, up as high as the knee.

From a careful study of the X-rays, it should be possible to reconstruct the mechanism of injury.

Treatment

To achieve a reduced ankle, four objectives must be met.

OBJECTIVES OF TREATMENT TO REDUCE THE ANKLE
The fibula must be restored to its full length. The talus must sit squarely in the mortise with no tilt. The medial joint space must be restored to its normal width. There must be no tibiofibular diastasis.

Swelling can be severe and may preclude surgery until improved enough that the surgeon is confident they can close primarily. If swelling is

Table 32.1 Danis–Weber classification of malleolar ankle fractures

Classification	Description	Mechanism of injury
Type A	Transverse fracture of the fibula below the tibiofibular syndesmosis, sometimes associated with an oblique or vertical fracture of the medial malleolus	Almost certainly an adduction (or adduction and internal rotation) injury
Type B	Oblique fracture of the fibula in the sagittal plane (and therefore better seen in the lateral X-ray) at the level of the syndesmosis Often accompanied by an avulsion injury on the medial side (a torn deltoid ligament or fracture of the medial malleolus)	Probably an external rotation injury
Type C	Fracture above the level of the syndesmosis, which means that the tibiofibular ligament and part of the interosseous membrane must have been torn Associated injuries are: • avulsion fracture of the medial malleolus • rupture of the medial collateral ligament • a posterior malleolar fracture • diastasis of the tibiofibular joint.	Severe abduction or a combination of abduction and external rotation

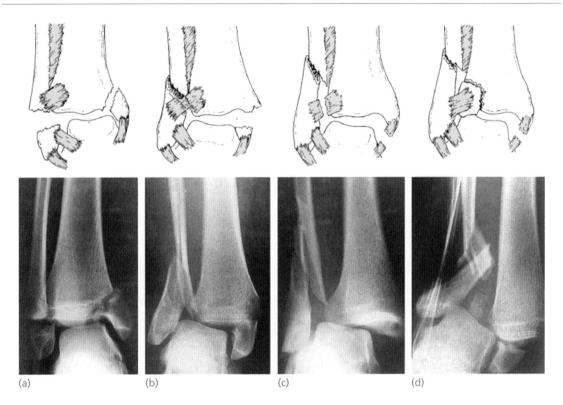

(a) (b) (c) (d)

32.3 Ankle fractures – classification The Danis–Weber classification is based on the level of the fibular fracture. **(a)** *Type A:* a fibular fracture below the syndesmosis and an oblique fracture of the medial malleolus (caused by forced supination and adduction of the foot). **(b)** *Type B:* a fracture at the syndesmosis often associated with disruption of the anterior fibres of the tibiofibular ligament and fracture of the posterior and/or medial malleolus, or disruption of the medial ligament (caused by forced supination and external rotation). **(c)** *Type C:* a fibular fracture above the syndesmosis; the tibiofibular ligament must be torn, or else **(d)** the ligament avulses a small piece of the tibia. Here, again, there must also be disruption on the medial side of the joint – either a medial malleolar fracture or rupture of the deltoid ligament.

not settling, it may be due to persistent subluxation or instability that needs to be addressed. Swelling will also occur postoperatively and elevation is required.

UNDISPLACED FRACTURES

The first step is to decide whether the injury is stable or unstable (**32.4**).

- *Isolated undisplaced Danis–Weber type A fractures* are stable and require only splintage for comfort.
- *Undisplaced type B fractures* are only unstable if the tibiofibular ligament is torn or avulsed, or if there is a significant medial-sided injury. Weight-bearing views can help determine

stability. If stable, the patient can mobilize full weight-bearing in a boot or cast and commence ankle range of motion exercises as soon as comfortable. Healing typically takes 6 weeks.

- *Undisplaced type C fractures* are innocent-looking but often accompanied by disruption of medial structures as well as the tibiofibular syndesmosis and interosseous membrane. Repeated checks to ensure no displacement are required and they may be easier to manage if fixed early.

DISPLACED FRACTURES

Reduction of these joint disruptions is a prerequisite to all further treatment. If satisfactory

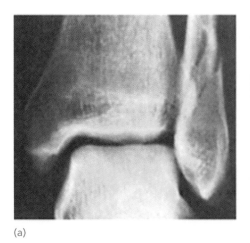

(a)

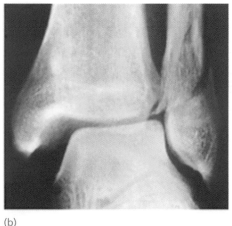

(b)

32.4 Ankle fractures – stable or unstable? **(a)** Stable fracture. In this Danis–Weber type B fracture, the tibiofibular syndesmosis has held; the surfaces of the tibia and talus are precisely parallel and the width of the joint space is regular both superiorly and medially. **(b)** Slight subluxation. The syndesmosis is intact but the talus has moved laterally with the distal fibular fragment; the medial joint space is too wide, signifying a deltoid ligament rupture. It is vital, after reduction of the fibular fracture, to check that the medial joint space is normal.

reduction can be achieved, even unstable fractures can be managed non-operatively. Recent randomized trial data has shown equivalent outcomes in the short to medium term in patients aged over 60.

- *Displaced Danis–Weber type A fractures* are usually accompanied by a nearly vertical medial malleolar fracture that tends to displace proximally and can be stabilized with screws or K-wires or, if comminuted, a tension-band wire or buttress plate. If the lateral malleolar fracture is reduced, it may not need fixing; if required, it is reduced and held with a plate and screws or intramedullary device.
- *Displaced type B fractures* are typically spiral and accompanied by an oblique medial malleolar fracture. If closed reduction is achieved, they can be managed conservatively, but imperfect reduction or further displacement requires fixation. Abduction injuries lead to a more transverse fibula fracture line and tend to be more unstable and more likely to require fixation.
- *Displaced type C fractures* occur above the syndesmosis and, frequently, there are associated medial and posterior malleolar fragments (**32.5**). Unstable fractures require restoration

of fibular length and fixation, often with fixation of the syndesmosis with screws or suspensory devices. Routine removal of syndesmotic fixation is not required in all cases. Aim to site hardware so it can be removed if it breaks. If the fracture is 1–2 weeks old, reduction may require opening and clearing out the syndesmosis.

Postoperative management Ankle range of motion exercises should be commenced early. Weight-bearing is dictated by the quality of the bone and fixation, but patients benefit from putting at least some weight through the ankle early.

OPEN FRACTURES

Open fractures of the ankle pose special problems due to the soft-tissue envelope. If the fracture is not reduced and stabilized at an early stage, it may prove impossible to restore the anatomy. Local soft-tissue reconstruction options include medial plantar flaps. The same principles as for the management of all open injuries need to be followed with expert assessment, thorough debridement, staged procedures where required and soft-tissue reconstruction playing an equally important role to fracture reduction and stabilization.

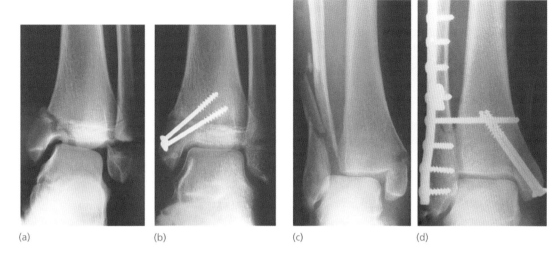

(a)   (b)   (c)   (d)

32.5 Ankle fractures – operative treatment (a,b) If the medial malleolar fragment involves a large segment of the articular surface, it is best treated by accurate open reduction and internal fixation with one or two screws. **(c,d)** An unstable fracture-dislocation almost always needs open reduction and internal fixation. The fibula must be restored to full length and fixed securely; in this case, the medial malleolus also needed internal fixation and the distal tibiofibular syndesmosis was disrupted, therefore secured with a tibiofibular screw.

Complications

VASCULAR INJURY

Neurovascular status must be checked pre and post any reduction manoeuvres. Reduction will often restore pulses but, if not, thorough vascular evaluation is called for.

WOUND BREAKDOWN AND INFECTION

The soft-tissue envelope is unforgiving. Diabetic patients are particularly at risk and fractures take longer to unite. The risks and benefits of conservative versus operative management need to be carefully weighed up.

STIFFNESS

Swelling and stiffness of the ankle are usually secondary to soft-tissue injury, including surgical approaches. Early range of motion helps reduce the incidence. Measures to reduce swelling and physiotherapy are helpful.

COMPLEX REGIONAL PAIN SYNDROME

This often follows fractures of the ankle. The patient complains of pain in the foot; there may be swelling and diffuse tenderness, with gradual development of trophic changes and severe osteoporosis. Management is discussed in Chapter 10.

OSTEOARTHRITIS

Malunion and/or incomplete reduction may lead to secondary osteoarthritis (OA) of the ankle in later years. Unless the ankle is unstable, symptoms can often be managed by judicious analgesic treatment and the use of firm, comfortable footwear. However, in the longer term, if symptoms become severe, arthrodesis may be necessary.

PILON FRACTURES

Pilon fractures occur when a large force drives the talus upwards against the tibial plafond. There is considerable damage to the articular cartilage and the subchondral bone may be broken into several pieces; in severe cases, the comminution extends some way up the shaft of the tibia.

SECTION 3 TRAUMA

Clinical features

Swelling usually becomes severe, fracture blisters are common and urgent reduction of dislocations is needed to help the soft tissues settle.

Imaging

This appears as a comminuted fracture of the distal end of the tibia, extending into the ankle joint. Sometimes the fibula also is fractured. The extent of the injury is usually not obvious in the plain *X-rays*; accurate definition of the fragments demands a *computed tomography (CT) scan* (**32.6**).

Treatment

The three points of early management are:

* span
* scan
* plan.

Judicious use of staged treatment may help reduce the complication rate in these complex injuries.

Control of swelling is a priority and best achieved by reduction and initial stabilization of the fracture, which may require a spanning

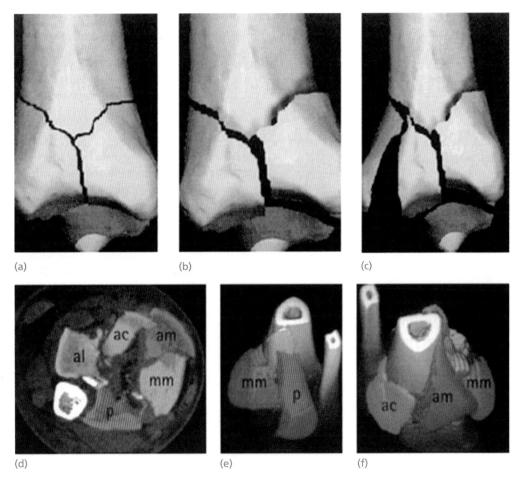

(a) (b) (c)

(d) (e) (f)

32.6 Pilon fractures – imaging These may be (a) undisplaced (type 1), (b) minimally displaced (type 2), (c) markedly displaced (type 3). CT (d) shows that there are usually five major tibial fragments: anterolateral (al), anterocentral (ac), anteromedial (am), the medial malleolus (mm) and the posterior fragment (p). These elements are usually clearly defined by 3D CT reconstruction (e,f).

external fixator. It can take 2–3 weeks before the soft tissues improve enough to allow definitive surgery.

Once the soft tissues allow, or using an approach that respects the zone of injury and pattern of vascularity, an open reduction and fixation with plates and screws may be possible. Severe injuries do not tolerate extensive exposures so indirect reduction techniques, percutaneous fixation and plating through limited exposures may be preferred. Circular frame and fine-wire fixation has also been successful.

The soft-tissue swelling following these injuries is substantial. After fixation, elevation and early movement help to reduce the oedema; arteriovenous impulse devices applied to the sole of the foot are also helpful.

Outcome

Pilon fractures usually take several months to heal. Physiotherapy focuses on joint movement and reduction of swelling. Although bony union may be achieved, the fate of the joint is decided by the degree of cartilage injury – the 'invisible' factor on X-rays. Secondary OA, stiffness and pain are frequent.

ANKLE FRACTURES IN CHILDREN

Physeal injuries are common in children and one-third occur around the ankle (32.7).

Mechanism of injury

A twisting injury occurs usually resulting in a *Salter–Harris type 1 or 2 fracture*. The fibula may also fracture more proximally. The tibial metaphyseal spike may come off posteriorly, laterally or posteromedially. With adduction injuries the tip of the fibula may be avulsed.

Type 3 and 4 fractures are uncommon and are due to a supination–adduction. The epiphysis is split vertically and part of the epiphysis (usually medial) may be displaced.

Two unusual variants are the Tillaux fracture and the notorious triplane fracture.

- *Tillaux fractures* are avulsions of a fragment of the tibia by the anterior tibiofibular ligament; in the child or adolescent, this fragment is the lateral part of the epiphysis and the injury is therefore a Salter–Harris type 3 fracture (32.8).

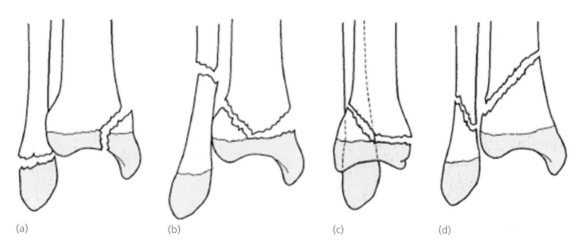

(a) (b) (c) (d)

32.7 Physeal injuries of the distal tibia The classification of Dias and Tachdjian points to the required reduction manoeuvre – reversing the causal mechanism. (a) *Supination–inversion:* the fibular fracture is usually an avulsion (Salter–Harris type 1) whereas the medial malleolar fracture can be variable. (b) *Pronation–eversion–external rotation:* the fibular fracture is often high and transverse. (c) *Supination–plantarflexion:* a fracture of the distal tibia only (Salter–Harris type 1 or 2) with posterior displacement. (d) *Supination–external rotation:* an oblique fibular fracture coupled with a fracture of the distal tibia.

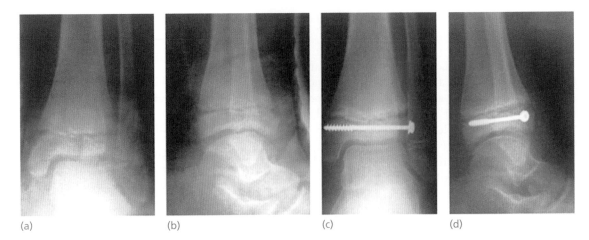

(a)   (b)   (c)   (d)

32.8 Tillaux fracture (a,b) This avulsion fracture of the lateral part of the physis was reduced and fixed percutaneously **(c,d)**.

- A *triplane fracture* occurs on the medial side of the tibia and is a combination of Salter–Harris type 2 and 3 injuries due to the pattern of fusion of the epiphysis. Fracture lines appear in the coronal, sagittal and transverse planes. Physeal injuries may result in asymmetrical or arrested growth.

Imaging

- Undisplaced physeal fractures are easily missed on X-ray and a hint of physeal widening should prompt repeat X-rays examination after 1 week if the diagnosis is not clear.
- Complex fracture patterns such as triplane fractures may need a CT scan to fully appreciate.

Treatment

- *Salter-Harris type 1 and 2 injuries* are treated closed with reduction under general anaesthesia if required followed by immobilization in a full-length cast for 3 weeks and then below-knee walking cast for a further 3 weeks. If irreducible, a periosteal flap may be blocking and need to be removed. *Undisplaced type 3 or 4 fractures* can be treated non-operatively with close monitoring to ensure no displacement occurs.
- *Displaced fractures* can sometimes be reduced closed. If the reduction is not anatomical, the fracture should be reduced open and fixed with interfragmentary screws, inserted parallel to the physis. Postoperatively the leg is typically immobilized for 6 weeks.
- *Tillaux fractures* are treated in the same way as type 3 fractures.
- *Triplane fractures,* if undisplaced, can be managed closed but require vigilant monitoring for late displacement. Displaced fractures must be reduced and fixed.

Complications

MALUNION

Imperfect reduction may result in angular deformity of the ankle – usually valgus.

- *In children under 10 years old,* mild deformities may correct.
- *In older children,* the deformity should be corrected by osteotomy.

ASYMMETRICAL GROWTH

Fractures through the epiphysis may result in fusion of part or all of the physis. The bony bridge is usually medial; the lateral half goes on growing and the distal tibia gradually veers into varus. *MRI* and *CT* are helpful in showing where it is.

- If the bridge is small (<30% of physeal width), it can be excised and replaced by a pad of fat in the hope that physeal growth may be restored.

- If more than half of the physis is involved, or the child is near the end of the growth period, supramalleolar osteotomy is indicated.

SHORTENING

Early physeal closure occurs in about 2% of children with distal tibial injuries. Fortunately, the resulting limb length discrepancy is usually mild. If it promises to be more than 2 cm and the child is young enough, proximal tibial epiphysiodesis in the opposite limb may restore equality.

INJURIES OF THE FOOT

Injuries of the foot are often followed by more severe effects than the initial injury suggests. The whole foot must be considered with the aim of restoring full weight-bearing without pain, with an appropriate propulsive gait.

Foot injuries are particularly easy to miss in the polytraumatized patient where they are common but initially underappreciated as the patient's symptoms are masked by injuries elsewhere or not apparent due to limited weight-bearing for other reasons.

Careful head-to-toe secondary and tertiary surveys are required in polytraumatized patients.

Clinical assessment

Examine the whole foot in a systematic manner as injuries are often multiple. Neurovascular assessment is critical.

Imaging

- Anteroposterior, lateral and oblique *X-rays* of the foot are required. Do not accept suboptimal views if suspicious of an injury. Weight-bearing views are useful to assess stability as long as the patient is able to apply weight to the foot.
- For irregular shaped bones such as the talus and calcaneum, *CT scans* are useful.

Treatment

Swelling is always a problem as it makes examination difficult and may lead to definitive treatment being delayed.

PRINCIPLES OF TREATMENT OF FOOT INJURIES

1 Realign and splint the foot, keep it elevated and apply CryoCuff or icepacks and intermittent pneumatic compression foot pumps.
2 Make the diagnosis, defining the extent of injury.
3 Start definitive treatment as soon as possible.

It is very important to commence range of motion and weight-bearing as soon as the treatment will permit. Prolonged immobilization can predispose to problems and must be avoided.

PROBLEMS ASSOCIATED WITH PROLONGED IMMOBILIZATION

Stiffness
Impaired function
Localized osteoporosis
Complex regional pain syndrome

FRACTURE OF THE TALUS

The talus is a vital structure for weight-bearing and has a vulnerable blood supply, particularly to the body, which is supplied mainly by vessels that enter the talar neck from the tarsal canal and then run retrograde from distal to proximal. Talar injuries are rare and due to high-energy injuries.

TYPES OF TALAR INJURY

Fractures of the neck, body, head or bony processes
Dislocations of the talus or the joints around it
Osteochondral fractures of the superior articular surface
Chip or avulsion fractures

Mechanism of injury

- *Talar neck fractures* are produced by forced ankle hyperextension with the neck coming into contact with the anterior edge of the tibia.
- *Talar body fractures* are usually axial compression injuries, or an eversion force fracturing the lateral process (snowboarder's fracture).
- *Avulsions* are associated with ligament strains around the ankle and hindfoot.

Clinical features

The foot and ankle are painful and swollen; if the fracture is displaced or the talus dislocated, there may be an obvious deformity or skin tenting or split.

> ⚠ Soft-tissue breakdown occurs rapidly if reduction is not achieved.

Imaging

Anteroposterior, lateral and oblique *X-ray* views are essential. *CT* helps define the fracture, displacement and associated injuries.

- *Talar neck fractures* are classified according to Hawkins (modified by Canale).

HAWKINS (MODIFIED BY CANALE) CLASSIFICATION OF TALAR NECK FRACTURES	
Type I	Undisplaced
Type II	Displaced with subtalar subluxation or dislocation
Type III	Displaced, with dislocation of the talar body
Type IV	Displaced vertical talar neck fracture with associated talonavicular joint disruption

- *Talar head fractures* are rare, usually involving the talonavicular joint.
- *Talar body fractures* are also rare and are difficult to fully appreciate without CT scan.
- *Lateral and posterior process fractures* are usually associated with ankle ligament strains. If

you are unsure whether it is a fracture or an ossicle, be guided by symptoms.
- *Osteochondral fractures* usually occur on the lateral dome and are frequently picked up late due to grumbling symptoms after an 'ankle sprain'.

Treatment

UNDISPLACED FRACTURES

Typically, undisplaced fractures of the neck or body are treated without weight-bearing for 4 weeks and then gradually built up. As swelling is often severe, split cast or removable boot are preferred in the early stages. It may be 8–12 weeks before splintage for walking can be discarded.

DISPLACED TALAR NECK FRACTURES

Type II fractures The slightest displacement makes it a type II fracture. Closed reduction can be attempted (traction is applied with the ankle in plantarflexion; the foot is then steered into inversion or eversion). If successful, a non-weight-bearing below-knee cast is applied. Weight-bearing is commenced when there are signs of union.

For those fractures that cannot be anatomically reduced, reduction and fixation is required, usually through an anteromedial approach that may be augmented by medial malleolar osteotomy.

Type III fracture-dislocations These require urgent open reduction and internal fixation with the approach determined by the fracture pattern and position of displaced fragments. Reduction of the talar body is difficult and may require a distractor to be placed across the joint.

DISPLACED TALAR BODY FRACTURES

Talar body fractures are usually displaced or comminuted involving the ankle and/or talocalcaneal joint, occasionally with dislocation.

- *Minimal displacement* can be accepted; a below-knee, non-weight-bearing cast is applied for 6–8 weeks; this is then replaced by a weight-bearing cast for another 4 weeks.
- *Displaced fractures* require reduction and fixation through exposures as described above

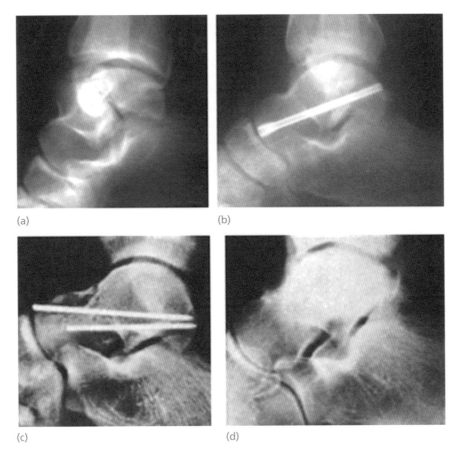

(a) (b)

(c) (d)

32.9 Fractures of the talus (a) This displaced fracture of the body of the talus was reduced and fixed with a counter-sunk screw **(b)** giving a perfect result. Fractures of the neck, even if well-reduced **(c)**, are still at risk of developing AVN **(d)**.

(**32.9**). The prognosis for these fractures is poor: there is a considerable incidence of mal-union, joint incongruity, avascular necrosis (AVN) and secondary OA of the ankle or talo-calcaneal joint.

DISPLACED TALAR HEAD FRACTURES

Treatment is guided by the state of the talona-vicular joint. Large fragments may be fixed and smaller ones excised if required.

TALAR PROCESS FRACTURES

Large fragments can be fixed with K-wires or small screws. Small fragments are left and can be excised later if symptomatic.

OSTEOCHONDRAL FRACTURES

These usually occur with severe ankle sprains or subtalar dislocations. Most acute lesions can be treated by immobilization for 4–6 weeks. Occasionally, large lesions warrant fixation but this is difficult and more often they are excised and microfracture performed.

OPEN FRACTURES

The general principles of open fractures apply.

 Urgent reduction of *injuries with threatened skin* to avoid them becoming open is vital.

SECTION 3 TRAUMA

Sometimes, in open injuries, the talus is completely detached and lying in the wound or extruded. After adequate debridement and cleansing, the talus should be replaced in the mortise and temporarily stabilized. Definitive fixation may need to be staged.

Complications

AVN

Talar body AVN can occur following displaced talar neck fractures. The incidence increases with severity of injury:

- *type I fractures* – less than 10%
- *type II fractures* – 30–40%
- *type III fractures* – more than 90%.

There is apparent increased density of the avascular segment by about 6 weeks; in reality, it is the rest of the tarsus that has become slightly porotic with disuse, but the avascular portion remains unaffected and therefore looks 'denser'. The opposite is also true: if the dome of the talus becomes osteoporotic, this means that it has a blood supply and it will not develop osteonecrosis. This is the basis of *Hawkins' sign*, which should be looked for 6–8 weeks after injury. Despite necrosis, the fracture may heal. If anything, weight-bearing should be delayed in the hope that the bone is not unduly flattened. However, if the talus becomes flattened or fragmented, or pain and disability are marked, the ankle may need to be arthrodesed.

FRACTURES OF THE CALCANEUM

Typically, the patient falls from a height onto one or both heels. The calcaneum is driven up against the talus and is split or crushed. Around 5–10% are bilateral and 20% suffer associated injuries of the spine, pelvis or hip. Avulsion fractures sometimes follow traction injuries of the tendo Achillis or the ankle ligaments. Occasionally, the bone is shattered by a direct blow.

EXTRA-ARTICULAR FRACTURES

Extra-articular fractures (**32.10**) account for around 25% and involve the calcaneal processes or the posterior part of the bone. In the tongue-type fracture, check the skin posteriorly: if there is pressure on the skin, urgent reduction may be required to prevent necrosis. Other than these, they are generally easy to manage and have a good prognosis. Treatment is 'closed' unless the fragment is large and badly displaced, in which case it will need to be fixed back in position.

INTRA-ARTICULAR FRACTURES

These fractures are much more complex and unpredictable. The primary fracture line runs obliquely across the posterior articular facet and the body from posteromedial to anterolateral. Posterior articular facet fracture lines depend upon the position of the foot at the time of impact.

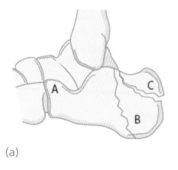
(a)

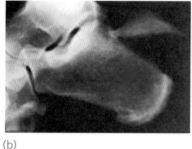
(b)

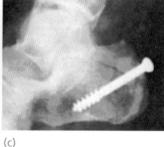
(c)

32.10 Extra-articular fractures of the calcaneum (a) Most extra-articular fractures occur through the anterior process (A), the body of calcaneum (B) or the tuberosity (C). Sometimes, the sustentaculum or the medial tubercle may fracture. (b) Avulsion fracture of the posterosuperior corner, which can be easily fixed by a screw (c).

- *If the heel is in valgus (abducted)*, the fracture is in the lateral part of the facet.
- *If the heel is in varus (adducted)*, the fracture is more medial.

The work of Sanders and Gregory has helped to define the intra-articular fracture pattern and the associated outcome and prognosis. The lateral joint fragment may sometimes be trapped within the body of the calcaneum and may require lateral wall osteotomy to reduce.

Clinical features

The foot is painful, swollen and bruised; the heel may look broad and squat. The normal concavity below the lateral malleolus is lacking. The subtalar joint cannot be moved but ankle movement is possible.

 Always check for signs of a *compartment syndrome of the foot* (intense pain, very extensive swelling and bruising and diminished sensation).

Imaging

Plain X-rays should include lateral views, but once a fracture has been identified, cross-sectional imaging (*CT scan*) is the standard of care. Extra-articular fractures are usually fairly obvious. Intra-articular fractures can also often be identified in the plain films and, if there is displacement of the fragments, the lateral view may show flattening of the tuber-joint angle (*Böhler's angle*) (**32.11**).

 With severe injuries – and especially with bilateral fractures – it is essential to assess the knees, the spine and the pelvis as well as the foot.

Treatment

Swelling is often severe so the patient usually requires admission for strict elevation and other measures to reduce swelling.

UNDISPLACED FRACTURES

These can be treated closed. Exercises are encouraged from the outset. When the swelling subsides, a firm bandage is applied and the patient is allowed up, non-weight-bearing on crutches for 6 weeks.

EXTRA-ARTICULAR FRACTURES

When they are threatening the skin, these may require reduction and fixation. Putting the foot into equinus can help reduce pressure on the skin posteriorly.

DISPLACED INTRA-ARTICULAR FRACTURES

These usually benefit from reduction and internal fixation. Fixation has traditionally been with plates and screws through an extensive lateral approach although percutaneous cannulated screw fixation from posterior to anterior is becoming more popular and has lower risks of wound breakdown. Postoperatively, the foot is lightly splinted and elevated. Exercises are begun as soon as pain subsides and, after 2–3 weeks, the

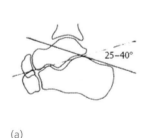
(a)

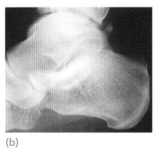
(b)   (c)

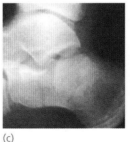

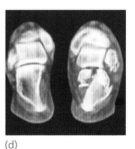
(d)

32.11 Fracture of the calcaneum – imaging (a,b) Measurement of Böhler's angle and the X-ray appearance in a normal foot. **(c)** Flattening of Böhler's angle in a fractured calcaneum. **(d)** The CT scan in this case shows how the articular fragments have been split apart.

patient can be allowed up, non-weight-bearing on crutches. Partial weight-bearing is permitted only when the fracture has healed (seldom before 8 weeks), and full weight-bearing about 4 weeks after that.

Complications

COMPARTMENT SYNDROME

Intense pressure symptoms develop in 10% of patients. The risk of compartment syndrome can be minimized by starting treatment early. If operative decompression is carried out, this will delay any definitive procedure for the fracture.

PERONEAL TENDON IMPINGEMENT

This may occur between the laterally displaced body of the calcaneum and lateral malleolus. Treatment consists of operative paring down of protuberant bone.

ACHILLES TENDON INSUFFICIENCY

Loss of heel height may result in diminished Achilles tendon action that may require subtalar arthrodesis with insertion of a bone block if persistently problematic.

TALOCALCANEAL STIFFNESS AND OA

Displaced intra-articular fractures may lead to joint stiffness and, eventually, OA. Persistent severe pain may necessitate subtalar arthrodesis or triple arthrodesis if the calcaneocuboid joint is also involved.

MIDTARSAL INJURIES

Injuries vary from minor sprains to severe fracture-dislocations which can threaten the survival of the foot. Isolated injuries of the navicular, cuneiform or cuboid bones are rare. Fractures in this region should be assumed to be 'combination' fractures or fracture-subluxations until proved otherwise.

Mechanism of injury

The Main and Jowett classification is useful (Table 32.2).

Clinical features

The foot is bruised and swollen with diffuse midfoot tenderness. Medial midtarsal dislocations look like an 'acute club foot' and lateral dislocations produce a valgus deformity. It is important to exclude distal ischaemia or a compartment syndrome.

Imaging

AP, lateral and oblique *X-rays* are required (**32.12**); weight-bearing views may demonstrate instability. *CT scans* are useful to delineate injury.

Treatment

LIGAMENTOUS STRAINS

The foot may be bandaged or supported until acute pain subsides. Movement is encouraged.

Table 32.2 Main and Jowett classification of midtarsal injuries

Classification	Description
Medial stress injury	Inversion of the foot If severe, can cause fracture-subluxation of the talonavicular or midtarsal joints
Longitudinal stress injury	Most common Caused by a severe longitudinal force with the foot in plantarflexion leading to fracture of the navicular and subluxation of the midtarsal joint
Lateral stress injury	Foot forced into valgus Causes fracture-subluxations of the cuboid and the anterior end of the calcaneum and medial avulsion injuries
Plantar stress injury	Foot twisted and trapped under the body Causes dorsal avulsion injuries or fracture-subluxation of the calcaneocuboid joint
Crush injury	Open comminuted midtarsal fracture

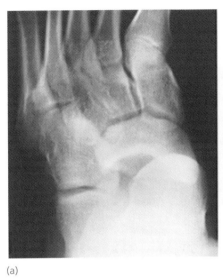
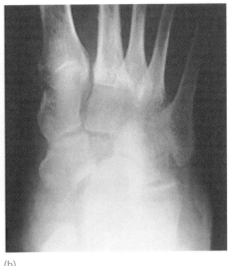

(a) (b)

32.12 Midtarsal injuries (a) X-ray showing dislocation of the talonavicular joint. (b) X-ray of another patient showing longitudinal compression fracture of the navicular bone and subluxation of the head of the talus. This injury is often difficult to demonstrate accurately on plain X-ray.

If symptoms do not settle within 2 weeks, check for a missed fracture.

UNDISPLACED FRACTURES

Elevate the foot. When swelling is improving, a below-knee cast or boot is applied and the patient commences protected weight-bearing. The support is retained for 6 weeks.

FRACTURE-DISLOCATIONS

Under general anaesthesia, the dislocation can usually be reduced by closed manipulation, but holding it is a problem. Open reduction is performed if necessary. Fixation can be achieved with K-wires or screws across the joints. Late diagnoses or severely damaged joints may benefit from spanning with a plate or arthrodesis.

The foot is immobilized in a below-knee cast for 6–12 weeks. Exercises are then begun and should be practised assiduously; it may be 6–8 months before function is regained.

TARSOMETATARSAL INJURIES

The five tarsometatarsal (TMT) joints form a structural complex that is held intact partly by

the interdigitating joints and partly by the strong ligaments that bind the metatarsal bones to each other and to the tarsal bones of the midfoot. Sprains are common, dislocations (e.g. *Lisfranc injury*) are rare but serious (**32.13**); twisting and crushing injuries are the usual causes.

> ⚠ A fracture-dislocation should always be suspected if the patient has pain, swelling and bruising of the foot after an accident, even if there is no obvious deformity.

Imaging

X-rays may be difficult to interpret; something looks wrong but it is often difficult to tell what. Concentrate on the second and fourth metatarsals in the oblique views: the medial edge of the second should be in line with the medial edge of the second cuneiform, and the medial edge of the fourth should line up with the medial side of the cuboid. A true lateral may show the dorsal displacement of the second metatarsal base. If a fracture-dislocation is suspected (the displacement may reduce spontaneously and not be immediately detectable), stress views may reveal the abnormality, but a *CT scan* is a more efficient way of showing the extent of injury.

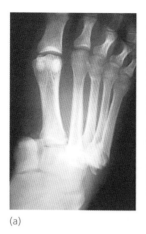
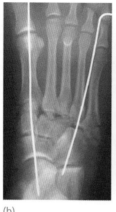
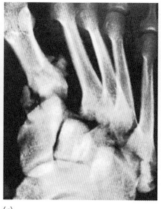
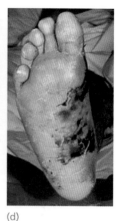

(a)   (b)   (c)   (d)

32.13 Tarsometatarsal injuries (a) Dislocation of the TMT joints. **(b)** X-ray after reduction and stabilization with Kirschner wires. **(c)** X-ray showing a high-energy fracture-dislocation involving the TMT joints. These are serious injuries which may be complicated by **(d)** compartment syndrome of the foot.

Treatment

UNDISPLACED SPRAINS

Undisplaced sprains require cast or boot immobilization for 4–6 weeks.

SUBLUXATION OR DISLOCATION INJURIES

These call for accurate reduction. Traction and manipulation under anaesthesia usually achieves reduction, and the position is then held with K-wires or screws and cast immobilization. When open reduction is required, it is usually to reduce the second metatarsal base through a longitudinal incision. A new cast is applied after the swelling has subsided and the patient is instructed to remain non-weight-bearing for 6–8 weeks before removal of wires.

METATARSAL FRACTURES

Metatarsal fractures are common.

COMMON CAUSES OF METATARSAL INJURIES
Crush injuries Spiral shaft fractures due to twisting Avulsion fractures Insufficiency fractures due to repetitive stress

In the usual case, there is a history of injury and the foot is painful and swollen but stress fractures have more insidious onset. Routine *X-ray* series will show the fracture or, for stress fractures, callus from healing after around 3 weeks.

Treatment

UNDISPLACED/MINIMALLY DISPLACED FRACTURES

For these fractures, a walking plaster or boot may be applied, mainly for comfort, and is retained for 3–6 weeks.

SEVERELY DISPLACED FRACTURES

In the unlikely event of severe displacement (particularly in the sagittal plane), reduction and fixation, may be justified. In that case, weight-bearing is avoided for 4 weeks and this is followed by a further 2–4 weeks in a weight-bearing cast.

FRACTURES OF THE BASE OF THE FIFTH METATARSAL

Forced inversion may lead to avulsion of the base of the fifth metatarsal. Most of these heal without any problem and the patient just needs to be protected against further inversion. There is, however, a watershed area in the blood supply at the metaphyseal–diaphyseal junction. Fractures in this area (*Jones fracture*) are at higher risk of non-union and therefore may justify a lower threshold for intervention.

STRESS INJURY (MARCH FRACTURE)

In a young adult (particularly a new army recruit or a sportsperson), the foot may become painful after overuse or sudden increase in activity. A tender lump is palpable just distal to the midshaft of a metatarsal bone, usually the second. The *X-ray* appearance may be normal at first. Later, a hairline crack may be visible and, after this, callus formation can be seen usually 3 weeks after symptom onset.

No displacement occurs and neither reduction nor splintage is necessary. The forefoot may be supported and normal walking is encouraged.

METATARSOPHALANGEAL JOINT INJURIES

Sprains and dislocations are common in dancers and athletes. Sprains require no more than light splinting such as buddy strapping. If the toe is dislocated, it should be reduced by traction and manipulation; the foot is then protected in a short walking cast for a few weeks.

FRACTURED TOES

A heavy object or stubbing the toe may fracture phalanges. If the skin is broken, the wound is cleaned (or debrided if contaminated), a sterile dressing applied and antibiotics given. The fracture is disregarded and the patient encouraged to walk wearing a supportive boot or shoe. Buddy strapping for 2–3 weeks may help.

FRACTURED SESAMOIDS

One of the sesamoids (usually the medial) may fracture from either a direct injury or sudden traction; chronic, repetitive stress is more often seen in dancers and runners.

The patient complains of pain directly over the sesamoid, and sometimes pain can be exacerbated by passively hyperextending the big toe. *X-rays* will usually show the fracture (which must be distinguished from a smooth-edged bipartite sesamoid).

Treatment is often unnecessary, although an injection of local analgesia and support in a boot or shoe for 2–3 weeks may help. Occasionally, intractable symptoms call for excision of the offending ossicle; care should be taken not to disrupt the flexor attachment to the proximal phalanx.

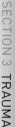

INDEX

Note: Page numbers in *italic* refer to figures.

ABC of trauma, 486–7
abduction, *9*, 10
accessory nerve, *see* spinal accessory nerve
acetabular fractures, 649–52
  associated fractures, 651
  complications, 652
  hip dislocation, *654*, 656
  Letournel classification, 649–51, *650*
  treatment, 651–2
acetabular implants, 416–18
  uncemented, 418, *418*
acetabuloplasty, *397*
acetylcholine, 227
Achilles' tendon, *see* tendo Achilles
achondroplasia, 137, 139, 329
acromioclavicular joint
  injuries, 553–5, *554*
  instability, 294
  osteoarthritis, 294–5, *295*, 555
acromion process, *276*, 277, *277*
acrylic cement, 269–70, 416
Actinomyces israelis, 47
action potential, 227
adduction, *9*, 10
adductor spasm (scissors stance), 207
adhesions, knee ligament injuries, 678
Adson's test, 244
adult respiratory distress syndrome (ARDS), 510–11, *510*

Advanced Trauma Life Support (ATLS®), 487–8
ageing; *see also* elderly
  and bone mass, 112, *112*
  fracture risk, *659*
  intervertebral disc degeneration, 375, 381–2, *381*
  osteoarthritis risk, 76, *76*, 77
  and tumours, 163
airway management (trauma), 486, 488, 490–3
airway obstruction, recognition, 491
albendazole, 48, 381
Albers-Schönberg disease (osteopetrosis), 139–40, *140*
alcohol intake, 94, 112, 116
alkaline phosphatase (ALP), 99, 102, 110, 117, 119, 166
allografts (bone), 258–9
allopurinol, 70
amniocentesis, 132
amputations, 264–6, *266*
  bone tumours, 167–8, 169
  fingers, 619
  indications (Apley's 'three Ds'), 264
  principles of technique, 266
  sites of election, 264–6, *266*
amyloidosis, in JIA, 63
amyoplasia, 223, 224, *224*
amyotrophic lateral sclerosis (motor neuron disease), 218

anatomical snuffbox, *310*
  swelling/tenderness, 599, *604*
Anderson/D'Alonzo classification (odontoid process fractures), 632
androgens, and bone metabolism, 107
aneurysmal bone cysts (ABCs), 162, 164, 176, *177*
angiosarcoma
  bone, 191
  soft-tissue, 195
ankle
  acute ligament injuries, 697–9
  examination, 454–7
  fractures in children, 705–7, *705*
  history, 453–4
  imaging, 457
  malleolar fractures, 700–3
  osteoarthritis, 474–5, 703, 712
  painful disorders, 477
  peroneal tendon dislocation, 699
  pilon fractures, 703–5
  recurrent instability, 699
  rheumatoid arthritis, 472–3, *473*
  stability testing, 456
  tuberculous arthritis, 472
ankle brachial pressure index (ABPI), 679
ankle jerk, 362

ankylosing spondylitis, 55, 57–60
  cause, 57
  cervical spine, 357
  clinical features, 58, *361*
  diagnosis, 58–9, 131
  and hip osteoarthritis, 414
  imaging, 58, *59*
  pathology, 57
  treatment, 59–60
antenatal screening, spina bifida,
  213
anterior cord syndrome, 640
anterior cruciate ligament (ACL),
  675
  assessment, 425–7, *427*, *429*
  bony avulsion, 678, *678*
  injury, 675–7
  reconstruction, 677
anterior drawer test
  ankle stability, 699
  knee stability, 676
anterior interosseous nerve, injury,
  569
anterior lumbar interbody fusion
  (ALIF), *387*
anterior superior iliac spine, 405
anterior talofibular ligament
  (ATFL), 697
anterior tibial (deep peroneal)
  nerve injury, 241, *241*
anterior (ventral), 8
antibiotic resistance, 24
antibiotics
  acute osteomyelitis, 30–1
  acute suppurative arthritis, 41
  chronic osteomyelitis, 35–6
  hand infections, 336, 339
  open fractures, 528, 530
  open tibial fractures, 693
  pyogenic spinal infection, 376–7
  subacute osteomyelitis, 33
antituberculous drugs, 46, 47, 380
AO/ASIF classification of spinal
  injuries, 625
AO/OTA classification,
  trochanteric region
  fractures, 658, *658*
aortic disruption, 496

Apert's syndrome, *156*
Apley's tests (knee), 428, 438
Apley's 'three Ds' (amputation),
  264
apophysitis, elbow, 572
apprehension test, 7, 549
  patellofemoral instability, 425,
  441, *442*
  shoulder stability, 287, *288*
Arnold–Chiari malformation, 214
arthritis; *see also* osteoarthritis;
  rheumatoid arthritis
  acute suppurative, 29, 31,
  38–42
  calcium pyrophosphate
  (pseudogout), 71–2, *72*
  gonococcal, 42
  reactive, 61–2
arthrodesis, 262
  DIP joint, *343*
  first CMC joint, *316*
  glenohumeral joint, 296
  knee arthritis, 452
  partial wrist, 317, *318*
  shoulder in poliomyelitis, *218*
  stages, 262, *262*
arthrography, hip, 407
arthrogryposis, distal, 223, 224
arthrogryposis multiplex
  congenita, 223–5, *224*
arthroplasty, 263–4, *263*; *see also*
  joint replacement; total
  hip arthroplasty
  excision, 263, *263*
  hip fractures, 660–1
  in osteoarthritis, 84
  partial replacement, 263, *263*
  shoulder, 295–6, *296*
  thromboprophylaxis, 252–4
  total replacement, 263, *263*
arthroscopy
  hip, 407–9, *409*
  knee, 429–30, *430*
  meniscectomy, 439
  shoulder, 277, 295
  wrist, 311
arthrotomy, 262
articular (hyaline) cartilage, 75, 98

loss/damage
  chondromalacia patellae,
  442–4
  osteoarthritis, 78, *78*, *79*
  osteonecrosis, 89, *89*
Aspergillosis, spinal, 380–1
aspirin, thromboprophylaxis, 253
ataxia, 203
athetosis, 207
atlantoaxial joint, 345, *348*
  instability, 136, 350
  rheumatoid arthritis, 355–6, *356*
  surgical stabilization, *356*, 357
atlantodental interval, *356*
atlanto-occipital erosion, 355–6,
  356
atlas (C1), 345, *345*
  imaging, 630–1, *631*
  ring fracture, 631–2
Austin Moore prosthesis, *263*
autonomic nervous system, 200,
  201
  dysfunction, 204–5
autosomal dominant inheritance,
  131
autosomal recessive inheritance,
  131
autosomes, 129
avascular necrosis, *see* osteonecrosis
avulsion, 548–9, *548*
  anterior/posterior cruciate
  ligaments, 678, *678*
  C7 spinous process, 635
  calcaneum, 710, *710*
  finger flexor tendons, 616, *616*
  lesser trochanter, 662
  pelvis, 644–5
  treatment, 549
axillary artery, injury, 557
axillary nerve, injury, 236, *236*,
  556
axis (C2), 345
  anomalies, 349–50
  imaging, 630–1, *631*
  injuries, 632, *633*
axonal regeneration, 229, *229*
axonotmesis, 229, *229*
axons, 199, *200*, 227–8, *228*

Babinski sign, 11
back disorders
    examination, 360–2, *360–2*
    history, 359–60
    imaging, 363–4, *365*
back pain; *see also* low back pain
    chronic syndrome, 391
Bacteroides fragilis, 25
Baker's cyst, *see* popliteal cyst
balance, sense of, 11
'bamboo spine', 58, *59*
Bankart lesion, 288, *288*, 542
'barbotage', 284
Barlow manoeuvre, 393, *394*
Barton's fracture, 591, *592*
baseball pitcher's elbow, 308
basic calcium phosphate (BCP)
        deposition disease, 72–4
Baumann's angle, 566, *566*
bed sores, 540
Beighton scores, 140
Bence–Jones proteins, 166
Bennet's fracture, 609, *610*
benzylpenicillin, 33
biceps tendon, *277, 279*
    distal tendinopathy, 308
    ruptured long head, 284–5,
        285
    tendinitis, 284
biochemical tests
    bone metabolic
        disorders, 110
    suspected tumours, 166
biofilms, 24, 34, 37–8
biological therapies, 56
biopsy, *see* bone biopsy; muscle
        biopsy
bisphosphonates, 114, 188
    adverse effects, 114
    osteogenesis imperfecta, 143
    osteoporosis, 114
    Paget's disease of bone, 128
bites, *338*, 339–40
bladder dysfunction, spinal lesions,
        212
bladder rupture, pelvic fractures,
        649
bladder training, 641

bleeding
    abdominal injuries, 504
    in closed fractures, *498*
    control of, 498–9
    hypovolaemic shock, 497, 498
    pelvic injuries, 504, 643, 648
blisters, fracture, 537
blood investigations
    acute osteomyelitis, 29
    RA, 54
'bloodless field', 249–50
blood transfusion, 499
Blount's disease, 434, *436*
body mass index (BMI), 112
bone
    age-related changes, 111–12, *111*
    blood supply, 101, *102*
    composition, 99–100, *100*
    mineral exchange, 105–6
    structure, 100–1, *101*
bone biopsy, 20–1, 110
    closed, 20
    open, 20
    osteomalacia, 110, *110*
    osteoporosis, 111, *111*
    osteosarcoma, 180
    precautions, 21
    principles, 166
    tumours, 166–7
bone cells, 99, *100*
bone cement, 269–70, 416
bone cement implantation
        syndrome, 661
bone cysts, 174–5
    aneurysmal, 162, 164, 176, *177*
    hydatid disease, 48
    osteoarthritis, 78, *78, 79*
    proximal humerus fracture,
        561, *562*
    radiographic appearance, *17*, 164
    simple, 164, 174, *176*
bone deformity, *13*, 14
bone development, 97–8, *98*,
        102–4
bone fixation
    external, 256, *258*, 526–8, *527*
    internal, 254, 256, *256*, 525–6,
        526

bone formation, 104–5
bone fragility, 112
bone grafts
    allografts, 259
    cancellous autografts, 36,
        257–8, *258*
    in chronic osteomyelitis, 36
    vascularized, 258–9
bone healing, *see* fracture healing
bone lesions
    imaging, 164–6, *165*
    investigation of 'suspicious',
        166
bone mass
    and age, 103–4, *104*, 112, *112*
    and bone strength, 112
    measurement, 109, *109*
    osteopenia, 109
    osteoporosis, 109
bone metabolic disorders
    assessment, 107–10
    bone mass measurement, 109,
        110
    chronic kidney disease, 122–3
    common presentations, 108
    examination, 108
    hypercalcaemia, 123–6
    hypocalcaemia, 116–17
    osteoporosis, 111–16
    rickets and osteomalacia,
        117–22
bone metabolism, 104–5
    and hormones, 106–7
    and mechanical stress, 107, *108*
    mineral exchange, 105–6
bone metastases, 125–6, 191–2
    clinical presentation, 163, 191
    imaging, *17, 19*, 126, *126*, 164,
        191, *192*
    pathological fractures, 546, *546*
bone mineral, 99
bone mineral density (BMD)
    and age, 103–4, *104*
    genetic factors, 104
    and osteoarthritis risk, 78
bone modelling, 103
bone morphogenetic proteins
        (BMPs), 104–5, 259

bone remodelling, 105
bone resorption, 104
bone substitutes, calcium-based
        synthetic, 259, *260*
bone 'transport', 37, *37*, 148
bone tumours; *see also* bone
        metastases
    benign, 169–79
    epidemiology, 161
    imaging, 164–6
    limb salvage, 167–8, *168*
    locally advanced, 169
    management principles, 167–9,
        168
    primary malignant, 179–91
    radionuclide scanning, 19, *19*
    staging, 162–3
    X-rays, 17, *17*
bone turnover, 105
    biochemical markers, 110
bony lumps, 14, *15*
    clinical features, 15
    knee, 432–3
Boston brace, 369
Boström–Karlsson operation, *699*
botulinum toxin, cerebral palsy,
        209
Bouchard's nodes, 342
boutonnière deformity, 334, *335*
bow legs, see genu varum
bowstring sign, 362, *363*
brachial artery, injuries, 569, 576
brachial neuritis, acute (neuralgic
        amyotrophy), 220–1,
        221, 351
brachial plexus, 232, *233*
brachial plexus injuries, 232–4,
        293, 557
    clinical features, 233–4
    management, 234
    obstetric, 234–5, *235*
bracing, scoliosis, 369
breathing management (trauma)
    at scene of accident, 486
    chest injuries, 493–7
    secondary survey, 488–9
brittle bones (osteogenesis
        imperfecta, 142–3, *143–5*
Brodie's abscess, 32, *32*

Brown-Séquard syndrome, 640
'brown tumours', 125, *125*, 164,
        166
buckle fractures, distal radius, 595,
        596
bulge test, 425, *426*
'bunions', 468, *470*
burns, 506–9
    assessment of extent and depth,
        506, *507*
    chemical, 508
    cold injury, 508–9, 623
    electrical, 508, 623
    hands, 623–4
    thermal, 506–8
bursae, semimembranosus, 432
bursitis
    calcaneal, 478, *478*
    knee, 432
    olecranon, 69, 305–6, *306*, *306*
burst fractures
    cervical spine, 633–4, *634*
    lumbar spine, 638–9, *639*
buttress plate, 685, *686*, *689*

café-au-lait spots, 144, *147*
Caisson disease, 92–3
calcaneal bursitis, 478, *478*
calcaneofibular ligament (CFL),
        697
calcaneonavicular bar, 463, *464*
calcaneum, fractures, 710–12,
        710–11
calcaneus, 457
calcific tendinitis, supraspinatus
        tendon, 73, *73*, 283–4,
        284
calcitonin, 107
calcitriol, 117
calcium, 105–6
    dietary sources, 105
    serum, 110, 119
    supplements, 113
    urinary, 110
calcium pyrophosphate dihydrate
        (CPPD) crystal-associated
        arthropathy, 70–2
calf squeeze test, 476, *477*
callosities, foot, 453–4, *455*, *481*

callus formation, 515, 516, *516*,
        517
camptodactyly, *330*
cancellous bone grafts, 36, 257–8,
        259
cancellous (trabecular) bone, 100,
        101
candidiasis, 47
Capener's sign, 402
capitellum
    fracture, 577–8
    osteochondritis dissecans, 305,
        306
capitulum, osteonecrosis, *88*
carbon fibre, 269
carbon monoxide poisoning, 506
carboxyhaemoglobin, 506, 507
cardiac disorders
    Ehlers–Danlos syndrome, 142
    in Paget's disease, 128
cardiac injury, blunt, 496
cardiac tamponade, 494
cardiogenic shock, 497
carpal injuries, 597–605
    clinical assessment, 597
    common, 597
    imaging, 597–8, *598*
    lunate and perilunate injury,
        603–4, *605*
    management principles, 598–9
    scaphoid fracture, 599–602,
        600–1
carpal instability, 318–19, *319*, 598
    chronic, 318–19, *319*
    traumatic, 598
    X-ray patterns, 598, *598*
carpal tunnel syndrome, 322–3,
        322, 328
carpectomy, proximal row, 317,
        318, *601*, 602
carpometacarpal boss, 321, *321*
carpometacarpal (CMC) joints
    dislocation, 608–9, *609*
    first, osteoarthritis, 315, *316*
cartilage calcification
        (chondrocalcinosis), 71, *71*
cast splintage, 524
    complications, 524, 537
    technique, 524

tibial fractures, 691
cauda equina, 640
    compression, 382, 383, 384
cauda equina syndrome, 205
cellulitis, 29
    anaerobic, 536
cement, acrylic, 269–70, 416
central cord syndrome, 640
central nervous system (CNS),
    199–200
cerclage wires, 525
cerebellar function, 11
cerebral palsy, 206–10
    causal factors, 207
    deformities, 207–8, *207*, 333,
        334
    early and late diagnosis, 207
    incidence, 206
    management, 208–10,
        209, 211
    posture and gait, 208
    types of motor dysfunction,
        207
cervical ribs, 244–5, *245*
cervical spine
    acute intervertebral disc
        prolapse, 350–2, *351*
    anatomy, 345–6, *345*
    ankylosing spondylitis, 357
    anomalies, 152, *153*, 349–50
    chronic disc degeneration
        (cervical spondylosis),
        352–4, *353*
    examination, 346, *347*
    history, 346
    imaging, 347–9, *348*
    immobilization, 490, 629–30,
        630
    normal range of motion, *348*
    operative stabilization, *356*, 357
    pyogenic infection, 354
    rheumatoid arthritis, 355–7,
        356
    tuberculosis, 354–5, *355*
    tumours, 352, 353
    vertebral spur, 352
cervical spine injuries, 630–6
    acute disc herniation, 635
    at more than one level, 635

avulsion of C7 spinous process,
    635
clinical features, 630
hyperextension, 635
imaging, 630–1, *631*
lower spine (C3 to C7), 632–5
methods of treatment,
    629–30
occipital condyle fracture, 631
occipitocervical dislocation, 631
operative fixation, 630
SLIC scoring system, 632–3
spinal cord injury, 640
sprains (whiplash injury),
    635–6
upper spine (C1 and C2),
    631–3, *632*
cervical spondylosis, 352–4, *353*
cervical–vertebral synostosis
    (Klippel–Feil syndrome),
    152, 293, *293*
Chance fracture, 636, 639
Charcot joints, 42, 77, 220, 475,
    475
Charnley total hip arthroplasty,
    417, *417*
chemical burns, 508, 623
chemotherapy
    antituberculous, 46, 47, 380
    neoadjuvant in bone tumours,
        168–9, 180, 188
chest drain, 494, 495
    insertion procedure, 495, *496*
chest expansion, assessment, 361
chest injuries, 493, 641
    immediately life-threatening,
        493–5
    mediastinal, 497, 641
    potentially life-threatening,
        495–7
    thoracic cage fractures, 495,
        521, 641
children
    acute haematogenous myelitis,
        25, 26–7, *27*, 30
    acute suppurative arthritis, 38,
        39–40
    ankle fractures, 705–7
    bone development, 97–8, *98*

distal humerus fractures,
    565–74
elbow fractures, 570–1, *571–2*
examination, 12
femoral fractures, 669–70, *670*
forearm fractures, 582–3, *583*
genetic disorders, 132
hip fractures, 663–4, *664*
knee deformities, 433–5, *433–5*
non-accidental injuries, 572–4,
    574, 670
normal developmental
    milestones, 12
olecranon fractures, 582
pes planus/pes valgus, 463–4,
    463
pulled elbow, 578
supracondylar fractures,
    566–70
Chinese, 77
chin lift, 491, *492*
Chlamydia trachomatis, 61
chloramphenicol, 30
chondroblastoma, 164, *165*, 172
chondrocalcinosis, 71, *71*
chondrolysis, 42
chondromalacia patellae, 442
chondromas, multiple, 171, *171*
chondro-osteodystrophies,
    134–40
chondroplasty, knee, 444
chondrosarcoma, 182–5
    primary central, 183, *183–4*
    secondary central, 184
    secondary peripheral,
        184, *185*
chordoma, 189, *190*
chorionic villus sampling, 132
chromosome disorders, 130, 134,
    150–1
chromosomes, 129–30
chronic back pain syndrome, 391
chronic kidney disease (CKD),
    122–3
Chvostek's sign, 117
circulation
    burns, 507
    major trauma, 486–7, 489
    shock, 498–9, *499*

clavicle
    congenital pseudarthrosis, 154,
        155, 294, *294*
    fractures, 232, 551–2, *552*
claw toes, 457, 465, *465*, 471–2,
        471
clay shoveller's fracture, 635
clinodactyly, *330*
Clostridium perfringens
        (*C. welchii*), 536
club foot
    arthrogryposis multiplex
        congenita, 224, *224*
    idiopathic (talipes equinovarus),
        457–61
Clutton's joints, 44
co-amoxiclav, 530
cobalt–chromium-based alloys,
        267
Cobb's angle, 366, *367*
coccyx, injuries, 652
cock-up deformity, 472
Codman's triangle, 180, *181*
colchicine, 70
cold injury, 508–9, 623, *623*
Coleman block test, 466, *466*
collagen, type I, 99
collagenase injections, 331, *333*
collagen disorders, 134
    Ehlers–Danlos syndrome,
        141–2
    generalized joint laxity, 140–1,
        141
    osteogenesis imperfecta, 142–3,
        143–5
collars, cervical spine, 629
collateral ligaments
    elbow, 306
    knee, 425, 675, 678
    thumb MCP joint, 611–12, *612*
Colles' fracture, 589–90, *591*
    impacted, 318
    risk and ageing, *659*
comminuted fractures, 519
    distal femur, 671, *672*
    distal tibia (pilon), 703–5
    femoral supracondylar fracture,
        672, *672*

middle phalanx, 613–14, *615*
olecranon, 580–1
patella, 682
proximal radius, 580
tibia, 691, 692, *693*
common peroneal nerve injury,
        240–1, *241*, 680
comorbidity, hip arthroplasty, 419
compact bone, 100, *101*
compartment syndrome, 535–6
    calcaneum fractures, 712
    clinical features, 535, 694
    crush syndrome, 509, 510
    forearm bone fractures, 583,
        585
    open fractures, 528
    prevention after distal radius
        fractures, 597
    supracondylar fractures, 569
    tibial plateau fractures, 688
    tibial shaft fractures, 694
    treatment, 535–6, 694
complex regional pain syndrome,
        286, 542
    after ankle fractures, 703
    after wrist fractures, 595
    shoulder, 286
    symptoms, 542
    tibial fractures, 695
    treatment, 542
    types, 542
compression stockings, 253
computed tomography (CT), 18
    3D reconstruction, 18, *18*
    acute osteomyelitis, 28
    calcaneum fracture, 711, *711*
    cervical spine, 349, 356, 628,
        634, *634*
    chronic osteomyelitis, 34–5
    elbow, 300
    foot/ankle, 457
    fractures, 519
    hip (adult), 406, *407*
    hip dislocation, 653, *654*
    pilon fractures, *704*
    proximal humerus fracture,
        560, *561*
    quantitative (QCT), 108

scaphoid fractures, 599, *600*
scapular fractures, 553, *553*
skull fractures, *502*
spinal injuries, 628, *629*
spinal stenosis, 389, *390*
spine, 364
tarsal coalition, 464, *464*
tibial plateau fractures, 685,
        685
trauma, 489, *490*
tumours, 165
wrist, 311
concussion, 501
Cone's callipers, 629, *630*
conjunctivitis, Reiter's disease,
        61, *61*
connective tissue disorders, 140–5
constriction bands, hands, 329,
        330
contrast radiography, 17
conus medullaris, 640
coracoacromial ligament, 277, *277*
    removal, 283, *283*
coracoclavicular ligaments, 553,
        554
coracoid process, 277
core needle biopsy, 166–7, *167*
corns, 453–4, *454*, 481
cortical function, 11
corticosteroids
    gout, 70
    muscular dystrophy, 225
    osteonecrosis, 91, 94
    and osteoporosis, 115
    RA, 56
    Reiter's disease, 62
    SLE, 64
Corynebacterium propinquum, 382
coxa vara
    developmental, 397, *398*
    in femoral dysplasia, 157
    following hip fracture, 664,
        664
Cozen's fracture, 690
CPPD, *see* calcium pyrophosphate
        dihydrate (CPPD) crystal-
        associated arthropathy
craniotabes, 118

crepitus, knee, 425
cricoid cartilage, 345
cricothyroidotomy
   needle, 491
   surgical, 492
CRITOE mnemonic, 566
cruciate ligaments
   bony avulsion, 678, *678*
   clinical assessment, 425–7, *427*
   imaging, 429, *429*
   injuries, 675–7
crush syndrome, 509–10
Cryptococcus, 381
crystal deposition disorders, 67
   basic calcium phosphate, 72–4
   calcium pyrophosphate
      dihydrate, 70–2, *71*, *72*
   gout, *54*, 55, 67–70, 306, 474,
      474
cubital tunnel, 238
cubitus valgus, 300, *302*
cubitus varus, 300, *301*, 569–70,
   570
Cushing's disease, 107, 115
cyclo-oxygenase, 2 (COX-2)
   inhibitors, 84
cyclophosphamide, 168–9
cytokines, synovial fluid, 75

dabigatran, 253
Danis–Weber classification (ankle
   fractures), 700, *701*
dead space, 36–7
debridement
   chronic osteomyelitis, 36
   open tibial fractures, 693
decompression disease, *see* Caisson
   disease
deep tendon reflex, 10
deep vein thrombosis (DVT), 252
   prevention, 252–4
   risk factors, 251
deformities, 5, *5*, 12–16; *see also*
   under the parts concerned
   back disorders, 359
   cerebral palsy, 207–8, *207*, 333,
      334
   common causes, 14

elbow, 297, 298, 300–1, *301–2*
   fixed, 13
   fixed flexion, 13
   fracture malunion, 539, *539*
   JIA, 62–3, *63*
   neuromuscular disorders, 202,
      203–4
   physeal injuries, 548
   postural, 13
   in spina bifida, 215–16, 458,
      459
   structural, 13
   surgical correction, 260, *261*
   valgus/varus, 13, *13*
delayed union, 517, 537–8
   femoral shaft fractures, 669
   forearm bone fractures, 584
   tibial shaft fractures, 695
deltoid ligament injury, 698–9
deltoid muscle
   examination, 274
   weakness, 238
demyelination, 219–20, 227
dendrites, 199, *200*
denosumab, 114, 174, *175*
deoxyribonucleic acid (DNA), 120
De Quervain's disease, 320, *320*
dermatofibroma, *344*
dermatomes, *204*
dermoid, implantation, *344*
developmental disorders; *see also*
   individual disorders
   classification, 134
   non-genetic, 130–1
developmental dysplasia of the hip
   (DDH), 393–7
   adult, 412, *412*
   classification, 393, 395
   diagnosis, 395
   and hip osteoarthritis, 412–13,
      412
   imaging, 395, *395*
   management, 395–7
   pathophysiology, 393–4
developmental milestones, 12
dexterity, 328
diabetes mellitus
   foot disorders, 475–6, *475*, *481*

neuropathy, 220
   and osteoporosis, 116
   vascular disease, 475
diagnostic imaging, 16–20
diaphragm, injury, 497
diaphysis, *98*
Dias and Tachdjian classification,
   705
diet
   calcium sources, 105
   and osteoarthritis, 77
   vitamin D deficiency, 117–18
DiGeorge syndrome, 116, 117
digital anomalies, 156, *156*
'dinner-fork' deformity, 589
diplegia, 203, 207, 210
direct anti-Xa inhibitors, 253
direct lateral interbody fusion
   (DLIF), 387
discectomy, 353, 384
discitis, pyogenic, 376–7, *377*
discography, MRI, *365*
discoligamentous complex (DLC),
   633
disease-modifying antirheumatic
   drugs (DMARDs), 56,
   414
dislocations, 549
   acromioclavicular joint, 553,
      554
   after fractures, 542
   clinical features, 549
   complications, 549
   elbow, 576–7, *577*
   habitual (voluntary), 549
   knee, 678–80, *679*
   midtarsal, 712, *713*
   radial head, 578
   recurrent, 549
   shoulder, 287, 556–9
   sternoclavicular, 555, *555*
   suppurative arthritis, 41, *41*
   treatment, 549
distal interphalangeal (DIP) joints
   arthrodesis, *343*
   flexor tendon avulsion,
      616, *616*
   osteoarthritis, 342, *342*

distal radioulnar joint (DRUJ)
  acute dissociation, 602
  arthritis, 316, *317*
  injuries, 587–8, 595, 602
  instability, 580
distal (term), 9
distraction osteogenesis, 259–61, *261*
dorsal intercalated segmental
    instability (DISI), *598*, 603
dorsal rhizotomy, 209
dorsiflexion, 10
  loss, 240–1, *241*
Down's syndrome (trisomy, 21), 130, 150, *151*
doxorubicin, 168
drapes, surgical, 250–1
drawer test
  ankle stability, 456
  knee stability, 426, *427*
  posterior (shoulder), 290
Drehmann's sign, 402
drop-foot gait, 203, 455
drop-wrist palsy, *10*, 237, *237*
drug-induced disorders, osteonecrosis, 94
DRUJ, *see* distal radioulnar joint
dual-energy X-ray absorptiometry
    (DEXA) scans, 103, 109
  indications, 110
  output, 109, *109*
Duchenne (pseudohypertrophic)
    muscular dystrophy, 225
Dunn osteotomy, 403
Dupuytren's contracture, 325, 331–2, *332–3*
Dupuytren's diathesis, 194
dysraphism, 212–16, *213*
dystonia, 203

Echinococcus granulosis, 48, 381
eFAST (extended focussed
    assessment with
    sonography), 490
Ehlers–Danlos syndrome, 141–2
elbow
  anatomy, 565–6, *566*

congenital radioulnar synostosis, 156, *156*, 300, *300*
deformities, 297, 298, 300–1, *301–2*
dislocation, 576–7, *577*
epiphyseal ossification, 300
examination, 297–9, *298–9*
history, 297
imaging, 299–300
loose bodies, 304–5, *305*
loss of function, 297
medial epicondylar apophysis
    separation, 571–2
medial epicondyle apophysitis, 572
movement, *298*, 299, *299*
olecranon bursitis, 69, 305–6, *306*
osteoarthritis, 82, 302–3, *305*
osteochondrosis
    (osteochondritis), *95*, 305, *306*
pulled (children), 578
radial head dislocation, 578
recurrent instability, 306, 580
rheumatoid arthritis, 302, *304*, 306
stiff, 301, *303*
tendinopathies, 307–8, *307*
tuberculosis, 301–2
ulnar nerve compression, 242–3
ulnar nerve injury, 238, 297
elbow fractures, 565, 565–80;
    see also humerus
    fractures, distal
  adults, 574–6
  capitellum, 577–8
  fracture–dislocation, 576
  fracture-separation of distal
    humerus epiphysis, 572–4, *574*
  lateral condyle (children), 570–1, *571*, *572*
  medial condyle (children), 572
  olecranon, 580–2, *581*
  proximal radius, *577–8*, 578–80
  supracondylar, *303*, 566–70, *567–8*

elderly
  acute osteomyelitis, 30
  back pain, 375, 386, 390
  fracture risk, *659*
  hip fractures, 657, 659, 660, *660*
    complications, 662
  kyphosis, 114, *114*, 374, 375
  proximal humerus fractures, 559
electrical burns, 508, 623
electrical stimulation, 253
electromyography (EMG), 21, 206, 231
Elmslie–Trillat procedure, *443*
embolization, pelvic fractures, 648
enchondroma, 164, 170, *171*
endochondral bone, 97–8
endochondral ossification, 102, *103*
endoneurium, 227–8, *228*
endosteal membrane, 101
Enneking staging system, 162
entonox, 490
enzyme defects, 134
  Gaucher's disease, 93–4, 130, 133, 149–50
  mucopolysaccharidoses, 145, 147–50
eosinophilic granuloma, 164
epidural abscess, 212, 376
epineurium, 228, *228*
epiphyseal dysplasia, multiple, 135, *135–6*
epiphysis, 97, *98*
  blood supply, *25*
epithelioid
    haemangioendothelioma, 191
epithelioid haemangioma, 191
equinovarus, 216, 457
equinus deformity, *207*
Erb's palsy, 234, *235*
erythema marginatum, 29
Escherichia coli, 376
Essex-Lopresti lesion, 580
etoposide, 169

Ewing's sarcoma, *17*, 163, 185
  diagnosis, 164, 185, *186*
  treatment, 168–9, *186–7*, 188
examination, 6–8, *8*
  in children, 12
  general observation, 6
  movement, 7, *9*
  neurological, *see* neurological
    examination
  routine for, 6–7
  terminology, 8–10, *9*
Exeter hip arthroplasty, 417, *417*
exostosis
  hereditary multiple (diaphyseal
    aclasis), 137, *138*
  subungual, 480
exsanguination, 249–50
extension, 9–10, *9*
extensor carpi radialis brevis
  release, *307*
  tenosynovitis, 320
extensor carpi ulnaris
  injury, 602
  tenosynovitis, 320
  weakness, 243, *244*
extensor pollicis brevis, *310*
extensor pollicis longus, *310*
  rupture, 334, *335*, 541, *594*,
    595
extensor retinaculum, 320–1
external fixation, 257, *257*, 526–8,
    527
  complications, 527–8
  femoral shaft fractures, 668
  indications, 526–7
  technique, 527, *527*
  tibial fractures, 692, *693*
extradural haematoma, *502*, 503
eye protection, 251

face mask, 251
facet joint arthritis, 388
facet joint dislocations, 630, 635
facial features
  achondroplasia, 137
  Down's syndrome, 150, *151*
familial hypocalciuric hypercalcaemia
    (FHH), 124

family history, 6
  genetic disorders, 132
fascial space infection, hands, 339
fasciotomy, 535–6, *536*, 694
fat embolism syndrome, 511
febuxostat, 70
felon (pulp-space infection), 338
femoral condyle, osteochondrosis,
    94, *95*
femoral epiphysis
  capital, slipped (SCFE),
    401–4
  distal, fracture-separation, 673,
    673
femoral head
  fractures, 656, *656*
  osteonecrosis, 87, *89*, *90*, *91*,
    93, 413–14, *413*
    after hip fracture, 661
    childhood hip fracture,
      663–4
femoral neck fractures, 657, *657*
  avascular necrosis, *540*
  combined with shaft fracture,
    668
  coxa vara deformity, 664, *664*
  hip dislocation, 654
  occult, *659*
  stress, 544
femoral nerve, injuries, 238
femoral shaft fractures, 504, *533*,
    665–70
  associated knee injuries, 667–8
  children, 669–70, *670*
  combined neck and shaft, 668
  complications, 668–9
  external fixation, 668
  initial treatment, 665
  internal fixation, 666–7, *667*
  intramedullary nailing, 667,
    667, 668
  non-operative management,
    665, *666*
  open, 667
  pathological, 668
  periprosthetic, 668, *669*
femoral shortening osteotomy,
    397, *397*

femoral stems, 416–18, *417*
femoral stretch test, 361, *362*
femoroacetabular impingement
    (FAI), 12, 410–12, *411*
femur
  deficiency (congenital short
    femur), 156–7, *157*
  distal replacement, 671, *672*
  Gaucher deposits, 93, *93*
  medial condyle osteonecrosis,
    88
  osteochondroma, 169, *169*
  osteosarcoma, *181–2*
  Paget's disease, *127*
  periprosthetic fractures, 420,
    668, *669*
  supracondylar/condylar
    fractures, 670–3,
    670–2
fibroblast growth factor receptor, 3
    (*FGFR3*), 137
fibrocartilage, 71, 98
fibroma, non-ossifying, 173–4,
    173
fibromatosis, palmar/plantar, 194
fibromyalgia, 64–5
fibrosarcoma, 194
fibrous dysplasia, 164, 178, *178*,
    179
fibrous tumours, 194–5
fibula
  deficiency (hemimelia), 157–9,
    158
  fractures, 692, 700, *701*
'fight bite', 340, 610, *611*
finger injuries
  closed tendon, 616, *616*
  distal phalanx, 614, *614*
  fractures, 612–14, *613*
  interphalangeal joint
    dislocation, 616
  joint sprains, 614–15
  MCP joint dislocation,
    615–16
  nail bed, 622
  open, 617–22, *619*
  pulp and fingertip, 622
  severe mutilation, 622, *623*

fingers
  amputations, 619
  congenital variations, 329, *330*
  'dropped', 334, *335, 341*
  in hyperparathyroidism, *125*
  movements, 326–7, *326*
  in osteoarthritis, *54, 82*
  pollicization, *331*, 622
  in psoriatic arthritis, 60, *60*
  replantation, 622–3, *623*
  in rheumatoid arthritis, *53*
  tasks, 328
  tendon lesions, 333–6, *335*
  ulnar deviation, *314, 341*
Finkelstein's test, 320, *320*
fixed flexion deformities
  definition, 13
  poliomyelitis, 217
  spina bifida, 215–16
flail chest, 488, 495, 641
flat foot, *see* pes planus/pes valgus
flexion, 9–10, *9*
flexor carpi radialis, tenosynovitis, 321
flexor carpi ulnaris, tenosynovitis, 321
flexor digitorum profundus (FDP)
  injuries, 621–2
  testing, 327, *327*, 617
flexor digitorum superficialis (FDS)
  injuries, 619, *619*, 621–2
  testing, 327–8, *327*, 617, *617*
flexor pollicis longus, testing, 328
flucloxacillin, 30, 33
fluids, intravascular, 498–9
folic acid, and neural tube defects, 214
foot
  arches, 457
  congenital abnormalities, 457–62
  deformity in spina bifida, 216, 458, *459*
  diabetic, 475–6, *475, 481*
  examination, 454–7
  gout, 69, *69*, 474, *474*
  hallux rigidus, 470–1, *470*
  hallux valgus, 467–70, *467–8*

history, 453–4
  imaging, 457
  lesser toe deformities, 471–2
  pes cavus, *454*, 457, 465–7, *465, 467*
  pes planus/pes valgus (flat foot), 462–5, *463–5*
  postures, 457
  rheumatoid arthritis, 472–3, *473*
  seronegative arthropathies, 473–4
  skin lesions, 480, *481*
  toenail disorders, 480, *481*
foot drop, 203, 240–1, *241*, 455
foot injuries, 707–15
  calcaneum fractures, 710–12, *710–11*
  imaging, 707
  metatarsal fractures, 714–15
  metatarsophalangeal (MTP) joints, 715
  midtarsal, 712–13
  sesamoid fractures, 715
  talus fractures, 707–10
  tarsometatarsal (TMT) joints, 713–14, *714*
  toe fractures, 715
foot pain, 453, *456*
  forefoot, 479–80, *479*
  heel, 478, *478*
  midfoot, 479
foraminotomy, 353
forearm, quadrilateral joint, 582, *582*
forearm fractures, 582–8
  five 'Ps', 582
  Galeazzi fracture, 587–8, *588*
  Monteggia fracture-dislocation, *303*, 586–7, *587*
  muscle contracture following, 541–2
  radius and ulna, 582–5, *583–5*
  single bone, 585–6
forearm muscles, ischaemic contracture, 332, *334*
Forestier's disease, 59
fracture blisters, 537
fracture-dislocation

  elbow, 576
  midtarsal, 713
  Monteggia (forearm), *303*, 586–7, *587*
  shoulder, 557, *557*
  thoracolumbar spine, 639–40
fracture fixation
  external, 257, *257*, 526–8, *527*
  internal, 254–7, *255, 256*, 525–6, *526*
  open fractures, 530–1
fracture healing, 515
  avascular necrosis, 540, *540*
  by callus (secondary healing), 516, *516, 517*
  delayed union, 517, 537–8
  direct union (primary healing), 515–16
  heterotopic ossification, 540–1
  malunion, 539
  non-union, 517, *518*, 538, *539*
  time to union, 516–17
  union, 517
fracture reduction, 521–2, *522*
  cast splintage, 524
  functional bracing, 524
  holding reduction, 522–8
  traction, 523–4, *523*
fracture risk
  and age, 112, *112, 659*
  assessment, 113
  metastatic bone disease, 192
  osteoporosis, 113, 114
fractures
  blood loss, *498*
  causes of, 513–14
  classification, 514–15, *515*
  clinical features, 518
  comminuted, *see* comminuted fractures
  compression, 514
  displacement, 520
  early complications, 533–7
  examination, 518–19
  greenstick, 514, 582, *583*, 595, *596*
  gunshot injuries, 532
  imaging, 519

involving physis, *see* physeal injuries
late complications, 537–43
long bones, 505–6
mechanisms of injury, *514*
open, *see* open fractures
osteogenesis imperfecta, 142, *143–5*
Paget's disease, 128
pathological, *see* pathological fractures
pelvis, *see* pelvic fractures
restoration of function, 528
rule of twos, 519
secondary injuries, 521
spiral, 519
transverse, 519
FREAS mnemonic, 243
Freiberg's disease, 94, 479, *479*
Friedreich's ataxia, 223
Froment's sign, *239*
frostbite, 508–9, 623, *623*
'frozen' shoulder, 285–6, *286*
functional bracing, 524
functional disability, 6
fungal infections, 47
    spinal, 380–1
'funny bone', 243
fusidic acid, 30

gait, 203
    antalgic, 405
    cerebral palsy, 208
    foot and ankle disorders, 454–5
    hip disorders, 405
    short leg, 405
    spastic, 203
    stiff leg, 405
    Trendelenburg, 203, 405
gait laboratory, 3D, 208, *209*
Galeazzi fracture, 587–8, *588*
Galeazzi test, 395
gamekeeper's thumb, 611–12
ganglion, wrist, 321, *321*
gangrene, 533, *533*
    diabetic foot, 476
    gas, 536–7
Ganz periacetabular osteotomy, 397

Garden classification, femoral neck fractures, 657, *657*
Garrod's pads, 194
gas gangrene, 536–7
Gaucher's disease, 30, 93–4, 133, 149–50
GCS, *see* Glasgow Coma Score
gender
    and bone mass, 104
    osteoarthritis risk, *76*, 77
gene mapping, 132
genes, 129, 130
gene therapy, 133
genetic counselling, 133
genetic disorders
    chromosomal, 130, 150–1
    diagnosis, 132–3
    mutations, 130
    patterns of inheritance, 131–2
    polygenic and multi-factorial, 130
    principles of management, 133–4
    single gene, 130
genetic heterogeneity, 131
genetic markers, 131
genome, 129–30
gentamicin, 530
genu recurvatum, 435, 437
genu valgum, 13, *13*
    adults, 435–7
    children, 433–5, *433–5*
genu varum, 13, *13*
    adults, 435–7
    children, 433
germ-line cells, 130
giant-cell tumour of bone, 164, 174, *175*
Girdlestone's arthroplasty, *263*
Glasgow Coma Score (GCS), 489
    classification of head injuries, 500
glenohumeral joint, 286, 290–2, 556
    anterior dislocation, 556–7
    arthrodesis, *218*, 296
    inferior dislocation, 558–9
    osteoarthritis, 291–2, *292*
    osteonecrosis, 292

posterior dislocation, 557–8
    rapidly destructive arthropathy (Milwaukee shoulder), 292, *292*
    tuberculous arthritis, 290, *290*
glenoid, *276*
    fracture, *553*
glomus tumour, 195, 343
gloves, surgical, 251
glucocerebrosidase, 149–50
glucocorticoids
    and bone metabolism, 107
    and osteoporosis, 115
glycocalyx, 24, 33
golfer's elbow, 307–8
gonadal hormones
    and bone metabolism, 106–7
    and osteoporosis, 115–16
goniometer, *9*
gonococcal arthritis, 42
Gonococcus, 41
gout, 54, 55, 67–70
    chronic, 70
    clinical features, 68–9, *69*, 306, *306*
    differential diagnosis, 69
    foot, 69, *69*, 474, *474*
    hands, *69*, *344*
    investigation, 69
    primary, 68
    risk factors, 67
    secondary, 68
gouty tophi, 54, *69*, *344*
Gower's sign, 225
gown, surgical, 251
granuloma, tuberculous, 44, *45*
greater trochanter, fracture, 662–3
greenstick fractures, 514
    distal radius, 595, *596*
    radius and ulna, 582, *583*
grinding test, 428
grip strength, 328
growth disturbance
    distal tibial physis fractures, 706–7
    in JIA, *63*
    physeal injuries, 540, 548
    proximal tibial epiphyseal injuries, 690

growth hormone (GH), 107
Guillain–Barré syndrome, 221–2
gummata, 44
gunshot injuries, 532
gunstock deformity, 300, *301*, *570*
Gustilo's classification (open
        fractures), 529, 691

haemangiomas, 190–1
haemarthrosis, 431, 536
haemochromatosis, 72
Haemophilus influenzae, 24–5,
        30, 41
haemothorax, 494, 495
hallux rigidus, 470–1, *470*
hallux valgus, 457, 467–70
halo ring, 630
hamate hook, fracture, *603*
hammer toe, 457, 471
hamstring power, assessment, 361,
        362
hand–arm vibration syndrome,
        343–4
hand injuries, 607
    assessment, 607
    burns, 623–4
    carpometacarpal (CMC) joint,
        608–9, *609*
    flexor tendon avulsion, 616, *616*
    metacarpal fractures, 609–11,
        611
    microsurgery, 263–4, *264*,
        622–3, *623*
    nail-bed, 622
    open, 617–22, *619–21*
    phalangeal fractures, 612–14, *613*
    pulp and fingertip, 622
    severe mutilation, *619*, 622, *623*
    skier's thumb, 611–12, *612*
    tendon repair, 619–22, *620*
    tendons (closed injuries),
        333–4, 616, *616*
    treatment principles, 608
    zones, 619, *619*
hands
    acute infections, 336–40
    bone lesions, 336
    congenital variations, 329,
        330–1

emboli, 342
examination, 325–8, *329*
failure of formation, 329, *330*
flexor tendons, 327, *327*, 617,
        617
functional tests, 328, *329*, 617,
        617
function loss, 325
general disorders, *69, 344*
history, 325
muscle contracture after injury,
        541
osteoarthritis, *54, 78, 82, 82*,
        85
'permissible' incisions, 618, *618*
rheumatoid arthritis, *53*, 334,
        335, 340, *341–2*
skin contracture, 330–1
spastic paresis, 333, *334*
splintage, 337, *337*, 608, *608*,
        620, *621*
hanging cast, 563
hangman's fracture, 632
Harms technique, 357
Harrison's sulcus, 118
Hartofilakidis classification, 412
haversian system, 101, *101*
Hawkins classification, talar neck
        fractures, 708
Hawkins–Kennedy test, 281
Hawkins' sign, 710
head injuries, 491, 499–503
    awareness, 500
    concussion, 501
    extradural haematoma, *502*,
        503
    GCS classification, 500
    management, 501–3
    recognition, 500–1
    severe brain contusion, 503
    skull fractures, 501, *502*
    spastic paresis of hand, 333,
        334
Heaf test, 46
Heberden's nodes, *54, 82*, 342,
        342
heel pain, 478, *478*
hemiarthroplasty, hip fracture,
        660

hemiplegia, 203, 207, 210
hemivertebrae, 152, *153*, 371, *372*
heparin, 253
hereditary motor and sensory
        neuropathy (HMSN),
        222–3
hereditary multiple exostosis
        (diaphyseal aclasis), 137,
        138
hereditary sensory neuropathy,
        222
heroin addicts, 31
Herring classification, Legg–
        Calvé–Perthes disease,
        400
heterotopic ossification, 540–1
    acetabular fractures, 652
    distal humerus fractures, 575
    elbow fracture-dislocation, 576
    fracture-dislocation of elbow,
        576
Hill–Sachs lesions, 288, *288*, 542
hip
    acute suppurative arthritis, *40, 41*
    arthroscopy, 407–9, *409*
    bony ankylosis, *59*
    chondrosarcoma, *183–4*
    developmental cox vara, 397,
        398
    developmental dysplasia, *see*
        developmental dysplasia
        of the hip (DDH)
    disorders in spina bifida, 215
    dysplasia in adult, 412, *412*
    examination, 405–6, *406*
    imaging, *18*, 406–7, *406–7*
    inflammatory arthritis, 414–15
    irritable (transient synovitis),
        397–9
    Legg–Calvé–Perthes disease,
        399–401
    osteoarthritis, *18, 78*, 81,
        409–15
        clinical features, 410
        investigations, 410, *410*
        mechanical causes, 77,
        410–13
        non-mechanical causes,
        413–15

non-operative management, 84–5, 415
post-traumatic, 413
rapidly destructive arthritis, 73, 74
septic arthritis, 398–9
slipped capital femoral epiphysis, 401–4
surgical planning tools/3D printing, 407, 408
symptoms, 404–5
total arthroplasty, 415–20
tuberculosis, 46
hip dislocation, 653
anterior, 655–6
central, 656
classification, 653
femoral head fractures, 656, 656
posterior, 653–5, 654–5
hip fractures, 657–64
in children, 663–4, 664
clinical features, 659
complications, 662
definition, 657
delays to surgery, 660
extracapsular, 658–9, 661–2
imaging, 659
intracapsular, 657, 660
isolated trochanteric, 662–3
occult, 659, 660
osteoporotic, 659
risk and age, 659
treatment, 659–62, 661
hip girdle pain, 404
Hippocratic method, 556
hip resurfacing, 418–19, 418
hip screw, sliding, 658, 660
histamine test, 233
history, 3–6
Hodgkin's lymphoma, 126
Hoffa fractures, 670
Horner's syndrome, 204–5
human immunodeficiency virus (HIV), 31, 380
human leucocyte antigen (HLA) system, 130
HLA-B27, 58, 61, 62, 131
humerus, osteochondroma, 170

humerus fractures
distal in adults, 574–6
distal in children, 565–74
fracture-separation of distal humerus epiphysis, 572–4, 574
malunion, 561
nerve injuries, 237
non-union, 539, 564
osteonecrosis, 561
proximal in adults, 559–62, 560
proximal in children, 561, 562
pseudarthrosis, 539
shaft, 562–4, 563
'hungry bone syndrome', 125
Hunter's syndrome, 147, 149
Hurler syndrome, 145, 147
Hutchinson's teeth, 44
hydatid disease, 48–9, 48, 49, 381
hydrocephalus, spina bifida, 213, 214–15
hydroxyapatite (HA), 104, 105
implant material, 270
hyoid bone, 345, 345
hypercalcaemia, 123–6
acute severe, 124
causes, 123
familial hypocalciuric (FHH), 124
of malignancy, 123, 125–6
in Paget's disease, 128
hypercortisonism, 108
hyperkyphosis, 360, 373
hypermobile joints, 14
hyperostosis, diffuse idiopathic (Forestier's disease), 59
hyperparathyroidism, 108, 123
primary, 124–5, 125
secondary, 118–19
hyperthyroidism, 116
hyperuricaemia, 68, 69
hypocalcaemia, 116–17, 125
hypoparathyroidism, 117
hypophosphataemia, familial, 118, 119–22, 120–1
hypothermia, 508
management, 509
hypovolaemic shock, 497, 498, 498

ifosfamide, 169
iliolumbar ligament, 644
iliotibial band, 675
Ilizarov method, 257, 259–61, 261
chronic osteomyelitis, 37, 37
'illness behaviour', 391
immobility, and osteoporosis risk, 116
immobilization
hands, 337, 337, 608, 608, 620, 621
pelvic injuries, 643
spinal injuries, 626–7, 627
trauma patient, 487
immunocompromised patients, acute osteomyelitis, 31
implant failure, 267–8, 267
implant materials, 267–70
acrylic cement, 269–70
carbon, 269
hydroxyapatite, 270
metals, 267–9
ultra-high molecular weight polyethylene, 269
impotence, following pelvic fractures, 649
inbreeding, 131
infants
acute haematogenous osteomyelitis, 25, 27, 30
acute suppurative arthritis, 38, 39
brachial plexus injuries, 234–5, 235
burns, 507
congenital torticollis, 349, 350
development milestones, 12
examination, 12
femoral fractures, 669–70, 670
infection, 23–4
acute haematogenous osteomyelitis, 24–31
acute pyogenic, 24
ankle fractures, 703
bacterial colonization/ resistance to antibiotics, 24
chronic non-pyogenic, 24
chronic pyogenic, 24

infection (*Continued*)
    femoral shaft fractures, 669
    hands, 336–40
    host susceptibility, 23–4
    inflammatory reaction, 23
    joints, 38–9
    mechanisms of, 23
    open fractures, 532, 536,
        694–5
    pelvic injuries, 649
    periprosthetic, 37–8, *38*, 420
    spinal, *see* spinal infections
    treatment, 24
inferior vena caval filters, 253
infrapatellar bursitis, 432
infraspinatus, 277
ingrown toenail, 480
inhalation injuries, 506
inheritance patterns, 131
instability, 5
intensity-modulated radiotherapy
        (IMRT), 169
interdigital nerve compression
        (Morton's metatarsalgia),
        480
interlocking bolts, 525
internal fixation, 254, 525–6, *526*
    complications, 525–6
    femoral shaft fracture, 665–7,
        666
    femoral supracondylar/condylar
        fractures, 671–2, *671–2*
    hip fractures, 660–1, *661*
    humeral shaft fracture, 563,
        563
    indications, 525
    intramedullary devices, 256–7,
        256, 525
    plates and screws, 256, 525, *526*
    screws, 254–5, *255*, 525
    tibial plateau fractures, 685–6,
        685, *688–9*
    types, 525
interphalangeal (IP) joints
    dislocation, 616
    osteoarthritis, 342, *342–3*
    replacement, *343*
intervertebral disc
    operative removal, 353, 384

replacement, 353, 387, *387*
intervertebral disc disease, 381–4,
        381
    acute herniation, 212, 382–4,
        383
        cervical spine, 350–2, *351*,
            635
        differential diagnosis, 384
        lumbar spine, 382–4
        treatment, 384
    chronic degeneration, 212,
        381–2, *381*
        cervical spine, 352–4, *353*
        lumbar spine, 381–2, *381*
    pathology, 381–2, *381*
intracompartmental pressures, 535
intramedullary nails, 256–7, 525
    femoral shaft fracture, 667, *667*
    interlocked, 256–7
    retrograde, 667
    tibial fractures, 691, *692*
    unlocked, *256*, 257
intraosseous cannulation, 498, *499*
intravenous fluids
    burn patients, 507
    shock, 498–9
intrinsic-minus deformity, 332
intrinsic-plus deformity, 332, 541
involucrum, 26, *26*, 34, *35*
iridocyclitis, JIA, 63
irritable hip, 397–9
ischaemia, clinical features, 535
ischaemic muscle, 332, *334*, 535,
        541

Jack-knife injury (Chance fracture),
        636, 639
Jack test (great toe extension), 463
Jamshidi needle, *167*
jaw thrust, 491, *492*
Jefferson's fracture, 631–2
JIA, *see* juvenile idiopathic arthritis
Jobe's test, 281
joint injections, 56
joint injuries, 548–9, *548*
    avulsions, 548–9, *548*
    dislocation, 549
    sprains/strains, 548
    subluxation, *548*, 549

joint instability, 5
    after injury, 542
joint laxity, 14, 16
    achondroplasia, 137, 139
    Down's syndrome, 150, *151*
    generalized, 140–1, *141*
    shoulder, 287
    tests (Beighton scores), 140
    versus joint instability, 287
joint locking, 4
    knee, 422, 438–9
joint posture, 11
joint replacement, 263, *263*
    first carpometacarpal joint, 315,
        316
    hands, 340, 342, *342*, *343*
    hip, *see* total hip arthroplasty
    implant materials, 266–9
    knee, 84, 450, 452
    osteoarthritis, 84
    thromboprophylaxis, 252–4
    VTE risk, 252
    wrist, *315*
joint shape, and osteoarthritis risk,
        77
joint space narrowing
    hip, 415, *415*
    knee, 428, *428*, *449*, 451, *451*
joint stiffness, 4–5
    after femoral shaft fracture, 669
    after femoral supracondylar/
        condylar fractures, 672
    after fractures, 542
    after hand injuries, 607
    after humeral shaft fracture,
        564
    after tibial shaft fracture, 695
    after wrist fractures, 595
    elbow, 302, *303*
        distal humerus fractures,
            575
        fracture-dislocation, 576
        supracondylar fracture, 570
    grades, 15
    hip, 404–5
    knee, 421, 450
        after dislocation, 680
        after femoral shaft fractures,
            669

after femoral supracondylar/ condylar fractures, 672
osteoarthritis, 81
proximal humerus fractures, 561
rheumatoid arthritis, 52, 53
shoulder, 285–6, 286
talocalcaneal, 712
Jones fracture, 715
juvenile idiopathic arthritis (JIA), 62–4
juxtapatellar hollow, 425, 426

Kanavel's signs, 339
Kaplan-Meier survival curve, 163, 163
Keller's operation, 470
keratoderma blennorrhagica, 481
Kienböck's disease, 94, 316–17, 318
Kingella kingae, 25, 41
Klein's line, 402, 402
Klinefelter's syndrome, 130, 151
Klippel–Feil syndrome, 152, 293, 293
Klumpke's palsy, 234, 235
knee
    acute ligament injuries, 675–8
    acute suppurative arthritis, 40, 40
    after femoral supracondylar/ condylar fractures, 672
    arthroscopy, 429–30, 430
    bony swellings, 432–3
    chronic ligamentous instability, 440–1
    complex ligament injuries, 427
    congenital dislocation, 435, 437, 437
    deformities, 13, 14
        in adults, 435–7
        in children, 433–5
        JIA, 63
    diagnostic calendar, 433
    dislocation, 678–80, 679
    disorders in spina bifida, 215
    examination, 422–8, 422–4
    extensor mechanism injuries, 680
    giving way, 422

history, 421
imaging, 20, 428–30, 428–30
injuries in children, 688–90
injury in femoral shaft fractures, 668
landmarks, 424
locking, 422, 438–9
loose bodies, 447, 448
meniscal lesions, 437–40, 680
movement, 424–5, 425
Osgood–Schlatter disease, 432, 445, 445
osteoarthritis, 18, 81–2, 81, 85, 422, 431, 435, 450–2, 451
osteochondrosis/ osteochondritis, 94, 95, 445–7, 446, 680
osteonecrosis, 452
patella dislocation, 441–2, 442, 682–4, 684
patella fracture, 681–2, 683
patellar tendinopathy, 445
patella tendon rupture, 681
patellofemoral pain syndrome, 442–5
plica syndrome, 448
quadriceps tendon rupture, 680–1
rheumatoid arthritis, 422, 449–50, 450
septic arthritis, 431
stabilizers, 675
stiffness, 421, 450, 669, 672, 680
swellings, 421, 430–3
synovial chondromatosis, 447–8
tests for intra-articular fluid, 425, 426
tests for ligamentous stability, 425–7, 427, 678
tests for meniscal injuries, 427–8
tibial plateau fractures, 685–8, 685, 687
tuberculosis, 45, 448
varus/valgus deformities, 13, 13
knee pain
    anterior, 433, 442–4

osteoarthritis, 450
knee replacement, 84, 450, 452
knock knees, see genu valgum
Kocher criteria, 399
Kocher–Langenbeck approach, 650, 651, 652
Köhler's disease, 479
Kramer osteotomy, 403
K-wire fixation, 525, 526
kyphoscoliosis, 137, 139
kyphos (gibbus), 360, 373, 373, 378, 378
kyphosis, 13–14, 360, 373–5, 373, 375
    adolescent (Scheuermann's disease), 373, 374, 375
    congenital, 374
    in elderly, 114, 114, 374, 375
    normal thoracic, 364
    postural, 373
    spina bifida, 215
    structural, 373–4, 373

Lachman test, 426–7, 427, 676
lag screws, 254–5, 255, 525
lamellar bone, 100
laminoplasty, cervical spine, 354
laryngeal mask airway, 491
laryngeal trauma, 491
Lasègue's test, 362
lateral (term), 9–10
lateral collateral ligament (elbow), 306
lateral collateral ligament (knee)
    injury, 675, 678
    testing, 425
lateral facet pressure syndrome, 444
Lauge–Hansen system (malleolar fractures), 700
Lautenbach approach, 37
Legg–Calvé–Perthes disease, 399–401, 400
leg length discrepancy
    ankle fractures, 707
    assessment, 405
    coxa vara, 397
    poliomyelitis, 217
    posterior hip dislocation, 655

leiomyosarcoma, 195–6
leprosy, 222, *222*
lesser trochanter, fractures, 662
Letournel classification, 649–51, *650*
lifestyle factors, and osteoporosis, 112, 113
ligament injuries
    ankle, 697–9
    knee, 427, 675–8
    MCP joints, 611–12, *612*
    midtarsal, 712–13
    rupture, 548–9, *548*
    sprains and strains, 548
    wrist, 602–3
limb anomalies, 153–9
    digits, 156, *156*, 329, *330*, 462, *462*
    lower limb, 156–9, *157–8*
    types, 153–4
    upper limb, 154–6, 311–13, *312*
limb replantation, 264, *265*
limb salvage, osteosarcoma, 167–8, *168*, 180
limb shortening, achondroplasia, 137, 139
lipomas, 193, *194*
liposarcomas, 193–4
Lisfranc injury, 713
log-rolling, 627, *627*
long extensors, hands, 328
long head of biceps, *277*, *279*
    rupture, 284–5, *285*
    tendinitis, 284
long thoracic nerve palsy, 235, *236*
loose bodies
    elbow joint, 304–5, *305*
    knee, 447, *448*
Looser's zones, 117, 119, *121*
lordosis, 14
    cervical, 345
    lumbar, 364
loupes, 249
low back pain, 384–7
    approach to diagnosis, 390–1
    causes, 384–5
    chronic syndrome, 391
    defined, 384

examination, 385
imaging, 386
incidence, 384
red flags, 385
referred, 359
treatment, 386–7
yellow flags, 385
lower limb anomalies, 156–9, *157–8*
lower motor neurons (LMN), 200, 201
low molecular weight heparin (LMWH), 253
low-to-middle-income countries (LMICs), 34, 47
lumbar spine; *see also* thoracolumbar spine injuries
    imaging, 363–4, *364–5*
    intervertebral disc disease, 381–4, *381*
    lordosis, 364
    movements, 360–1, *361*
    stiffness, 359, *361*
lumbar stenosis, achondroplasia, 139
lunate, *311*
    avascular necrosis, 317–18, *318*, 604
    injuries, 603–4, *605*
    Kienböck's disease, 316–17, *318*
lunotriquetral ligament, tear, 604, *605*
luxatio erecta, 558–9, *559*

McCune–Albright syndrome, 178, *179*
McMurray test, 427, 438
macrodactyly, foot, 462, *462*
Madelung's deformity, 312–13, *312*
Maffucci's syndrome, 171, *171*, 184, *344*
Magerl technique, *356*, 357
magnetic resonance imaging (MRI), 19–20, *20*
    chondrosarcoma, *183*
    elbow, 300, *305*
    Ewing's sarcoma, *187*

foot/ankle, 457
fractures, 519
hip, 406–7
knee, 429, *429*, 676
metastatic bone disease, 191, *192*
neuromuscular disorders, 205
osteomyelitis, 29, 134–5
osteonecrosis, 90, *91*, 413
osteosarcoma, *181*
patellar dislocation, 684
pyogenic spinal infection, 376, *377*
shoulder, 275, *276*, 285, 288, *288*
    rotator cuff pathology, 282, *282*
spine, 364
    cervical, 349, 356, *634*
    injuries, 628
    intervertebral disc disease, 365, 382, *383*
    tuberculosis, 379, *379*
    tumours, 165–6, *181*, *187*
    wrist, 311
Main and Jowett classification (midtarsal injuries), 712
Maisonneuve injury, 698
major histocompatibility complex (MHC), 130
malleolar fractures, 700–3
    complications, 541, 703
mallet finger, 333, *335*, 616, *616*
mallet toe, 472
malunion, 539
    ankle fractures in children, 706
    causes, 539
    clinical features, 539
    distal radius fracture (children), 597
    distal radius fractures (adults), 595
    femoral shaft fractures, 669
    femoral supracondylar/condylar fractures, 672
    forearm fractures, 584
    proximal humerus fracture, 561
    supracondylar fractures (elbow), 300, 569–70, *570*

tibial shaft fractures, 695
treatment, 539
Mantoux test, 46
Maquet's tibial tubercle
    advancement, 444
marble bones (osteopetrosis),
    139–40, *140*
march fractures, 715
Marfan's syndrome, 16, 141, *141*,
    329
Maroteaux Lamy syndrome, 149
medial collateral ligament (knee)
    injury, 675, 678
    testing, 425
median nerve
    compression, 322–3, *322*, 328
    injuries, 238, *240*, 575, 595
mediastinal injuries, 497, 641
meningocele, 213, *213*
meniscus
    clinical assessment, 427–8
    cysts, 432, 440, *440*
    degeneration, 439–40
    discoid lateral, 440
    imaging, *429*
    roles of, 437
    tears, 437–9, *438*, 680
meniscectomy, 437, 439
menopause
    and bone loss, 107, 111–12, *111*
    osteoporosis, 113–15, 375
metacarpal bones, fractures,
    609–11, *611*
metacarpophalangeal (MCP) joints
    dislocation, 615, *615*
    replacement, *342*, *343*
    rheumatoid arthritis, 340, *341*
    ulnar collateral ligament tear,
    611–12, *612*
metal implants, 267–9
    cobalt-chromium alloys, 267
    corrosion, 267–8
    dissimilar metals, 268
    failure, 267, *267*
    friction and wear, 268–9
    hip arthroplasty, 418
    stainless steel, 267–8
metaphysis, *25*, *98*, 102, *102*
metastasis

bone, *see* bone metastases
    definition, 191
metastatic infection, acute
    osteomyelitis, 31
metatarsal bone fractures, 480,
    714–15
    causes, 714
    fifth metatarsal base, 714–15
    stress fractures, *479*, 480, 715
metatarsalgia, 453, 479
metatarsophalangeal (MTP) joints
    injuries, 715
    osteochondritis (Freiberg's
        disease), 479
    valgus deformity, 467–70,
        467–8
metatarsus adductus, 461, *461*
methicillin-resistant *Staphylococcus
    aureus* (MRSA), 31
methoxyflurane, 490
metronidazole, 33
microscope, operative, 249
microsurgery, 264
    hand, *265*, 622–3, *623*
midtarsal injuries, 712–13, *713*
Milwaukee brace, 369
Milwaukee shoulder, *73*, *74*, 82,
    292, *292*
Mirel's score, 192, 668
mirror hand (ulnar dimelia), *330*
Moberg procedure, 641
Moberg's pickup test, 328
monoplegia, 203
Monteggia fracture–dislocation,
    303, 586–7, *587*
Morquio–Brailsford syndrome,
    149, *149*
Morton's metatarsalgia, 480
motor neuron disease
        (amyotrophic lateral
        sclerosis), 218
motor vehicle accidents, 635–6,
    650
movement, examination, 7, *9*
mucopolysaccharidoses, 145,
    147–50
Mulder's click, 480
Müller's classification of fractures,
    514–15, *515*

multiple endocrine neoplasia
        (MEN) syndromes, 126
multiple epiphyseal dysplasia, 135,
    135–6
multiple myeloma, 116, 126, 188,
    189
multiple organ failure, 510–11
muscle
    fibre types, 202
    nerve supply, 204, 227
    structure, 201–2
muscle biopsy, 205
muscle charting, 203
    poliomyelitis, 217
muscle contraction, 202
muscle contracture
    after fractures, 541
    definition, 202
    joint deformity, 14
    spinal injuries, 641
muscle fasciculation, 202
muscle flap transfer, chronic
        osteomyelitis, 36–7
muscle ischaemia, 332, *334*, 535,
    541
muscle power, 10
    MRC scale, 10, 203, 230
    testing, 11, 230
    testing distal, 361
muscle tone, 202
muscle tumours
    skeletal muscle, 197
    smooth muscle, 195–6
muscle wasting, 202
muscle weakness, 202, 203
    flaccid, 203
    poliomyelitis, 217
    spastic, 203
muscular dystrophy, 225
mycobacterial infections, atypical,
    380
Mycobacterium tuberculosis, 44
mycoses
    deep, 47
    superficial, 47
myelin, 199, *200*, *201*, 227, *228*
myelomeningocele, 213, *213*, *214*
myositis, streptococcal necrotizing,
    29

'myositis ossificans', 576
myxofibrosarcoma, 195

nail-bed injuries, 622
nail disorders, 480, *481*
nasopharyngeal airway, 491
natriuretic peptide, therapeutic, 139
navicular bone, injuries, 712–13, *713*
neck; *see also* cervical spine
    accessory nerve injuries, 236, *236*
    hyperextension injuries, 626, *626*
    normal range of motion, *348*
    wry (torticollis), 349, *350*
neck pain, differential diagnosis, 352–3
Neer's classification, proximal humerus fractures, 559–60
Neer's impingement sign, 281
Neisseria gonorrhoeae, 42
neoadjuvant chemotherapy, 168–9, 180, 188
nerve compression; *see also* nerve entrapment syndromes
    acute, 534–5
    after fractures, 541
    interdigital (Morton's metatarsalgia), 480
    in Paget's disease, 128
nerve conduction studies, 21, 205–6, 231
nerve entrapment syndromes, 242–5
    clinical features, 242
    common sites, 242
    differentiation from cervical spondylosis, 353
    median nerve (carpal tunnel syndrome), 322–3, *323*, 328
    radial nerve, 243–4, *244*
    tarsal tunnel, 242, 480
    thoracic outlet syndrome, 244–5
    treatment, 242

ulnar nerve, 242–3, 300, *302*
nerve grafts, 231, 618
nerve injuries, 228–30, 534–5
    acetabular fractures, 652
    acute, 230
    care of paralysed parts, 232
    classification, 229
    closed, 231–2, 534
    common injuries, 534
    diagnosis, 230–1
    distal humerus fractures, 575
    distal radius fractures, 595
    forearm bone fractures, 583
    fracture-dislocation of elbow, 576
    hip dislocation, 654–5
    humeral shaft fractures, 562, 564
    indications for early exploration, 534
    lower limb, 238–42
    open, 231, 534
    pelvic fractures, 649
    shoulder dislocation, 556–7
    supracondylar fractures, 569
    upper limb, 232–8, *239–40*
nerve regeneration, 229, *229*
nerve repair, 231, *231*
    delayed, 232
    hand injuries, 618
nerve root supply, 204
nerve-sheath tumours, 196–7, *196*
nervous pathways, 199–200, *200*
neuralgic amyotrophy (acute brachial neuritis), 220–1, *221*, 351
neurapraxia, 228–9, 640
neurilemma, 199
neurofibromata, 144, *147*, 196–7
neurofibromatosis (NF), 143
    congenital pseudarthrosis, 144–5, *147–8*
    scoliosis, *372*, 373
    type, 1 (NF1/von Recklinghausen's disease), 143–4, *147*, 196–7
    type, 2 (NF2), 144
neurogenic shock, 505

neurological examination, 9–11, 202–5
    acute intervertebral disc prolapse, 383
    appearance, 9–10
    back disorders, 362–3
    low back pain, 385
    neck disorders, 346
    pelvic fractures, 644
    reflexes, 10–11
    routine for, 9
    spinal injuries, 521, 628
    tone and power, 10
neuroma, 196, 230
neuromuscular disorders
    causing pes cavus, 466
    examination, 202–5
    hands, 332–3, *333*
    history, 202
    investigation, 205–6
neurons, 227–8, *228*
    structure, 199, *200, 201*, 227–8, *228*
neuropathic joint disease, 475, 476
neurophysiological tests, 205–6
neurotmesis, 229–30
neurotransmitters, 199
new bone formation
    acute osteomyelitis, 26
    chronic osteomyelitis, 34
NICE guidelines, osteoarthritis management, 83
non-accidental injuries
    femoral shaft fracture, 670
    fracture-separation of distal humerus epiphysis, 572–4, *574*
'non-organic' physical signs, 391
non-ossifying fibroma, 173–4, *173*
nonsteroidal anti-inflammatory drugs (NSAIDs), 60, 70, 84
non-union, 517, 538
    atrophic, *518*, 538, *539*
    causes, 517
    femoral shaft fractures, 669
    femoral supracondylar/condylar fractures, 672–3
    forearm fractures, 584

hip fractures, 662
    humeral shaft fractures, *539*,
       564
    hypertrophic, *518*, 538
    olecranon fracture, 581
    tibial shaft fractures, 695
numbness (paraesthesia), 5–6,
      202, 359
nutriceuticals, 84

OA, *see* osteoarthritis
obesity, osteoarthritis risk, 77, 78,
      85
occipital condyle fracture, 631
occipitocervical dislocation, 631
occupation, and osteoarthritis
      risk, 78
occupational disorders, wrist/
      hand, 321
odontoid process (dens), 345, *348*
    absence/hypoplasia, 349–50
    fractures, 632, *633*
oedema, after fractures, 528
oestrogen
    and bone metabolism, 107
    and osteoporosis, 113, 115–16
1,25-OHD, 117, 119
olecranon
    bursitis, *69*, 305–6, *306*
    fractures, 580–2, *581*
Ollier's disease, 171, 184
onychogryphosis, 480
open fractures, 33, 528–32
    ankle, 702
    antibiotics, 528, 530
    classification, 529
    debridement, 529–30, *531*
    delivery of the fracture, 529,
      531
    femoral shaft, 668
    gunshot injuries, 532
    initial management, 528
    nerve injuries, 534
    sequels, 531–2
    stabilizing, 530
    tibial shaft, 692–3
    wound closure, 530
oropharyngeal airway, 491, *492*
orthopaedic operations

amputations, 264–6
bloodless field, 249–50
bone fixation, 254–6, *255*, *257*
bone grafts/substitutes, 257–9,
    259–60
correction of bone deformities,
    260, *261*
distraction osteogenesis,
    259–61, *261*
equipment, 247, 248
hand/digit replantation, 622–3,
    622–3
incidence of thromboembolic
    events, 252
infection risk reduction, 250–1
intraoperative X-rays, 248–9,
    248
on joints, 262–4, *262–3*
limb replantation, 264, *265*
osteotomy, 254
planning, 247
shoulder, 295–6, *296*
surgical attire, 251
thromboprophylaxis, 251–4
Ortolani manoeuvre, 393, *394*
Osgood–Schlatter disease, 432,
    445, *445*
ossification
    endochondral, 102, *103*
    heterotopic after injury, 540–1,
      575
    intramembranous, 102–3
ossification centres, 97, *98*
    elbow, 300
osteitis fibrosa cystica, 124, *125*
osteoarthritis (OA), 75
    acromioclavicular joint, 294–5,
      295, 555
    aetiology and risk factors, 76–8,
      76
    after acetabular fractures, 652
    after ankle fractures, 703
    after elbow injuries, 576, 581
    after femoral supracondylar
      fractures, 673
    after hip dislocation, 655
    after hip fracture, 662
    after joint fractures, 542–3
    after scaphoid fracture, 602

after tibial plateau fracture, 688
after wrist fracture, 595
ankle, 474–5, 703, 712
assessment, 82
cardinal signs, 83
CPPD in, 72
distal radioulnar joint, 317, *317*
distinction from rheumatoid
    arthritis, 342
elbow, 302–3, *305*
first carpometacarpal joint, 315,
    316
hands, *54*, 78, 82, *82*, 85, 342,
    342–3
hip, *18*, *78*, 81, 84–5, 409–15
knee, *13*, *18*, *78*, 81–2, 84, 85,
    422, 431, 435, 450–2
management, 83–5, *83*
natural history and outcomes,
    78–80
in Paget's disease, 128
pathology, 78, *78*
prevalence and distribution,
    76, *76*
radiocapitellar joint, 580
shoulder, *73*, *74*, 82, 286,
    291–2, *292*
symptoms and signs, 80–2, *81*
wrist, 314–17, *315–17*
osteoblastoma, 164, 173
osteoblasts, 99, *100*, 104–5
osteochondral fragments, 446,
    446–7, 447, 680
osteochondritis dissecans, 94, *95*
    elbow, 305, *306*
    knee, 445–7, *446*, 680
    talus, 477
osteochondroma, *15*, 169–70, *169*,
    170
osteochondrosis
    ('osteochondritis'), 94–5,
      95, 479, *479*
osteoclasts, 99, *100*, 104
osteocytes, 99, *100*
osteogenesis, 257–8
osteogenesis imperfecta (brittle
    bones), 142–3, *143–5*
osteoid, 99, 104
osteoid osteoma, *165*, 172, *172*

osteolysis, hip arthroplasty, 419
osteolytic lesions, multiple
          myeloma, 188, *189*
osteomalacia, 108, *110*, 117–19,
          121
osteomyelitis
    acute haematogenous, 24–31
    chronic, 26, 33–7
    post-traumatic, 33
    proximal femur, 399
    spinal, 375–7, *377*
    subacute haematogenous, 32–3
osteonecrosis, 87–91
    acetabular fractures, 652
    after fractures, 540, *540*
    aseptic, 87
    in Caisson disease, 92–3
    clinical features, 89–90
    common sites, 87, *88*
    diagnosis of underlying
          disorder, 91
    drug-induced, 94
    factors causing, 87–8
    femoral head, 87, *89, 90, 91, 93*,
          413–14, *413*
       after hip fracture, 662
       childhood hip fracture,
          663–4
    imaging, 90, *91*
    knee, 452
    lunate, 317–18, *318*, 604
    non-traumatic, 88
    pathology, 89–91, *90–1*
    posterior hip dislocation, 655
    proximal humerus fractures,
          561
    scaphoid fractures, 602
    shoulder, 292
    in sickle-cell disease, 92, *92*,
          414
    in SLE, 64
    staging, 90–1
    talus, *88*, 477, 710
    traumatic, 88
    treatment, 91
osteopenia, WHO bone mass
          definitions, 109
osteopetrosis, 139–40, *140*
osteophytes, 78, *78*

osteoporosis, 78, 111–16
    assessment of fracture risk, 113
    comparison with osteomalacia,
          117
    diabetic foot, 475
    fracture risk, 113, 114, *659*
    in men, 115
    post-menopausal, 107, 113–15,
          375
    risk factors, 112
    secondary, 115–16
    tibial plateau fractures, 686
    treatment, 114–15
    vertebral, 108, *125*
    WHO bone mass definitions,
          109
osteosarcoma, 179–82
    clinical presentation, 179–80
    histological appearance, *181*
    investigations, 164, 180, *181*
    mistaken diagnosis, 544, *544*
    neoadjuvant chemotherapy,
          168, *168*, 180
    in Paget's disease, 128, 180,
          182
    treatment, 164, 180, *182*
osteotomy, 254
    developmental dysplasia of the
          hip, 396–7
    genu varum/genu valgum, 434,
          435–6
    knee arthritis, 452
    metatarsal, *469*, 470
    slipped capital femoral
          epiphysis, 403–4
    subtrochanteric valgus, 664,
          664
Ottawa ankle rules, 697–8
'overbone', 479

Paget's disease of bone, *17*, 126–8
    clinical features, *13*, 126–7
    complications, 128
    imaging, 127–8, *127*
    osteosarcoma, 128, 180, 182
    pathological fractures, 545, *546*
    pathology, 126
    treatment, 128
pain, 3–4

    autonomic, 4
    back disorders, 359
    complex regional syndrome,
          286, 542, 595, 703
    foot, 453, *456*, 478–80, *478–9*
    hip girdle, 404
    osteoarthritis, 81
    referred, *see* referred pain
    shoulder, 273
pain management
    low back pain, 386
    trauma, 490
Pancoast's syndrome, 245
Panner's disease, 94
Papineau technique, 36
paraesthesia, 202, 359
    spinal disorders, 359
paralysis
    balanced, 203
    care of paralysed parts, 232,
          641
    spinal cord injuries, 640, 641
    unbalanced, 203–4
paraplegia
    management, 641
    spinal tuberculosis, 380
parasitic infections, 48–9, *48, 49*,
          381
parasympathetic nervous system,
          200, 201
parathyroidectomy, 125
parathyroid glands, adenoma,
          124–5
parathyroid hormone (PTH), 104,
          105, 106, 166
    CKD, 122, 123
    hypercalcaemia, 124
    role, 107
    testing, 110
Parkland formula, 507
paronychia, 337–8, *338*
patella
    acute dislocation, 682–4, *684*
    alignment assessment, 423, *423*
    congenital bipartite, 682
    fractures, 681–2, *683*
    recurrent dislocation, 441–2, *443*
patella alta, 423, 683, 684, 685,
          688

patellar apprehension test, 425, 441, *442*

patellar sleeve fractures, 688

patellar tap test, 425, *426*

patellar tendon (ligament)
rupture, 681
tendinopathy, 445

patellofemoral joint, 424

patellofemoral pain syndrome, 442–5

pathological fractures, 163–4, 514
acute osteomyelitis, 31
causes, 545
compression of the spine, 546
examination, 544–5
femoral shaft, 668
history, 544
imaging and investigations, 545
metastasis, 546, *546*
treatment, 545–6, *546*

Pavlik harness
developmental dysplasia of the hip, 395–6
femoral fracture, 670, *670*

pectoralis major, testing, 274

pelvic binders, 504, *504*, 643, 648

pelvic fractures, 504–5
acetabulum, 649–52
avulsion fractures, 644–5
bleeding, 643, 648
clinical assessment, 643–4
complications, 649
direct fractures, 645
imaging, 644, 645–6
initial management, 504–5, *504*, 648
operative management, 648–9, *648*
pelvic ring, 645–9, *646–7*
secondary injuries, 521, 649
stress fractures, 645

pelvis, ligamentous stabilizers, 643, *644*

Pemberton osteotomy, 397

penetrating injuries
abdomen, 503, *503*
gunshot, 532
neck, 236

pentasaccharide, 253

periacetabular osteotomy, 397

perilunate dislocation, 603–4, *605*

perineurium, 228, *228*

periosteal bone formation, 98

periosteal reaction, *17*

periosteum, 101, 516

peripheral nerves, 201, *201*
blood supply, 228
pathology of injuries, 228–30
signal (action potential), 227
spinal monitoring, 206
structure, 199, *200*, *201*, 227–8, *228*
testing, 205–6

peripheral nervous system, 199–200

peripheral neuropathies, 219–25
classification, 219
clinical features, 219–20
demyelinating, 219–20
diabetic, 220, 475
Guillain–Barré syndrome, 221–2
hereditary, 222–3
leprosy, 222, *222*
neuralgic amyotrophy (acute brachial neuritis), 220–1
pathology, 219

peripheral vascular disease, diabetes, 475

periprosthetic fractures
after hip arthroplasty, 420, 668, *669*
femur, 668, *669*
Vancouver classification, 668

periprosthetic joint infection (PJI), 37–8, *38*
hip arthroplasty, 420, 668, *669*
prevention, 420

peroneal muscular atrophy, 222, *223*

peroneal nerves, injuries, 240–2, *241*, 679, 680

peroneal tendon
dislocation, 699
impingement, 712

Perthes' disease, 87

pes cavus (high-arched foot), 454, 457, 465–7, *465*, *467*

pes planus/pes valgus (flat foot), 454, 457, 462
in adults, 464–5, *465*
in children/adolescents, 463–4, *463*

Phalen's test, 322–3, *322*

phosphate, 106, 110, 122

phosphorus, 106

physeal injuries, 546–8
ankle, 705–7, *705*
causing knee deformity, 434, *436*
complications, 547–8
distal femur, 673, *673*
distal humerus, 572–4, *574*
distal radius fractures, 595
distal tibia, 705–7, *705*
growth disturbance, 540, 548, 706–7
imaging, 547
lateral condyle, 570–1, *571*
proximal tibia, 680, 688
Salter–Harris classification, 547, *547*
suppurative arthritis, 42
treatment, 547
wrist, 313

physiotherapy, 56–7, 231, 337

physis (growth plate), 97, *98*
acute osteomyelitis, 31
injuries, *see* physeal injuries
involvement in chronic osteomyelitis, 34, *35*
zones, 102

'piano-key' sign, 602

Picture Archiving and Communications System (PACS), 16

pigmented villonodular synovitis, 195

pilon fractures
ankle, 703–5
middle phalanx, 613–14, *615*

pinch grip, restoration in spinal cord injury, 641

Pipkin classification, femoral head fractures, *656*

pisiform, *311*

pivot shift test, 427

planes of the body, 8–9, *9*

plantar fasciitis, 61, 478, *478*

plantar flexion, 10

plantaris, 457

plantar reflex, 11

plantar venous compression, intermittent, 253

plantigrade stance, 457

plaster casts, 524, 537

plates (bone fixation), 256, 525, *526*
    complications, 525–6, 584, *585*
    types, 256

plexopathy, 219

plica syndrome, 448

pneumatic compression of the leg, 253

pneumothorax
    open, 494
    simple, 495
    tension, 486, 488, 493–4, *494*, 641

podagra, 68

'pointing index sign', *240*

poliomyelitis, 216–17, *216*
    paralytic scoliosis, *372*
    treatment, 217, *218*

polydactyly
    foot, 462, *462*
    hand, 329

polymethylmethacrylate (PMMA), 269, 416, *417*

polymyalgia rheumatica, 55

Ponseti technique, 458
    reverse, 462

popliteal aneurysm, 432

popliteal artery, injuries, 679, 694

popliteal 'cyst', 428, 432

popliteal pterygium, 224, *224*

position sense, 11

posterior cord syndrome, 640

posterior cruciate ligament (PCL)
    assessment, 425–7, *427*, *429*
    bony avulsion, 678, *678*
    injury, 675, 677

posterior drawer test
    knee, 676
    shoulder, 290

posterior interosseous nerve
    compression, 243–4, *244*
    injuries, 305, 583

posterior ligament complex (PLC), injury, 634–5, 638, 639

posterior sag test, 426

posterior tibial nerve
    compression, 242, 480
    injury, 241, *241*

posture
    cerebral palsy, 208
    neurological disorders, 9–10, *10*

Pott's paraplegia, 380

power, *see* muscle power

preotact, 114

prepatellar bursitis, 432

pressure sores, 524, 537

PRICER regimen, 698

primary survey, 488–9

Propionibacterium acnes, 38, *377*, 382

prostate cancer, 166

prostheses, 266–7
    lower limb, 157, *157*, 266–7
    upper limb, 266

Proteus mirabilis, 25

provocative movement, 7

proximal (term), 9

proximal femoral varus derotation osteotomy, 397

proximal interphalangeal (PIP) joints
    dislocation, 616
    osteoarthritis, 342, *343*

pseudarthrosis
    congenital of clavicle, 154, *155*, 294, *294*
    congenital of tibia, 144–5, *147–8*, 159
    humerus fracture, *539*

pseudoclaudication, back pain, 391

pseudogout, 69, 71–2

pseudomeningoceles, 233

Pseudomonas spp., 376, 532

Pseudomonas aeruginosa, 25

'pseudoparesis', 40

psoriasis, *344*

psoriatic arthritis, 60–1, *60*, 474

pterygia syndromes, 223, 224, *224*

pubic rami, stress fractures, *544*, 645

pubic symphysis, plate fixation, 648–9, *648*

pulmonary contusion, 496

pulmonary embolism, 252
    pathophysiology, 251
    prevention, 252–4
    risk in orthopaedic operations, 252

pulmonary function, scoliosis, 367

punching injuries, 610, *611*

pyrocarbon, 269

pyrophosphate crystal deposition, 69, *70*

quadriceps angle (Q-angle), 423, *423*

quadriceps tendon, rupture, 680–1

quadriceps wasting, 424, *424*

quadriplegia, 203
    management, 641

'raccoon eyes' sign, 500, *501*

radial club hand, 311–12, *312*, 330

radial head, isolated dislocation, 578

radial nerve
    compression, 243–4, *244*
    injuries, 237, *237–8*, 305, 562, 564

radial tunnel syndrome, 242, 244

radiation exposure, intraoperative radiography, 249

radiculopathy, 219

radiocapitellar joint, osteoarthritis, 580

radiocarpal joint, osteoarthritis, 314–15, *315*

radionuclide scanning, 18–19, *19*
    acute osteomyelitis, 28
    chronic osteomyelitis, 34
    hypercalcaemia of malignancy, 126, *126*
    osteonecrosis, 90
    Paget's disease, *127*, 128
    spine, 364
    tumours, 165

radiotherapy, high-energy, 169

radioulnar discrepancy, 597
radioulnar joint, 582, *582*
  distal, *see* distal radioulnar joint (DRUJ)
  injuries, 582, 595
  testing, 299, *299*
radioulnar synostosis, 156, *156*, 300, *300*
radius
  congenital deficiency, 154–5, *155*
  distal dislocation/subluxation (Galeazzi fracture), 587–8, *588*
  distal fractures in adults, 589–95
  distal fractures in children, 595–7
  fractures with ulna, 582–5
  isolated fracture, 585–6
  proximal end fractures, 578–80, *578–9*
  styloid process fracture, 592, *593*
'raft' screws, 686, *688*
raloxifene, 114
RANKL antagonists, 114, 174, *175*
Ranvier's nodes, *200*, 227
Raynaud's phenomenon, 343
Raynaud's syndrome, 343
red flags
  bony swellings around knee, 433
  low back pain, 385
referred pain, 5, *5*
  shoulder, 273
reflexes, 10–11, 200–1
  lower limbs, 362–3
rehabilitation
  fractures, 528
  open hand injuries, 621
  open tibial fractures, 693
  total hip arthroplasty, 419
Reiter's disease, 55, 61–2, *61*
renal failure, crush syndrome, 509, 510
repetitive stress injury, 321
replantation

hands/digits, 622–3, *623*
  limbs, 263–4, *264*
respiratory dysfunction, 510–11, *510*
  signs of, 493
rhabdomyosarcoma, 197
rheumatoid arthritis (RA), 51–7
  aetiology, 51
  ankle and foot, 472–3, *473*
  cervical spine, 355–7, *356*
  clinical features, 52–3, *53*
  complications, 55
  differential diagnosis, 54–5, *54*
  distinction from osteoarthritis, 342
  elbow, 302, *304*
  hands, *53*, 334, *335*, 340, *341–2*
  hip, 414–15
  knee, *13*, *422*, 449–50, *450*
  pathology, 51–2, *52*
  prognosis, 55–6
  shoulder, 286, 290–1, *291*
  treatment, 56–7
  wrist, 314, *314*
  X-ray changes, 53–4, *54*
rheumatoid nodules, 52, *53*
rib excursion, 361
rib fractures, 495, 521, 641
rib hump, 366, *366*, 370
rickets, 108, 117–22
  assessment, 118–19
  clinical features, 118, 434, *436*
  hypophosphataemic, *118*, 119–22, *120–1*
  pathology, 118
  vitamin D-deficiency, 117–18, *120*
  vitamin D-resistant, 118
'rickety rosary', 118
rigidity, 10
Risser sign, 366, *367*
rivaroxaban, 253
robot-assisted surgery, 249
Romberg's sign, 11
rotation, *9*
rotator cuff, anatomy, 277, *277*
rotator cuff disorders, 277–84
  calcific tendinitis, 283–4, *284*

imaging, 281–2, *282*
  impingement syndrome, 278–9, *278*, 282–3, *283*
  tears, 279, 280–1, 282, *282*, 556
    repair, 283
  treatment, 282–3, *283*
Roux–Goldthwait procedure, *443*
'rugby jersey finger', 616
'rule of nines', *507*
'rule of twos', 519

sabre tibia, 44
sacral agenesis, 153, *154*
sacroiliac joints, 385
sacroiliac ligament, *644*
sacrospinous ligament, *644*
sacrotuberous ligament, *644*
sacrum, injuries, 652
Salmonella spp., 61
Salter–Harris classification, 547, *547*
Salter osteotomy, 396
SAM Sling™, 504, *504*
Sanfilippo syndrome, 147, 149
'Sarmiento' cast, 691
Saturday night palsy, 237
scalp wounds, 501
scaphocapitate fusion, *318*
scaphoid, *311*
scaphoid fractures, 599–602, *600–1*
scapholunate ligament, rupture, 318, *319*, 592, 602–3, *604*
scaphotrapeziotrapezoid joint, arthritis, 315–16, *316*
scapula, 293–5
  failure of descent, 152, *153*, 293, *293*
  fractures, 552–3, *553*
  grating, 294
  winging, 220, *221*, 235, *236*, 274, 293–4, *293*
scapulothoracic dissociation, 553
scars, *8*
SCFE, *see* slipped capital femoral epiphysis
Schatzker classification (tibial plateau fractures), 685, 686, *687*

Scheie syndrome, 149
Scheuermann's disease, *373*,
　　374–5, *375*
Schmorl's nodes, 374, *375*
Schwann cells, *200*, *201*, 227, 230
schwannoma, 196, *196*
sciatica, 359, 362, 382, 390
sciatic nerve injuries, 239–40
　　clinical features, 239, *241*
　　hip arthroplasty, 240
　　hip dislocation, 652, 654–5
sciatic stretch tests, 362, *363*
sclera, blue, 142, *143*
scleroderma, *344*
scoliosis, 13, 365–73
　　adolescent idiopathic, 367–70,
　　　367
　　congenital, 152, *153*, 371–2,
　　　372
　　infantile, *368*, 371
　　juvenile idiopathic, 370–1
　　and neurofibromatosis, 373
　　neuropathic and myopathic,
　　　372–3, *372*
　　operative treatment, 269–70,
　　　370–1
　　　complications, 370
　　patterns of idiopathic, *368*
　　poliomyelitis, 216, *216*
　　postural, 365
　　structural, 365–7
screws (bone fixation), 254, 525,
　　526
　　cannulated variable pitch, 255
　　lag, 254–5, *255*, *526*
seat-belt injuries, 636, 639
Secretan's syndrome, *344*
selective oestrogen receptor
　　　modulators (SERMs),
　　　114
semimembranosus bursa, 432
sensibility
　　changes in, 5–6
　　deep, 11
　　testing, 11, 230
sensory nerve dermatomes, *204*
sensory neuropathy, hereditary,
　　222
septic arthritis

hip, 398–9
knee, 431
sequestra, bone, 26, *26*, 34, *35*
seronegative arthropathies, 55,
　　60–2, 473–4
serratus anterior
　　long thoracic nerve palsy, 235,
　　　236
　　testing, 274
　　weakness, 293
sesamoid fractures, 715
sesamoiditis, 479
Sever's disease, 478, *478*
Shigella spp., 61
shock, 497–8
short femur, 156–7, *157*
short stature, 137, 139
shoulder; *see also* glenohumeral
　　　joint; scapula
　　adhesive capsulitis (frozen
　　　shoulder), 285–6, *286*
　　anatomy, 277, *277*
　　anterior instability, 286–9
　　arthrodesis, *218*, 296
　　arthroplasty, 295–6, *296*
　　arthroscopy, 295
　　congenital elevation, 293, *293*
　　dislocation, 287
　　　after proximal humerus
　　　　fracture, 561
　　　anterior, 556–7, *557*
　　　inferior, 558–9, *559*
　　　posterior, 289–90, *289*,
　　　　557–8, *558*
　　　recurrent, 287, 557, *557*
　　examination, 274–5, *275*, *276*
　　history of disorder, 273
　　imaging, 275–7, *276*
　　joint laxity, 287
　　movements, 274, *275*
　　osteoarthritis, 82
　　osteonecrosis, 292
　　painful arc syndrome, 279–80,
　　　280
　　posterior instability, 289–90
　　rapidly destructive arthropathy
　　　(Milwaukee shoulder),
　　　73, 74, 292, *292*
　　rotator cuff disorders, 277–84

SLAP lesions, 285
Sprengel's deformity, 152, *153*,
　　293, *293*
　　subluxation, 287, 288
sickle-cell disease, 29–30, 92, *92*,
　　414
Simmonds' test (Achilles' tendon
　　rupture), 476, *477*
simple bone cysts, 164, 174, *176*
Sinding-Larsen–Johansson
　　　syndrome, 445
single gene disorders, 130
single photon emission
　　　tomography (SPECT), 29
skeleton, primary foles, 107
skier's thumb, 611–12, *612*
skin contracture, hands, 330–1
skin grafts, open fractures, 531
skin preparation, 249, 250
skin traction, 523
skull, 'pepper-pot' osteolytic
　　　lesions, 188, *189*
skull fractures, 501, *502*
　　basal, 500, *501*
slipped capital femoral epiphysis
　　　(SCFE), 401–4
Smith's fracture, 591, *591*
social background, 6
SOCRATES, 404
soft-tissue tumours, 161, 164,
　　192–3
　　age-related variations, 193
　　fibrous, 194–5
　　imaging, 193
　　lipomatous, 193–4, *194*
　　muscle, 197
　　nerve sheath, 196–7, *196*
　　smooth muscle, 195–6
　　synovial, 195
　　vascular, 195
somatic nervous system, 200
somatosensory-evoked responses
　　　(SSEPs), 206
Southwick angle, 402
Southwick osteotomy, 403
spasticity, 10, 203
spastic paresis
　　acquired adult, 210, *334*
　　cerebral palsy, 207, 208

hands, 333, *334*
treatment, *211*
spina bifida, 133, 213–16
  clinical features, 213–14, *214*
  definitions, 212–13, *213–14*
  foot deformities, 216, 458, *459*
  hydrocephalus, 213
  incidence and screening, 213
  joint deformities, 215–16
  management, 214–16
  spinal deformity, 215
spinal accessory nerve, injuries,
      235–6, *236*
'spinal claudication', 389
spinal cord injury without obvious
      radiographic abnormality
      (SCHIWORA), 631
spinal cord lesions, 210–12,
      640–1
  acute compression, 212
  anatomical levels, 211, 640
  common causes, 211
  diagnosis, 211–12
  features suggestive of, 628
  incomplete injury syndromes,
      640
  intrinsic, 212
  paraplegia and quadriplegia
      management, 641
  patterns of cord dysfunction,
      210, 211
  tumours, 212
spinal cord monitoring, 206, 370
spinal extension, testing, 58, *58*
spinal fusion, 386–7, *387*
spinal infections, 375–81
  cervical spine, 354, *354*
  fungal, 380–1
  parasitic, 381
  pyogenic, 354, *354*
  tuberculosis, *46*, 354–5, *355*,
      378–80, *378–9*
spinal injuries, 505
  AO/ASIF classification, 625
  cervical spine, 630–6, *630*
  early management, 626
  history, 627
  imaging, 628, *629*
  mechanisms, 626, *626*

neural, 628, 629, 640–1
neurological examination, 521,
      628
pathological fractures, 546
physical examination, 627–8
primary pathophysiological
      changes, 625
secondary pathophysiological
      changes, 625
stability, 625
thoracolumbar spine, 636–40
transfer of patient, 626–7, *627*
treatment, 628–30
spinal muscular atrophy, 217–18
spinal stenosis, 212
  achondroplasia, 137, 139
  acquired, 389
  clinical features, 389
  congenital, 389
  imaging, 389, *390*
  in Paget's disease, 128
  treatment, 389–90
splintage
  acute osteomyelitis, 31
  acute suppurative arthritis, 41
  cerebral palsy, 210
  fractures, 515, 524, 537
  hands, 337, *337*, 608, *608*, 620,
      621
  in JIA, 63
spondyloepiphyseal dysplasia,
      135–7
spondylolisthesis, 387–9, *388*
  degenerative, 388, *388*
  dysplastic, 388
  lytic/isthmic, 388, *388*
  Wiltse–Newman classification,
      388
spontaneous osteonecrosis of the
      knee (SONK), 452
sprains, 548
  ankle, 697, 699
  finger joints, 614–15
  neck (whiplash injury), 635–6
  wrist, 320, 598–9, *598*
Sprengel's shoulder, 152, *153*, 293,
      293
Spurling's test of neck movement,
      346

stab injuries, neck, 236
staging systems
  basis, 162
  osteonecrosis, 90–1
  Perthes disease, 400, *400*
  tumours, 162–3
stainless steel implants, 266–7
Staphylococcus aureus, 24, 30, 532
  methicillin-resistant, 31
  spinal infections, 354, 376
steal syndromes, 127
Steel sign, 402
stereognosis, 11, 12, 231, 328
sternoclavicular dislocation, 555,
      555
sternomastoid tumour, 349, *350*
sternum fractures, 641
stiffness, 4–5; *see also* joint
      stiffness
  lumbar spine, 359, *361*
  neck disorders, 346
Still's disease, 55, 62
Stimson's method, 556
straight-leg raise test, 362, *363*
strains, 548
Streptococcus pyogenes, 24
stress fractures, 543–4
  causes, 543
  clinical features, 543
  femoral neck, 544
  imaging, 543–4, *544*
  mechanisms, 513–14
  metatarsal bones, *479*, 480, 715
  in Paget's disease, 128
  pubic rami, 645
  sites affected, 543
  treatment, 544
stretch reflex, 200
strontium ranelate, 114
Subaxial Cervical Spine Injury
      Classification (SLIC)
      scoring system, 632–3
subchondral bone, 75
  sclerosis, 78, *79*
subluxation, *548*, 549
  hip sepsis, 41, *41*
  radioulnar joint, 587–8, *588*
  shoulder, 287, 288
subscapularis, 277, *277*

suppurative arthritis, 29, 31, 38
　causes, 38–9
　clinical features, 39–40
　complications, 41–2, *41*
　pathology, 39, *39*
supracondylar fractures
　elbow, *303*, 566–70, *567–8*
　femur, 670–3, *670*, *672*
supraglottic airway, 491
supraspinatus
　examination, *275*
　imaging, *276*
supraspinatus tendinitis, 279
　calcific, 73, *73*, 283–4, *284*
　chronic, 280
　clinical tests, 281
　imaging, 281, *282*
　pathology, 279
　subacute (painful arc
　　syndrome), 279–80, *281*
　treatment, 282–3
surgical drainage
　acute osteomyelitis, 31
　acute suppurative arthritis, 41
　hand infections, 336, *337*
swan-neck deformity, 334, *335*,
　341
sweating, absence, 230
swelling, 5
sympathetic nervous system, 200,
　201
symptoms, 3–6
synapse, 199
synarthroses, 98
syndactyly, 156, *156*, 329, *330*
syndesmophytes, 58, *59*
synovial effusions, knee, 431–2
synovial fluid
　cytokines, 75
　pyrophosphate crystals, *70*, *72*
　urate crystals, 69, *70*
synovial thickening, knee, 424
synovitis
　knee, 431
　pigmented villonodular, 195
　rheumatoid arthritis, 52, *52*,
　　340
syphilis, 42–4, *43*
syringomyelia, 212

systemic lupus erythematosus
　　(SLE), 64, 414

tabes dorsalis, 212
tailor's bunion, 472
talar tilt test, 699
talipes calcaneovalgus, 461, *461*
talipes equinovarus (idiopathic
　　club foot), 457–61
talocalcaneal joint, stiffness/OA,
　　712
talonavicular joint, dislocation, *713*
talus
　congenital vertical, 462, *462*
　fractures, 707–10, *709*
　osteochondrosis/osteochondritis,
　　95, 477
　osteonecrosis, 88, 477, 710
tarsal bones, injuries, 712–13, *713*
tarsal coalition, 463, *464*
tarsal tunnel syndrome, 242, 480
tarsometatarsal (TMT) joint
　　injuries, 713–14, *714*
temperature recognition, 11
tenderness, examination for, 7, *8*
tendinitis
　after fractures, 541
　biceps tendon, 284
　calcific, 73, *73*, 283–4, *284*
　rotator cuff, 279–84
　supraspinatus, 280
　tendo Achilles, 476
　tibialis posterior, 541
tendo Achilles
　insufficiency after calcaneum
　　fracture, 712
　rupture, 476–7, *477*
　tenderness in Reiter's disease,
　　61
　tendinitis, 476
tendon injuries
　distal radius fractures, 541,
　　594, 595
　hands/fingers, repair, 618–19,
　　619–20
　hands/fingers (closed), 333–4,
　　616, *616*
　hands/fingers (open), 617–22
　rheumatoid arthritis, *53*, 55

tendon necrosis, 339
tendon reflexes, 10–11, 200,
　　362–3
tendon repair, 618–19, *619–20*
tendon-sheath infections, hands,
　　339
tendon transfers
　cerebral palsy, 210, 211
　nerve injuries, 232
　poliomyelitis, 217, *218*
　principles, 232
　spinal cord injuries, 641
tennis elbow, 307–8, *307*
tenosynovitis
　ankle, 477
　suppurative of hand/digits, 339
　wrist, 319–21, *320*
tension-band fixation, 525, 581,
　　581
teratogens, 130–1
teres minor, 277
teriparatide, 114
terminology, 8–10, *9*
'terrible triad', 576
testicular atrophy, 108
TFCC, *see* triangular fibrocartilage
　　complex
thenar eminence, wasting, 238,
　　240, *322*
Thessaly test, 428, 438
Thomas splint, 537, 666
Thompson and Epstein
　　classification, hip
　　dislocation, 653
thoracic cage injuries
　complex, 641
　rib fractures, 495, 521, 641
　sternal fracture, 641
thoracic outlet syndrome, 244–5,
　　245
　differential diagnosis, 245
thoracolumbar spine injuries, 630,
　　636–40
　axial compression/burst injury,
　　638–9, *639*
　examination, 637
　flexion-compression injury, 638
　fracture-dislocation, 639–40
　imaging, 637

jack-knife injury (Chance fracture), 636, 639
pars interarticularis fractures, 638
pathogenic mechanisms, 636, 637
transverse process fractures, 638
treatment, 638
thoracospinal anomalies, 152, 153
3D modelling, 407, 408
thrombin inhibitors, direct, 253
thromboprophylaxis, 252–4
pelvic fractures, 649
thumb-in-palm, 333
thumbs
absence, 330
congenital variations, 329, 330–1
infantile 'trigger', 335
movements, 326–7, 327
osteoarthritis of the CMC joint, 315, 316
replantation/replacement, 331, 622, 623
testing abduction power, 240
ulnar collateral ligament tear (skier's thumb), 611–12, 612
thyroid cartilage, 345, 345
thyroxine, 107, 116
tibia
congenital pseudarthrosis, 159
deficiency (hemimelia), 157, 158
distal comminuted fracture, 703–5
distal physeal injuries, 705–7, 705
non-ossifying fibroma, 173
Paget's disease, 127
proximal epiphyseal injuries, 680, 688
proximal metaphyseal injuries, 690
tibialis posterior tendon
rupture, 477
tendinitis, 541
tibial plateau fractures, 685–8, 685, 687–8

classification, 686, 687
clinical features, 685
complications, 688
imaging, 685
mechanism, 685
treatment, 685–8, 685, 688–9
tibial shaft fractures, 690–5
clinical features, 690
complications, 694–5
management, 691–2, 693
open, 531, 692–3
tibial spine fracture, 678, 678
tibial tubercle
'apophysitis' (Osgood–Schlatter disease), 432, 445, 445
Maquet's advancement operation, 444–5
tibiofemoral alignment, 429
tibiofibular ligament, injuries, 700, 701
tibiofibular syndesmosis, 700, 701, 702
Tile classification, pelvic ring fractures, 647
Tillaux fracture, 705–6, 706
Tinel's sign, 11, 196, 231, 322–3, 322
tip–apex distance, 661, 661
tissue cavitation, 503, 503, 532
titanium alloys, 267
toes
claw, 457, 465, 465, 471–2, 471
fractures, 715
lesser toe deformities, 471–2, 471
nail disorders, 480, 481
tone, 10
tophi, 54, 69, 344, 474, 474
torticollis (wry/skew neck), 349, 350
torus fractures, 595
total disc replacement (TDR), 387, 387
total hip arthroplasty (THA), 263–4, 263, 415–20
cemented, 416–17, 417
complications, 406, 419–20
contraindications, 420
hip fractures, 660–1

hip resurfacing, 418–19, 418
implant types, 416
indications, 415–16
rehabilitation, 419
revision, 420
sciatic nerve injury, 240
surgical approaches, 416
surgical planning tools/3D printing, 407, 408
thromboprophylaxis, 252–4
uncemented, 417–18, 418
tourniquet, 249, 250
tourniquet time (ischaemia time), 250
tracheal intubation, 486, 491
tracheobronchial tree, injury, 495, 496
traction, 523–4, 523
cervical spine injuries, 635
femoral shaft fractures, 666, 666
supracondylar elbow fractures, 569
trapeziectomy, 315, 316
trapezium
anatomy, 311
fracture, 602, 603
trapezoid, 311
trauma
ABC, 486–7
abdominal, 503–4
ATLS® concept, 487–8
burns, 506–9
crush syndrome, 509–10
death rates, 485, 485
head injuries, 499–503
intrahospital/interhospital transfer, 490
long bone injuries, 505–6
management at scene of accident, 485–7
management stages, 485
multiple organ failure, 510–11
pain management, 490
pelvic fractures, 504–5
primary survey, 488–9
secondary survey, 489–90
spinal, 505–6
transfer to hospital, 487

trauma teams, 487
Trendelenburg gait, 203, 405
Trendelenburg test, 405
Treponema pallidum, 42
Trethowan sign, 402, *402*
triage, 486
triangular fibrocartilage complex
(TFCC)
anatomy, 317, *318*
chronic degeneration, 317–18
tears, 317, 602
'trigger finger', 334–6
triplane fractures, 706
triquetrum, *311*
'triscaphe joint', arthritis, 315–16,
316
trochanteric hip fractures, 658–9,
658
isolated, 662–3
treatment, 661, *661*
Trousseau sign, 117
Tscherne classification (closed
fractures), 521
skin lesions, 690
tuberculosis, 44–7
ankle joint, 472
elbow, 301–2
knee, 431, 448–9, *449*
shoulder, 290, *290*
spinal, 354–5, *355*, 378–80,
378–9
treatment, 46–7
wrist, 313, *313*
tuft fracture, 614, *614*
tumour necrosis factor (TNF)
inhibitors, 56, 60, 415,
450
tumour–node–metastasis (TNM)
staging, 162–3
tumours
benign, 161–2, 169–79
biopsies, 166–7, *167*
cervical spine, 352, 353
classification, 161–2
clinical presentation, 163–4
epidemiology, 161
imaging, 164–6
intermediate, 162
malignant bone, 162, 179–91

metastatic bone, 191–2
potential diagnosis by age
group/radiographic
appearance, 164
potential diagnosis by site, *165*
soft-tissue, 192–7
spinal cord, 212
staging, 162–3
Turner's syndrome, 115–16, 130,
150–1
two-point discrimination, 11, 231

ulceration
diabetic foot, *475*, 476, *481*
sciatic nerve injuries, *241*
ulna
congenital deficiency, 156
fracture-dislocation (Monteggia
fracture), 586–7, *587*
fractures with radius, 582–5
isolated fracture, 585–6
shortening, 318, *319*
ulnar 'claw hand' (intrinsic-minus
deformity), 332, *333*
ulnar collateral ligament (MCP
joint), tear, 611–12, *612*
ulnar dimelia (mirror hand), *156*,
330
ulnar head, replacement, *317*
ulnar nerve
compression, 242–3
injuries, 237–8, *239*, 569, 575
testing, *205*
ulnar nerve palsy
cubitus valgus, 300, *302*
leprosy, 222, *222*
'ulnar paradox', 238
ulnar styloid injury, 602
ulnocarpal impaction, 317–18, *319*
ultra-high molecular weight
polyethylene
(UHMWPE), 269, 416,
419
ultrasonography
acute osteomyelitis, 28
adult hip, 407
developmental dysplasia of the
hip, 20, 395, *395*
principles, 20

rotator cuff tears, 282
shoulder, 277, 282
trauma, 490
upper limb anomalies, 311
incidence, 311
Madelung's deformity, 312–13,
312
radial longitudinal deficiency,
311–12, *312*
transverse deficiency, 154, 311
upper motor neurons (UMN),
200, 201
urate crystals
deposition, 68, *69*
synovial fluid, 69, *70*
urate-lowering therapy, 70
urethral injuries, 649
urethritis, Reiter's disease, 61
uric acid, serum levels, 68
urinary symptoms, back disorders,
360
urogenital injuries, in pelvic
fractures, 649

valgus deformity, 9, 13, *14*
elbow (cubitus valgus), 300, *302*
first MTP joint (hallux valgus),
467–70, *467–8*
knee, *422*, 433–7, *433–5*
Vancouver classification
(periprosthetic femur
fracture), 668
varus deformity, 13, *14*
elbow (cubitus varus), 300, *301*,
569–70, *570*
hip (coxa vara), 167, 397, *397*,
664, *664*
knee (genu varum), 13, *13*, *422*,
433–7
vascular access, trauma, 498, *499*
vascular injuries, 533–4, *533*
common injuries, 534
femoral shaft fracture, 668
fracture-dislocation of elbow,
576
knee dislocation, 679
malleolar fractures, 703
supracondylar elbow fracture,
569

tibial shaft fractures, 694
treatment, 534
vascular tumours
    bone, 190–1
    soft tissue, 195
venous thromboembolism (VTE)
    femoral shaft fractures, 669
    pathophysiology, 251
    pelvic fractures, 649
    prevention, 252–4
    risk factors, 251
    risk in orthopaedic operations,
        252
ventriculoperitoneal (VP) shunt,
    214–15
vertebrae, biconcave, *121*
vertebral anomalies, 152–3, *153*,
    349–50, *350*
vertebral fractures
    cervical spine, 630–6
    imaging, *19*
    mechanisms, 626, *626*
    osteomalacia, 119
    osteoporotic, 113, *113*, 114–15,
        659
    thoracolumbar spine, 636–40
    treatment, 628–30
vibration test, 11
vincristine, 168
visceral injuries, 503–4, *503*, 533
    pelvic fractures, 643
vitamin D, 106, *106*
    assessment of activity, 110
    deficiency, 116, 117–18, 119,
        120
    metabolites, 106, *106*
    supplementation, 113
volar intercalated segmental
    instability (VISI), *598*, 604
Volkmann canals, 101
Volkmann's ischaemic contracture,
    535, 541

Waldenström staging (Legg–
    Calvé–Perthes disease),
    400, *400*
Wallerian degeneration, 229
wall test (spinal extension), 58, *58*,
    361

warfarin, 254
Watson's test, 602
weakness, 5, 202, 203
Weaver Dunn operation, modified,
    554–5, *555*
wedge compression fractures
    cervical spine, 633
    thoracolumbar spine,
        636, *637*
weight loss, and osteoarthritis, 85
wide awake local anaesthetic no
    tourniquet (WALANT),
    249
Wiltse–Newman classification, 388
Wolff's law, 107, *108*, 513
Wormian bones, 142–3
wound dressings, 620, *621*
wound management
    hand injuries, 618–20
    open fractures, 529–30
Wright's test, 244
wrist
    acquired deformity, 313
    carpal injuries, *see* carpal
        injuries
    clinical assessment, 309–11
    congenital variations/
        deformities, 311–13, *312*
    distal radius fractures (adults),
        589–95
    fusion, *315*
    ganglia, 321, *321*
    imaging, 311, *311*, 597–8, *598*
    instability, 318–19, *319*, 598,
        598
    median nerve entrapment,
        322–4, *323*
    movements, 310–11, *310*
    occupational disorders, 321
    osteoarthritis, 314–17, *315–17*,
        595
    replacement, *315*
    rheumatoid arthritis, 314, *314*,
        341
    scapholunate ligament rupture,
        318, *319*, 592, 602–3,
        604
    'sprains', 320, 598–9, *598*
    tender points, *310*

tenosynovitis/tenovaginitis,
    319–21, *320*
TFCC degeneration, 317–18
TFCC tears, 317, 602
tuberculosis, 313, *313*
ulnar nerve compression, 243
ulnar nerve injury, 237–8, *239*
ulnar-sided injuries, 602
ulnocarpal impaction, 317–18,
    319
wry neck (torticollis), 349, *350*

X-linked disorders, 131
X-rays, 16–18
    acute osteomyelitis, 28, *28*
    ankle ligament injuries, 697–8
    ankylosing spondylitis, 58, *59*
    cartilage calcification, 71, *71*
    cervical spine, *345*, 347–9, *348*
    cervical spine injuries, 630–1,
        631
    chronic destructive arthritis,
        73, 74
    chronic osteomyelitis, 34, *35*
    contrast, 17
    femoral head AVN, 413, *413*
    femoral shaft fracture, 664–5,
        665
    fractures, 519, *520*
    gout, 69, *69*
    head injuries, *502*
    hip, *18*, 406, *406*, 410, *410*,
        657, 658–9
    hydatid bone disease, 48, *49*
    hyperparathyroidism, 125, *125*
    intervertebral disc disease, 382
    intraoperative, 248–9, *248*, 249
    joints, 18, *18*
    knee, 428–9, *428*, 451, *451*
    Legg–Calvé–Perthes disease,
        400, *400*
    low back pain, 386
    lumbar spine, 363–4, *364*
    major trauma, 490, *494*
    metastatic bone disease, 191,
        192
    osteoarthritis, 78, *78*
    osteochondrosis, 95
    osteomalacia, *121*

X-rays (*Continued*)
osteonecrosis, *88*, 90, *90*
osteoporosis, 113, *113*
PACS, 16
Paget's disease of bone, 127–8, *127*
plain film, 16
pyogenic spinal infection, 376, *377*
reading, 16–17, *17*
rheumatoid arthritis, 53, *54*

rickets, 118–19, *118–19*, *120–1*
scoliosis, 366, *367*
shoulder, 275, *276*, 281, *282*
slipped capital femoral epiphysis, 402, *402*
spinal injuries, 628, *629*
spinal stenosis, 389, *390*
spinal tuberculosis, 378–9, *379*
stress fractures, 543, *544*
supracondylar fractures, 566–7, *566–7*

tumours, 164–6, *165*, 180, *181*
wrist, 311, *311*, 598, *598*

yellow flags, low back pain, 385
Yersinia enterocolitica, 61
Young and Burgess classification, pelvic ring fractures, 646–7

zoledronate, IV, 128
Z-plasty, *333*